$ 225.00

FRACTURES

Diagnosis and Treatment

NOTICE

FRACTURES

Diagnosis and Treatment

Edited by

H. David Moehring, MD
Associate Professor
Department of Orthopedic Surgery
University of California, Davis
Co-Director of Orthopedic Trauma
University of California, Davis Medical Center
Sacramento, California

Adam Greenspan, MD, FACR
Professor of Radiology
University of California, Davis
Chief of Musculoskeletal Radiology
University of California, Davis Medical Center
Sacramento, California

With 45 contributors

Developed by Current Medicine, Inc.
Philadelphia

McGraw-Hill
Health Professions Division
New York St. Louis San Francisco Auckland Bogotá Caracas Lisbon London
Madrid Mexico City Milan Montreal New Delhi San Juan
Singapore Sydney Tokyo Toronto

McGraw-Hill

A Division of The **McGraw·Hill** *Companies*

CM
CURRENT
MEDICINE

Current Medicine, Inc.
400 Market Street
Suite 700
Philadelphia, PA 19106

Fractures: Diagnosis and Treatment

ISBN 0-0713-5902-8

1 2 3 4 5 6 7 8 9 0 EBREBR 99

Director of Product Development: Mary Kinsella
Editorial Supervisor: Susan L. Hunsberger
Developmental Editor: Jennifer Wood
Editorial Assistant: Forrest Rian Perry
Art Director: Jerilyn Kauffman
Cover Design: Christine Keller-Quirk
Design and Layout: Christine Keller-Quirk
Illustration Director: Debra Wertz
Illustrators: Wieslawa Langenfeld, Marie Dean, and Paul Schiffmacher
Production Manager: Lori Holland
Production Associate: Peter O'Steen
Indexing: Holly Lukens

Printed and bound in the United States by Edwards Brothers.

This book was printed on acid-free paper.

Fractures: diagnosis and treatment / edited by H. David Moehring, Adam Greenspan.

p.cm.
Includes bibliographical references and index.
ISBN 0-0713-5902-8 (hardcover: alk. paper)
1. Fractures. 2. Bones—Wounds and injuries. I. Moehring, H. David, 1936- II. Greenspan, Adam. III. Title: Fractures
RD101 .C8925 1999
617.1'5--dc21
99-29747

CIP

CONTENTS

Section I—Imaging

Chapter 1
Radiologic Evaluation of Fractures 3
Adam Greenspan
Conventional Radiography and Tomography 3
Computed Tomography 7
Skeletal Scintigraphy 8
Magnetic Resonance Imaging 9

Chapter 2
Imaging of Fractures and Dislocations of the Spine 13
Pasquale Montesano, Elvert F. Nelson, and Adam Greenspan
General Principles 13
Imaging of Cervical Injuries 14
Imaging of Thoracic and Lumbar Trauma 16

Chapter 3
Imaging of Fractures of the Pelvis and Lower Extremities 21
Eric A. Brandser
Radiography 21
Computed Tomography 22
Magnetic Resonance Imaging 22

Chapter 4
Imaging of Fractures of the Shoulder Girdle and Upper Extremities 33
Ronald W. Hendrix
Picture Archiving and Communication System and Computed Radiography 34
Plain Radiographs 35
Skeletal Scintigraphy 40
Computed Tomography 40
Magnetic Resonance Imaging 41
Ultrasonography 43
Fracture Healing 43

Section II—Fracture-Dislocations of the Spine

Chapter 5
Cervical Spine Fractures 49
Robert F. McLain
Classification of Injuries 50
Criteria for Instability and Surgical Indications 51
Subluxation and Dislocation 51
Fracture of the Anterior Elements 52
Fracture of the Posterior Elements 55
Fractures of the Lateral Masses 56
Spinal Cord and Root Injury 56

Chapter 6
Thoracolumbar Fractures and Fracture-Dislocations 59
Munish C. Gupta and Daniel R. Benson
Patient Evaluation 59
Concept of Stability and Classification 60
Diagnosis and Treatment 62

Section III—Fractures of the Pelvis and Acetabulum

Chapter 7
Current Diagnosis and Management of Pelvic Ring Fractures 71
Kenneth A. Egol and James F. Kellam
Diagnosis 71
Management 73

Chapter 8
Fractures of the Acetabulum 79
H. David Moehring
Diagnosis 79
Classification 80
Treatment 80
Reduction and Fixation 81
Adjunctive Techniques 81
Percutaneous Screws 82
Postoperative Care 87
Prevention of Complications and Caveats 87
Prognosis 87

Section IV—Fractures of the Hip and Femur

Chapter 9
Femoral Neck Fractures 91
David C. Teague and Marc F. Swiontkowski
Anatomy 91
Pathophysiology 92
Surgical Management 92
Hemiarthroplasty 93
Current Debates 93
New Materials and Techniques 95

Chapter 10
Intertrochanteric Hip Fractures 99
Richard F. Kyle and Thomas J. Ellis
Epidemiology 99
Anatomy 99
Biomechanics of the Hip 100
Classification 101
Clinical Signs 101
Radiographic Evaluation 102
Surgical Technique 102
Postoperative Care 104
Prosthetic Replacement 104
Complications 105

Chapter 11

SUBTROCHANTERIC FRACTURES OF THE FEMUR 107

Ronald W. Lindsey and Zbigniew Gugala

Subtrochanteric Region 107
Epidemiology 108
Biologic and Biomechanical Considerations of Subtrochanteric Fractures 108
Classification 109
Diagnosis 109
Imaging 109
Definitive Treatment Options 110
Authors' Preferred Treatment Method and Possible Complications 115

Chapter 12

FRACTURES OF THE FEMORAL SHAFT 121

Todd O. McKinley

Preoperative Evaluation and Treatment 121
Operative Treatment 122
Segmental Fractures 124
Open Fractures 125
Retrograde Intramedullary Nailing 126
Critically Injured Patients 127
Reamed Versus Unreamed Nailing 127
Current Recommendations 127

Section V—Fracture-Dislocations and Fractures of the Lower Limbs

Chapter 13

SUPRACONDYLAR FRACTURES OF THE FEMUR 131

Christopher G. Finkemeier

Classification 131
History and Evolution of Treatment Philosophy 132
Relevant Surgical Anatomy 132
Treatment Methods 134

Chapter 14

PATELLA FRACTURES 143

William I. Sterett and John M. Wright

Classification and Mechanism 143
Clinical and Radiographic Evaluation 143
Nonoperative Treatment 144
Operative Treatment 144
Transverse Fractures 144
Polar Fractures 147
Longitudinal Fractures 149
Stellate Fractures 149
Open Fractures 150
Osteochondral Fractures 150
Patella Fracture Following Anterior Cruciate Ligament Graft Harvest 150
Periprosthetic Fractures 151
Patellectomy 151
Patellar Nonunion 153

Chapter 15

FRACTURES OF THE TIBIAL PLATEAU 155

Edward A. Perez and Paul J. Duwelius

Anatomy 155
Associated Injuries 156
Classification 156
Clinical Evaluation 157
Treatment 157
Arthroscopy 157
Our Preferred Surgical Technique 158
Type I or Split Fractures 158
Type II or Split-Central Depression Fractures 158
Type III or Central Depression Fractures 159
Type IV or Medial Plateau Fractures 159
Type V or Bicondylar Fractures 161
Type VI Fractures 161
Results 161
Complications 162

Chapter 16

FRACTURES OF THE TIBIAL SHAFT 165

Thomas A. Russell

Pertinent Anatomy 165
Fracture Classifications 166
Initial Injury Assessment....
Treatment Options for Closed Diaphyseal Fractures 168
Open Fractures 170
Complications 171

Chapter 17

PILON FRACTURES 175

Vasilios Mathews and Lon S. Weiner

Principles of Treatment 175
Classification 176
Associated Injuries 176
Imaging 176
Analysis Checklist 177
Nondisplaced Fractures 177
Unreconstructable Fractures 178
Principles of Operative Treatment 178
Authors' Preferred Method of Management 180
Closure 181
Postoperative Care 181
Complications 181

Chapter 18

ANKLE FRACTURES AND ANKLE FRACTURE-DISLOCATION 185

Bruce H. Ziran and Franklin D. Shuler

Ankle Fracture Evaluation 186
Management of Specific Fractures 186
Special Considerations 192

Chapter 19
Foot Fractures 197
David S. Levine and Sigvard T. Hansen, Jr
Calcaneus Fractures 198
Talus Fractures 198
Midfoot Fractures 200
Lisfranc Fracture-Dislocations 200
Metatarsal Fractures 201
Phalangeal Fractures 201

Section VI—Fractures of the Upper Extremities

Chapter 20
Fractures of the Scapula 207
Thomas P. Goss
Incidence and Mechanisms of Injury 207
Diagnosis and Nonoperative Treatment 208
Operative Indications 209
Fractures of the Glenoid Process 209
Double Disruptions of the Superior Shoulder Suspensory Complex with Significant Displacement of One or More Scapular Elements 214
Postoperative Management and Rehabilitation 215

Chapter 21
Fractures of the Humeral Head and Neck 217
Michael E. Torchia
Surgical Indications 217
Anatomic Considerations 218
Surgical Approach 219

Chapter 22
Functional Bracing of Diaphyseal Humeral Fractures and Operative Management of Humeral Shaft Fractures 225
Augusto Sarmiento and J. Tracy Watson
Rationale 225
Indications 226
Management Protocol 226
Results 229
Operative Management of Humeral Shaft Fractures 230
Surgical Anatomy 231
Surgical Approaches 232
Surgical Treatment 233
Intramedullary Nailing 234
Interlocking Nails 237
External Fixation 239

Chapter 23
Supracondylar Fractures of the Humerus 243
Mark S. Vrahas and Michael J. Leddy, III
Anatomy 243
Mechanism of Injury and Associated Injuries 244
Classification 244
Approaches to the Distal Humerus 246

Chapter 24
Fracture-Dislocations of the Elbow 249
David Ring and Jesse B. Jupiter
Anatomy and Mechanics 249
Patterns of Injury 251
Operative Tactics 253

Chapter 25
Fractures of the Radius and Ulna 257
Lawrence E. Weiss and A. Lee Osterman
Evaluation 257
Surgical Anatomy and Operative Approaches 258
Isolated Fractures of the Ulna (Night-Stick Fractures) 260
Fractures of the Ulna with Dislocation of the Radial Head (Monteggia Fractures) 260
Fractures of Both the Radius and Ulna (Both-Bones Fractures) 262
Fractures of the Radius With and Without Distal Radioulnar Joint Dislocation (Galeazzi, Essex-Lopresti, and Isolated Radius Fractures) 264
Specific Issues 266

Chapter 26
Distal Radius Fractures 269
Larry R. Padgett and Terry L. Whipple
Anatomy 270
Mechanism of Injury 270
Classification 270
Treatment Options 272

Chapter 27
Fracture-Dislocations of the Wrist 281
Robert R. Slater, Jr
Anatomy and Biomechanics: Injury Patterns Explained 281
Diagnosis 283
Classification 285
Treatment 286

Chapter 28
Current Management of Selected Problem Fractures of the Phalanges and Metacarpals 293
Dean S. Louis and Peter J. L. Jebson
Specific Fracture Types 294
Multiple Fractures: Polytrauma 295
Fractures and Fracture-Dislocations of the Proximal Interphalangeal Joint 297

Index 299

PREFACE

Because of the advances in orthopedic surgery, it has become necessary for the surgeon to be familiar not only with current treatment options and surgical techniques but also with contemporary imaging modalities. Radiologic imaging plays a pivotal role in fracture detection and classification and treatment monitoring. The rapid changes in the field of radiology and recent technological progress significantly improved our ability in all three of these venues. Computed tomography (CT) provides excellent cross-sectional osseous details; multiplanar reformation, including three-dimensional images, can enhance surgical fracture classification and surgical planning. Magnetic resonance imaging (MRI) has excellent contrast resolution and is the screening procedure for some traumatic problems. However, everyday use of CT and MRI, which has become a primary diagnostic tool, do not diminish the role of conventional radiography as an effective modality for diagnosing fracture and monitoring the results of treatment.

This text represents an effort to update the areas of diagnosis and treatment of various fractures and dislocations. The goal is to provide graphic sound bites in succinct and compact chapters that can be rapidly referenced and used to complement standard orthopedic texts. The emphasis is on the effectiveness of new imaging techniques and current orthopedic approaches to treatment of the various fractures. We have compiled a group of national experts to discuss the effectiveness of imaging and treatment of fractures of the axial skeleton and extremities. The content of this book is divided into six sections; the first section is solely devoted to contemporary imaging, and the five other sections systematically discuss fractures and their treatment in the spine, pelvis and acetabulum, hip and femur, lower limbs, and upper extremities. The text is generously supplemented with line drawings and schematics to clarify the various surgical approaches to fracture treatment.

This book is designed primarily for orthopedic surgeons subspecializing in trauma, but general surgeons and even radiologists may find this publication useful in their clinical practice.

H. David Moehring, MD
Adam Greenspan, MD

CONTRIBUTORS

Daniel R. Benson, MD
Professor
Department of Orthopedic Surgery
University of California, Davis
Professor and Chief of Spine Service
University of California, Davis Medical Center
Sacramento, California

Eric A. Brandser, MD
Associate Professor
Department of Radiology
University of Iowa
Iowa City, Iowa

Paul J. Duwelius, MD
Adjunct Associate Professor
Department of Orthopedic Surgery
Oregon Health Sciences University
Portland, Oregon

Kenneth A. Egol, MD
Clinical Instructor
Department of Orthopedic Surgery and Joint Diseases
New York University Hospital
New York, New York

Thomas J. Ellis, MD
Assistant Professor
Department of Orthopedic Surgery
University of Oregon Health Sciences Center
Portland, Oregon

Christopher G. Finkemeier, MD, MBA
Assistant Professor
Department of Orthopedic Surgery
University of California, Davis
Sacramento, California

Thomas P. Goss, MD
Professor
Department of Orthopedic Surgery
University of Massachusetts Medical School
Attending Orthopedic Surgeon
University of Massachusetts—Memorial Health Care
Worcester, Massachusetts

Zbigniew Gugala, MD
Department of Orthopedic Surgery
Baylor College of Medicine
Houston, Texas

Munish C. Gupta, MD
Assistant Professor
Department of Orthopedic Surgery
University of California, Davis
Assistant Professor
University of California, Davis Medical Center
Sacramento, California

Sigvard T. Hansen, Jr, MD
Professor
Department of Orthopedics
University of Washington
Chief
Foot, Ankle Amputee
Harborview Medical Center
Seattle, Washington

Ronald W. Hendrix, MD
Associate Professor
Department of Radiology
Northwestern University Medical School
Co-Director
Department of Musculoskeletal Radiology
Northwestern Memorial Hospital
Chicago, Illinois

Peter J. L. Jebson, MD
Assistant Professor
Department of Orthopedic Surgery
University of Michigan
Assistant Professor
University of Michigan Hospitals and Health System
Ann Arbor, Michigan

Jesse B. Jupiter, MD
Professor
Department of Orthopedic Surgery
Harvard Medical School
Chief, Hand Surgery Service
Department of Orthopedic Surgery
Massachusetts General Hospital
Boston, Massachusetts

James F. Kellam, MD
Vice Chairman
Department of Orthopedic Surgery
Carolinas Medical Center
Charlotte, North Carolina

Richard F. Kyle, MD
Associate Professor
Department of Orthopedic Surgery
University of Minnesota Medical School
Chairman
Department of Orthopedic Surgery
Hennepin County Medical Center
Minneapolis, Minnesota

Michael J. Leddy, III, MD
Resident
Department of Orthopedics
Louisiana State University Health Sciences Center
New Orleans, Louisiana

David S. Levine, MD
Instructor
Department of Orthopedic Surgery
Cornell University Medical College
Assistant Attending Orthopedic Surgeon
Hospital for Special Surgery
New York, New York

Ronald W. Lindsey, MD
Professor
Department of Orthopedic Surgery
Baylor College of Medicine
Houston, Texas

Dean S. Louis, MD
Professor of Surgery
Department of Orthopedic Surgery
University of Michigan
Professor of Surgery
University of Michigan Hospitals and Health System
Ann Arbor, Michigan

Vasilios Mathews, MD
Resident in Orthopedic Surgery
Lenox Hill Hospital
New York, New York

Todd O. McKinley, MD
Fellow
Department of Orthopedic Surgery
University of Maryland Shock Trauma Center
Baltimore, Maryland

Robert F. McLain, MD
Director of Spine Research
Department of Orthopedic Surgery
The Cleveland Clinic Foundation
Cleveland, Ohio

Pasquale Montesano, MD
Mercy Hospitals of Sacramento
Sacramento, California

Elvert F. Nelson, MD
Orthopedic Spine Surgeon
Sacramento, California

A. Lee Osterman, MD
Professor and Section Chief of Hand Surgery
Department of Orthopedic Surgery
Thomas Jefferson University
Director
Philadelphia Hand Center
Philadelphia, Pennsylvania

Larry R. Padgett, MD
Director of Sports Medicine
Gessler Clinic
Winter Haven, Florida

Edward A. Perez, MD
Department of Orthopedic Surgery
Oregon Health Sciences University
Portland, Oregon

David Ring, MD
Fellow, Hand Surgery Service
Department of Orthopedic Surgery
Harvard Medical School
Fellow, Hand Surgery Service
Department of Orthopedic Surgery
Massachusetts General Hospital
Boston, Massachusetts

Thomas A. Russell, MD
Professor
Department of Orthopedic Surgery
University of Tennessee
Memphis Orthopedic Group, Inc
Memphis, Tennessee

Augusto Sarmiento, MD
Professor and Chairman Emeritus
Department of Orthopedics and Rehabilitation
University of Miami
Miami, Florida
Director
Arthritis and Joint Replacement Institute
HealthSouth Doctor's Hospital
Coral Gables, Florida

Franklin D. Shuler, MD
Resident
Department of Orthopedic Surgery
University of Pittsburgh
Pittsburgh, Pennsylvania

Robert R. Slater, Jr
Assistant Professor
Department of Orthopedic Surgery
University of California, Davis
Sacramento, California

William I. Sterett, MD
Orthopedic Surgeon
Steadman Hawkins Clinic
Vail, Colorado

Marc F. Swiontkowski, MD
Professor and Chairman
Department of Orthopedic Surgery
University of Southern California
Los Angeles, California
University of Minnesota Physicians
Minneapolis, Minnesota

David C. Teague, MD
Assistant Professor
Department of Orthopedic Surgery and Rehabilitation
University of Oklahoma
Assistant Professor
University Physicians Medical Group
Oklahoma City, Oklahoma

Michael E. Torchia, MD
Associate Professor
Department of Orthopedic Surgery
Mayo Medical School
Consultant
Mayo Clinic
Rochester, Minnesota

Mark S. Vrahas, MD
Visiting Assistant Professor
Department of Orthopedic Surgery
Harvard Medical School
Partners Chief of Orthopedic Trauma
Massachusetts General Hospital
Brigham and Women's Hospital
Boston, Massachusetts

J. Tracy Watson, MD
Professor
Department of Orthopedic Surgery
Wayne State University School of Medicine
Vice Chief
Division of Orthopedic Trauma
University Health Center
Detroit Receiving Hospital
Detroit, Michigan

Lon S. Weiner, MD
Chief
Trauma Section
Department of Orthopedic Surgery
Lenox Hill Hospital
New York, New York

Lawrence E. Weiss, MD
Director of Hand and Upper Extremity Surgery
North Shore University Hospital at Forest Hills
Forest Hills, New York

Terry Whipple, MD
Professor
Department of Orthopedic Surgery
Bowman Gray School of Medicine
Winston-Salem, North Carolina
Associate Clinical Professor of Orthopedics
University of Virginia
Charlottesville, Virginia

John M. Wright, MD
Orthopedic Surgeon
Steadman Hawkins Clinic
Vail, Colorado

Bruce H. Ziran, MD
Assistant Professor
Department of Orthopedic Surgery
University of Pittsburgh
Pittsburgh, Pennsylvania

SECTION I

Imaging

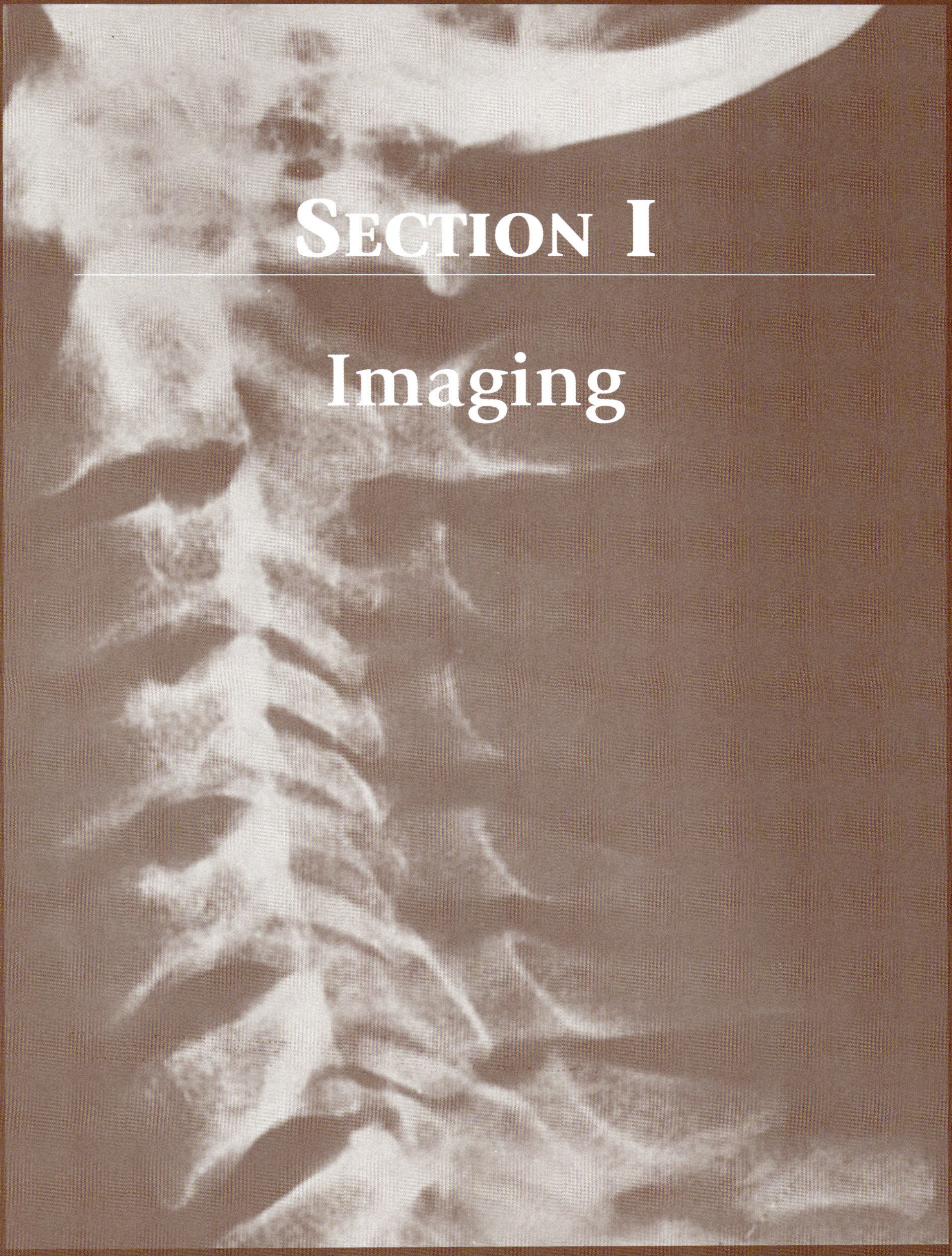

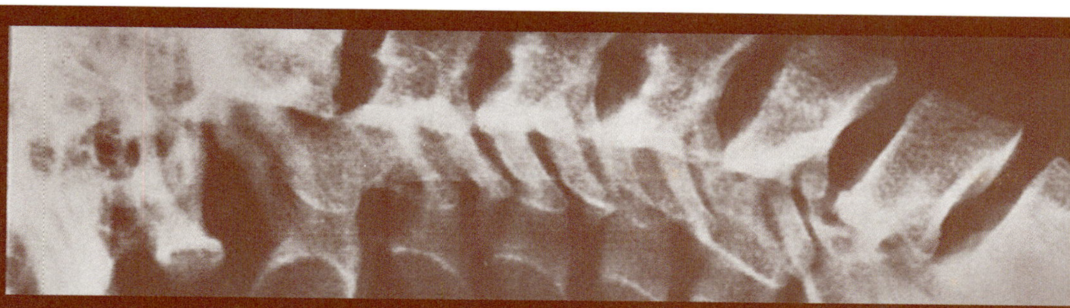

1

Radiologic Evaluation of Fractures

Adam Greenspan

Continued progress in radiology and the introduction of new imaging modalities have significantly improved our capabilities for diagnosing and evaluating traumatic abnormalities. Clinical information and physical examination findings are effective in making a presumptive diagnosis in a patient who has sustained injury to the musculoskeletal system. Conventional radiography in most instances reveals the type of fracture. However, occult and nondisplaced fractures may be missed and misdiagnosed. Likewise, fractures in severely osteopenic patients may be difficult to identify. Recent applications of computed tomography (CT) and magnetic resonance imaging (MRI) have facilitated the process of diagnosis, and hence, the treatment of various fractures [1,2]. It must be stressed, however, that conventional radiography remains the primary tool in the diagnosis and evaluation of various fractures and should always be obtained first, before more sophisticated (and more costly) modalities are considered [3•].

CONVENTIONAL RADIOGRAPHY AND TOMOGRAPHY

In most instances, radiographs obtained in two orthogonal projections—usually anteroposterior (AP) (or posteroanterior) and lateral—at 90° to each other are sufficient to demonstrate the fracture. Occasionally, oblique and special views are necessary, particularly in evaluating fractures of complex structures, such as the spine, pelvis, elbow, wrist, and ankle.

Tomography, particularly that which employs multidirectional movements (hypocycloidal or trispiral) by producing a blurring effect outside the field of interest and therefore yielding sharp focal plane images, is very effective in demonstrating anatomic details otherwise obscured by overlying structures. Hence, tomography is effective in diagnosing a subtle fracture that may be missed on conventional radiography [4]. It is used in demonstrating fractures of small bones of the hand and foot as well as the cervical spine. It is superior to conventional radiography for delineating the extent of fracture line, evaluating the healing process, and evaluating nonunions.

Radiographic examination of a patient with cervical spine trauma may be difficult when the patient is unconscious, because it is limited to one or two projections; in the presence of associated injuries; and when unnecessary movement risks damage to the cervical cord. It is not so uncommon in these circumstances, for instance, to miss a fracture at the level of occipitoatlantal junction, odontoid, or C7 vertebra. Fractures of the occipital condyles are almost impossible to detect on radiography; therefore, if such is suspected, either conventional tomography or CT with coronal reformation should be performed. Fracture of C1 vertebra, conversely, should not create a problem with diagnosis on the standard lateral and open-mouth AP radiographs. A characteristic lateral displacement of the lateral masses of C1 over cranial aspect of C2, even if actual fracture line can not be seen, is diagnostic of Jefferson's fracture (Figure 1-1). Odontoid fracture can be missed if proper radiographs are not obtained. The best techniques for demonstrating fractures of the dens are the lateral radiograph (Figure 1-2), the open-mouth AP radiograph, and Fuchs' projection [5]. If fracture is suspected but not clearly demonstrated on conventional radiography, either thin-section trispiral tomography (Figure 1-3) or CT with coronal and sagittal reformation should be performed.

The C7 vertebra must be visualized on any standard projections of the cervical spine, because fracture of C7 can easily be overlooked. This is particularly true about a fracture of the spinous process (clay-shoveler's fracture). If C7 cannot be visualized despite good positioning and technique because of a patient's short, thick neck or wide shoulders, for example, the swimmer's view should be obtained. The clinician should be aware of a possibility to diagnose clay-shoveler's fracture on an AP radiograph by the "ghost sign" (Figure 1-4), which is produced by displacement of the fractured spinous process.

In the lower thoracic and lumbar spine, it is easy to overlook the seat belt (or Chance) fracture, particularly if the injury mainly affects ligaments and intervertebral disk with minimal or no involvement of the vertebra. It is recognized on the AP radiograph by an increased distance between affected spinous processes (Figure 1-5). Bilateral traumatic or stress fractures of pars interarticularis associated with spondylolisthesis can be diagnosed on the lateral radiographs alone. This type of spondylolisthesis can be

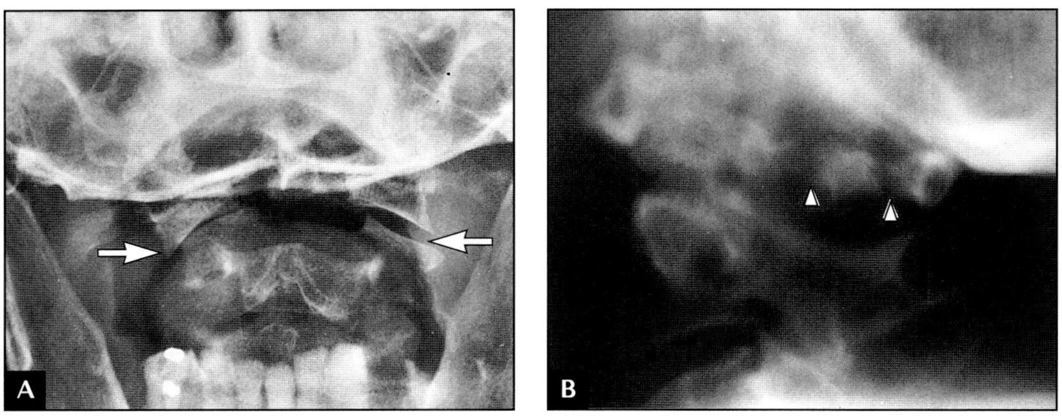

FIGURE 1-1. **A**, Open-mouth anteroposterior radiograph of the cervical spine shows malalignment of the lateral masses of the atlas (*arrows*). **B**, Lateral radiograph demonstrates fracture lines of the posterior arch of C1 (*arrowheads*). These findings are diagnostic of Jefferson fracture.

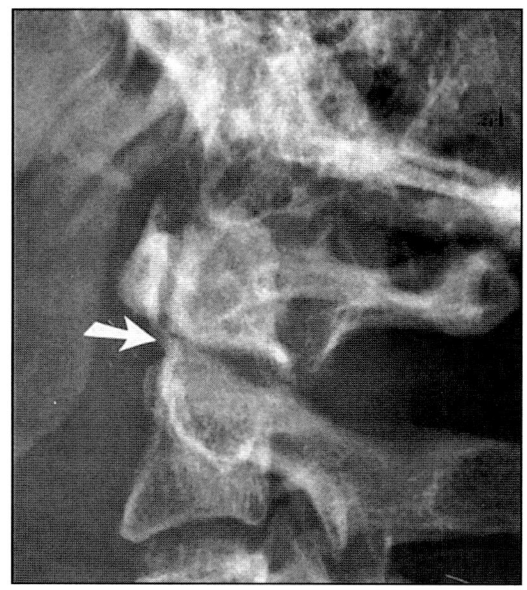

FIGURE 1-2. Lateral radiograph shows a Type II odontoid fracture (*arrow*).

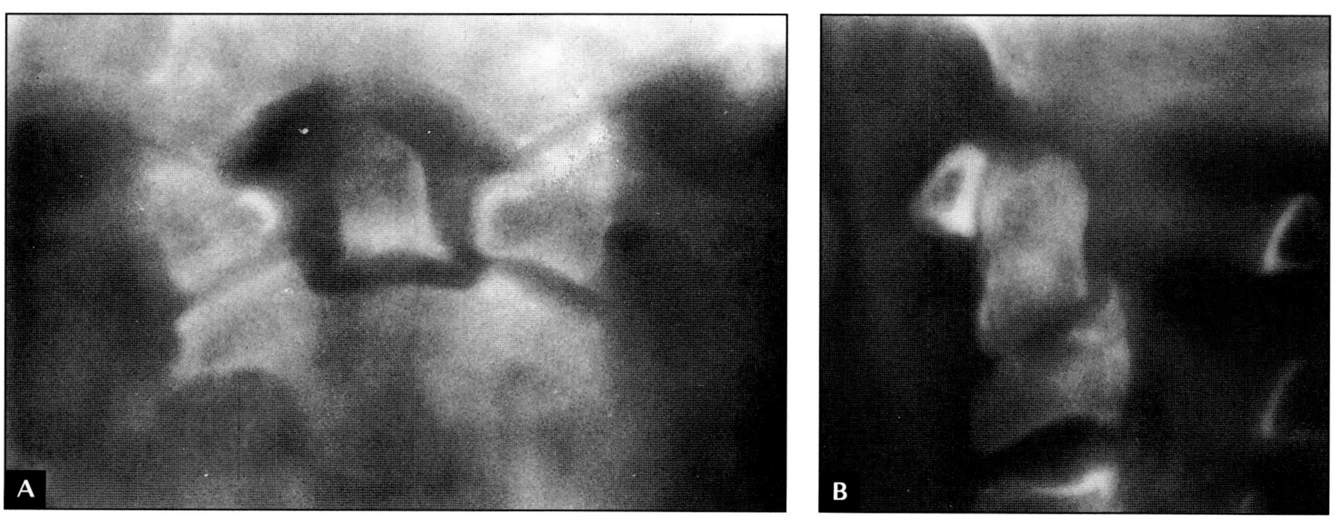

FIGURE 1-3. Trispiral tomograms in anteroposterior (**A**) and lateral (**B**) projections show a Type II odontoid fracture.

distinguished from the degenerative spondylolisthesis without the defect in the isthmus by the spinous process sign. The sign is a logical outgrowth of the different processes at work. In spondylolisthesis associated with spondylolysis, a bilateral defect in the pars interarticularis leads to ventral slippage of the body, pedicles, and superior articular process of the involved vertebra, whereas the spinous process, laminae, and inferior articular process remain in normal position. Therefore, study of the most dorsal aspects of the spinous processes reveals a step-off at the interspace above the level of the slip. On the other hand, in degenerative spondylolisthesis (without pars defect), the entire vertebra, including the spinous process, moves forward. In this situation, the most dorsal aspects of the spinous processes exhibit a step-off at the interspace below the level of the slipped vertebra [6]. Application of this sign allows a correct diagnosis to be made on a single lateral film; oblique projections are frequently not necessary.

Trauma to the elbow may, at times, create diagnostic difficulties. In particular, a subtle fracture of the radial head or coronoid process may not be visualized on the standard projections of the elbow joint because of the overlap of the anatomic structures. The radial head–capitellum view, a variant of the lateral projection, overcomes the major limitations of the standard lateral view by projecting the radial head ventrad, free of the overlap of the coronoid process [7]. This view has proved to be a particularly effective technique to demonstrate fractures of the posterior aspect of the radial head and fractures of the coronoid process (Figure 1-6).

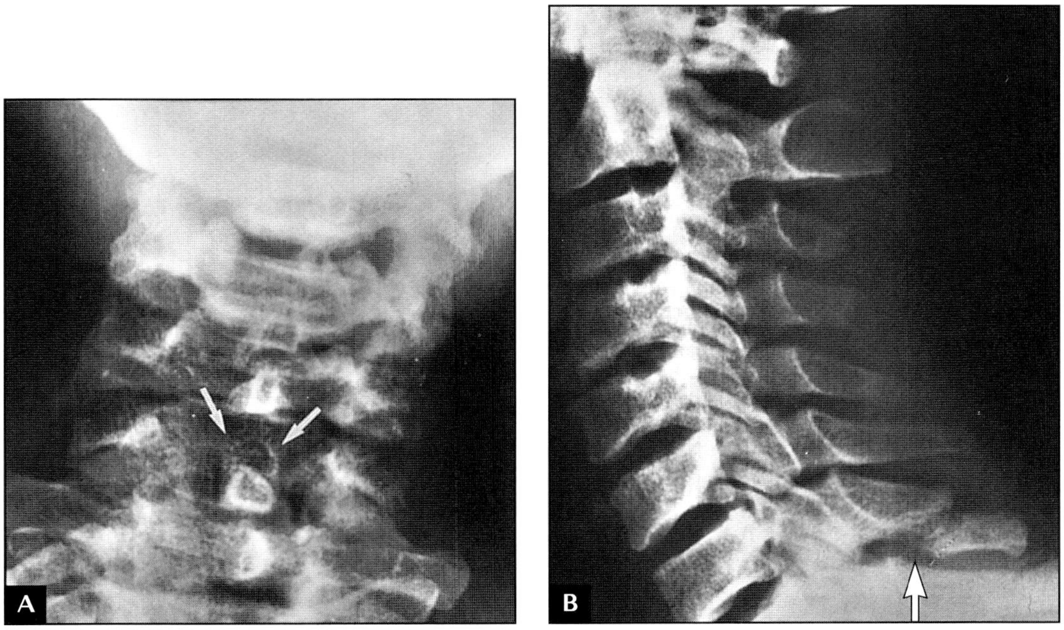

FIGURE 1-4. A, Anteroposterior radiograph of the cervical spine shows a "ghost sign" (double outline of the spinous process of C7) (*arrows*) secondary to slight caudal displacement of the fractured tip of the spinous process. **B**, "Clay-shoveler's" fracture of C7 is confirmed on the lateral radiograph (*arrow*).

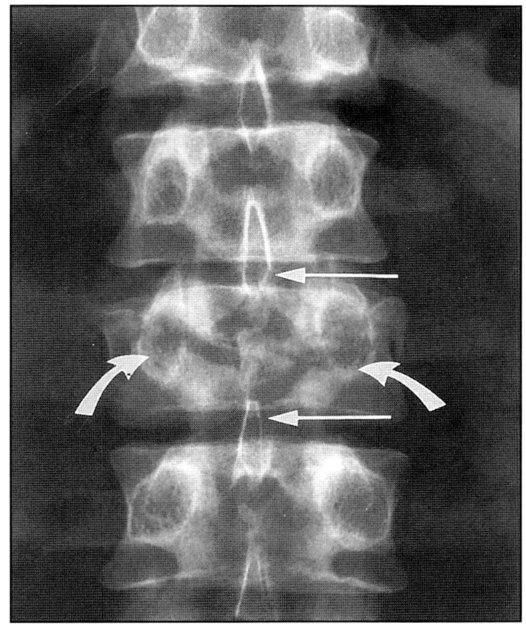

FIGURE 1-5. Anteroposterior radiograph of the lumbar spine shows increased distance between spinous processes of L1 and L2 (*arrows*), a characteristic sign of a Chance fracture. A faint radiolucent line through the body of L2 is also present (*curved arrows*).

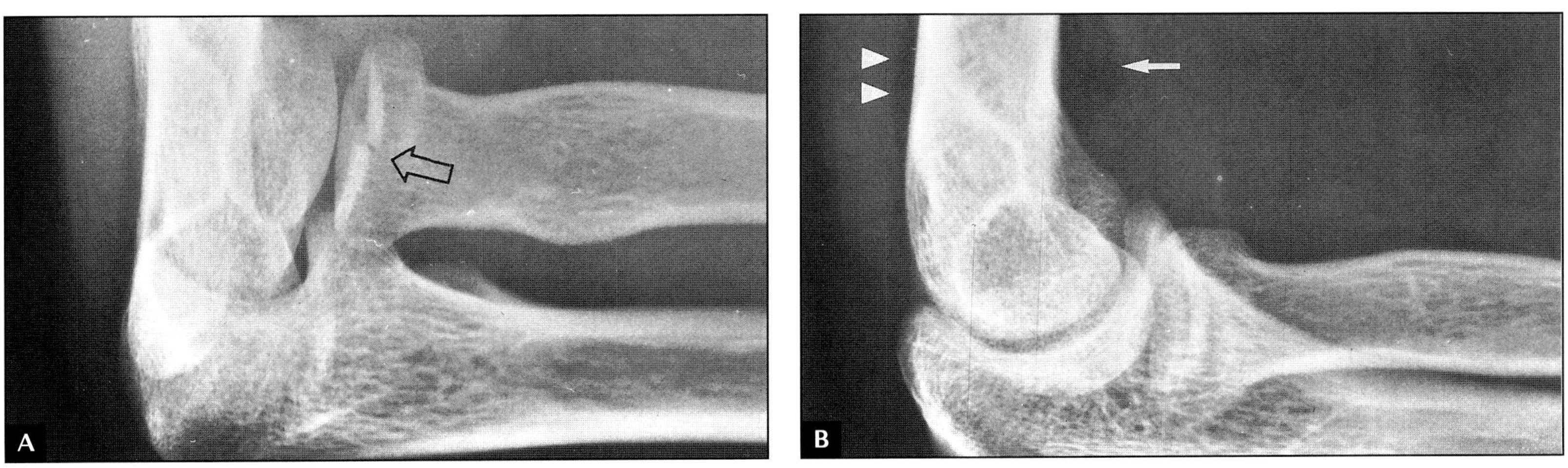

FIGURE 1-6. A, Radial head–capitellum view shows a fracture of the radial head (*open arrow*) not clearly demonstrated on the conventional radiographs of the elbow joint. **B**, The lateral radiograph showed only positive anterior (*arrow*) and posterior (*arrowheads*) fat-pad sign, but the radial head fracture was not apparent because of the overlap of the bones.

Fractures of the scaphoid occasionally may be difficult to diagnose on the standard projections of the wrist [8••]. When there is strong clinical suspicion for a fracture and routine films fail to visualize a fracture line, thin-section trispiral tomography has proven to be effective (Figure 1-7). This technique is equally helpful in monitoring the progress of scaphoid fracture healing and in detecting posttraumatic complications.

Fractures of the hook of the hamate are not apparent on conventional radiographs and consequently may go undiagnosed. As an aid to recognizing hamulus fracture on a standard dorsovolar projection of the hand, the clinician should be familiar with the "eye sign" [9], which derives its name from the dense, oval cortical ring shadow, representing the hook of the hamate seen on end, that is normally seen over the hamate on the dorsovolar view. The absence or indistinct outline of the cortical shadow suggests the diagnosis of hamulus fracture. Confirmation of the diagnosis can be made on the carpal-tunnel projection or on trispiral tomography (Figure 1-8).

Regarding trauma to the lower extremities, Lisfranc's fracture-dislocation may occasionally be so subtle that it can easily be missed on the standard views of the foot. If it is suspected, but AP, lateral, and oblique views of the foot appear normal, then radiographs of the contralateral foot should be obtained for comparison, and, if the diagnosis is still in doubt, conventional tomography in AP and lateral projections may reveal the abnormality.

Subtle fractures around the knee joint may be missed on conventional radiography. Lipohemarthrosis, which is identified on the cross-table lateral radiographs by the fat–blood interface (FBI) sign [10,11], is an important clue to the presence of an intra-articular fracture (Figure 1-9). Radiologic evaluation of depressed tibial plateau fractures is essential for determining the method of treatment. Assessment of the amount of displacement and depression is not accurate from the conventional radiographs but may be achieved more effectively using trispiral tomography in AP and lateral projections (Figure 1-10).

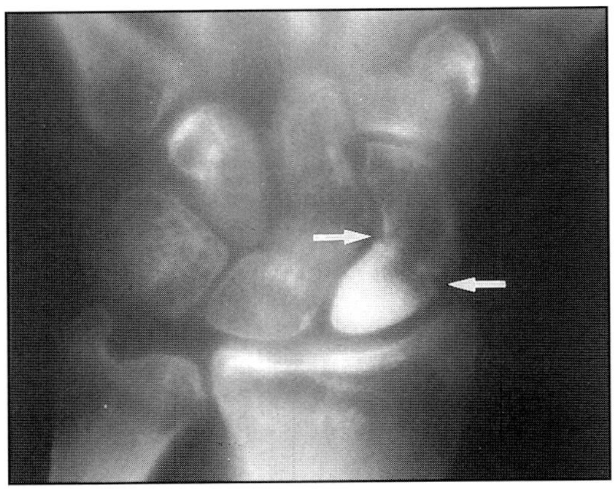

FIGURE 1-7. Trispiral tomogram of the wrist demonstrates a nonunited fracture of the scaphoid (*arrows*) and osteonecrosis of the proximal fragment.

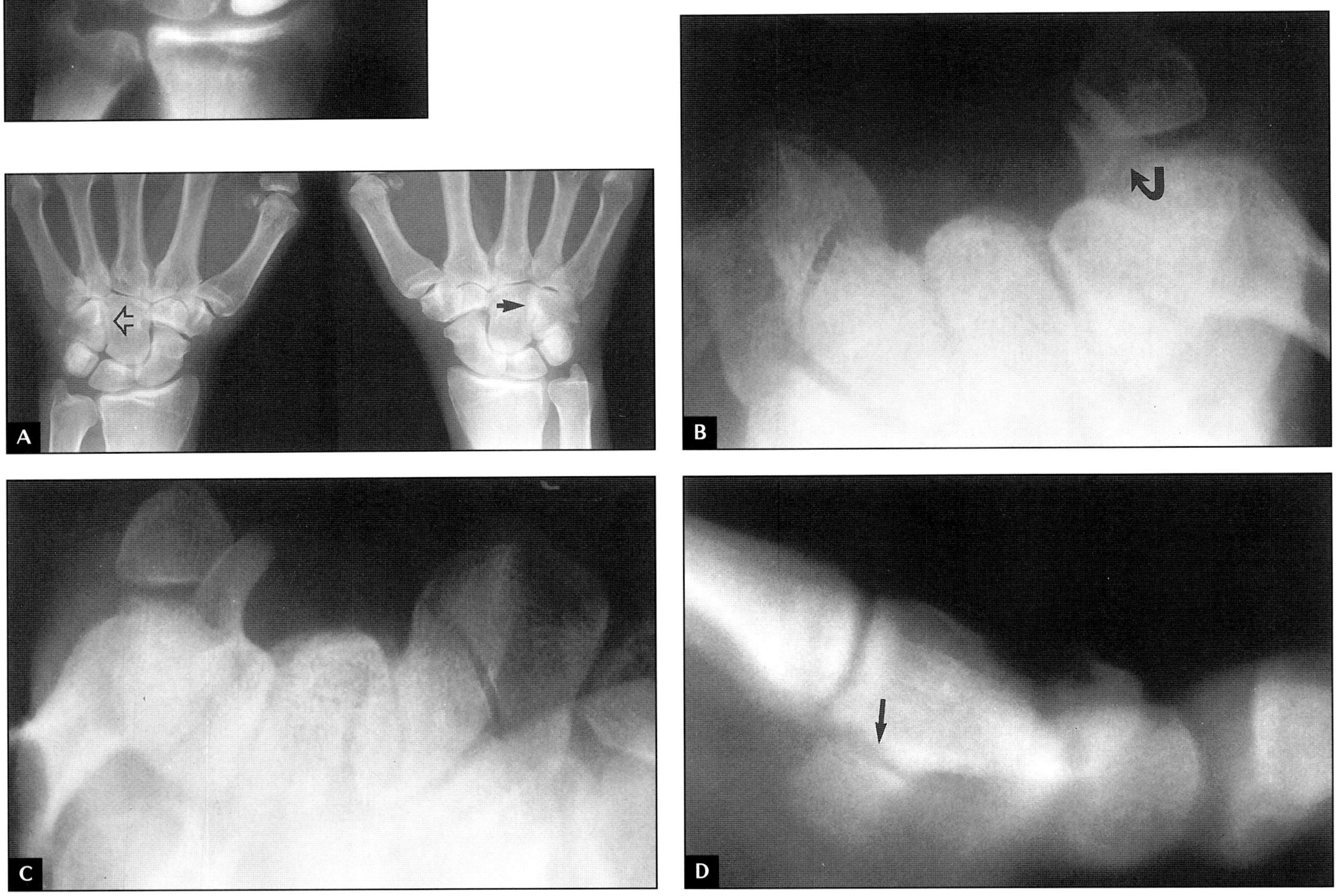

FIGURE 1-8. A, Dorsovolar radiograph of both wrists shows that the oval cortical shadow normally seen projecting over the hamate is not visible on the left wrist (*arrow*), suggesting fracture. Note normal eye sign of the right wrist (*open arrow*). **B**, Carpal projection shows a radiolucent line at the base of the hook (*curved arrow*). Compare with a normal opposite site (**C**). **D**, Trispiral tomogram in the lateral projection confirms the fracture of the hook of the hamate (*arrow*).

COMPUTED TOMOGRAPHY

Computed tomography is an indispensable modality in the evaluation of many fractures, particularly those involving the spine. It is effective for detecting small bony fragments displaced into the joint after trauma. An advantage of CT over conventional radiography and tomography is its ability to image the bone not only in axial plane, but also in coronal, sagittal, and oblique planes using the reformation technique. In trauma to the spine, this multiplanar reconstruction is particularly helpful in evaluating occipital condyle fractures (Figure 1-11), odontoid fractures (Figure 1-12), evaluating vertebral alignment, and demonstrating horizontally

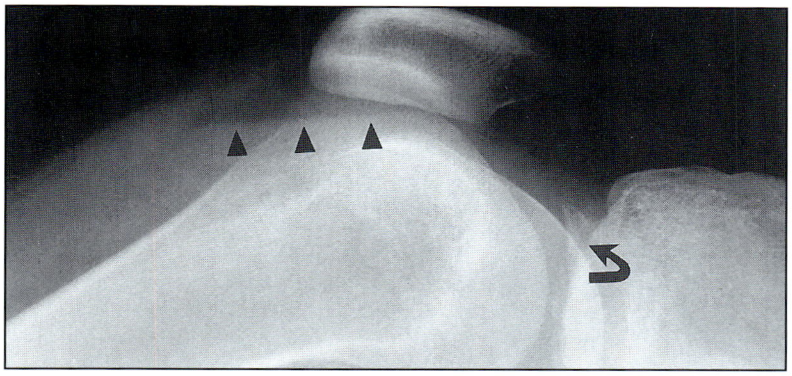

FIGURE 1-9. Cross-table lateral radiograph of the knee shows a fat–fluid level (fat-blood-interface, or FBI sign) in the joint (*arrowheads*), indicative of an intra-articular fracture. The fracture of the tibial plateau is not clearly seen (*curved arrow*).

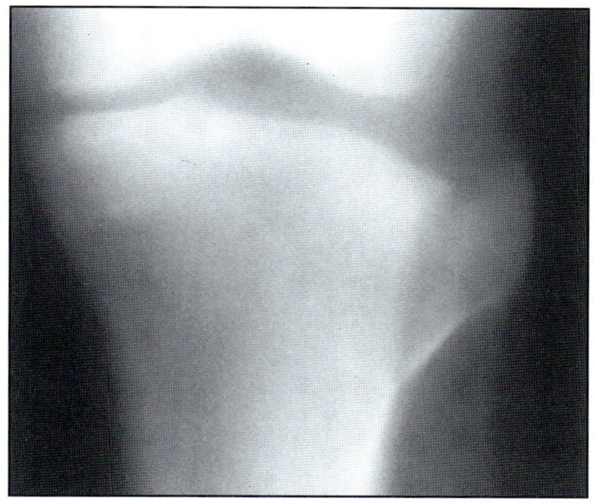

FIGURE 1-10. Frontal trispiral tomogram shows a displaced local split type of a tibial plateau fracture.

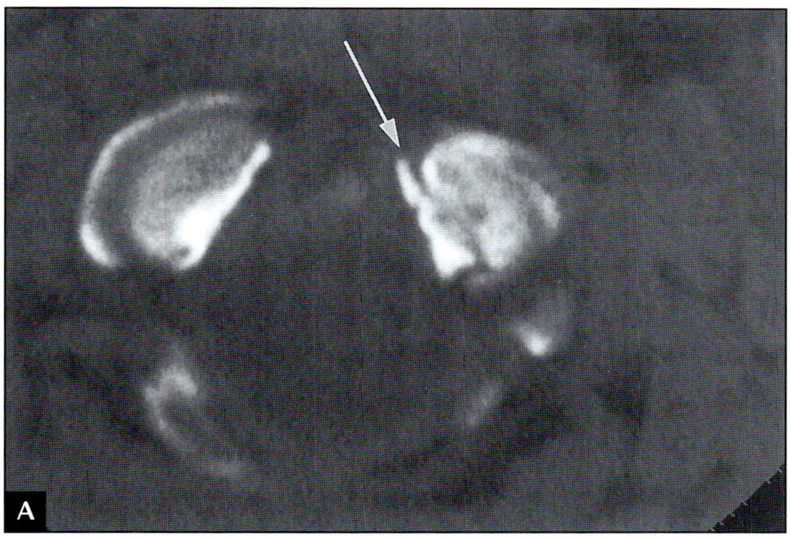

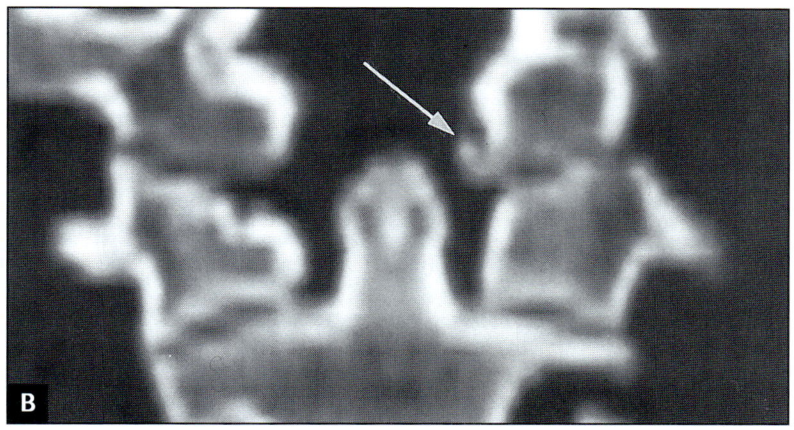

FIGURE 1-11. Axial (A) and coronal (B) reformatted computed tomography images demonstrate a fracture of the left occipital condyle (*arrows*).

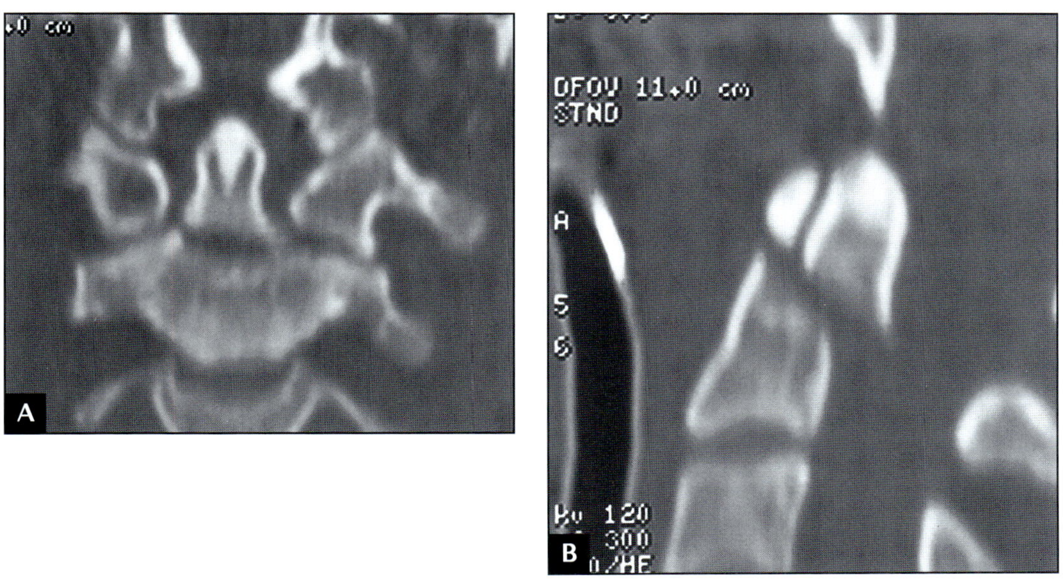

FIGURE 1-12. Coronal (A) and sagittal (B) reformatted computed tomography images show a Type II odontoid fracture.

oriented fractures of the vertebrae (Figure 1-13). This technique is also effective in evaluating complex fractures of the pelvis, knee, or calcaneus. The role of CT in evaluating tibial plateau fractures has been well established. CT provides optimal visualization of the plateau depression, articular defects, and split fragments. It has also been proven more accurate than conventional tomography in assessing depressed and split fractures when they involve the anterior and posterior border of the plateau and in demonstrating the extent of fracture comminution. For the latter, reformatted images in various planes are particularly helpful [12,13]. To evaluate trauma to the ankle joint, CT is especially useful when the fracture extends into the tibial plafond and the tibiotalar joint is involved. Although most talar fractures can be identified on conventional radiography, a nondisplaced fracture of the lateral process may be overlooked. CT is invariably more effective in this respect. Likewise, most fractures of the calcaneus should be evaluated by CT for assessment of the number and location of various fragments [14•]. CT is also indispensable in evaluating acetabular fractures. This technique is more sensitive than conventional radiography in detecting fractures of the acetabular roof, quadrilateral plate, and posterior wall of the acetabulum (Figure 1-14) [15]. It also can more accurately assess the degree of comminution of the acetabular dome and the configuration of fracture fragments [16]. The intra-articular loose fragments are also better delineated.

A recently developed modality, spiral (helical) scanning, permits three-dimensional reconstruction for analysis of regions with complex anatomy, such as the pelvis, vertebral column, wrist, foot, and ankle [17,18]. The three-dimensional CT images are obtained from the data of the contiguous thin axial sections, which are reformatted by computer programs [19,20]. The advantage of three-dimensional imaging lies not only in the ability to globally visualize anatomic structures under consideration, but also its ability to subtract parts of the images as well as rotate the image on the monitor to display the area of interest in any plane or degree of angulation (Figure 1-15).

SKELETAL SCINTIGRAPHY

One major advantage of radionuclide bone scanning over all other imaging techniques is its ability to image the entire skeleton simultaneously [21•]. Although specificity of the radionuclide bone scan is low, its sensitivity is extremely high and the fracture may be detected before it is seen on conventional radiography, tomography, or CT scan [22]. This technique may also exclude the fracture in cases in which conventional radiographs are equivocal. Skeletal scintigraphy is extremely helpful in the early diagnosis of stress fractures (Figure 1-16) [23,24]. It is also valuable in diagnosing fractures of the scaphoid and the femoral neck in elderly patients with osteoporosis, if the standard radiographic examination appears normal [25]. Single photon emission computed

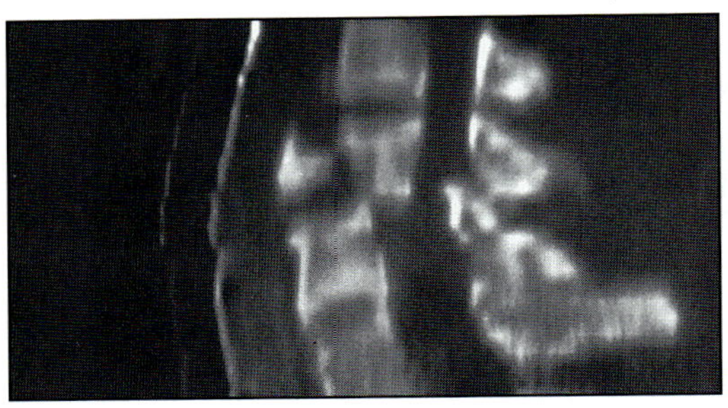

FIGURE 1-13. Sagittal reformatted computed tomography image of the cervical spine shows a tear-drop fracture of C5. The vertebral body is posteriorly displaced, and compromise of the spinal canal at this level is clearly demonstrated.

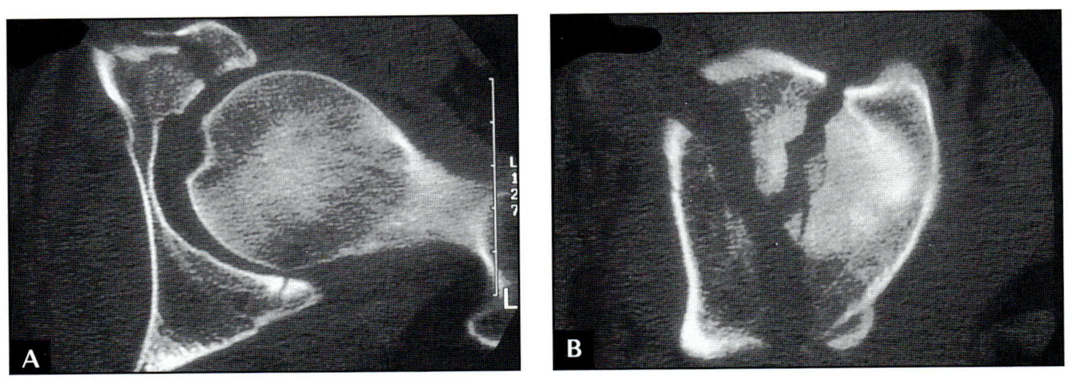

FIGURE 1-14. Two computed tomography sections, one at the midlevel of the hip joint (A) and the other through the acetabular roof (B), clearly demonstrate the extent of the acetabular fracture.

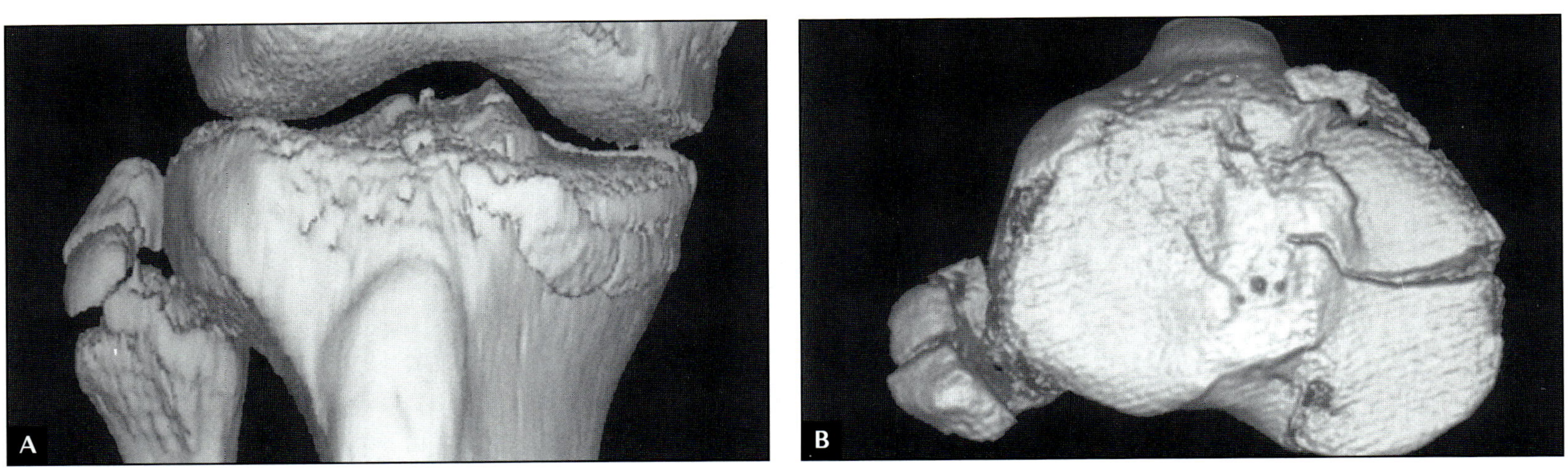

FIGURE 1-15. Frontal (A) and bird's-eye (B) view of the three-dimensional reformatted computed tomography images of the knee demonstrate the spatial orientation of the fracture lines in a patient with a comminuted fracture of the tibial plateau and proximal fibula.

tomography (SPECT) has, in the past decade, established a critical role in diagnosing traumatic conditions of bone [26].

MAGNETIC RESONANCE IMAGING

Recently, MRI became widely used in various traumatic conditions [27]. In most examinations, at least two orthogonal planes should be obtained (axial and either coronal or sagittal), and on many occasions all three planes are imaged. For adequate MRI, surface coils are necessary, because they provide improved spatial resolution. Because of high sensitivity and good specificity of MRI, occult fractures that often are missed on standard radiography and even CT can be well demonstrated (Figure 1-17) [28,29,30•,31••]. Some abnormalities, such as trabecular microfractures, that cannot be diagnosed on other imaging modalities are well depicted by this technique (Figure 1-18) [32]. MRI is frequently used to diagnose or exclude a hip fracture when the initial radiographs are equivocal on negative [33–36]. Moreover, MRI has proved to be a cost-effective alternative to bone scintigraphy in the evaluation of patients with suspected hip fractures [35,37•]. Recently, MRI was used in children with suspected injury to the growth plate and in patients with osteoporosis with suspected occult fracture [36].

Magnetic resonance imaging plays the leading role in evaluating fractures and fracture-dislocations of the spine in which injury to the spinal cord is suspected. This modality appears to be clearly superior to CT for assessing the soft tissues (*eg*, hematoma) and is particularly useful in patients with neurologic deficit. Both T1- and T2-weighted sequences are essential for adequate detection and characterization of bone and soft tissue injury [38]. Associated ligamentous injury can be identified by the presence of ligamentous discontinuity and vertebral malalignment [39]. MRI is extremely sensitive in the detection of pathophysiologic changes associated with stress injuries [40••]. Typical findings in early stress reactions include areas of low signal intensity in the marrow on T1-weighted images that increase in signal intensity with T2 weighting. Fat-saturation techniques, such as inversion-recovery or fast spin echo (FSE) T2-weighted imaging with frequency-selective fat saturation, are especially useful for identifying these

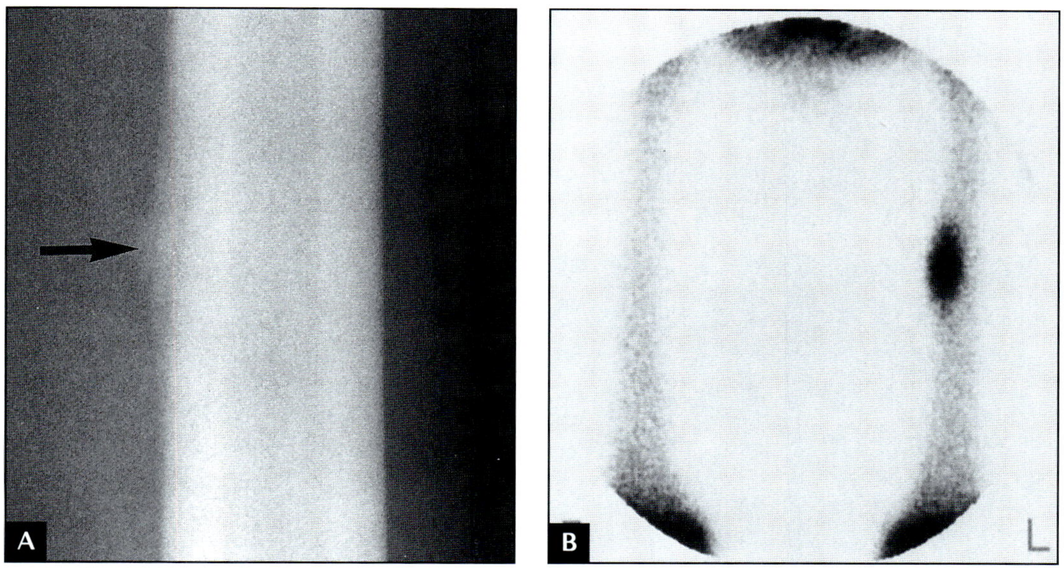

FIGURE 1-16. A, Conventional radiograph of the midportion of the left femur shows ill-defined radiolucent line and shaggy periosteal reaction (*arrow*) suggestive of a stress fracture. B, Radionuclide bone scan shows a fusiform area of increased uptake of a radiopharmaceutical tracer in the medial cortex, characteristic for a stress fracture.

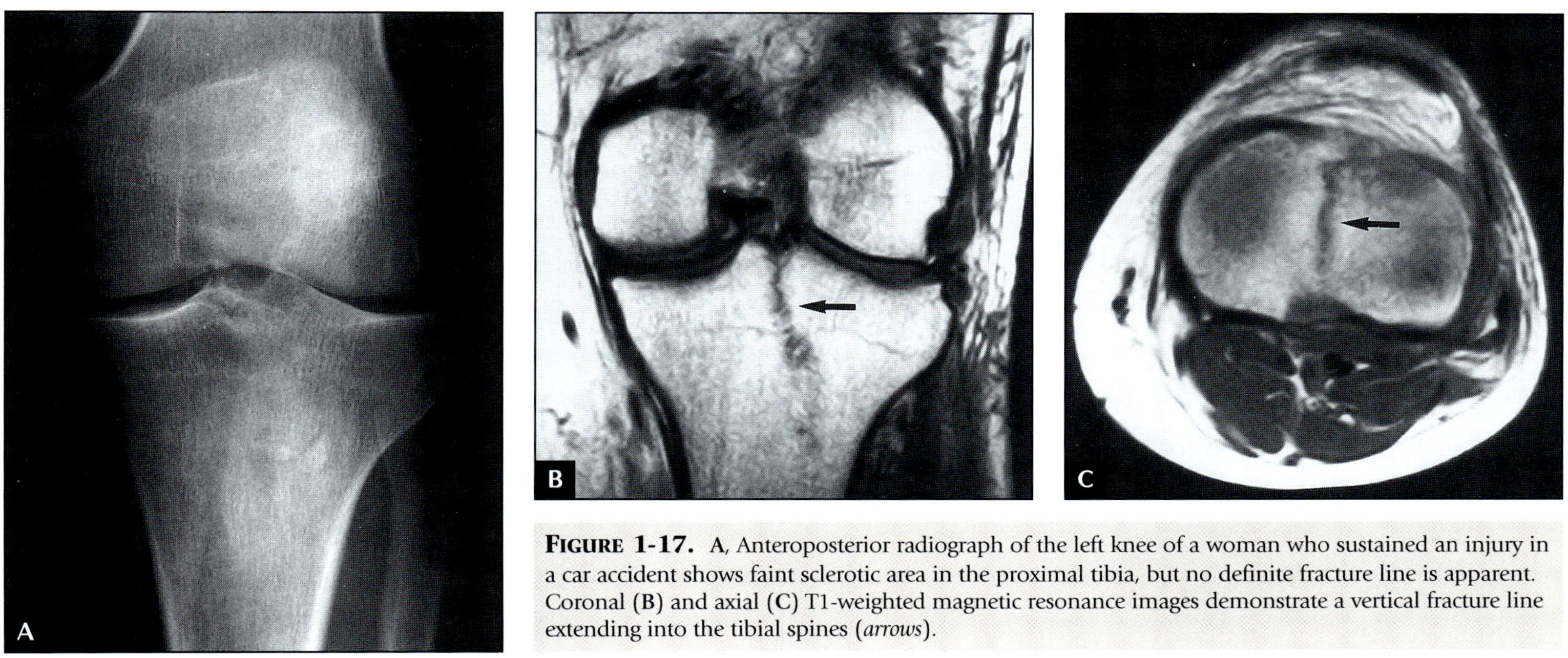

FIGURE 1-17. A, Anteroposterior radiograph of the left knee of a woman who sustained an injury in a car accident shows faint sclerotic area in the proximal tibia, but no definite fracture line is apparent. Coronal (B) and axial (C) T1-weighted magnetic resonance images demonstrate a vertical fracture line extending into the tibial spines (*arrows*).

injuries (Figure 1-19). The increased water content of the associated medullary edema or hemorrhage results in high signal intensity against the dark background of suppressed fat such that these sequences should maximize sensitivity [41,42]. On T2-weighted images of more advanced lesions, low intensity bands—contiguous with the cortex—have been seen within the marrow edema; these presumably represent fracture lines. The multiplanar capability of MRI provides a further advantage by allowing for optimal demonstration of the fracture line. In some cases, increased signal intensity has also been observed in a juxtacortical, subperiosteal location [43,44]. MRI has been advocated as a problem-solving modality, such as in a patient with negative conventional radiographs and an equivocal or confusing bone scan. It may secure the diagnosis if the fracture line is identified.

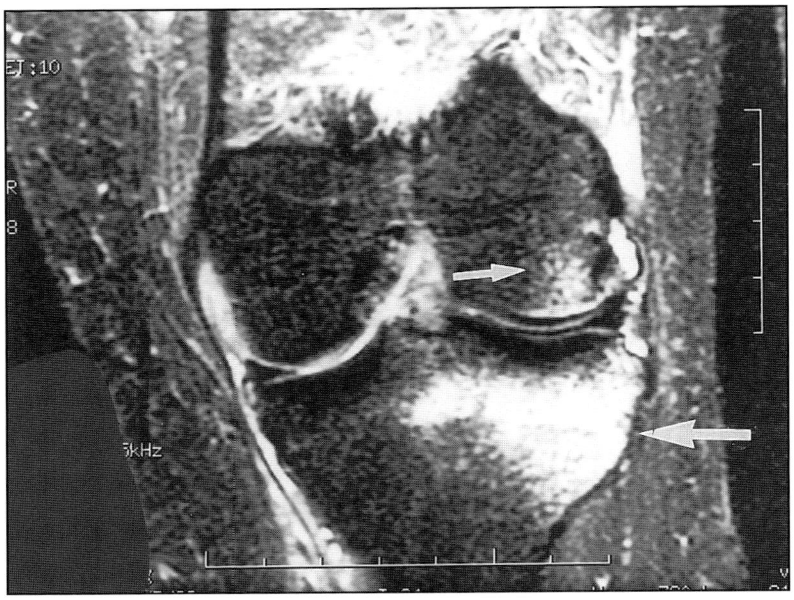

FIGURE 1-18. Coronal T2-weighted inversion recovery with fat saturation technique magnetic resonance image of the knee shows trabecular injury (a bone "bruise") in the lateral tibial plateau and lateral femoral condyle (*arrows*).

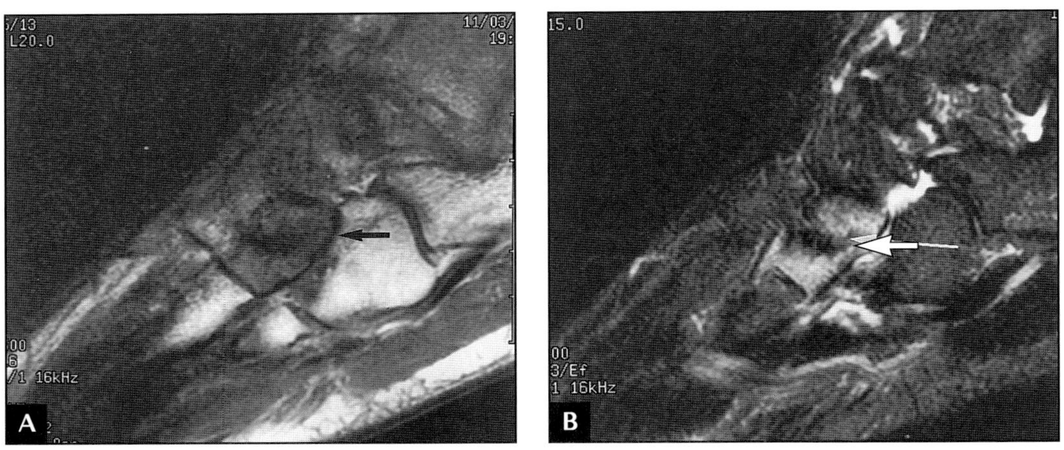

FIGURE 1-19. **A**, Sagittal T1-weighted magnetic resonance imaging (MRI) scan shows diffuse low signal intensity in the lateral cuneiform bone with central area of signal void (*arrow*). **B**, Sagittal T2-weighted MRI shows bright signal within the cuneiform bone due to marrow edema and hemorrhage. Central band of low signal intensity (*arrow*) represents a stress fracture.

REFERENCES AND RECOMMENDED READING

Recently published papers of particular interest have been highlighted as:
- • Of interest
- •• Of outstanding interest

1. Deutsch AL, Mink JH: Magnetic resonance imaging of musculoskeletal injuries. *Radiol Clin North Am* 1989, 27:983–1002.
2. McEnery KW, Wilson AJ, Pilgram TK, *et al.*: Fractures of the tibial plateau: value of spiral CT coronal plane reconstructions for detecting displacement in vitro. *Am J Roentgenol* 1994, 163:1177–1181.
3. • Pettersson H, Resnick D: Musculoskeletal imaging. *Radiology* 1998, 208:561–562.

The current status and future directions of imaging of the musculoskeletal system are discussed in this article.

4. Ho C, Sartoris DJ, Resnick D: Conventional tomography in musculoskeletal trauma. *Radiol Clin North Am* 1989, 27:929–932.
5. Ballinger PW: *Merrill's Atlas of Radiographic Positions and Radiologic Procedures* vol 1, edn 3. St. Louis: Mosby; 1986.
6. Bryk D, Rosenkranz W: True spondylolisthesis and pseudospondylolisthesis: the spinous process sign. *J Can Assoc Radiol* 1969, 20:53–56.
7. Greenspan A, Norman A: The radial head-capittellum view: useful technique in elbow trauma. *Am J Roentgenol* 1982, 138:1186–1188.
8. •• Munk PL, Lee MJ, Logan PM, *et al.*: Scaphoid bone waist fractures, acute and chronic: imaging with different techniques. *Am J Roentgenol* 1997, 168:779–786.

This article provides algorithms for imaging suspected scaphoid bone fractures and for evaluating avascular necrosis or delayed and nonunion of this bone. The roles of MRI and CT are stressed.

9. Norman A, Nelson JM, Green SM: Fractures of the hook of hamate: radiographic signs. *Radiology* 1985, 154:49–53.
10. Mitchell MJ, Ho C, Resnick D, *et al.*: Diagnostic imaging of lower extremity trauma. *Radiol Clin North Am* 1989, 27:909–928.
11. Wenzel WW: The FBI sign. *Rocky Mount Med J* 1972, 69:71–72.
12. Rafii M, Firooznia H, Golimbu C, *et al.*: Computed tomography of tibial plateau fractures. *Am J Roentgenol* 1984, 142:1181–1186.
13. Rafii M, Lamont JG, Firooznia H: Tibial plateau fractures: CT evaluation and classification. *Crit Rev Diagn Imaging* 1987, 27:91–112.
14. • Prokuski LJ, Saltzman CL: Challenging fractures of the foot and ankle. *Radiol Clin North Am* 1997, 35:655–670.

Radiologic evaluation of pilon fractures, fractures of the talus and calcaneus, and dislocations in the subtalar joint are discussed. Radiographic findings of Lisfranc's fracture-dislocation are provided.

15. Kricun M: Fractures of the pelvis. *Orthop Clin North Am* 1990, 21:573–590.
16. Rubenstein J, Kellam J, McGonigal D: Acetabular fracture assessment with computerized tomography. *J Can Assoc Radiol* 1982, 33:139–141.
17. Fishman EK: Spiral CT evaluation of the musculoskeletal system. In *Spiral CT: Principles, Techniques, and Clinical Applications*. Edited by Fishman EK, Jeffrey RB Jr. New York: Raven Press; 1995:141–158.
18. Fishman EK, Wyatt SH, Bluemke DE, *et al.*: Spiral CT of musculoskeletal pathology: preliminary observations. *Skeletal Radiol* 1993, 22:253–256.
19. Burk DL Jr, Mears DC, Cooperstein LA, *et al.*: Acetabular fractures: three-dimensional computed tomographic imaging and interactive surgical planning. *J Comput Tomogr* 1986, 10:1–10.
20. Magid D, Fishman EK: Imaging of musculoskeletal trauma in three dimensions: an integrated two-dimensional/three-dimensional approach with computed tomography. *Radiol Clin North Am* 1989, 27:945–956.
21. • Johnson RP: The role of bone imaging in orthopedic practice. *Semin Nucl Med* 1997, 27:386–389.

Bone scintigraphy is valuable in uncovering skeletal lesions that are obscure on other imaging studies. Its high sensitivity makes this technique an extremely useful tool in the diagnosis and management of a wide variety of skeletal disorders.

22. McDougall IR, Rieser RP: Scintigraphic techniques in musculoskeletal trauma. *Radiol Clin North Am* 1989, 27:1003–1011.
23. Ammann W, Matheson GO: Radionuclide bone imaging in the detection of stress fractures. *Clin J Sport Med* 1991, 1:115–122.
24. Daffner RH, Pavlov H: Stress fractures: current concepts. *Am J Roentgenol* 1992, 159:245–252.
25. Holder LE, Schwarz C, Wernicke PG, *et al.*: Radionuclide bone imaging in the early detection of fractures of the proximal femur (hip): multifactorial analysis. *Radiology* 1990, 174:509–515.
26. Murray PC: The role of SPECT in the evaluation of skeletal trauma. *Ann Nucl Med* 1993, 7:1–9.
27. Meyers SP, Weiner SN: Magnetic resonance imaging features of fractures using the short tau inversion recovery (STIR) sequence: correlation with radiographic findings. *Skeletal Radiol* 1991, 20:499–507.
28. Berger PE, Ofstein RA, Jackson DW, *et al.*: MRI demonstration of radiographically occult fractures: what have we been missing? *RadioGraphics* 1989, 9:407–436.
29. Yao L, Lee JK: Occult intraosseous fracture: detection with MR imaging. *Radiology* 1988, 167:749–751.
30. • Hunter JC, Escobedo EM, Wilson AJ, *et al.*: MR imaging of clinically suspected scaphoid fractures. *Am J Roentgenol* 1997, 168:1287–1293.

MRI can reveal occult scaphoid fractures when findings on radiographs are normal or equivocal.

31. •• Breitenseher MJ, Metz VM, Gilula LA, *et al.*: Radiographically occult scaphoid fractures: values of MR imaging in detection. *Radiology* 1997, 203:245–250.

MRI has a high sensitivity for detection of fractures of the scaphoid bone not evident on conventional radiographs and may enable early diagnosis and treatment.

32. Arndt WF III, Truax AL, Barnett FM, *et al.*: MR diagnosis of bone contusions of the knee: comparison of coronal T2-weighted fast spin-echo with fat saturation and fast spin-echo STIR images with conventional STIR images. *Am J Roentgenol* 1996, 166:119–124.
33. Deutsch AL, Mink JH, Waxman AD: Occult fractures of the proximal femur: MR imaging. *Radiology* 1989, 170:113–116.
34. Quinn SF, McCarthy JL: Prospective evaluation of patients with suspected hip fracture and indeterminate radiographs: use of T1-weighted MR images. *Radiology* 1993, 187:469.
35. Rizzo PF, Gould ES, Lyden JP, *et al.*: Diagnosis of occult fractures about the hip: magnetic resonance imaging compared with bone scanning. *J Bone Joint Surg Am* 1993, 75:395–401.
36. Ohashi K, Brandser EA, El-Khoury G: Role of MR imaging in acute injuries to the appendicular skeleton. *Imag Orthop Trauma* 1997, 35:591–613.
37. • Rubin SJ, Marquardt JD, Gottlieb RH, *et al.*: Magnetic resonance imaging: a cost-effective alternative to bone scintigraphy in the evaluation of patients with suspected hip fractures. *Skeletal Radiol* 1998, 27:199–204.

In the evaluation of patients with suspected hip fractures, early examination with MRI is more cost effective than delayed bone scanning. MRI has additional value in obtaining information about the exact site of the fracture and its extent.

38. Pathria MN, Petersilge CA: Spinal trauma. *Radiol Clin North Am* 1991, 29:847–865.
39. Emery SE, Pathria MN, Wilber RG, *et al.*: Magnetic resonance imaging of posttraumatic spinal ligament injury. *J Spinal Dis* 1989, 2:229–233.
40. •• Anderson MW, Greenspan A: State of the art: stress fractures. *Radiology* 1996, 199:1–12.

This is an in-depth discussion of the imaging features of stress fractures. An algorithm is suggested on the use of diagnostic imaging modalities if a stress fracture is suspected.

41. Lee JK, Yao L: Stress fractures: MR imaging. *Radiology* 1988, 169:217–220.
42. Martin SD, Healy JH, Horowitz S: Stress fracture MRI. *Orthopaedics* 1993, 16:75–78.
43. Stafford SA, Rosenthal DI, Gebhardt MC, *et al.*: MRI in stress fracture. *Am J Roentgenol* 1986, 147:553–556.
44. Steinbronn DJ, Bennett GL, Kay DB: The use of magnetic resonance imaging in the diagnosis of stress fractures of the foot and ankle: four case reports. *Foot Ankle Int* 1994, 15:80–83.

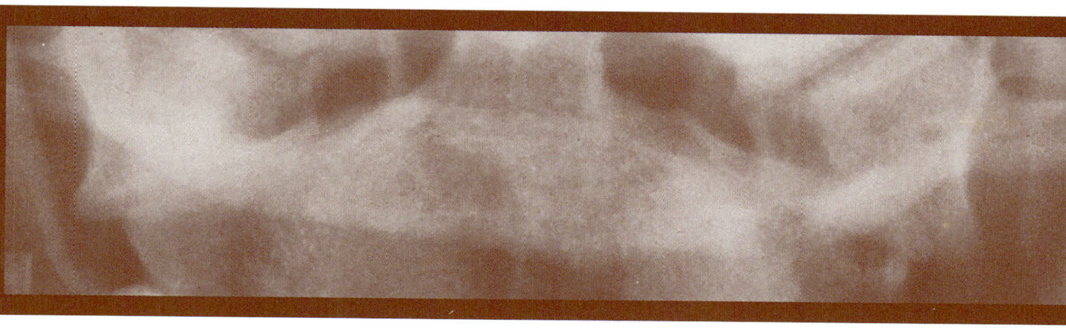

2

Imaging of Fractures and Dislocations of the Spine

Pasquale Montesano
Elvert F. Nelson
Adam Greenspan

GENERAL PRINCIPLES

Conventional radiography remains the primary modality in the initial evaluation of spinal injuries. By localizing the area of concern, radiographic films assist in decision making for more comprehensive imaging. When choosing a particular imaging protocol, numerous factors must be taken into consideration, including the patient's neurologic status, the site and age of the injury, the size of the patient, and the potential benefit unique to each imaging modality. For patients with head or spinal cord injuries, anteroposterior (AP) and lateral radiographs should be obtained in all areas below the level of injury including the pelvis.

Computed tomography (CT) directly visualizes the spine in the axial plane, identifying fractures and fracture patterns not seen on conventional radiographs. It has better spatial and contrast resolution, which is particularly important when visualizing the spinal canal (Figure 2-1). CT is noninvasive, has minimal ionizing radiation, and is often unsurpassed in the definition of bony pathology in the spinal canal and articular pillars. It remains the standard technique for assessing fractures at the thoracolumbar junction. Imaging problems in the uncooperative or severely traumatized patient have been addressed with the development of spiral (helical) CT scanning. The speed of the spiral CT, often less than 1 minute, has helped deal with patient positioning or repositioning problems, cost, and ability to rapidly scan many areas of the spine. The role of two-dimensional versus three-dimensional reformatted images is unclear. Although beautiful images are possible under ideal conditions, the quality of the reconstructions is vulnerable to patient movement and postprocessing time and is operator dependent [1].

Magnetic resonance imaging (MRI) has been an exciting addition to the evaluation of spinal trauma. Its signal intensity is a result of the property of the hydrogen protons within the nucleus. The nucleus is perturbed in the presence of a superimposed magnetic field and external radio frequency pulse. MRI enhances soft tissue visualization, allowing demonstration of intramedullary contusions, hematomas, ligament tears, disk herniations, and fluid accumulations (Figure 2-2). MRI is the only imaging modality that provides global fine detail in the coronal and sagittal planes.

Detection of disruption of the anterior or posterior longitudinal ligaments and hemorrhage in the posterior ligaments can identify underlying subtle or gross instability patterns. In spinal cord injuries, identification of blood within the cord substance or spinal cord edema has prognostic value. Disadvantages of MRI include cost, marginal bony detail, the typical contraindications for scanning, and the inaccessibility for patients with bulky life-support systems [2,3].

Conventional tomography has recently been replaced by CT (Figure 2-3) and MRI scanning. However, it can still be helpful in isolated situations. Axial CT sections may miss a Type II odontoid fracture, particularly in the osteoporotic spine, whereas lateral conventional tomography effectively shows this injury (Figure 2-4). Complex cervical lateral mass fracture-dislocation patterns are easier to understand and identify with two-plane tomography. Tomography may also be useful to diagnose and evaluate the Chance fracture, in which the minimally displaced horizontal fracture line extends into the pedicles.

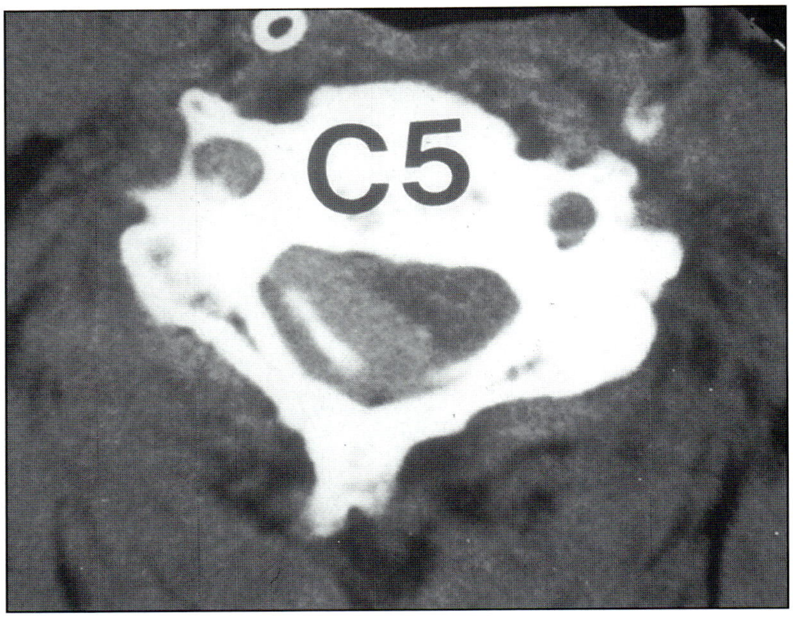

FIGURE 2-1. Computed tomography section showing a fracture of the lamina of C5 and a large hematoma compressing the spinal cord.

IMAGING OF CERVICAL INJURIES

GENERAL CONSIDERATIONS

In general, the trauma patient without neck pain or tenderness who is neurologically intact and has a full cervical range of motion does not need cervical radiographs. The trauma patient with subjective neck pain who is alert and neurologically intact requires a lateral cervical radiograph, an open-mouth anteroposterior (AP) view, and a radiograph to visualize the cervicothoracic junction. If C7 cannot be clearly seen, the swimmer's view should be obtained and frequently augmented with CT scans. In the patient with neck pain, altered mental status, and neurologic deficit, the workup must include AP and lateral radiographs and a CT scan of the entire cervical spine. A cross-table lateral radiograph will demonstrate 77% of cervical pathology. The accuracy increases to 84% when an open-mouth odontoid view is added [4].

In the acute phase, flexion-extension lateral radiographs have not statistically improved the identification of subtle or gross abnormalities. They are contraindicated in patients with neurologic deficits. A special normal variant known as pseudosubluxation at C2-C3 attributed to ligamentous laxity occurs in up to 25% of children up to age 8 years [5].

Loss of cervical lordosis has been overrated as an important sign of pathology. Normal cervical lordosis can be diminished with muscular spasm, prior trauma, preexisting degenerative changes, wearing a hard collar, flexion of the spine, and radiographic positioning.

The value of retropharyngeal soft tissue swelling is frequently of limited diagnostic value. Reported measurements of normal and abnormal values are variable and depend on age, radiographic techniques, position, and time interval between injury and radiographic examination. In the upper cervical spine (C3), measure-

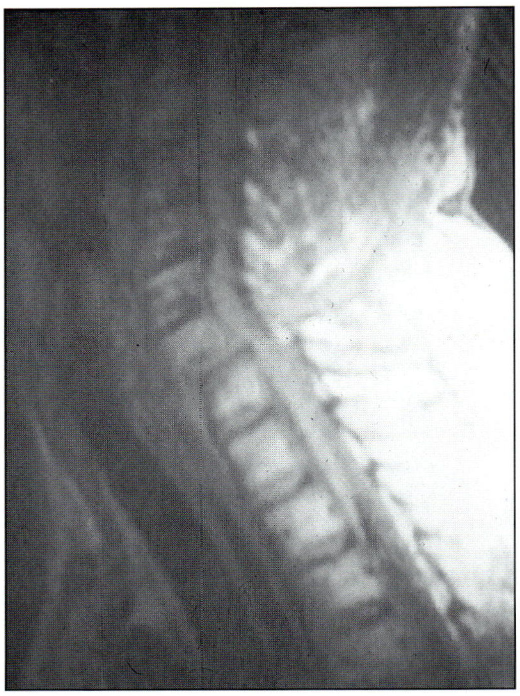

FIGURE 2-2. Sagittal spin-echo proton-density magnetic resonance imaging scan demonstrating a fracture-subluxation at C6-C7 with spinal cord compression.

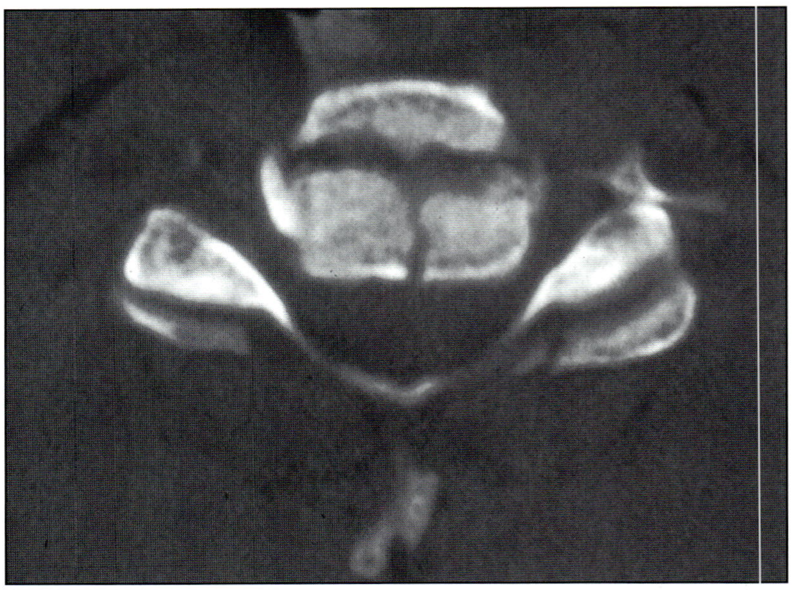

FIGURE 2-3. Axial computed tomography scan demonstrating all components of a burst fracture of C5.

ments above 7 mm indicate a statistical probability of injury, rising significantly with the measurements over 10 mm [6].

Determining spinal stability is frequently difficult except with obvious complete dislocations or fracture dislocations. Radiographic findings suggestive of instability include a combination of 3.5-mm horizontal translation and greater than 11° localized kyphosis [7], spinous process splaying, widening of the disk space, and vertebral body bidirectional displacement. Determining stability in compression fractures and burst fractures is not always feasible. The three-column concept of stability established by Denis [8] usually requires a CT scan to determine the integrity of the middle column.

Injury to the Occipitocervical Region and C1-C2

Recognition of occipitocervical pathology requires a high index of suspicion. Conventional cross-table lateral radiographs may be difficult to interpret or inconclusive, particularly in the severely traumatized patient with endotracheal and nasogastric tubes. Replacing standard open-mouth views with CT scans at the cervicocranial junction identifies occipital condyles, C1, and C2 fractures not seen on routine radiographs [9,10].

Injuries to the atlas can be diagnosed on conventional radiographs (Figure 2-5). Thin-section CT with the gantry angle parallel to the equator of the atlas defines the nature of the injury. Injury to the transverse ligament is suspected if the total lateral mass separation relative to the body of C2 is greater than 8 mm on the open-mouth view.

Rare transverse ligament tears with an intact atlas are considered unstable if the interval between the odontoid process and the arch of C1 is greater than 3 mm in adults and 4 to 5 mm in children. There is usually anterior soft tissue swelling. A CT scan may show an avulsion of the lateral mass of the atlas.

Radiographic understanding and recognition of rotary subluxation of C1-C2 has many pitfalls. A true lateral view of the skull and AP and lateral views of C1 and C2 are difficult to obtain, but are mandatory to diagnose this abnormality. The lateral mass asymmetry on the open-mouth view is characteristic. If improperly done, a CT scan may not be helpful. Tomography may be easier to interpret. A thin-cut CT scan with the patient's head turned to one side and then the other has been reported to be useful in diagnosing rotary subluxation. A MRI would be useful to rule out neoplasm or infection as an etiologic factor of rotary subluxation [11].

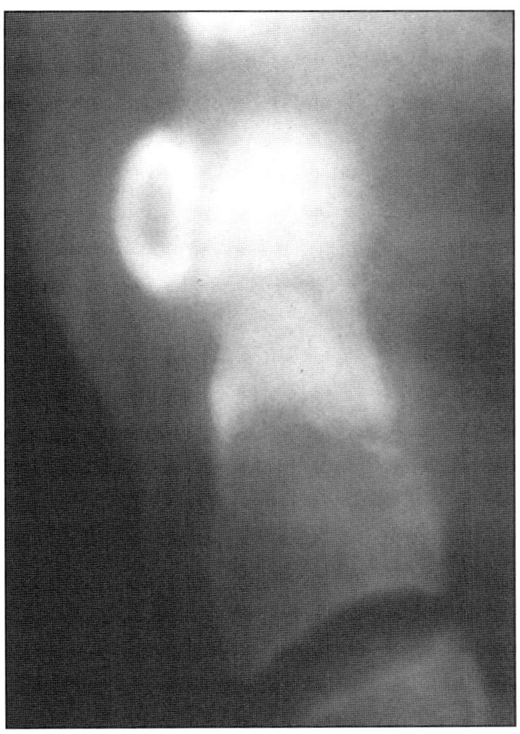

Figure 2-4. Lateral trispiral tomograph demonstrating a Type II odontoid fracture.

Imaging of Odontoid Fractures

Odontoid fractures are among the most frequently missed spinal fractures, particularly in elderly persons with osteopenic bone. Undisplaced fractures may be difficult to identify, even on the open-mouth view. If the CT section misses the axially orientated fracture line, it may be overlooked. For this reason, reformatted images in coronal and sagittal planes are mandatory (Figure 2-6). Occasionally, the sagittal reformation lacks fine detail. This is one situation in which conventional polytomography seems to be superior to CT. Static or dynamic MRI not only identifies spinal cord pathology but also may determine instability patterns and confirm the suspicion of a fracture or the presence of os odontoideum [12].

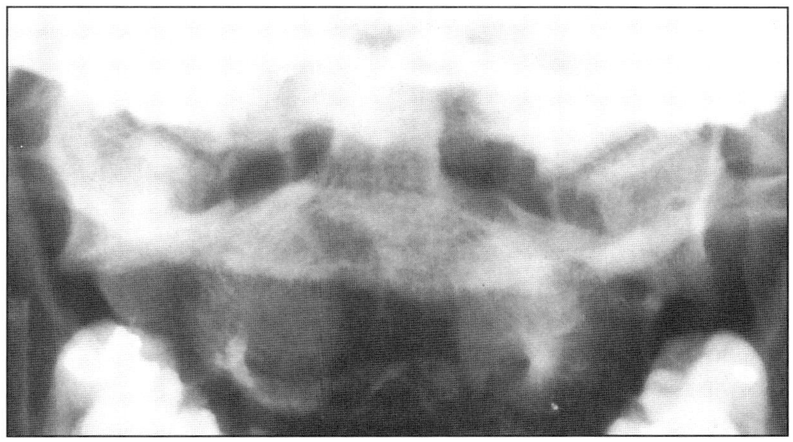

Figure 2-5. A Jefferson fracture is identified on this open-mouth anteroposterior radiograph by lateral displacement of lateral masses of C1 vertebra.

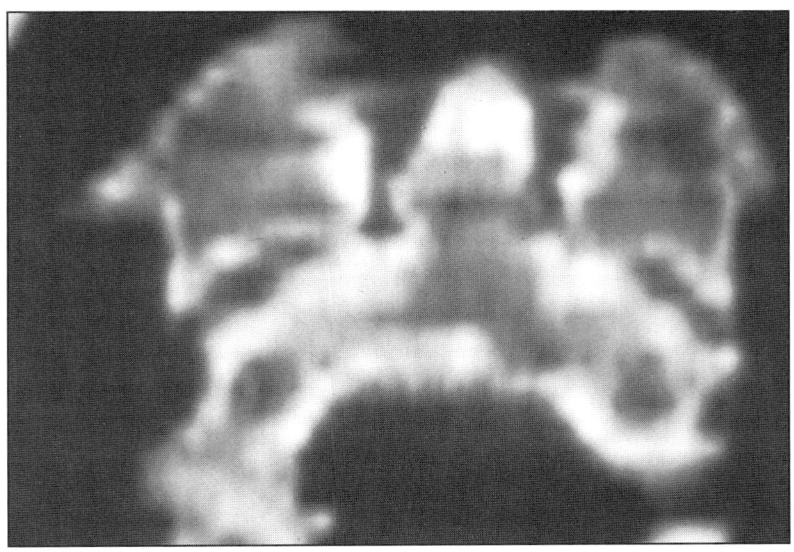

Figure 2-6. Reformatted coronal computed tomography (CT) image showing a Type II odontoid fracture that was not seen on axial CT images.

Facet Dislocation in the Lower Cervical Spine

These unilateral or bilateral injuries represent a flexion-distraction mechanism. There is a continuum in every pattern with facet subluxation and unilateral facet dislocation. The injury pattern depends on the position of the head at the moment of impact.

The radiographic patterns are clearly established and well recognized on conventional radiographs (Figure 2-7) and CT and MRI scans. Because prompt reduction is necessary, recognition of an associated disk herniation is essential (incidence 8% to 50%). Neurologic deterioration following reduction is preventable. Myelography has been replaced with MRI. A large disk fragment behind the vertebral body will dictate the operative approach. In patients with severe immediate neurologic compromise (Frankel A or B), one may weigh the risk–benefit ratio and perform an immediate reduction prior to more elaborate imaging. This would not be a viable option in the patient who is neurologically intact or minimally compromised with a great deal to lose [13].

IMAGING OF THORACIC AND LUMBAR TRAUMA

There are unique local features that make the thoracolumbar junction the most common site of vertebral column injury. In the sagittal plane, this junction lies between the kyphotic thoracic spine and lordotic lumbar area. It remains the junction between the rigid thoracic and mobile lumbar spine. The facet joint orientation changes from the overlapping coronal thoracic segments to the loose sagittal lumbar joints. The unique neuroanatomy gives rise to a wide variety of neurologic presentations. In this delicate hypermobile T12-L1 junction with the cauda equina and conus medullaris, the mixture of upper motor neurons (conus medullaris cord segment S1-S3) and lower motor neurons (cauda equina) make neurologic prognosis unpredictable.

Identification and recognition of the unstable spine injury is a formidable challenge, even to the experienced clinician. Obtaining an accurate history of the mechanism of injury is frequently difficult in the multiply injured patient. The physical examination at best may give some indirect clues as to the mechanism of injury and severity of the spinal damage. The middle and anterior column are inaccessible to palpation. The neurologic picture is frequently confused, with associated head trauma or extremity musculoskeletal injuries. Rectal tone and perianal sensation determine the integrity of the sacral plexus (conus medullaris). The unstable spine, once recognized, may present with bony instability, neurologic instability, or both.

Surgery to realign the unstable spine and clear the spinal canal has been enhanced by experience with improving internal fixation both anteriorly and posteriorly. Presently, it appears the ultimate neurologic function is the by-product of the moment of injury rather than the degree of canal restoration [14]. Imaging plays a vital role in evaluating these injuries precisely.

Anteroposterior and lateral views of the thoracolumbar spine begin the investigative process; however, when used alone, their evaluation of these unique three-dimensional osteoligamentous structures is incomplete. Recognition of subtle variations in normal soft tissue and bony anatomy on conventional radiographs, however, can assist in determining spinal stability. There must be a high index of suspicion for contiguous injuries [15]. In the large, polytraumatized patient, obtaining useful information on the AP view may be difficult. The lateral spine radiograph is superior to all other views in localizing the level of spinal injury [16]. Cross-table lateral radiography at several locations may be necessary due to the divergence of the x-ray beam. The lateral radiographs easily demonstrate the dimensions of the disk space, the vertebral body height, and the sagittal alignment. In the thoracic spine, accurate recognition of an injury pattern on the AP view can be problematic by overlapping cardiac and mediastinal shadows.

Careful attention to the AP radiographs may offer useful information about the mechanism of injury and instability patterns. Rotation of spinous processes suggest a torsional injury. Splaying of the vertebral body and posterior elements denote energy absorption from an axial load. If displaced, flexion-distraction injuries will show widening of the pedicles, or an increased distance between the pedicles or spinous process. Discontinuity of the facet joints are easily recognized in the lumbar spine. Fractures of the lumbar transverse process, often considered benign, require significant mechanical force and are frequently accompanied by other spinal injuries [17]. The experienced clinician must imagine the radiographic appearance of the spine at the moment of impact. Frequently, static radiographs underestimate the severity of the soft tissue and bony damage. The role of dynamic loading radiographs in identifying soft tissue instability in the neurologically intact patient is not clearly defined.

Computed tomography is indispensable in accurately assessing the integrity of the spinal canal (Figure 2-8). With high resolution of bony anatomy, the size of cortical and cancellous fragments can

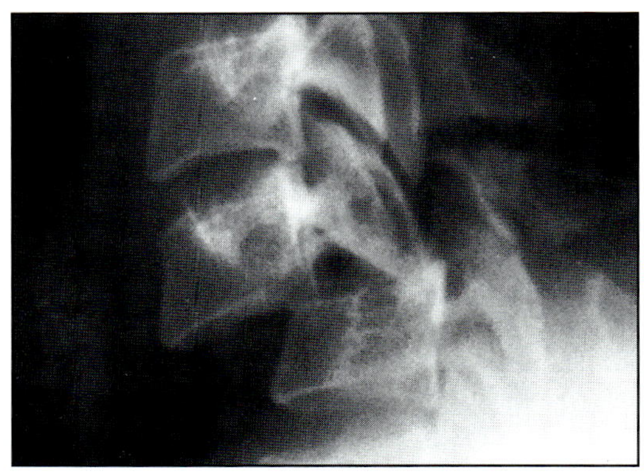

Figure 2-7. Lateral radiograph of the cervical spine shows typical appearance of bilateral locked facets at C5-C6.

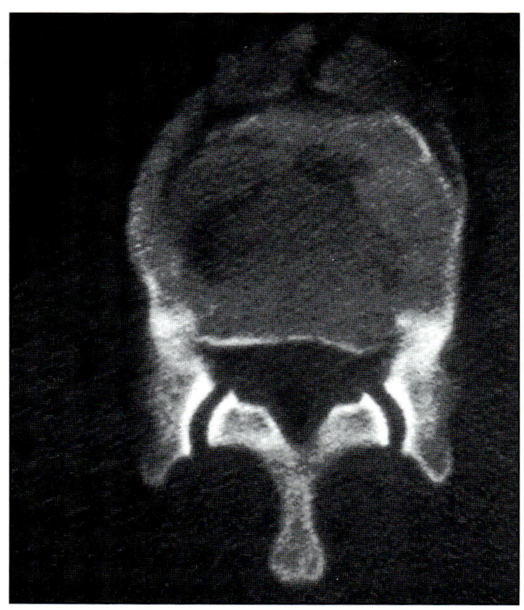

Figure 2-8. Burst fracture of L2 is well imaged with computed tomography. Comminution of the vertebral body and compromise of the spinal canal is effectively demonstrated.

be measured. The CT scan can also determine injuries to other organ systems. No other imaging modality more clearly defines the middle column described by Denis [8]. Along with radiography, CT has been used to better classify thoracolumbar injuries based upon fracture mechanism [18]. Implant failure can be prevented by understanding the non–load-sharing classification outlined by Gaines *et al.* [19]. They stressed the importance of calibrating the fracture comminution, apposition of fragments seen on the CT scan, the degree of kyphosis in determining the length of posterior instrumentation, and whether anterior load sharing is necessary. Disadvantages of CT include the inability to identify noncontiguous fractures or detect fractures orientated horizontally, the less-than-ideal soft tissue visualization, and the occasional partial volume averaging that simulate fractures.

The use of MRI adds another dimension in our understanding of thoracic lumbar injuries. It offers clear soft tissue images, helps identify soft intervertebral disk herniations, and quantitates neural tissue damage such as hemorrhage, edema, or contusion (Figure 2-8). In the presence of normal bony anatomy, MRI may identify occult ligamentous instability. The highly sensitive, variable, large field of view occasionally identifies noncontiguous injuries. MRI can localize the level of the conus medullaris and assist in determining operative approach. The quality of this modality depends on patient cooperation, lack of metallic interference, and availability in the acute or subacute setting.

Imaging of Fracture-Dislocations of the Thoracic Spine

Fracture-dislocations of the thoracic spine result from various forces—flexion, rotation, distraction, or anteroposterior or posteroanterior shear—and cause failure of all three columns of the spine. These are unstable injuries usually associated with severe neurologic complications. In the flexion-rotation type of injury, the posterior and middle columns are completely disrupted. The anterior column may show anterior wedging of the vertebral body on lateral radiographs (Figure 2-10). The posterior wall of the vertebral body may be intact if the dislocation occurs at the level of the intervertebral disk. In the shear type of fracture-dislocation, all three columns are disrupted. In the anteroposterior shear type, the spinal segment above the point of shear is dislocated posteriorly to the segment below (Figure 2-11), and there may be associated fracture of the spinous process. The posteroanterior shear type is characterized by forward displacement of the spinal segment onto the vertebra below at the point of shear. The vertebral bodies are intact; however, the posterior elements of the dislocated vertebral segment, including the laminae, articular facets, and spinous processes, are usually fractured at several levels (Figure 2-12). Fracture-dislocation of the flexion-distraction type resembles seat belt injuries, involving failure of the posterior and middle columns (Figure 2-13).

Imaging of Distraction Injuries

Distraction injuries of the lumbar spine are also called *seat belt fractures* because they frequently occur in individuals involved in automobile accidents who were wearing only lap seat belts. Acute forward flexion of the spine across a restraining lap seat belt during sudden deceleration causes the spine above the belt to be pushed forward and distracted from the lower, fixed part of the spine. The classic Chance fracture results in a horizontal splitting of the vertebra, beginning in the spinous process or lamina and extending through the pedicles and the vertebral body (Figure 2-14). In addition to bone abnormalities, CT and MRI demonstrate injury to the soft tissues, such as anterior and posterior longitudinal ligament tear as well as tear of interspinous segment. Associated intervertebral disk rupture may also be effectively imaged.

Imaging of Burst Fractures

Radiologic imaging assists in determining the nature of each unique fracture pattern. Awareness of burst fractures, which are high-energy injuries, have increased with the availability of CT

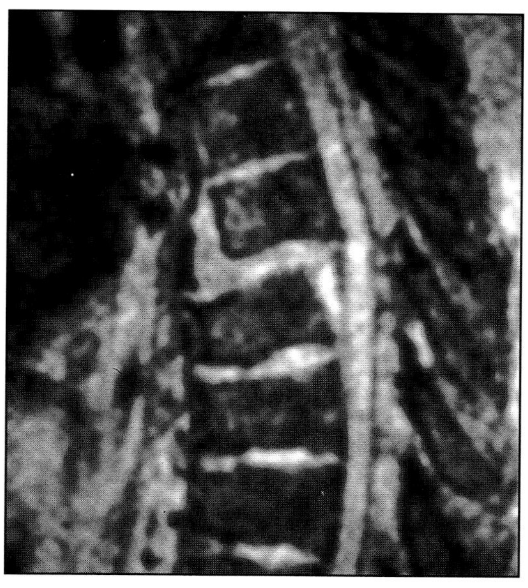

Figure 2-9. Sagittal T2-weighted multiplanar gradient recalled (MPGR) magnetic resonance imaging scan showing fracture-dislocation at T2. The injury to the anterior and posterior longitudinal ligaments and the spinal cord are well demonstrated.

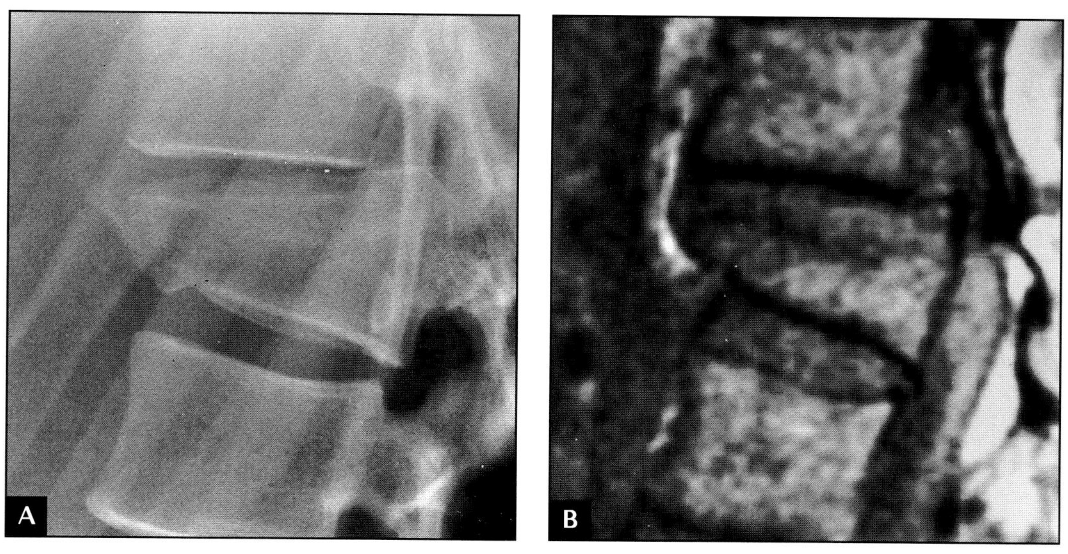

Figure 2-10. **A**, Lateral radiograph in a man who sustained a flexion-rotation type of fracture-dislocation at the T12-L1 level shows anterior wedging of the body of L1 and disruption of the middle column associated with slight anterior displacement of vertebra T12. **B**, Sagittal T2-weighted magnetic resonance image shows additional disruption of the middle and posterior columns and compression of the thecal sac.

scanning. Posterior vertebral body-wall disruption differentiates the burst fracture from the compression fracture. Prior to CT scanning, burst fractures were frequently underestimated or misdiagnosed with conventional radiography [9]. AP radiographs may show splayed pedicles, vertebral body collapse, and fractures through the transverse process. The lateral view shows loss of vertebral height, segmental kyphosis, and possible posterior superior body displacement associated with rotation. The CT scan evaluates much more than the status of the spinal canal. Burst, as the word suggests, involves a radial disruption of the vertebral body.

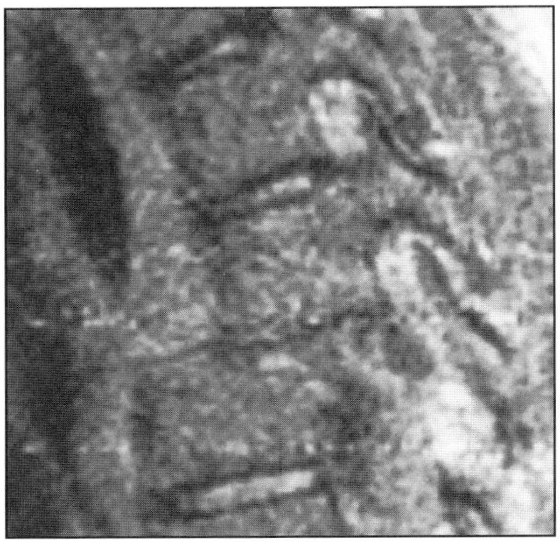

FIGURE 2-11. Sagittal T2-weighted magnetic resonance image shows anteroposterior shear type of fracture-dislocation at the lower thoracic level. Note posterior displacement of the upper segment of thoracic spine in relation to the lower segment.

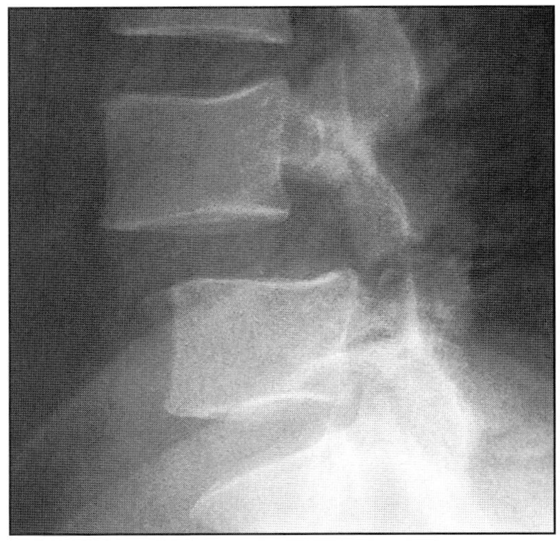

FIGURE 2-12. Lateral radiograph of the lumbar spine demonstrating posteroanterior shear type of fracture-dislocation. The vertebral bodies are intact, but there are fractures of the posterior elements of the affected vertebrae.

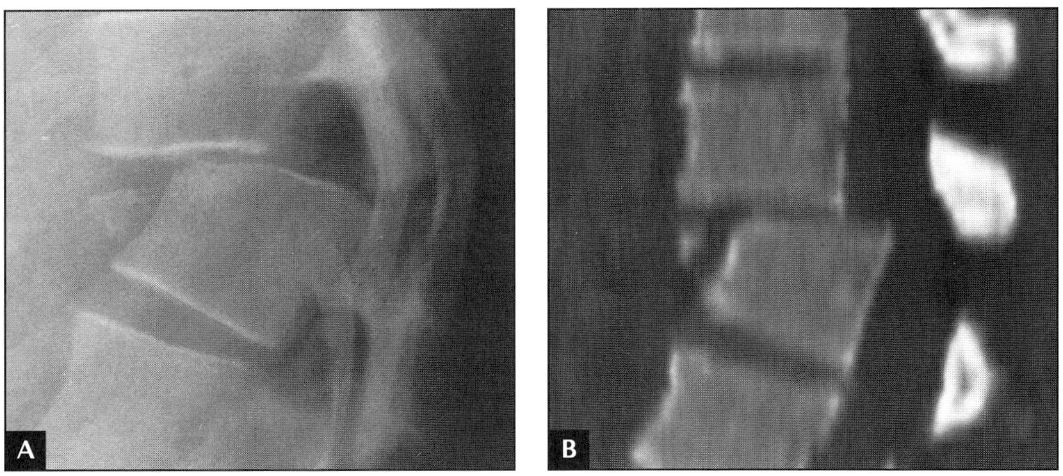

FIGURE 2-13. **A**, Lateral radiograph of the thoracolumbar spine and **B**, sagittal reformatted computed tomography scan show characteristic features of a flexion-distraction type of fracture-dislocation.

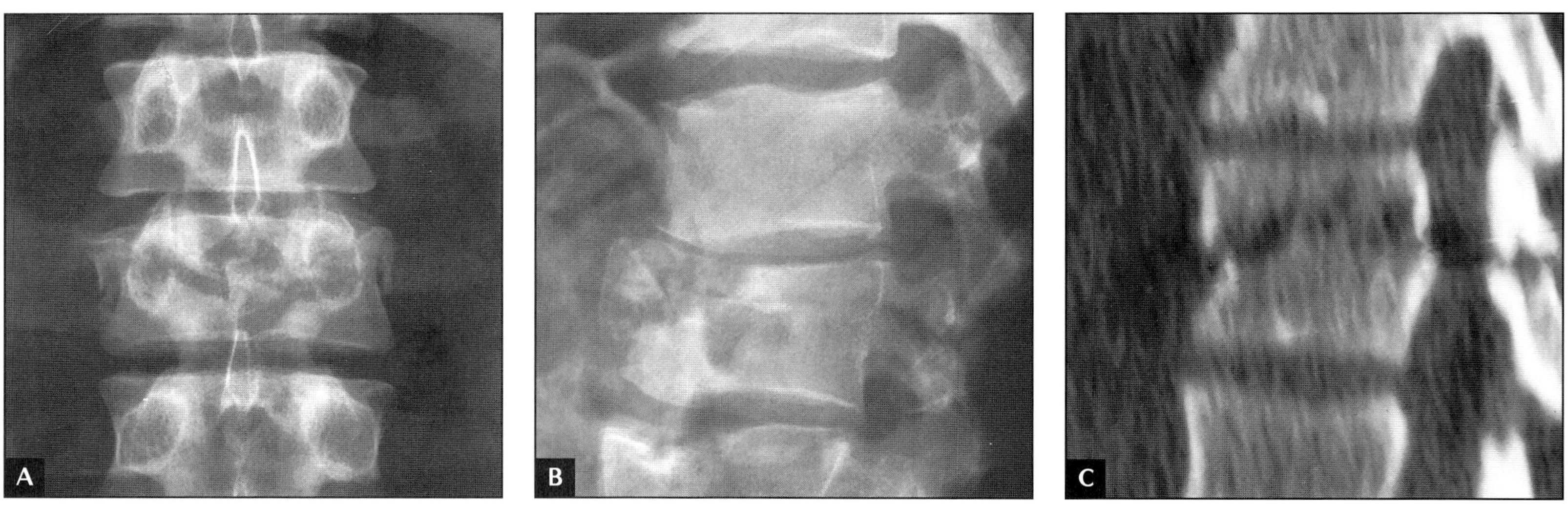

FIGURE 2-14. **A**, Anteroposterior radiograph of the lumbar spine showing a radiolucent line traversing horizontally through the vertebral body of L2. **B**, Lateral radiograph showing additional horizontal splitting of the lamina of L2. **C**, Reformatted sagittal computed tomography scan showing classic appearance of Chance fracture.

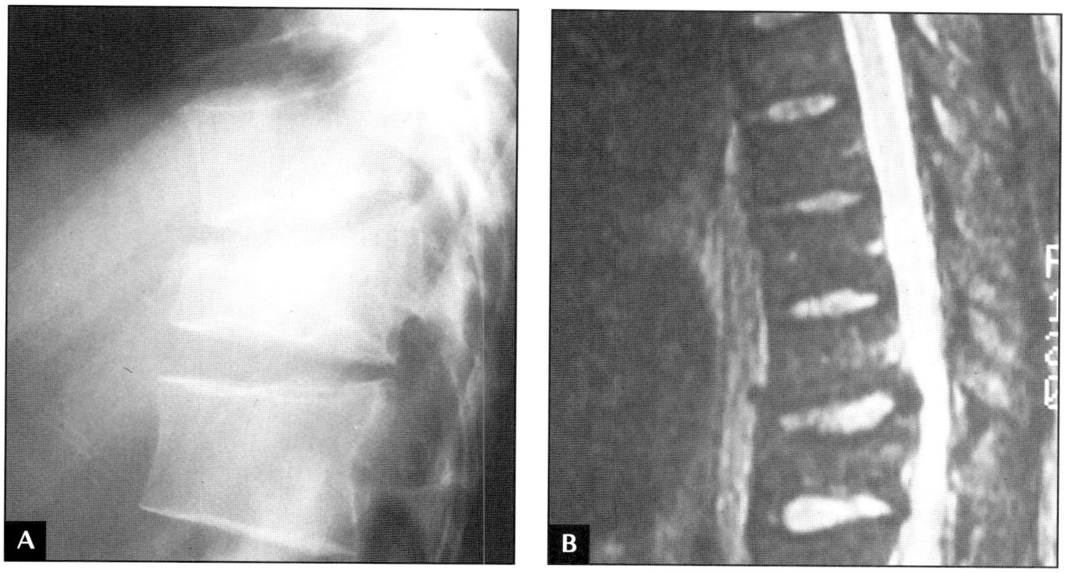

FIGURE 2-15. **A**, Lateral radiograph showing a burst fracture of T12. The status of the spinal canal cannot be adequately evaluated. **B**, Sagittal T2-weighted multiplanar gradient recalled (MPGR) magnetic resonance imaging scan showing posterior displacement of the vertebral body, tear of the posterior longitudinal ligament, and compression of the spinal cord.

The CT scan shows the degree of disruption and comminution of the injured vertebrae (Figure 2-8), thus predicting the future load-sharing capacity even after posterior stabilization. The CT scan assists in evaluating the posterior arch. Laminar, facet, or pars interarticularis fractures suggest a more unstable burst fracture pattern [11]. The inconsistent correlation between the degree of canal compromise seen on the CT scan in burst fractures and the severity of the neurologic injury is not well understood. Likely explanations include the proximity of the conus medullaris to the injured segment and the presence of preexisting relative congenital spinal canal stenosis [12].

Use of MRI in burst fractures adds additional insight, understanding to these complex injuries (Figure 2-15). MRI may quantitate the hydration of adjacent noninjured intervertebral disks, show underestimated posterior ligamentous disruptions, and better define the soft tissue components inside the spinal canal. The integrity of the posterior longitudinal ligament occasionally seen on sagittal images may assist in determining operative approach. In pathologic burst fractures, the MRI is invaluable for evaluating the metabolic bone condition or extent of neoplastic process.

REFERENCES AND RECOMMENDED READING

Recently published papers of particular interest have been highlighted as:

- • Of interest
- •• Of outstanding interest

1. McEvery KW, Wilson AJ, Murphy WA: Comparison of spinal CT versus conventional CT multiplanar reconstructions of a fracture displacement. *Invest Radiol* 1994, 29:665–670.
2. Beers GJ, Rague GH, Wagner GG, *et al.*: MRI of acute cervical spine trauma. *J Comput Assist Tomograph* 1988, 12:755–761.
3. Marvis SE, Gersler FH, Jslinck JJ, *et al.*: Acute cervical spine trauma: evaluation with 1.5 T MR imaging. *Radiology* 1988, 166:807–816.
4. Streitwieser DR, Knopp R, Wales LR, *et al.*: Accuracy of standard radiographic views in detecting cervical spine fractures. *Ann Emerg Med* 1983, 12:538–542.
5. Cattell HS, Filtzer DL: Pseudosubluxation and other normal variations of the cervical spine in children: a study of one hundred and sixty children. *J Bone Joint Surg* 1965, 47:1295–1309.
6. Templeton PA, Young JW, Mirvis SE, *et al.*: The value of retropharyngeal soft tissue measurements in trauma of the adult cervical spine: cervical spine soft tissue measurements. *Skeletal Radiol* 1987, 16:98–104.
7. White, Johnson, Panjab, *et al.*: Biomedical analysis of clinical stability in the cervical spine. *Clin Orthop* 1975, 109:85–93.
8. Denis F: The three column spine and its significance in classification of acute thoracolumbar spinal injuries. *Spine* 1983, 8:817–831.
9. Blacksin MF, Lee HJ: Frequency and significance of fractures of the upper cervical spine detected by CT in patients with severe neck trauma. *Am J Roentgenol* 1995, 165:1201–1204.
10. Link TM, Schuierer G, Hufendiek A, *et al.*: Substantial head trauma: value of routine CT examination of the cervicocranium. *Radiology* 1995, 196:741–745.
11. Kowalski HM, Cohen WA, Cooper P, Wisoff JH: Pitfalls in the CT diagnosis of atlantoaxial rotary subluxation. *Am J Roentgenol* 1987, 149:595–600.
12. Sutterlin CE, Gutentag I, Martinez CR, Rechtine GR: False-positive diagnosis of an odontoid fracture by CT scan. *J Orthop Trauma* 1989, 3:348–351.
13. Eismont FJ, Arena MJ, Green BA: Extrusion of an interverteral disc associated with traumatic subluxation or dislocation of cervical facets: a case report. *J Bone Joint Surg* 1991, 73:1555–1560.
14. Gertzbein SD: Scoliosis Research Society: Multicenter Spine Fracture Study. *Spine* 1992, 17:528–540.
15. Reid DC, Henderson R, Saboe L, *et al.*: Etiology and clinical course of missed spine fractures. *J Trauma* 1987, 27:980.
16. Keene JS: Radiographic evaluation of thoracolumbar fractures. *Clin Orthop* 1984, 198:158.
17. Krueger MA, Green DA, Hoyt D, Garfin SR: Overlooked spine injuries associated with lumbar transverse process fractures. *Clin Orthop* 1996, 327:191–198.
18. Gertzbein SD: Spine update: classification of thoracic and lumbar fractures. *Spine* 1999, 19:626–628.
19. Gaines RW, Holt B, McCormack T: A classification to predict screw breakage when using short segment instrumentation and pedicle screws: the load sharing classification of spinal fractures [abstract]. *J Orthop Trauma* 1994, 18:103.

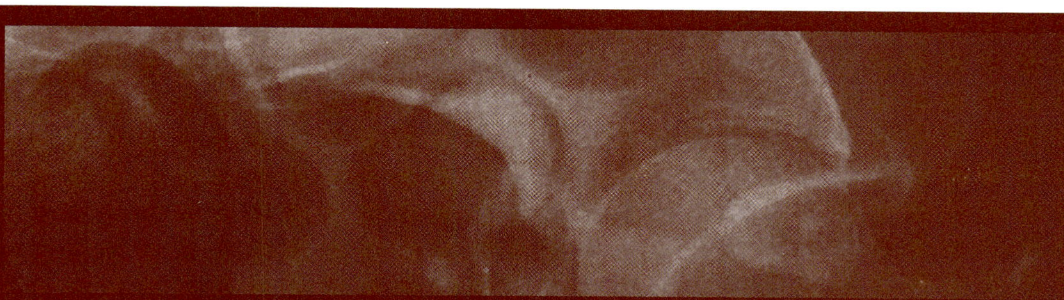

3

Imaging of Fractures of the Pelvis and Lower Extremities

Eric A. Brandser

Fractures of the pelvis and lower extremities are common; many are life threatening and require immediate attention. Proper and prompt characterization of the extent of injury and type of fracture is critical to patient care and management. Imaging plays an increasingly pivotal role in the detection, classification, and staging of fractures. Standard radiographs continue to be the mainstay of screening and remain the method of choice for characterization of some fractures. Computed tomography (CT) provides excellent cross-sectional osseous detail; multiplanar reconstructions can enhance surgical planning and fracture classification. Magnetic resonance imaging (MRI) has excellent contrast resolution and is the screening procedure of choice for some acute trauma settings.

Fractures of the pelvis and lower extremities differ from one another based on biomechanics, deforming forces, and resultant fracture patterns. Optimal imaging for these fractures often requires different algorithms and choice of imaging tests. This chapter reviews the advantages of several imaging modalities and offers a framework for imaging evaluation of patients with pelvic and lower-extremity trauma.

RADIOGRAPHY

Conventional radiographs are the mainstay for evaluating trauma. Radiographs are familiar to physicians, are readily available in emergency departments, and can be obtained rapidly. High-quality radiographs are critical for initial patient evaluation and often are sufficient to guide initial treatment. If further imaging is required, radiographs often dictate which subsequent imaging studies should be obtained. In general, two views of an area with suspected fracture are required, because fractures can be difficult to see on a single projection. Dedicated trauma radiography rooms in the emergency department greatly facilitate the speed and quality of radiographs in the trauma setting.

COMPUTED TOMOGRAPHY

The use of CT has greatly enhanced imaging of skeletal trauma. Conventional CT consists of alternating radiographic acquisition of a slice in the patient followed by translation of the patient into the CT machine. A newer technique, now standard in many hospitals, is called helical or spiral CT. Spiral CT differs from conventional CT in that patient translation and data collection through radiographs occur simultaneously (Figure 3-1) [1]. The advantages of spiral CT are shorter examination times as well as the ability to reconstruct as many overlapping slices from the volume of data as necessary [2,3]. Increasing the amount of slice overlap improves fracture detection by decreasing volume averaging. This is especially true for fractures that run in the plane of the CT gantry.

A new technology just being introduced clinically is a modification of spiral CT called *limited cone-beam CT* [4]. This technique uses a cone-shaped beam of x-rays directed through a patient to multiple rows of detectors. This differs from current spiral CT, in which a fan-shaped beam and a single row of detectors are used. The advantage of cone-beam CT is a dramatic decrease in scan times. A brain CT scan may be done in as little as three seconds, a chest CT scan in 13 seconds, and a scan of the entire body in under 1 minute. This new technology may revolutionize the use of CT for evaluation of trauma, with patients being scanned virtually from head to toe with specific multiplanar reconstructions to better delineate any fractures that are detected.

MAGNETIC RESONANCE IMAGING

Magnetic resonance imaging is a powerful modality in the setting of trauma. MRI generates images with radio waves and strong magnetic fields. The signal from hydrogen protons are collected and processed to generate the MRI images with which we are familiar. By varying computer parameters and timing the radio waves, differences in the magnetic and chemical properties of tissues of interest can be accentuated to yield excellent differentiation of these tissues on images [5,6]. Many MRI images are made with a technique called *fast spin echo*, and it is important to be aware that with this technique, fat signal stays relatively bright on T2-weighted images, similar to T1-weighted sequences [7,8]. As a result, detection of edema within osseous structures can be difficult with a fast spin echo T2-weighted sequence. Therefore, to improve detection of bone marrow edema, suppression of fat signal, either through chemical selective radio frequency presaturation or inversion recovery, is important [7,8]. Advances in MRI technology include very rapid scanners that allow near real-time magnetic resonance fluoroscopy evaluation.

PELVIC FRACTURES

The pelvis is a ring composed of three bones, including the sacrum and two innominate bones. These bones connect posteriorly at the sacroiliac joints and anteriorly at the symphysis pubis. The posterior and interosseous sacroiliac ligaments are strong and very important for pelvic stability because they resist vertical translation. The sacrotuberous ligament also resists vertical translation. The anterior sacroiliac, symphyseal, and sacrospinous ligaments resist "open-book" rotation of the pelvis [9,10].

Pelvic ring disruptions are caused by deforming force in one or more of three directions, including anteroposterior (AP) compression, lateral compression, and vertical shear. Imaging can reveal the mechanism of injury if radiographic clues are recognized at evaluation [11]. For example, diastasis of the symphysis pubis and sacroiliac joint is a hallmark of the AP compression pattern. CT scans of the sacroiliac joints may reveal disruption anteriorly with intact posterior articulation in the more stable types. Widening of the posterior sacroiliac joints implies disruption of the posterior sacroiliac ligaments and a more unstable injury [9,11–13].

IMAGING APPROACH FOR PELVIC TRAUMA

Radiographs are the initial studies used to evaluate a patient with suspected pelvic fracture; an AP view of the pelvis is obtained on nearly every trauma patient (Figure 3-2). Pelvic inlet and outlet views are added when a pelvic fracture is detected; Judet oblique views are obtained with acetabular fractures [9,11,14–17].

Computed tomography is an important tool for diagnosis and preoperative planning of pelvic, sacral, and acetabular fractures.

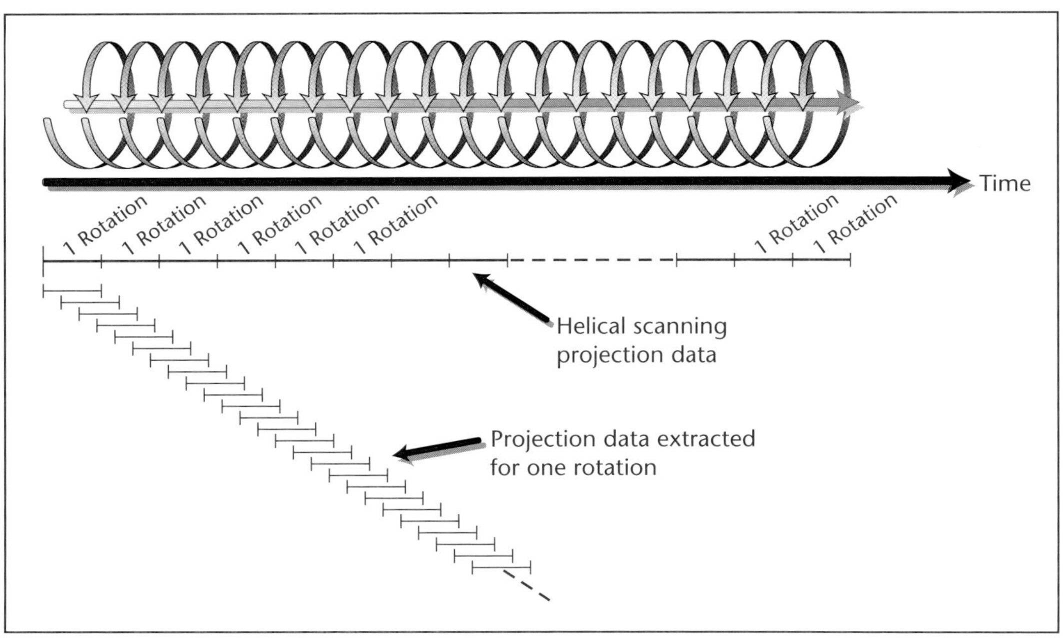

FIGURE 3-1. Spiral computed tomography scan. Diagram illustrates how x-ray tube rotation and patient translation occur simultaneously (*top*), resulting in a volume of data that can be reconstructed into contiguous slices (*middle*). The data can also be reconstructed into multiple overlapping slices at no additional radiation or data collection time cost (*bottom*). (*Adapted from* Tokhi *et al.* [2].)

CT is more sensitive than plain radiographs for detecting pelvic disruptions; in a published study, plain films failed to diagnose 29% of sacroiliac diastasis, 57% of acetabular rim fractures, and 34% of vertical shear fractures [18]. Up to one third of pelvic fractures detected by CT are missed on radiographs [16]. With helical CT, multiple overlapping slices can be reconstructed into multiplanar two-dimensional images or three-dimensional reconstructions. These images are useful in selected cases in which multiple displaced fracture fragments are present. Such images serve as a surgical planning tool to improve the understanding of complex anatomic relationships [19–23].

When performing CT of the pelvis, images should be obtained from the iliac crest through the level of the ischial tuberosities. The typical abdomen and pelvis CT to image trauma usually ends at the level of the symphysis pubis, and thus a number of fractures can be overlooked [24]. We typically use 5- to 7-mm thick slices in the upper pelvis, and thinner slices through the acetabulum if acetabular fracture is suspected or known.

Classifications of pelvic fractures are important because they address issues of stability, associated injuries, complications, and outcomes [25]. Several classifications for pelvic fractures have been developed. Pennal *et al.* [26] demonstrated the relationship between direction of force and reproducible patterns of injury. Tile [10,27,28] combined directional patterns of injury with radiographic signs of stability or instability. Young *et al.* [12,13] further refined this approach by combining directional patterns of injury with radiographic grading of severity, correlating with the level of energy imparted. Both the Tile [10,27,28] and Young *et al.* [12,13] classifications incorporate the basic mechanisms of pelvic ring disruption: AP compression, lateral compression, and vertical sheer forces [9,13,17,26–28]. In addition to the direction of force, the Tile classification emphasizes stability, whereas the Young *et al.* classification grades the magnitude of the injury [9,13,25].

Tile's classification includes major categories (A, B, and C) with numeric subtypes to cover most fracture patterns (Table 3-1 and Figure 3-3) [26,29]. Type A injuries are stable pelvic fractures that

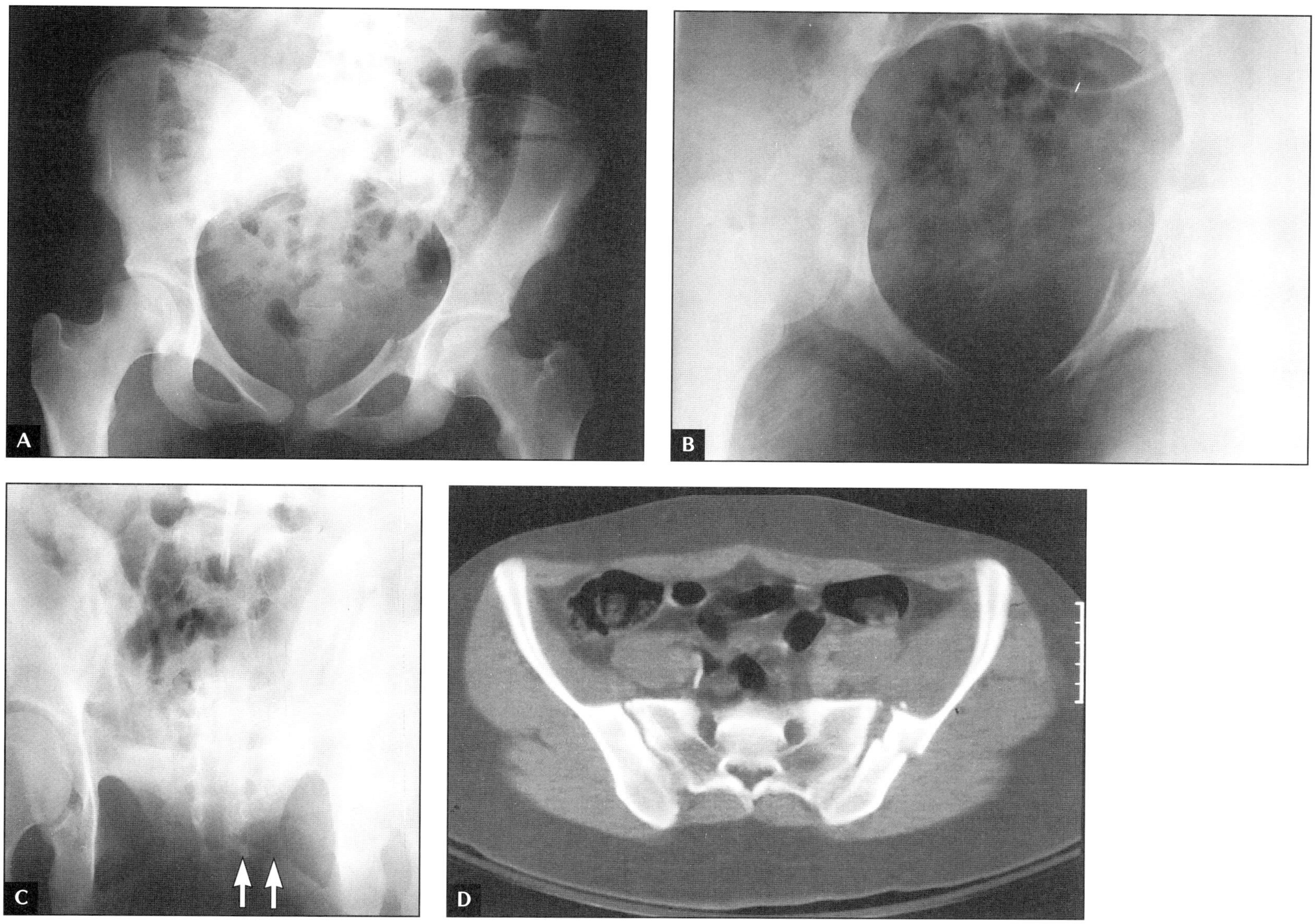

FIGURE 3-2. Evaluation of pelvic fracture. **A**, Anteroposterior (AP) radiograph of a woman aged 17 years who was involved in a motor vehicle accident with lateral compression injury to pelvis. Note the fractures of the inferior and superior left pubic rami and the left iliac wing. Status of the left sacroiliac joint is difficult to assess. **B**, Inlet view shows disruption at the left sacroiliac joint and the anterior fractures of the pubic rami. **C**, Outlet view better shows that the pubic fractures have a horizontal orientation (*arrows*), characteristic of lateral compression injuries. **D**, Computed tomography scan at the level of the sacroiliac joints shows that the iliac wing fracture extends into the sacroiliac joint; however, more typically, a buckle fracture of the sacral ala occurs.

TABLE 3-1. TILE CLASSIFICATION OF PELVIC FRACTURES

Type	Description
A	Stable
A1	Fractures of the pelvis not involving the ring
A2	Stable, minimally displaced ring fractures
B	Rotationally unstable, vertically stable
B1	Open book
B2	Lateral compression—ipsilateral
B3	Lateral compression—contralateral (bucket-handle)
C	Rotationally and vertically unstable
C1	Rotationally and vertically unstable
C2	Bilateral
C3	Associated with acetabuar fracture

Adapted from Tile [10].

do not disrupt the pelvic ring. Type B injuries are rotationally unstable but vertically and posteriorly stable—the anterior pelvic ligaments are disrupted but the posterior hinge is preserved. Type C injuries describe the vertical shear pattern and are vertically, posteriorly, and rotationally unstable; one subtype (Type C3) includes pelvic ring injury with associated acetabular fracture [17,26–28].

Acetabulum

Fractures of the acetabulum have varied fracture lines traversing complex three-dimensional anatomy that makes them difficult to describe. Acetabular fractures are almost universally classified by the method described by Letournel and Judet [14]. This classification is the first step in surgical decision making. For inexperienced observers, it is complicated; however, a systematic analysis of radiographs and CT scans has been described that allows classification in most fractures [24].

The acetabulum is made up of two columns and two walls, each termed anterior or posterior [30,31]. The walls stabilize the hip

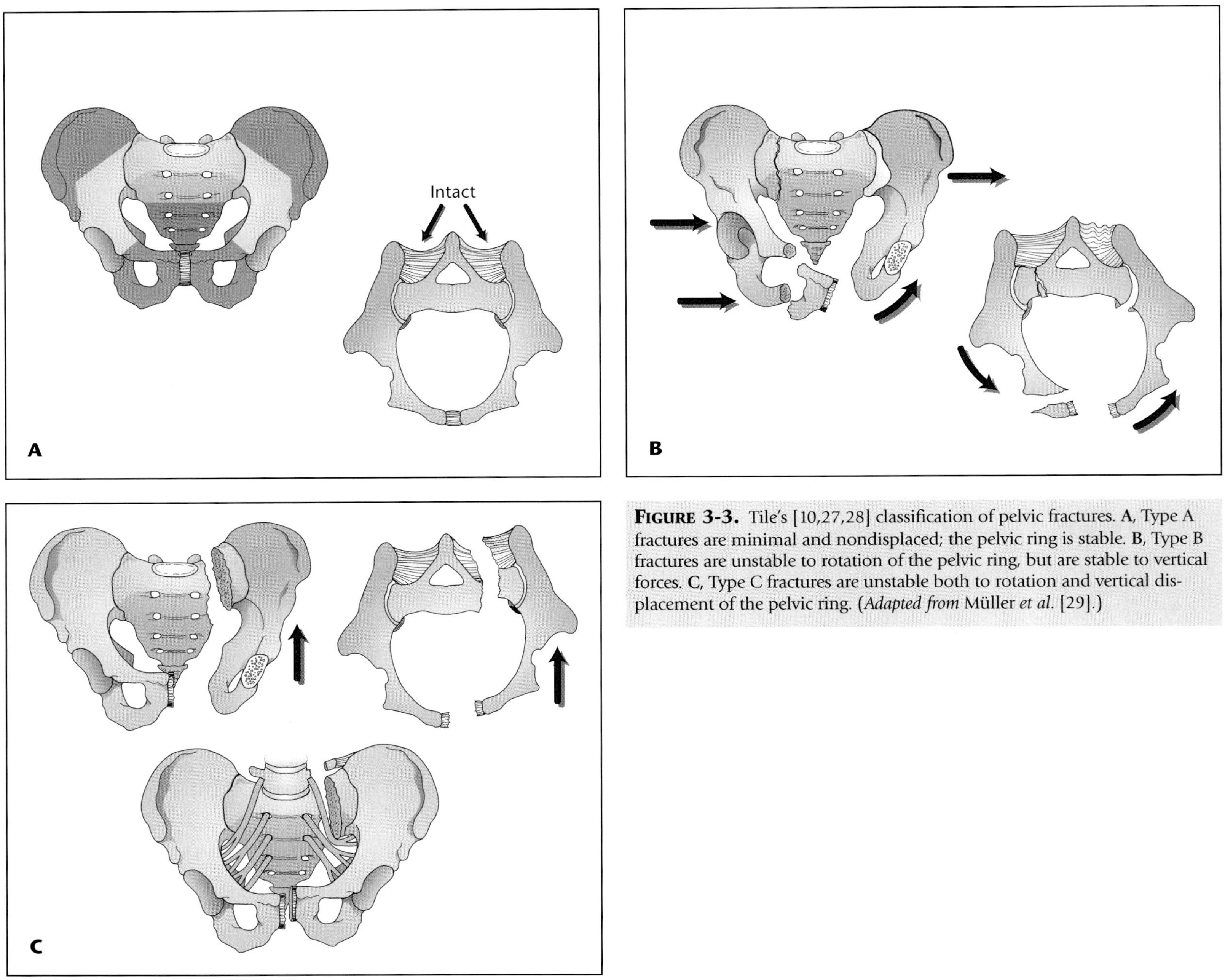

Figure 3-3. Tile's [10,27,28] classification of pelvic fractures. **A**, Type A fractures are minimal and nondisplaced; the pelvic ring is stable. **B**, Type B fractures are unstable to rotation of the pelvic ring, but are stable to vertical forces. **C**, Type C fractures are unstable both to rotation and vertical displacement of the pelvic ring. (*Adapted from* Müller *et al.* [29].)

joint in the anterior and posterior directions. The posterior wall is larger in size and is more commonly fractured than the anterior wall [4,31,32]. The anterior and posterior columns are unequal in size; the anterior column is larger than the posterior column [29]. The column orientation resembles the lower-case Greek letter lambda (λ), with the longer limb of the letter representing the anterior column and the smaller limb the posterior column (Figure 3-4). Both columns are connected to the axial skeleton through the sciatic buttress, a strut of bone that transfers forces from weight bearing to the axial skeleton [30,31].

The standard radiographic examination for a suspected acetabular fracture consists of an AP radiograph and two oblique views called Judet views. These oblique radiographs are taken with the patient turned 45° and are called right and left posterior oblique views. In clinical practice, these images are often called the obturator and iliac oblique views, referring to whichever portion of the injured side of the pelvis is best visualized. The radiographic anatomy of both the normal and fractured acetabulum has been described [31–35]. Several structures on the AP radiograph are important for fracture classification (Figure 3-4) [30,35].

Most orthopedic surgeons classify acetabular fractures with the system developed by Letournel and Judet [14], in which fractures are divided into elementary and associated patterns. Elementary fractures consist of a single main fracture line, whereas associated fractures involve combinations of elementary fractures (Table 3-2) [30,31]. An illustration of the types of acetabular fractures can be found in Chapter 8. Rote memorization of the ten elementary and associated fractures is difficult, and another way to organize the

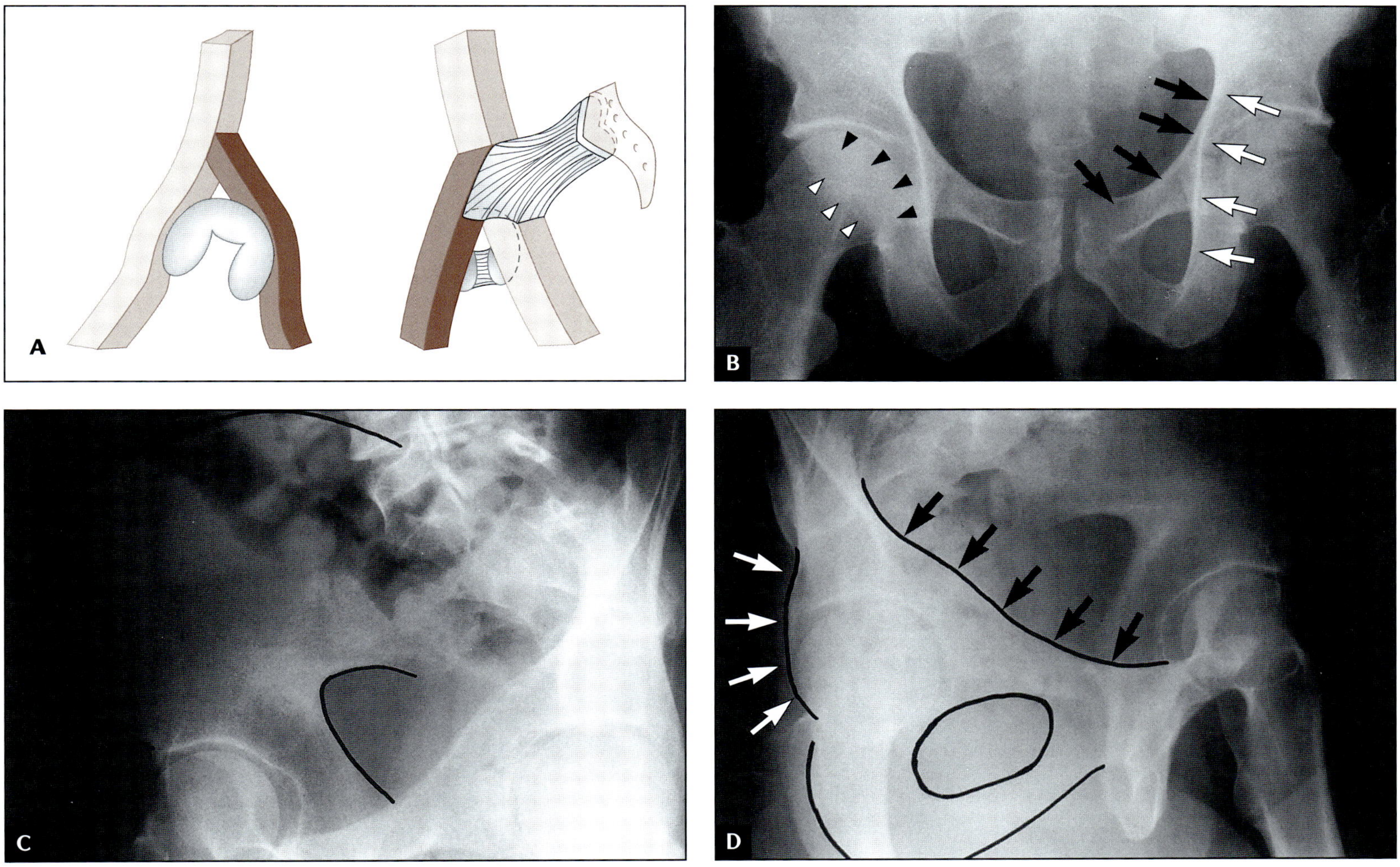

FIGURE 3-4. Acetabular anatomy. **A**, Acetabular columns. *Left*, diagram of left acetabulum viewed from outside. Note that the anterior column (*light*) is larger than the posterior column (*dark*), and that both columns support the horseshoe-shaped articular surface. *Right*, view of the left acetabulum viewed from inside the pelvis. The sciatic buttress (stippled) connects both columns to the axial skeleton through the sacroiliac joint. **B**, Anteroposterior (AP) view of the pelvis has the ilioischial (*white arrows*) and iliopectineal (*black arrows*) lines outlined on the left acetabulum, and the lateral margins of the anterior (*black arrowheads*) and posterior (*white arrowheads*) walls on the right acetabulum. The obturator ring is visible on this view but is better evaluated on the obturator oblique view. The iliac wing is viewed obliquely on the AP view and is better demonstrated on the iliac oblique view. **C**, Right posterior oblique view with right acetabulum highlighted. This view is also called the iliac oblique view, and shows the posterior part of the acetabulum and greater sciatic notch to advantage, facilitating evaluation of fractures that extend into this region. The edge of the anterior wall can be seen on this view, especially with steeper degrees of rotation. The iliac wing is seen en face and it is therefore the best view for detecting fractures that extend proximally into the iliac wing. The obturator ring is poorly seen on this view. **D**, Left posterior oblique, also called the obturator oblique for the right acetabulum. Note that the obturator ring is well seen; the anterior portion of the iliopectineal line (*black arrows*) and the posterior wall (*white arrows*) are seen to advantage. In the setting of a both column fracture, this is the best view to demonstrate the spur sign. Obturator ring fractures can occur in several places, usually the inferior portion of the ring at the ischiopubic junction or the anterior and superior portion of the ring, at the puboacetabular junction. (Panel A *adapted from* Letournel and Judet [14].)

fracture types is to divide them into those that are predominantly column-type, transverse-type, or wall-type fractures. Learning the imaging features that differentiate these groups is easier than memorizing the ten patterns (Table 3-3) [32].

Computed tomography is useful for evaluating patients with acetabular fractures [35–41]. It detects intra-articular fragments and shows articular discontinuity better than plain film [41–44]. Between 30% and 40% of intra-articular fragments and up to 50% of femoral head fractures seen with CT are missed on plain radiographs [37,45]. Rotation of fragments can also be difficult to assess by plain film and may be better evaluated with CT. The CT appearances of the fracture types of the Letournel and Judet [14] classification have been described [32,35,37,43,46]. For column-type fractures, the main fracture plane on CT is from medial to lateral, producing a horizontal fracture on the CT image (Figure 3-5). Transverse type fractures have an anterior-to-posterior fracture line that is vertical on the CT image, and wall fractures have an oblique fracture orientation (Figure 3-6).

When performing acetabular CT, scanning should begin at the iliac crest and continue through the ischial tuberosities, extending beyond the symphysis pubis, similar to scans made to assess pelvic fractures. Scanning with thin slices through the articular surface improves detection of nondisplaced fractures and leads to better reconstructions than when thicker slices are used. We typically use 5-mm–thick slices obtained from the iliac crest to 1 cm above the acetabular dome with 3-mm slices for the remainder of the study through the ischial tuberosities, but significant interinstitutional variation exists in actual scan parameters. Helical or spiral technique is recommended if available because it allows faster examination times, decreased motion artifact, and improved reconstructions [3]. However, if a patient is large, using spiral technique may yield images with an unacceptable level of noise; in this circumstance, conventional scanning with overlapping slices is preferred.

Three-dimensional reconstructions are helpful for surgical planning [39,47,48]. Preoperative assessment of predominant fracture orientation may direct lag screw or malleable plate placement, and displacement or rotation of fragments may alter reduction methods. Techniques that improve fracture visualization include disarticulating the ipsilateral hip (by region of interest subtraction) and reconstructing only the fractured hemipelvis.

TABLE 3-2. LETOURNEL AND JUDET'S CLASSIFICATION OF ACETABULAR FRACTURES

Elementary Types	Associated Types
Anterior column	Both column
Posterior column	Transverse with posterior wall
Anterior wall	Posterior column with posterior wall
Posterior wall	Anterior column with posterior hemitransverse
Transverse	T-shaped

Adapted from Letournel and Judet [14].

Femur

Fractures of the proximal femur are fairly common and can be devastating. These include not only posttraumatic fractures but also insufficiency fractures in the setting of osteoporosis. Fracture of the femoral neck and intertrochanteric region occurs mainly in elderly patients and is more common in women [49,50]. These fractures most commonly occur during a fall from a standing position, and are considered low-energy fractures. The most commonly used classification of femoral neck fractures is the Garden classification system [51]. This classification divides fractures into incomplete (Type I), complete nondisplaced (Type II), incomplete displaced (Type III), and complete displaced (Type IV). For intertrochanteric fractures, Evans' classification [52] is commonly used. Fractures are divided into five types, based on displacement and number of fracture parts; a reverse oblique pattern is also described.

For radiographic evaluation of suspected femoral fracture, an AP radiograph is required along with either a shoot-through or frog-leg lateral radiograph. However, many patients have decreased bone density, and radiographs may show only subtle abnormalities or seem normal [53]. If the clinical suspicion for fracture is high (*eg*, the patient is unable to bear weight) and radiographs are negative, other imaging tests should be considered. Both MRI and bone scanning are more sensitive than radiography for detecting femoral neck fracture; MRI has the advantages of showing fractures earlier than bone scan, providing better anatomic information, and having better specificity than scintigraphy. For these reasons, MRI is the preferred imaging test to obtain when radiographs are negative (Figure 3-7).

When using MRI to detect femoral neck fracture, coronal T1-weighted images show fractures occult on radiographs. However, the addition of fat-suppressed T2-weighted sequences dramatically increases the visibility of fractures and better shows other abnormalities that can be responsible for posttraumatic hip pain, such as muscle tears [54•]. The MRI study should extend from the posterior sacrum anterior to the symphysis pubis, because pelvic insufficiency fractures may mimic the clinical presentation of femoral neck fracture.

TABLE 3-3. GROUPED FRACTURE TYPES

Wall Fractures	Column Fractures	Transverse Fractures
Posterior wall	Both column	Transverse
Anterior wall	Anterior column	T-shaped
	Posterior column	
Transverse with posterior wall		Transverse with posterior wall
Posterior column with posterior wall	Posterior column with posterior wall	
	Anterior column with posterior hemitransverse	Anterior column with posterior hemitransverse

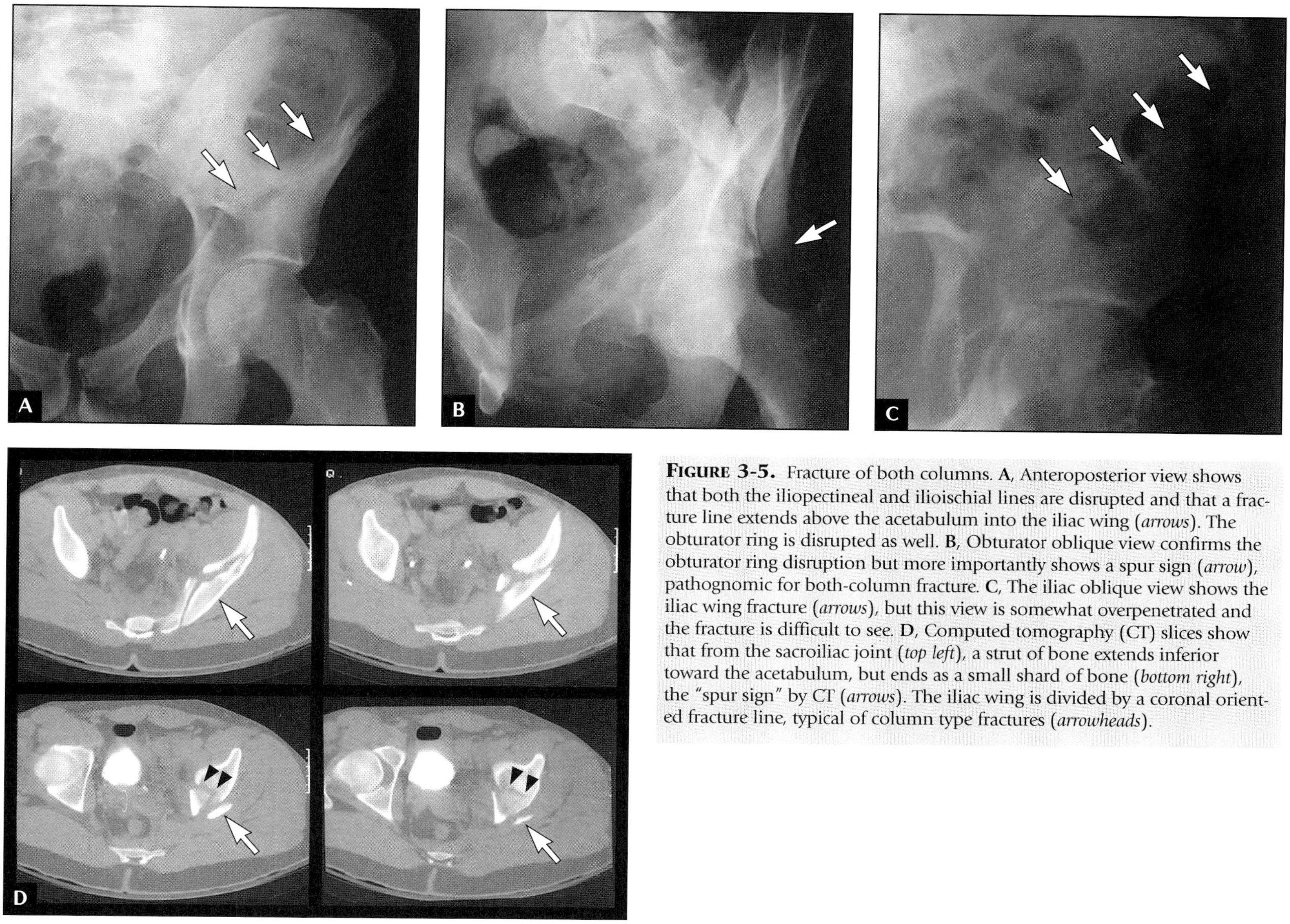

FIGURE 3-5. Fracture of both columns. **A**, Anteroposterior view shows that both the iliopectineal and ilioischial lines are disrupted and that a fracture line extends above the acetabulum into the iliac wing (*arrows*). The obturator ring is disrupted as well. **B**, Obturator oblique view confirms the obturator ring disruption but more importantly shows a spur sign (*arrow*), pathognomic for both-column fracture. **C**, The iliac oblique view shows the iliac wing fracture (*arrows*), but this view is somewhat overpenetrated and the fracture is difficult to see. **D**, Computed tomography (CT) slices show that from the sacroiliac joint (*top left*), a strut of bone extends inferior toward the acetabulum, but ends as a small shard of bone (*bottom right*), the "spur sign" by CT (*arrows*). The iliac wing is divided by a coronal oriented fracture line, typical of column type fractures (*arrowheads*).

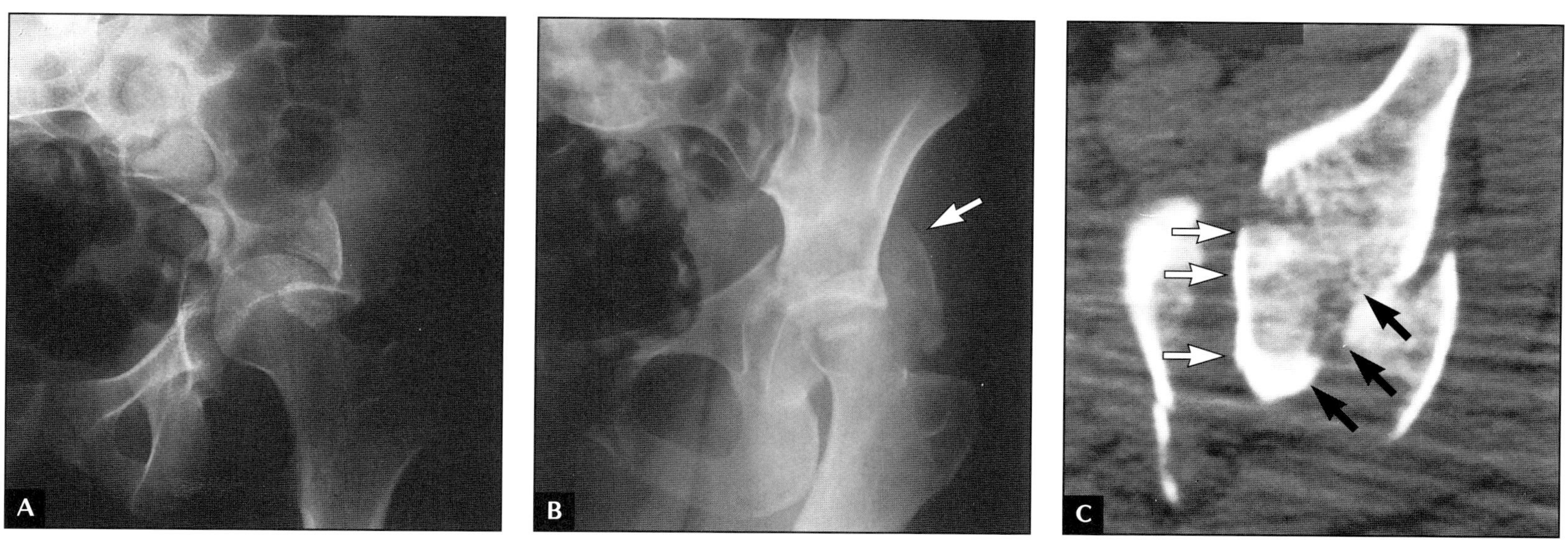

FIGURE 3-6. Transverse with posterior wall fracture. **A**, Anteroposterior view shows disruption of both the iliopectineal and ilioischial lines; the lateral margin of the posterior wall is absent and the femoral head is posteriorly dislocated. **B**, Obturator oblique view (underrotated due to patient discomfort) more clearly shows the position of the posterior wall fragment (*arrow*). The obturator ring is intact, despite a fracture adjacent to the symphysis pubis that does not enter the ring. **C**, Computed tomography scan shows a vertical lucent line representing the transverse part of the fracture (*white arrows*). The posterior wall fragment is noted, and the fracture plane of this fragment is oblique, typical for wall fractures (*black arrows*).

Knee and Proximal Tibia

Fractures of the distal femur are usually the result of high-energy trauma and are evaluated using AP and lateral radiographs. Fractures of the patella are also typically evaluated with AP, lateral, and occasionally Merchant view radiographs. CT can be done if detailed anatomy of the degree of articular disruption or fracture comminution is needed. If posterior dislocation of the knee is identified, angiography is indicated to search for vascular injury. Injury to the popliteal artery occurs in between 25% and 40% of knee dislocations [55]. Ligamentous damage also is common with knee dislocations and is best evaluated by MRI.

Fractures of the tibial plateau occur from either a varus or valgus stress, an axial load of the tibia into the femur, or a combination of these forces. The plateau fractures as a single split, a depression of the articular surface, or a combined split-depression fracture. The Schatzker [56] classification is widely used for tibial plateau fractures. This classification divides fractures into six types. The AO classification [57], similar to the Schatzker classification, is also available.

Imaging of patients with suspected tibial plateau fracture consists of AP and lateral radiographs. If a fracture is detected, oblique radiographs define articular depression better than standard views. However, CT is far better than radiographs for characterizing fracture fragment position and number and is now almost considered routine for evaluating these fractures. When using CT in this setting, it is important to collect slices with adequate overlap to generate optimal reconstructions, because coronal and sagittal images are valuable for characterizing the amount

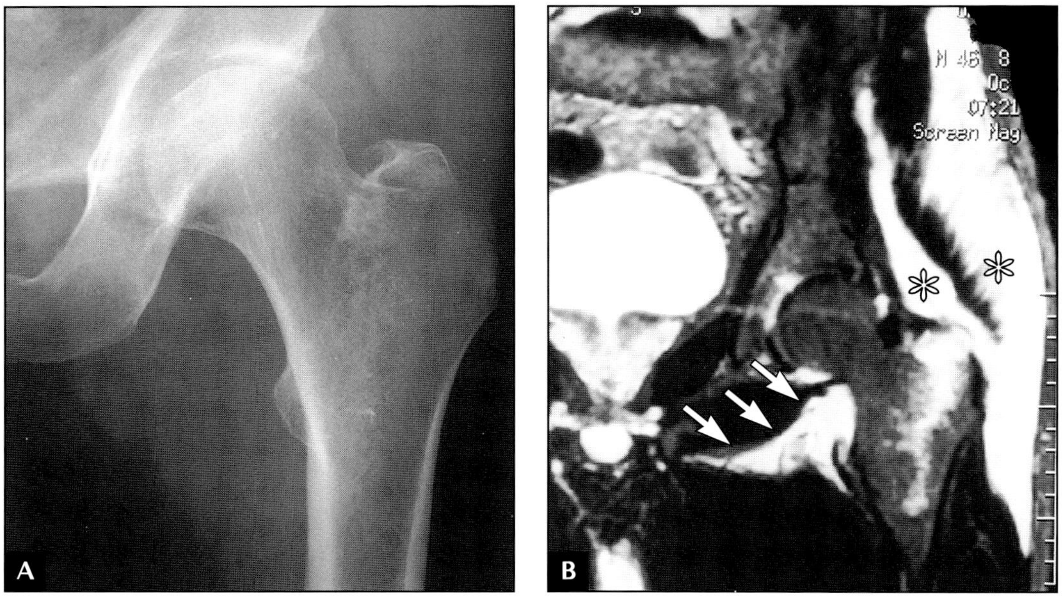

Figure 3-7. Occult hip fracture in a man aged 46 years. **A**, Anteroposterior radiograph shows a fracture of the greater trochanter but is indeterminate for fracture extending into the intertrochanteric region. **B**, Coronal T2-weighted magnetic resonance images with fat suppression show the fracture line as a bright linear area extending into the intertrochanteric region. Note also the bleeding along obturator externus (*white arrows*) and adjacent to gluteus medius and minimus (*asterisks*).

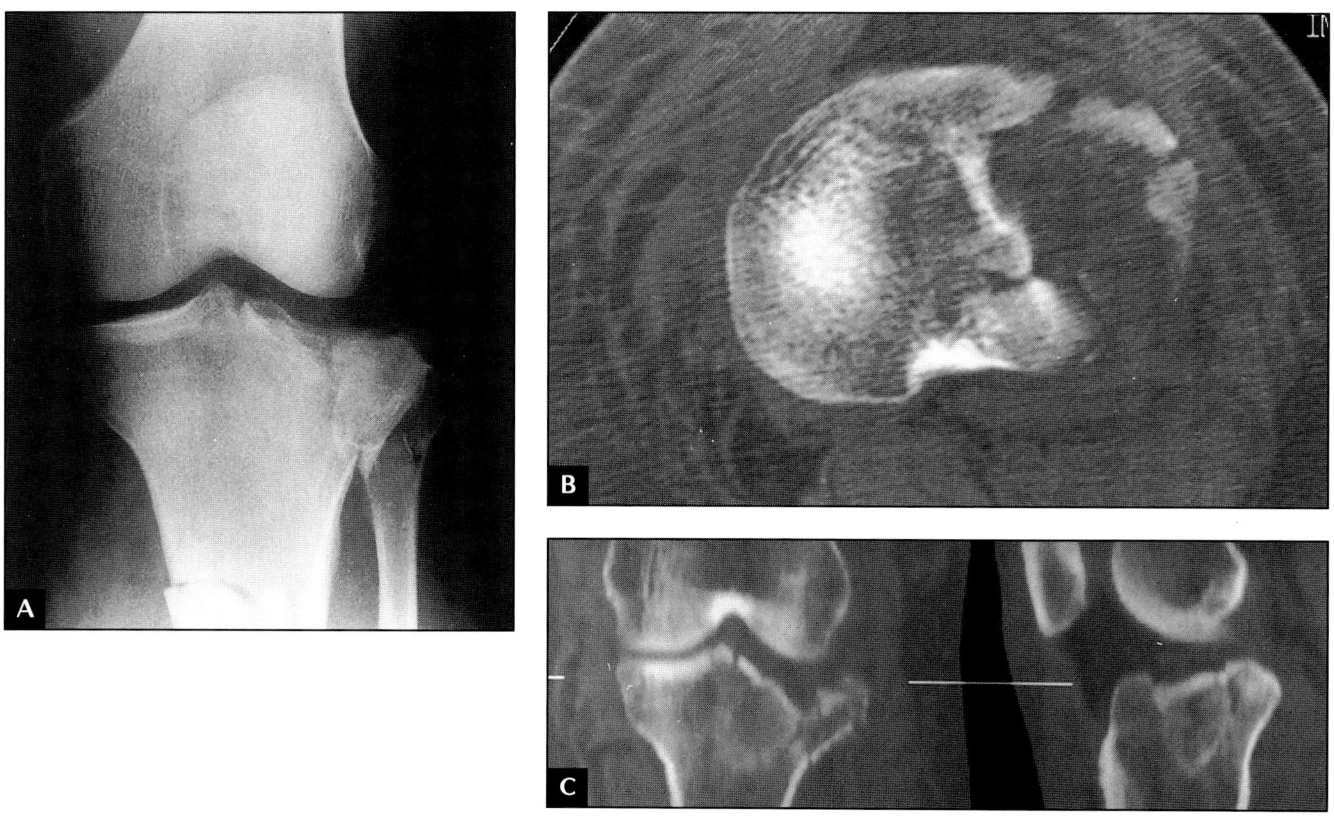

Figure 3-8. Tibial plateau fracture. **A**, Anteroposterior radiograph shows split depression fracture of the lateral tibial plateau. Note also fractures of the proximal fibula and tibial shaft. **B**, Axial computed tomography image at level of plateau shows that much of the lateral plateau is depressed; the medial plateau remains intact. **C**, Reconstructions in the coronal and sagittal planes define the extent and depth of depression better than the radiographs do. Also note that the anterolateral corner shows significant comminution.

of depression of the articular surfaces (Figure 3-8). Axial slices with 3-mm thickness obtained at 1.5-mm increments yield good reconstructed images. MRI is not considered a routine study for the evaluation of tibial fractures but may show occult fractures on patients suspected of internal derangement of the knee following trauma (Figure 3-9). In some instances, MRI may show entrapment of a meniscus within an articular depression, which could alter surgical management.

Ankle Fractures

Fractures of the ankle are typically assessed with conventional radiographs. AP, mortice, and lateral views are those most often applied during traditional radiographic examination of the ankle. One paper has suggested that the mortice and lateral views may be sufficient to detect ankle fractures [58]. Several different classifications are commonly used to characterize ankle fractures, including the Lauge-Hansen [59] and the Danis-Weber/AO [57,60] classifications. The Lauge-Hansen classification [59] describes fracture patterns based on the position of the foot and direction of deforming force at the time of injury. Ligaments and bones fail in a predictable order, leading to characteristic fracture patterns. The Danis-Weber/AO [57,60] classifications are based on the shape and position of fracture of the distal fibula grouped into three types.

Although most ankle fractures are sufficiently evaluated with radiographs, comminuted fractures of the distal tibia, called *pilon fractures*, require a more thorough imaging evaluation. Pilon fractures are most commonly classified using either the AO [57,60] or Rüedi and Allgöwer [61] classifications. The Rüedi and Allgöwer classification [61] divides pilon fractures into three types: nondisplaced fractures (Type I) , fractures with some articular disruption (Type II), and fractures with significant articular disruption (Type III). The AO classification [57,60] divides fractures initially as extra-articular, partial articular, or total articular types. This distinction is particularly useful because it guides surgical management. Beyond the initial fracture types, the AO classification is comprehensive but complex. Each of the main fracture groups is further subdivided into subgroups. Interobserver agreement is good at the initial level (type A, B, or C), but agreement drops to unacceptable levels when the full classification is used [62].

Imaging evaluation of pilon fractures begins with AP, mortice, and lateral radiographs. Assessment of fracture comminution can be made, but CT is better than radiographs for characterizing fracture fragment size, number, and displacement. CT has become a common examination modality for patients with pilon fractures. As with fractures of the tibial plateau, thin (3-mm) slices with overlapping images allow for multiplanar reconstructions, which are helpful for surgical planning.

Foot Fractures

The calcaneus is the most commonly injured bone of the foot and is bilateral in 5% to 9% of cases [63,64]. Calcaneal fractures are associated with other injuries; a fracture of the thoracolumbar spine is present 10% of the time [65] and lower extremity injuries can be seen in between 26% and 70% of cases [65–67]. Fractures of the calcaneus are divided into intra-articular and extra-articular types. Moreover, 75% of calcaneal fractures are intra-articular, whereas extra-articular fractures make up 25% of cases [63]. Extra-articular fractures include fractures of the anterior process, the tuberosity, the medial process, the body, and, uncommonly, isolated fracture of the sustentaculum tali. More serious intra-articular fractures involve the subtalar joint and are further subdivided by the Essex-Lopresti [68] classification into joint depression and tongue types.

Axial loading is the usual cause of intra-articular fractures, with force being transmitted through the talus into the calcaneus. As the lateral process of the talus is driven down through the crucial angle of Gissane, the primary fracture line occurs [64]. This fracture extends from plantarmedial to dorsolateral and includes an anteromedial (sustentacular) fragment as well as a posterolateral fragment. A secondary fracture line occurs as fracture energy is dissipated through the posterior calcaneus. If a fracture line extends back to the tuberosity, a tongue-type fracture results. In this setting, the posterior facet of the subtalar joint is often intact. With joint depression fractures, the secondary fracture line extends cephalad just behind the posterior facet of the subtalar joint, resulting in comminution and incongruency of that facet.

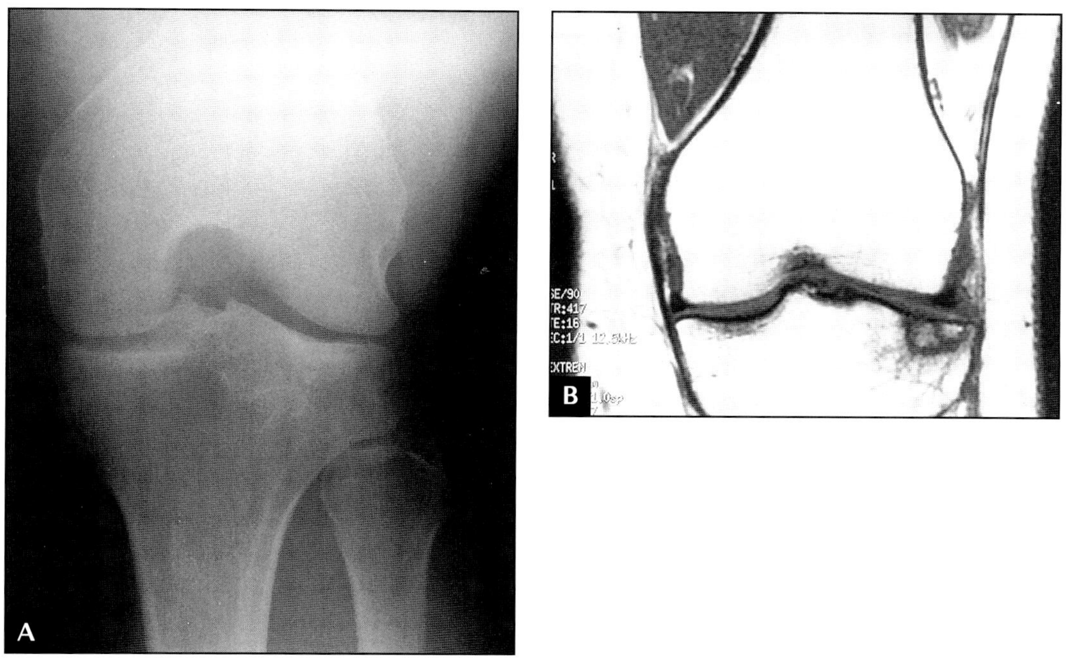

Figure 3-9. Occult tibial plateau fracture. **A**, Anteroposterior radiograph of a patient who fell 1 month previously and was experiencing continued pain. Subtle sclerosis was noted in the lateral plateau, but fracture was not suspected. **B**, Coronal T1-weighted magnetic resonance image shows nondisplaced depression-type fracture of lateral plateau.

Imaging evaluation of patients with suspected calcaneal fractures begins with radiographs (Figure 3-10). The lateral view is the most helpful for assessing calcaneal integrity. Böhler's angle is normally 25° to 40°; an angle of less than 20° indicates a fracture [63]. The crucial angle of Gissane is normally visible as a V-shaped projection of dense subchondral bone in the calcaneus below the lateral process of the talus. Disruption of this angle indicates a fracture of the calcaneus. Additional radiographic views, including Harris and axial, can be obtained for better evaluation of the posterior and middle facets of the subtalar joint [64].

Computed tomography is valuable for assessment of the severity of calcaneal fractures and as a preoperative planning tool [69,70]. The amount of comminution and articular incongruency of the posterior facet of the subtalar joint is the primary determinant of risk for accelerated osteoarthritis [63]. Open reduction and internal fixation to restore alignment of the subtalar joint decreases risk of accelerated osteoarthritis. The goals of operative intervention are to restore the height and congruency of the posterior facet of the subtalar joint and to restore the length of the calcaneus. When fractured, the calcaneus usually foreshortens as compared with normal, especially when longitudinally oriented fractures are present. Thus, it is important to extend CT scans of the calcaneus anterior to the level of the calcaneocuboid joint.

With the detail that CT provides of the posterior facet, classifications beyond the Essex-Lopresti [68] system were needed. Crosby and Fitzgibbons [71] as well as Sanders *et al.* [70] have developed classifications of intra-articular calcaneal fractures. In the Crosby and Fitzgibbons classification [71], fractures are classified into three types based on the status of the posterior facet of the subtalar joint: Type I fractures have small nondisplaced fragments, Type II fractures have a displaced single fracture line, and Type III fractures are comminuted. The classification by Sanders *et al.* [70] is divided into four types. Type I represents a nondisplaced fracture (less than or equal to 2 mm of joint widening or articular step off). Type II fractures consist of a two-part fracture with a split in the posterior facet of subtalar joint, whereas Type III fractures are three-part fractures with two fracture lines in a split-depression configuration. Type IV injuries are severely comminuted fractures of the posterior facet. These types are further subdivided based on where the fracture lines enter the subtalar joint. Fracture lines are graded as lateral, central, medial, or sustentacular with respect to the subtalar joint [70•].

When performing CT of the calcaneus, we usually obtain two scans. For the first, the patient and gantry are positioned so that images obtained are oriented perpendicular to the posterior facet of the subtalar joint. We obtain 3-mm slices at 1.5-mm increments. The second scan is in the axial plane, parallel to the longitudinal axis of the calcaneus and perpendicular to the calcaneocuboid joint. Scan parameters are the same as the oblique coronal images. From the oblique coronal study, we usually generate sagittal reconstructions. If needed for preoperative planning, reconstructions can be made parallel to the plane of the posterior facet of the subtalar joint to show any incongruity of the joint en face.

Various fractures and dislocations can occur through the midfoot. Some of these are adequately evaluated with radiographs, but others require the cross-sectional detail that CT provides. For example, midfoot dislocations can be very difficult to detect and characterize with radiographs alone [72,73]. CT scanning is a more sensitive and specific method to characterize midfoot fracture dislocations than radiographs [74•,75–77). Lu *et al.* [74•] studied small (1 to 2 mm) displacements at the tarsometatarsal joints and noted that 2-mm displacements are not detected on plain radiographs yet are well seen with CT. In this study, the CT gantry plane was perpendicular to the long axis of the metatarsal shafts. Images parallel and perpendicular to the long axis of the metatarsals have been suggested as optimal planes for imaging midfoot fracture dislocations [74•,77,78].

CONCLUSIONS

Imaging plays an important part in the evaluation of trauma patients; it often dictates initial therapy or guides the decision

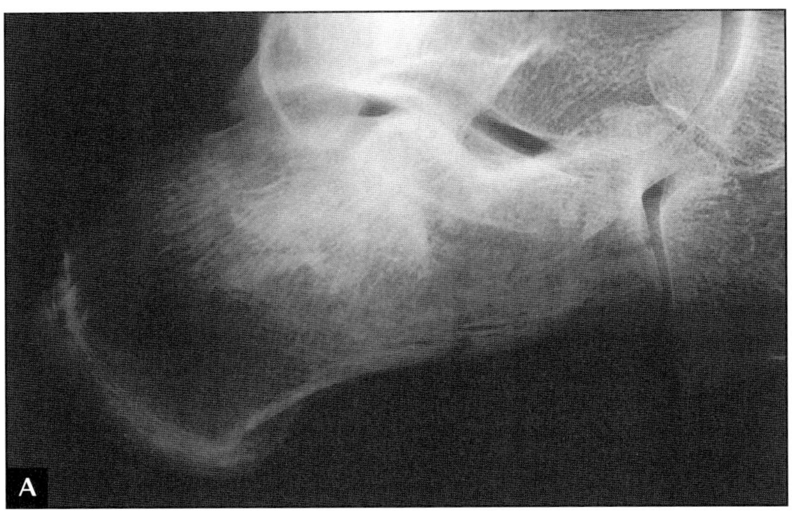

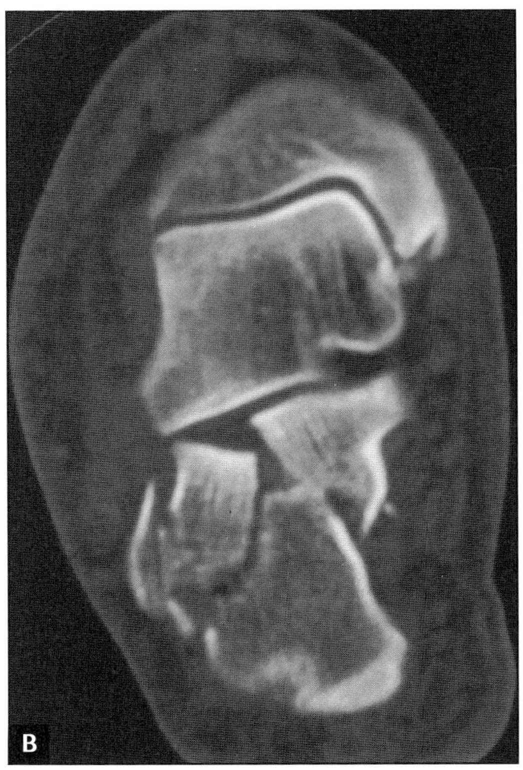

FIGURE 3-10. Joint depression calcaneal fracture. **A**, Lateral radiograph shows depression of Böhler's angle and lack of visualization of the crucial angle of Gissane. **B**, Computed tomography image obtained with the gantry oriented perpendicular to the posterior facet of the subtalar joint shows that two fracture lines result in a split depression type of fracture, which would be classified as a Type III under the Sanders *et al.* [70] classification. The degree of joint disruption is far better defined than on the radiograph.

between conservative and operative treatment. Radiographs remain the standard examination for trauma, but many other imaging tests can be done to supplement radiographs or to provide further evaluation. Choosing which imaging study to obtain depends on the type of injury present or suspected, the clinical circumstances of the injury, and how that imaging test alters patient care. A thorough understanding of the advantages and limitations of each modality allows the treating physician to choose optimal imaging tests for accurate and efficient diagnoses.

REFERENCES AND RECOMMENDED READING

Recently published papers of particular interest have been highlighted as:
- • Of interest
- •• Of outstanding interest

1. Crawford C, King K: Computed tomography scanning with simultaneous patient translation. *Med Phys* 1990, 17:967–982.
2. Tohki Y: Principles of helical scan. In *Basic Principles and Clinical Applications of Helical Scan*. Edited by Kimura K, Koga S. Tokyo: Iryokagakusha; 1993:110–120.
3. Fishman E: Spiral CT evaluation of the musculoskeletal system. In *Spiral CT: Principles, Techniques and Clinical Application*. Edited by Fishman EK, Jeffrey RB. New York: Raven Press; 1995:141–158.
4. Silver MD: High-helical-pitch, cone-beam computed tomography. *Phys Med Biol* 1998, 43:847–855.
5. Horowitz AL: *MRI Physics for Radiologists: A Visual Approach* edn 2. New York: Springer-Verlag; 1991.
6. Newhouse JH, Wiener JI: *Understanding MRI*. Boston: Little, Brown & Co; 1991.
7. Gregory BA, Hesselink JR, Meddleton MS: Fat-suppression contrast-enhanced MRI in the failed back surgery syndrome: a prospective study. *Neuroradiology* 1995, 37:51–57.
8. Schick F, Bongers H, Aicher K, *et al.*: Subtle bone marrow edema assessed by frequency selective shift MRI. *J Comput Assist Tomogr* 1992, 16:454–460.
9. Kellam JF, Browner BD: Fractures of the pelvic ring. In *Skeletal Trauma: Fractures, Dislocations, Ligmentous Injuries* edn 2. Edited by Browner BD, Jupiter JB, Levine AM, *et al.* Philadelphia: WB Saunders; 1992:849–897.
10. Tile M: *Fractures of the Pelvis and Acetabulum*. Philadelphia, Williams & Wilkins; 1995.
11. Daffner RH: Pelvic trauma. In *Trauma Radiology*. Edited by McCort JJ, Mindelzun RE. New York: Churchill Livingstone; 1990:339–380.
12. Young JWR, Burgess AR: *Radiological Management of Pelvic Ring Fractures*. Baltimore: Urban & Schwarzenberg; 1987.
13. Young JWR, Burgess AR, Brumbach RJ, *et al.*: Pelvic fractures: value of plain radiography in early assessment and management. *Radiology* 1986, 160:445–451.
14. Letournel E, Judet R: *Fractures of the Acetabulum*, edn 2. New York: Springer-Verlag; 1993.
15. Mayo KA: Hip joint: Acetabular fractures. In *Orthopaedic Trauma Protocols*. Edited by Hansen ST, Swiontkowski MF. New York: Raven Press; 1993: 243–254.
16. Rogers LF: *Radiology of Skeletal Trauma* edn 2. New York: Churchill Livingstone; 1992:991–1105.
17. Routt ML: Pelvic fractures. In *Orthopaedic Trauma Protocols*. Edited by Hansen ST, Swiontkowski MF. New York: Raven Press; 1993:225–236.
18. Montana MA, Richardson ML, Kilcoyne RF, *et al.*: CT of sacral injury. *Radiology* 1986, 161:499–503.
19. Guy RL, Butler MPA, Holder P, *et al.*: The role of 3D CT in the assessment of acetabular fractures. *Br J Radiol* 1992, 65:384–389.
20. Howie JL: Computed tomography of the bony pelvis: a protocol for multiplanar imaging. Part II: trauma. *J Can Assoc Radiol* 1985, 36:287–295.
21. Kuhlman JE, Fishman EK, Ney DR, *et al.*: Nonunion of acetabular fractures: evaluation with interactive multiplanar CT. *J Orthop Trauma* 1989, 3:33–40.
22. Vannier MW, Hildebolt CF, Gilula LA, *et al.*: Calcaneal and pelvic fractures: diagnostic evaluation by three-dimensional computed tomography scans. *J Digit Imaging* 1991, 4:143–52.
23. White MS: Three-dimensional computed tomography in the assessment of fractures of the acetabulum. *Injury* 1991, 22:13–19.
24. Brandser EA, Marsh JL: Acetabular fractures: easier classification with a systematic approach. *Am J Roentgenol* 1998, 171:1217–1228.
25. Burgess AR, Tile M: Fractures of the pelvis. In *Fractures in Adults*. Edited by Rockwood CA, Green DP, Bucholz RW. Philadelphia: JB Lippincott; 1991:1399–1479.
26. Pennal GF, Tile M, Waddell JP, *et al.*: Pelvic disruption: assessment and classification. *Clin Orthop*1980, 151:12–21.
27. Tile M: *Fractures of the Pelvis and Acetabulum*. Baltimore: Williams & Wilkins; 1984.
28. Tile M: Pelvic ring fractures: should they be fixed? *J Bone Joint Surg Br* 1988, 70:1–12.
29. Müller ME, Allgöwer M, Schneider R, *et al.*: *Manual of Internal Fixation: Techniques Recommended by the AO-ASIF Group* edn 3. Berlin: Springer-Verlag; 1977.
30. Judet R, Judet J, Letournel E: Fractures of the acetabulum: classification and surgical approaches for open reduction. *J Bone Joint Surg Am* 1964, 46:1615–1638.
31. Letournel E: *Fractures of the Acetabulum* edn 2. New York: Springer-Verlag; 1993.
32. Brandser E, El-Khoury G, Marsh JL: Acetabular fractures: a systematic approach to classification. *Emerg Radiol* 1995, 2:18–28.
33. Armbuster TG, Guerra J, Resnick D, *et al.*: The adult hip: an anatomic study. *Radiology* 1978, 128:1–10.
34. Saks BJ: Normal acetabular anatomy for acetabular fracture assessment: CT and plain film correlation. *Radiology* 1986, 159:139–145.
35. Olson SA, Matta JM: The computerized tomography subchondral arc: a new method of assessing acetabular articular continuity after fracture (a preliminary report). *J Orthop Trauma* 1993, 7:402–413.
36. Shirkhoda A, Brashear H, Staab E: Computed tomography of acetabular fractures. *Radiology* 1980, 134:683–688.
37. Mack L, Harley J, Linquist R: CT analysis of acetabular fractures: analysis of fracture patterns. *Am J Roentgenol* 1982, 138:407–412.
38. Harley J, Mack L, Linquist R: CT of acetabular fractures: comparison with conventional radiography. *Am J Roentgenol* 1982, 138:413–417.
39. Burk DL, Mears DC, Kennedy WH, *et al.*: Three dimensional computed tomography of acetabular fractures. *Radiology* 1985, 155:183–185.
40. Calkins MS, Zych G, Latta L, *et al.*: Computerized tomography evaluation of stability in posterior fracture dislocations of the hip. *Clin Orthop Rel Res* 1988, 227:152–163.
41. Keith JE, Brashear HR, Guilford WB: Stability of posterior fracture dislocations of the hip: quantitative assessment using computed tomography. *J Bone Joint Surg Am* 1988, 70:711–714.
42. Mayo K: Fractures of the acetabulum. *Orthop Clin North Am* 1987, 18:43–57.
43. Brandser EA, El-Khoury GY, Marsh JL: Utility of roof arc measurements in acetabular fractures. *Emerg Radiol* 1995, 2:323–330.
44. Griffiths HJ, Standertskjold-Nordenstam CG, Burke J, *et al.*: Computed tomography in the management of acetabular fractures. *Skeletal Radiol* 1984, 11:22–31.
45. Vas WG, Wolverson MK, Sundaram M, *et al.*: The role of computed tomography in pelvic fractures. *J Comput Assist Tomogr* 1982, 6:796–801.
46. Martinez C, DiPasquale T, Helfet D, *et al.*: Evaluation of acetabular fractures with two and three dimension CT. *Radiographics* 1992, 12:227–242.
47. Scott WW, Fishman EK, Magid D, *et al.*: Acetabular fractures: optimal imaging. *Radiology* 1987, 165:537–539.
48. Fishman EK, Brebin B, Magid D, *et al.*: Volumetric rendering techniques: applications for three-dimensional imaging of the hip. *Radiology* 1987, 163:737–738.

49. Zetterberg CH, Elmerson S, Andersson G: Epidemiology of hip fractures in Gotegorg, Sweden, 1940–1983. *Clin Orthop* 1984, 191:43–52.
50. Melton LJ, Ilstrup DM, Rigs BL, *et al.*: Fifty-year trend in hip fracture incidence. *Clin Orthop* 1982, 162:144–149.
51. Swiontkowski MF: Intracapsular hip fractures. In *Skeletal Trauma: Fractures, Dislocations, Ligamentous Injuries* edn 2. Edited by Browner BD, Jupiter JB, Levine AM, *et al.*: Philadelphia: WB Saunders; 1992:1369–1442.
52. Evans EM: Trochanteric fractures. *J Bone Joint Surg Br* 1951, 33:192–204.
53. Haramati N, Staron RB, Barax C, *et al.*: Magnetic resonance imaging of occult fractures of the proximal femur. *Skeletal Radiol* 1994, 23:19–22.
54.• Bogost GA, Crues JV: Postraumatic hip pain: the role of magnetic resonance imaging in the emergency setting. *Emerg Radiol* 1998, 5:368–374.

This discussion and pictorial essay demonstrates that MRI is not only useful for diagnosing occult femoral neck fractures. Many patients with posttraumatic hip pain who do not have a fracture by MRI *are* shown to have muscle tears or hematoma. Pelvic insufficiency fractures can also be revealed because they may mimic the clinical presentation of femoral neck fracture.

55. Leffers D: Dislocations and soft tissue injuries of the knee. In *Skeletal Trauma: Fractures, Dislocations, Ligamentous Injuries* edn 2. Edited by Browner BD, Jupiter JB, Levine AM, *et al.* Philadelphia: WB Saunders; 1992:1717–1744.
56. Schatzker J: Tibial plateau fractures. In *Skeletal Trauma: Fractures, Dislocations, Ligamentous Injuries* edn 2. Edited by Browner BD, Jupiter JB, Levine AM, *et al.* Philadelphia: WB Saunders; 1992:1745–1770.
57. Mueller ME, Nazarian S, Koch P, *et al.*: *The Comprehensive Classification of Fractures of Long Bones*. Berlin: Springer-Verlag; 1990.
58. Vangsness CT, Carter V, Hunt T, *et al.*: Radiographic diagnosis of ankle fractures: are three views necessary? *Foot Ankle Int* 1994, 15:172–174.
59. Lauge-Hansen N: Fractures of the ankle: analytic historic survey as basis of new experimental roentgenologic and clinical investigations. *Arch Surg* 1948, 56:259–317.
60. Lindsjö U: Classification of ankle fractures: the Lauge-Hansen or AO system? *Clin Orthop* 1985, 199:12–16.
61. Rüedi TP, Allgöwer M: The operative treatment of intraarticular fractures of the lower end of the tibia. *Clin Orthop* 1979, 138:105–110.
62. Martin JG, Marsh JL, Bonar SK, *et al.*: Assessment of the AO/ASIF fracture classification for the distal tibia. *J Orthop Trauma* 1997, 11:477–483.
63. Rogers LF: The foot. In *Radiology of Skeletal Trauma* vol 2. Edited by Rogers LF. New York: Churchill Livingstone; 1992:1429–1521.
64. Heckman JD: Fractures and dislocations of the foot. In *Rockwood and Green's Fractures in Adults.* Edited by Rockwood CA, Green DP, Bucholz RW. Philadelphia: JB Lippincott; 1991:2041–2182.
65. Cave EF: Fracture of the os calcis: the problem in general. *Clin Orthop* 1963, 30:64–66.
66. Lance EM, Carey EJ, Wade PA: Fractures of the os calcis: treatment by early mobilization. *Clin Orthop* 1963, 30:76–90.
67. Lance EM, Carey EJ, Wade PA: Fractures of the os calcis: a follow-up study. *J Trauma* 1964, 4:15–56.
68. Essex-Lopresti P: The mechanism, reduction technique, and results in fractures of the os calcis. *Br J Surg* 1952, 39:395–419.
69. Hindman BW, Ross SD, Sowerby MR: Fractures of the talus and calcaneus: evaluation by computed tomography. *J Comput Tomogr* 1986, 10:191–196.
70. Sanders R, Fortin P, DiPasquale T, *et al.*: Operative treatment in 120 displaced intraarticular calcaneal fractures. *Clin Orthop* 1993, 290:87–95.
71. Crosby LA, Fitzgibbons T: Intraarticular calcaneal fractures: results of closed treatment. *Clin Orthop* 1993, 290:46–54.
72. Schiller MG, Ray RD: Isolated dislocation of the medial cuneiform bone: a rare injury of the tarsus. *J Bone Joint Surg Am* 1970, 52:1632–1636.
73. Lynch JR, Cooperstein LA, DiGioia AM: Plantar medial subluxation of the medial cuneiform: case report of an uncommon variant of the Lisfranc injury: *Foot Ankle Int* 1995, 16:299–301.
74.• Lu J, Ebraheim NA, Skie M, *et al.*: Radiographic and computed tomographic evaluation of Lisfranc dislocation: a cadaver study. *Foot Ankle Int* 1997, 18:351–355.

The authors studied six cadaver feet with 1- or 2-mm stepoffs at the Lisfranc joint and demonstrated that CT is superior to radiographs for detection of small displacements. The authors used CT images obtained perpendicular to the long axis of the metatarsals; images can also be obtained parallel to the long axis of the metatarsals.

75. Brandser EA, Henrichsen TA, El-Khoury GY, *et al.*: Combined Lisfranc and medial cuneiform fracture dislocation. *Emerg Radiol* 1999, 6:32–35.
76. Goiney RC, Connell DG, Nichols DM: CT evaluation of tarsometatarsal fracture-dislocation injuries. *Am J Roentgenol* 1985, 144:985–990.
77. Seltzer SE, Weissman BN, Braunstein EM, *et al.*: Computed tomography of the hindfoot. *J Comput Aid Tomogr* 1984, 8:488–497.
78. Leenen LPH, van der Werken C: Fracture-dislocations of the tarsometatarsal joint: a combined anatomical and computed tomographic study. *Br J Accident Surg* 1992, 23:51–55.

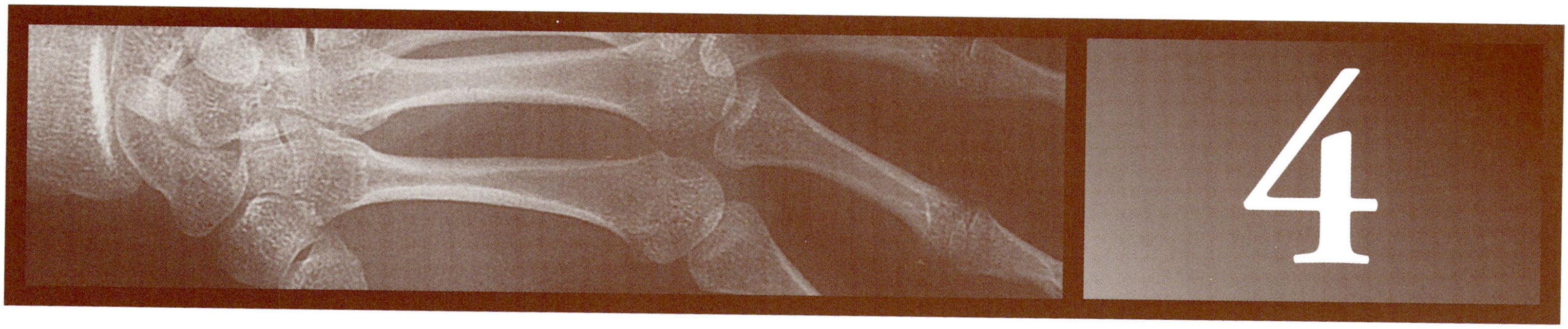

Imaging of Fractures of the Shoulder Girdle and Upper Extremities

Ronald W. Hendrix

Imaging provides four categories of information about fractures: fracture detection, fracture position, fracture healing, and viability of fracture fragments. The information in any one of these categories may change as time passes. Initially, radiographic images should be obtained to confirm that a clinical suspicion of a fracture is correct. In cases of negative plain radiographs and a strong clinical suspicion of fracture, scintigraphy or magnetic resonance imaging (MRI) should be used to detect occult fractures. Immobilization with repeat radiographs in 10 to 14 days for possible fracture (*eg*, in the scaphoid) has been a less aggressive way to proceed but is not always acceptable to the patient (*eg*, a competitive athlete) who needs or demands an immediate and definitive answer. Establishing bone fragment position of complicated fractures is necessary to plan surgical reduction or to decide whether surgery is needed. More sophisticated studies, such as computed tomography (CT) or conventional tomography (a modality totally superseded by CT at many institutions), are employed to provide this information. When preoperative assessment of vascular integrity of a fracture fragment is needed, MRI is used [1•]. Fracture fragment position, fracture alignment, bone bridging across the fracture, and demonstration of complications are determined using imaging to document progression of appropriate fracture healing. In most cases, plain radiographs provide completely adequate information for fracture detection, position evaluation, and healing assessment to provide optimal patient management. However, additional imaging will sometimes be needed to identify an occult fracture [2], evaluate adjacent soft tissues for injury [3•], determine vascular integrity of a bone fragment [1•], evaluate for physeal injury in children [4], or to assess fracture extent to speed up patient treatment or to determine patient management. Occult fractures refer to those fractures that are not detected or are below the threshold of detection using plain radiographic imaging. How occult they are has some relation to the perceptive abilities of the individual interpreting the study. They may not be at all occult when imaged by other modalities, such as bone scintigraphy or MRI. This chapter reviews imaging of routine fractures, not-so-routine fractures, and special imaging problems in the upper extremity. Most images contain fractures to demonstrate how a particular view or study can be used to describe pathology.

PICTURE ARCHIVING AND COMMUNICATION SYSTEM AND COMPUTED RADIOGRAPHY

Large changes are being made in the way radiographic images are obtained, stored, handled, manipulated, and viewed at most large medical facilities [5•]. With time, this shift to computed radiography (CR) is expected to filter throughout the medical community with economics as the driving force, because it is less expensive in the long term than current film-screen systems [5•]. CT, MRI, and ultrasound images have been in digital format in the past, but film-screen systems used for plain radiographs remained in an analog format. The recent advent of CR with digital images for plain radiography (Figures 4-1 and 4-2) now makes it possible for all images in a radiology department to be digitized. This allows extensive image manipulation, compact storage, display on video monitors, viewing at multiple sites simultaneously, decreased repeat studies, rapid retrieval, and rapid transmittal of images to remote sites, which affects everyone using such images. This should end the bane of every radiology department—lost films. Many radiology departments either have become or are in the process of becoming "filmless." This saves the cost of film, film processing, film handling,

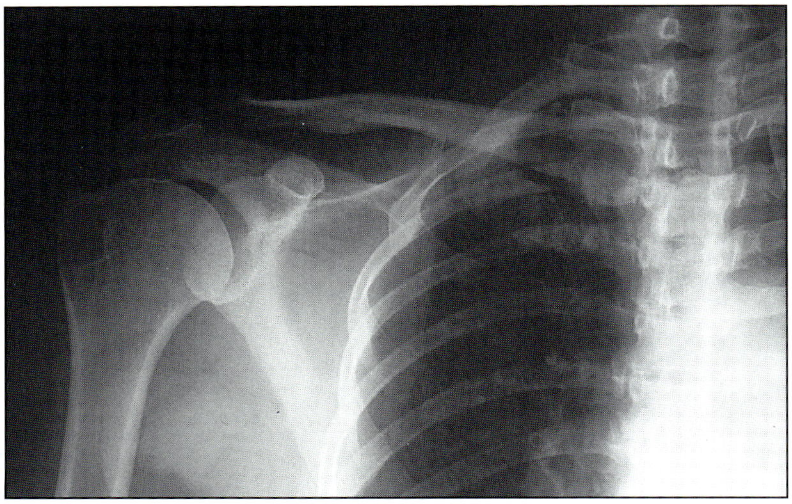

FIGURE 4-1. Digital radiograph of a normal shoulder demonstrates the extensive latitude of computed radiography. The area from the proximal end of the clavicle to the lateral soft tissues over the acromion is all clearly seen. Both thick and thin areas and dense and lucent areas are visible on the same film, unlike the more limited area visible with an analog film.

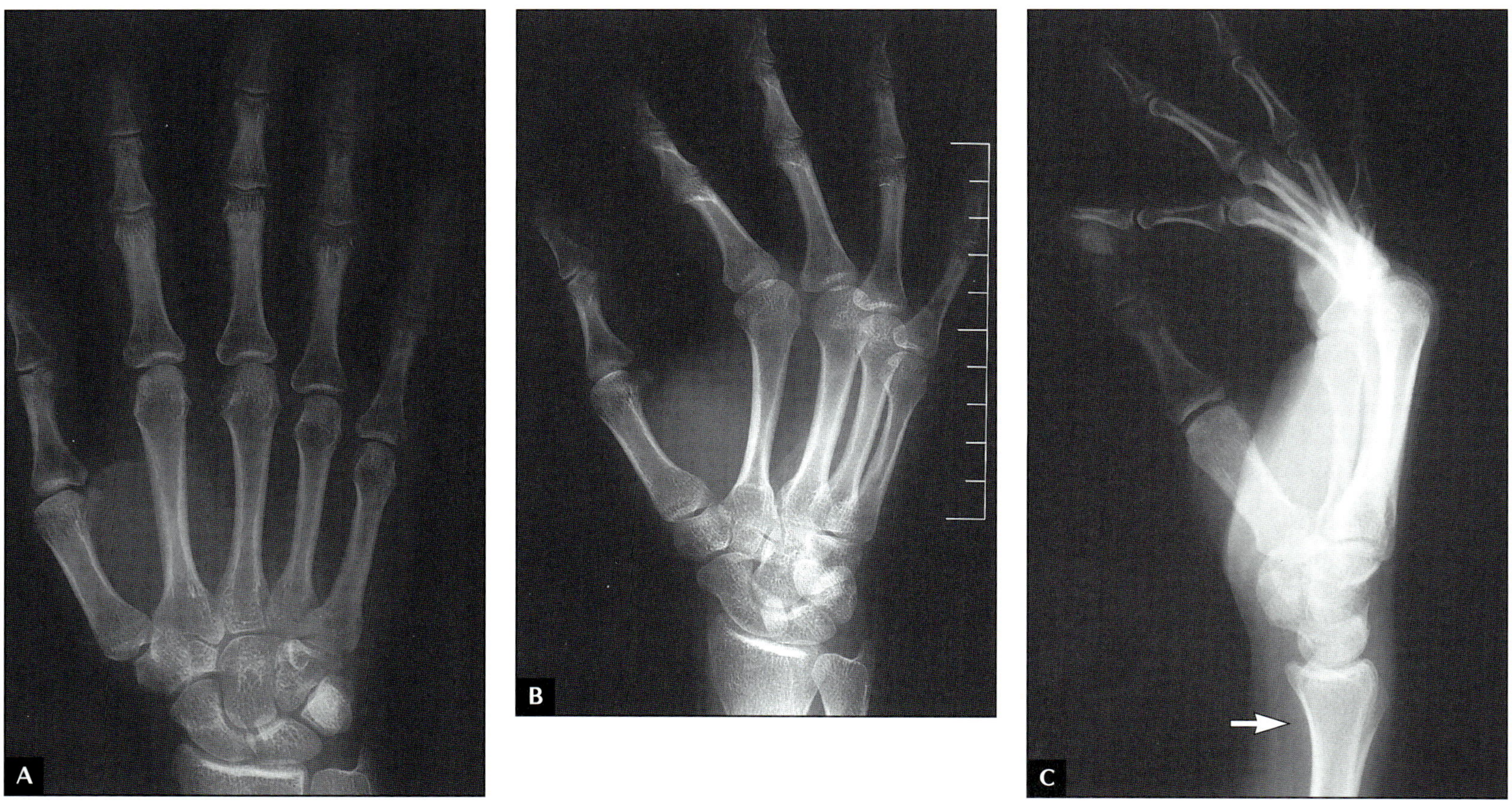

FIGURE 4-2. Digital radiographic study of a normal hand and wrist in a woman aged 23 years. **A**, Posteroanterior view demonstrates excellent detail in bone, joints, and soft tissues. **B**, Oblique view shows the metacarpal heads, phalangeal condyles, the scaphoid, and the radial styloid well. **C**, Lateral view clearly shows the interphalangeal joints, first metacarpal phalangeal joint, and the pronator quadratus fat plane (*arrow*).

and film storage amounting to nearly $20 per examination at present over the life of the examination. These future savings are counterbalanced, however, by a large initial investment and expensive maintenance [5•]. The images are digitally obtained and are viewed on cathode ray tube (CRT) monitors. Physicians at short or long distances from the radiology department can simultaneously look at the same films, point to abnormalities with an on-screen pointer, and discuss the findings by telephone instead of in person. At those institutions using soft-copy viewing on CRT monitors, hard copies can be printed as desired.

Computed radiography has a wider dynamic range by two to three orders of magnitude than film-screen systems in current use [6•]. What this means to anyone viewing a film is that CR allows bone and soft tissue detail to be seen clearly at the same time on the same image instead of one or the other being too light or too dark when the first is clearly visible, which occurs with screen-film systems (as seen in Figures 4-1 and 4-2). This wide dynamic range allows clear visualization of dense tissues (*eg*, bone) at the same time as radiolucent ones (*eg*, subcutaneous fat) or thick and thin areas simultaneously. The tip of the acromion and adjacent soft tissues can be seen at the same time as the humeral head and shoulder joint, or the sternoclavicular and acromioclavicular joints are clearly visualized simultaneously on the same image. Unlike analog films, additional information cannot be obtained from viewing a digital film with a bright light. An additional advantage of the wide dynamic range of CR is that the radiographic technologists have a much greater latitude for image exposure. A poorly exposed image can be adjusted electronically into a diagnostic image instead of repeating an exposure. This saves time, expense, and patient radiation exposure.

A picture archiving and communication (PAC) system stores images, allows them to be retrieved at any time, retrieved from sites distant from the radiology department by several persons simultaneously, and permits the images to be sent almost anywhere.

Image quality is dependent on contrast resolution and spatial resolution [7•]. Spatial resolution involves the ability to distinguish small objects that are in close proximity. Contrast resolution has the ability to differentiate two different normal tissues or normal from abnormal tissue. CR has a slightly decreased spatial resolution compared with analog film-screen systems in current use but has an increased contrast resolution that mostly compensates for the former (as seen in Figure 4-1).

PLAIN RADIOGRAPHS

Plain radiographs are the initial, and in most cases the only, imaging modality used to demonstrate the presence and position of most fractures of the upper extremities as well as the imaging modality used to monitor the healing process. In most cases, they are entirely sufficient. They are quickly and easily obtained, inexpensive, and most clinicians are comfortable with them. The maxim to obtain at least two films at 90° to one another is a starting place. However, when the study is obtained particularly to search for fractures, oblique views are so often necessary that it is wise for them to be part of the routine examination. Standard anteroposterior (AP), lateral, and oblique views are adequate to diagnose a fracture in most patients but at times they will reveal nothing despite a high clinical suspicion of fracture. Additional views specific to a given area must be tailored to the clinical situation for detecting subtle fractures (Figure 4-3). At times these will be normal, and thus CT, scintigraphy, or MRI examination will be needed.

Hand and Wrist

The routine radiographic study of the hand consists of three views: AP, lateral, and oblique (as seen in Figure 4-2). Standard views include the digits, the metacarpals, the wrist, and the distal 2 to 3 cm of the forearm. The thumb is seen in lateral view with the pos-

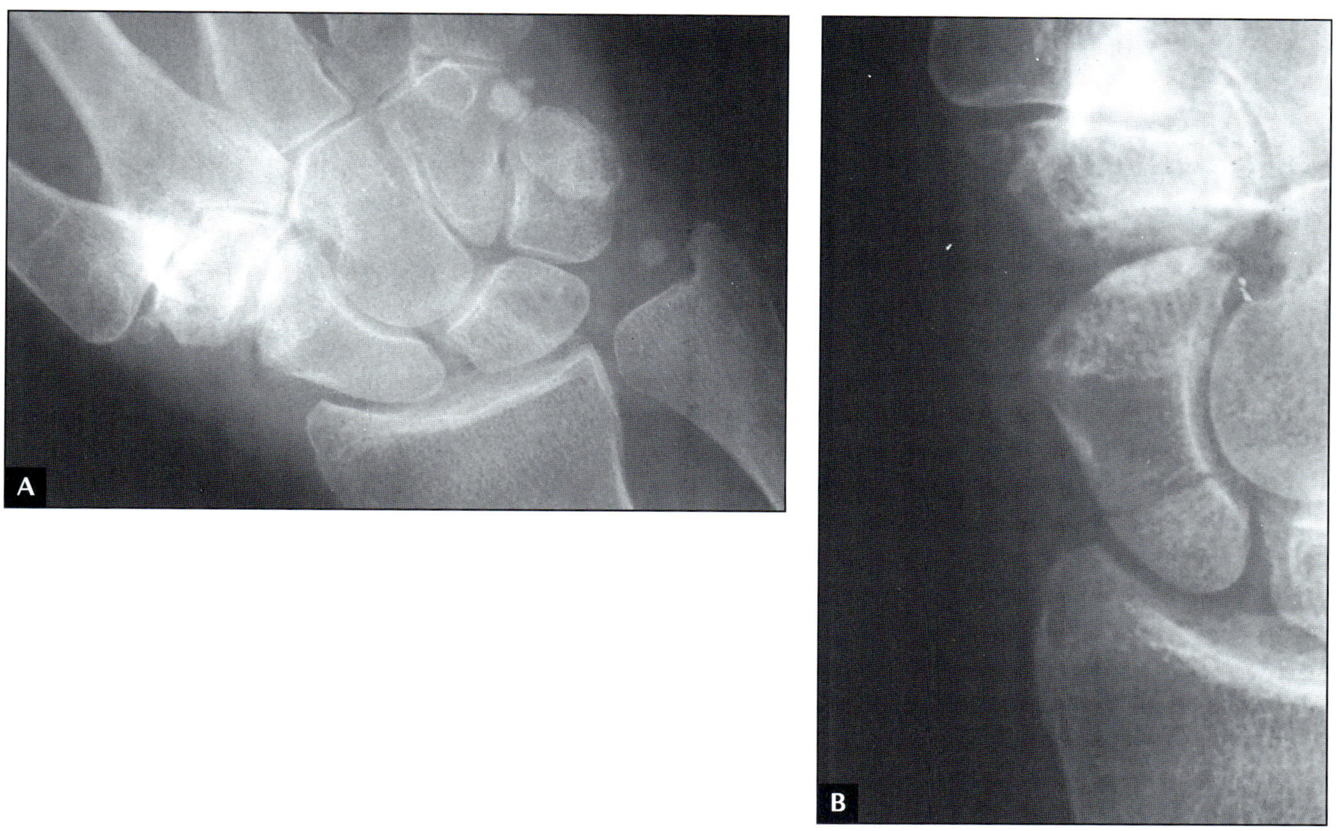

Figure 4-3. Scaphoid fracture only seen with a scaphoid view following a fall in a woman aged 78 years. **A**, Routine posteroanterior view of the wrist is normal. **B**, Scaphoid view taken as part of the same study as *panel A* shows a scaphoid fracture.

teroanterior (PA) view of the hand and in PA view with the lateral hand view. The lateral view of the hand superimposes the metacarpal bones (2 to 5), which allows an angulated fracture or a carpometacarpal dislocation to be detected. Individual digits at times are imaged singly to provide better detail if uncertainty exists about an area or no abnormality is seen on the standard whole-hand views and suspicion of a fracture persists. AP, lateral, and oblique views of individual digits typically are obtained.

The three routine views of the wrist are positioned the same as for the hand except the center of the x-ray beam is aimed at the radioulnar joint instead of the third metacarpal head as in the hand views. The images are coned down so that 2 to 3 cm of the forearm and most of the metacarpal shafts are imaged. In addition, a fourth view of the wrist, a scaphoid view, is obtained (as in Figure 4-3, *panel B*). This is obtained by maximally deviating the hand and wrist in the ulnar direction with the palm flat on the film cassette and angling the x-ray tube 25° toward the elbow. Normal radiocarpal, intercarpal, and carpometacarpal joint spaces measure approximately 2 mm wide or less. Opposing articular surfaces are parallel when a joint is seen in profile (as in Figure 4-2). Overlapping of articular surfaces indicates that subluxation or dislocation is present.

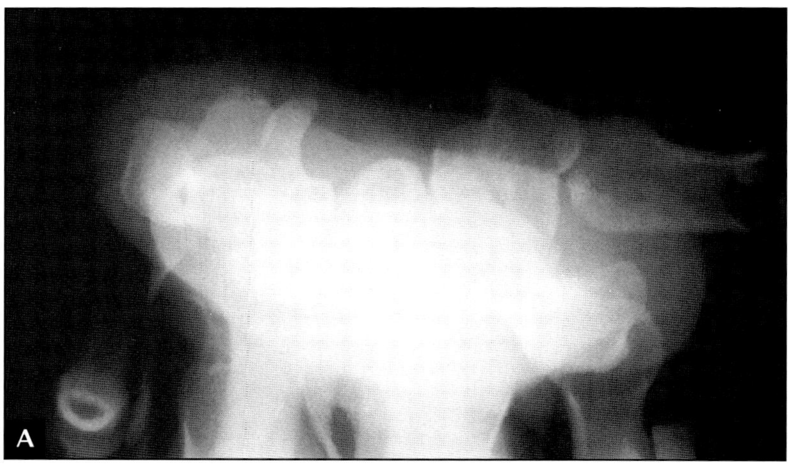

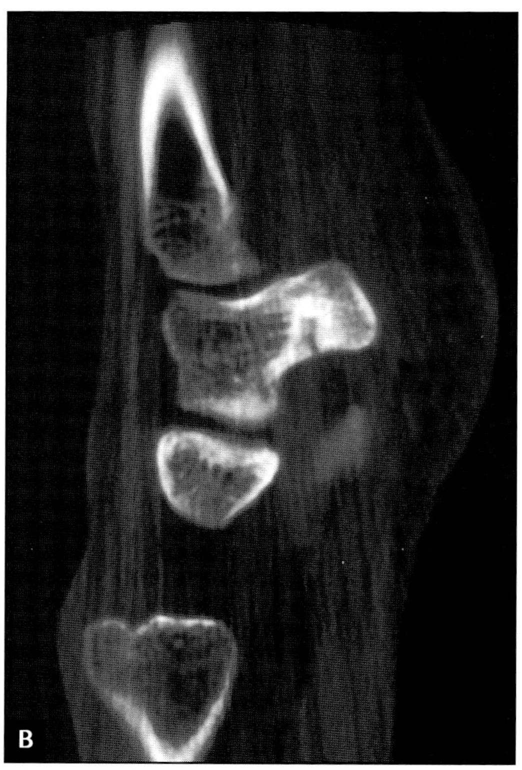

FIGURE 4-4. Stress fracture of the hook of the hamate in a professional baseball player aged 27 years from repetitive trauma of "check swings" during batting. He had increasing pain in his wrist for 4 months until he could no longer swing a bat. **A**, Carpal tunnel view of the wrist 2 months after onset of pain fails to demonstrate a fracture. **B**, Sagittal computed tomography image demonstrates a fracture line incompletely crossing the hook of the hamate with adjacent sclerotic bone. The same area 2 months earlier in *panel A* was normal.

Three roughly concentric articular surface arcs are formed in the normal PA wrist view, which are diagnostically useful when evaluating wrist trauma (*see* Figure 4-2, *panel A*). The first arc consists of a line joining the proximal articular surfaces of the scaphoid, lunate, and triquetrum. The second arc consists of the distal articular surfaces of the same three bones. The third arc consists of the proximal articular surfaces of the capitate and hamate. Disruption of or loss of parallelism of one or more of these arcs indicates that a fracture, dislocation, or a fracture-dislocation is present.

A fat plane outlines the margin of the pronator quadratus muscle along the volar surface of the distal radius (*see* Figure 4-2, *panel C*). Obliteration or displacement of this fat plane (more than 1 cm from the anterior radial surface) may be the only sign of a subtle distal radial fracture.

Hamate hook fractures are usually difficult to identify using plain radiography because of overlapping bones on the lateral view or the impossibility of the patient placing a painful hand in the needed position for special views to show the hamate in profile. A CT scan is typically resorted to at this point (Figure 4-4). A wrist view described by Bhalla *et al.* [8•] is quickly obtained (Figure 4-5) and may make a CT scan unnecessary. The patient is positioned with the ulnar side of the hand and wrist against the film cassette with 5° to 10° of supination. The thumb is maximally abducted and extended so that it is nearly perpendicular to the palm. The x-ray beam is angled 10° toward the patient. The hook of the hamate clearly is seen in profile (as in Figure 4-5).

ELBOW AND FOREARM

A standard examination of the elbow in some radiology departments consists of AP and lateral views (Figure 4-6), although this is an inadequate initial examination to locate fractures in a trauma patient. A significant number of additional fractures may be identified only by adding an external oblique view. When these three views fail to

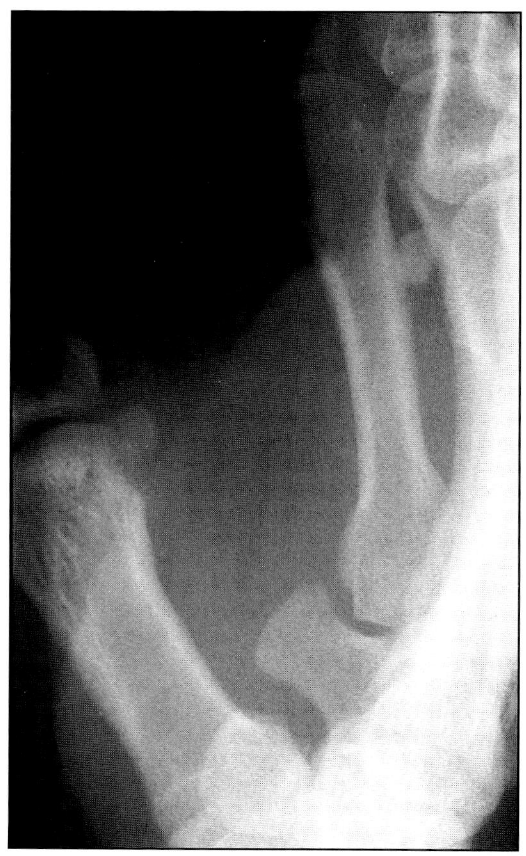

FIGURE 4-5. Supinated, thumb-extended view of the hamate hook provides excellent visualization of the hook but is much easier to obtain in an injured patient than the carpal tunnel view that gives much the same diagnostic information.

demonstrate a fracture but a joint effusion is present and a strong clinical suspicion for a fracture exists, a capitellum view may be of value. It is a modified lateral view obtained by positioning the patient for a lateral view of the elbow but then angling the x-ray beam 45° toward the patient [9]. It throws the radial head and neck clear of the ulna (Figure 4-7), thus showing fractures of the posterior radial head and neck and the capitellum not visible with other views. When dealing with a skeletally immature patient, comparison views of the opposite side should be obtained if concern is present about the position of an apophyseal or epiphyseal growth center.

Irshad *et al.* [10•] found that the fat-pad sign, any visualization of the posterior fat pad or elevation of the anterior fat pad, had a highly negative (87%) predictive value. The absence of a positive fat-pad sign is a reliable, although not an absolute, indicator that no fracture is present. The radial neck normally has a gentle curve with any angulation or discontinuity in it being indicative of a fracture (as in Figures 4-6 and 4-7). The radial head and neck are the most likely sites of subtle, missed fractures in the elbow although occasional subtle olecranon fractures are difficult to identify.

Several important radiographic relationships in the elbow ought be remembered. The normal radial head and capitellum retain the same alignment on all views. The posterior fat pad is only seen in the presence of a joint effusion, which could be a hemarthrosis from a fracture. An imaginary line contiguous with the anterior cortex of the humeral shaft, if extended into the elbow joint, should pass through the middle third of the capitellum. This is useful for detecting subtle supracondylar fractures in children.

The standard forearm radiographic examination includes AP and lateral views. The wrist and elbow joints are included on both views. Almost all forearm fractures are exceedingly obvious.

Shoulder Girdle

No consensus exists about the ideal way to image the shoulder with plain radiographs primarily because of the many overlapping structures. AP (Figure 4-8) views in internal and external rotation long were the standard examination of the shoulder but are often inadequate. Obtaining views at 90° to one another in the shoulder is difficult but necessary. The transthoracic view is almost useless because of poor detail from overlapping ribs but the axillary view can be used along with the AP view. An axillary view (Figure 4-9) typically is obtained using a curved cassette in the axilla with the shoulder

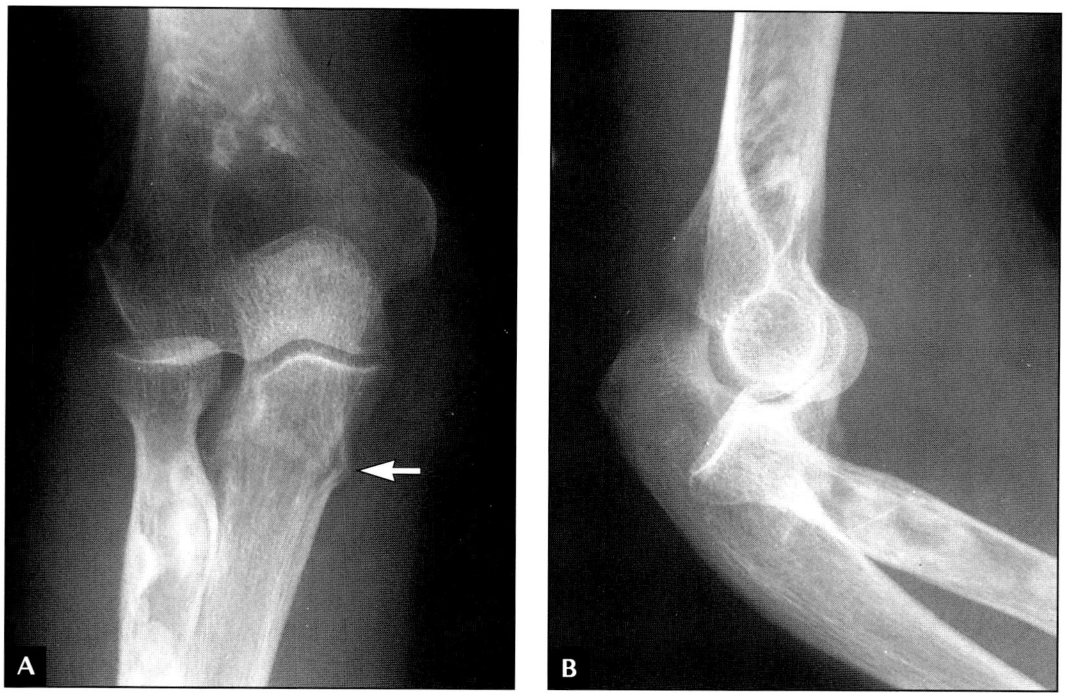

Figure 4-6. Fracture of the proximal ulna and posterior dislocation of the radial head (Monteggia fracture) in a woman aged 65 years following a fall on ice. **A**, Anteroposterior view with overlap of the radial and capitellar articular surfaces from dislocation. The medial ulnar cortex is buckled (*arrow*) from a fracture. **B**, Lateral view best visualizes the loss of normal alignment of the radial head and capitellum. Tunnel vision may lead to overlooking the sclerotic metastases in the radius and humerus from a transitional cell carcinoma of the bladder.

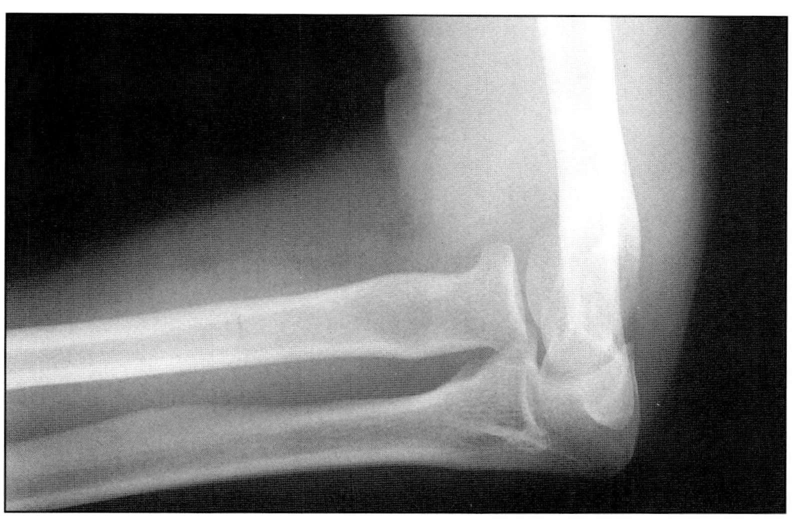

Figure 4-7. Radial head, capitellum view of the elbow throws the radial head and neck free from the ulna, making it useful in detecting some otherwise obscure fractures.

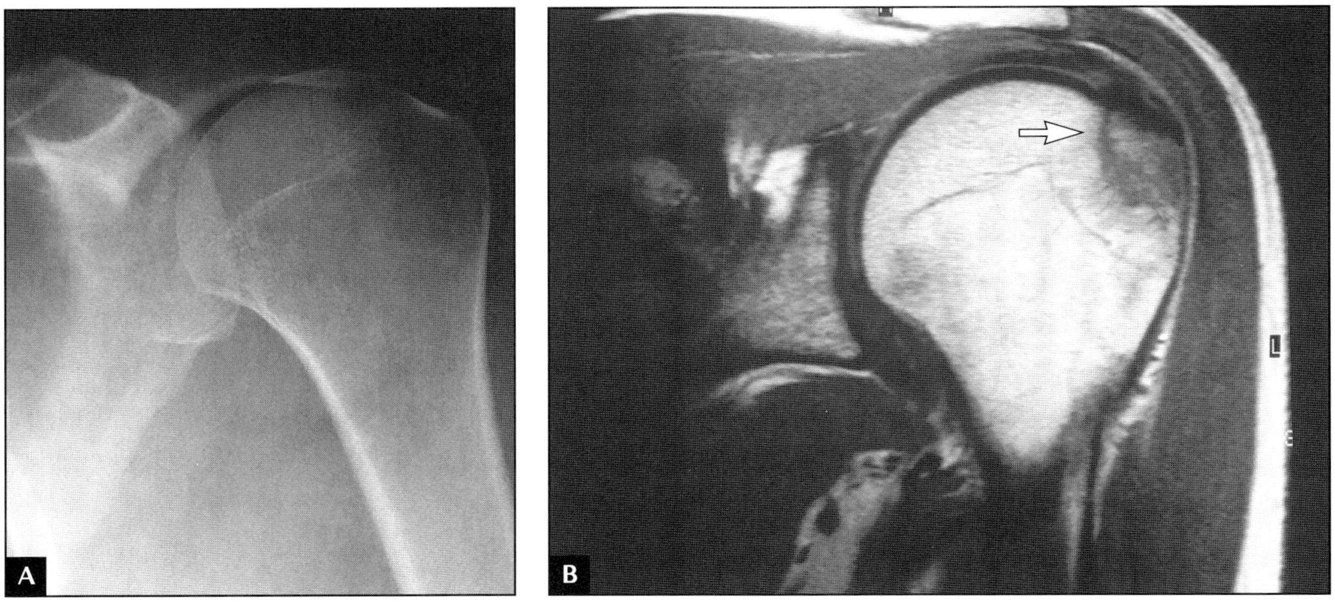

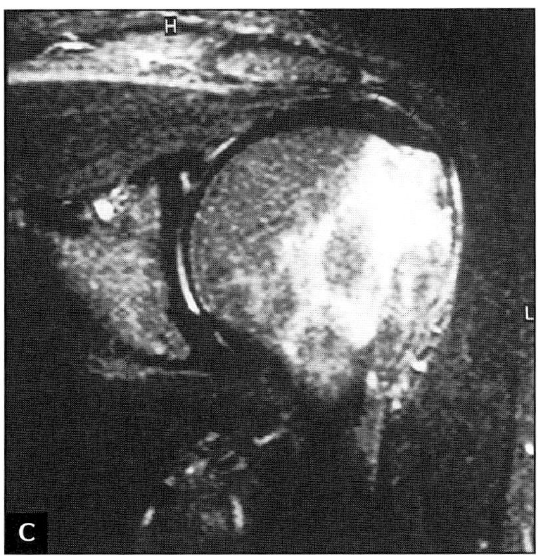

FIGURE 4-8. Fracture, occult to plain radiographic examination, of the greater tuberosity in a man aged 51 years who fell on ice and thereby sustained a direct blow to the shoulder. **A**, Anterposterior radiograph in partial external rotation shows no abnormality. Additional plain radiographs were also normal. The patient had continued unexplained pain leading to a magnetic resonance imaging study to rule out a rotator cuff tear. **B**, A turbo spin-echo proton-density (TR/TE, 1700/17) sequence demonstrates a nondisplaced greater tuberosity fracture (*arrow*). **C**, Short inversion time inversion recovery sequence (2600/60; inversion time, 150) with fat suppression shows part of the fracture line and high signal intensity from surrounding bone marrow edema resulting from the acute fracture.

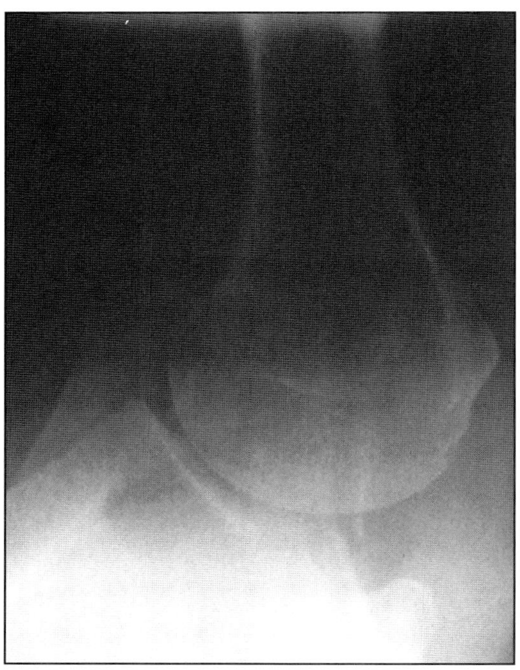

FIGURE 4-9. A man aged 51 years fell directly onto his shoulder while skiing. Axillary view demonstrates the shoulder joint, coracoid, acromion, and distal clavicle. A fracture of the distal clavicle was not visible with multiple other views.

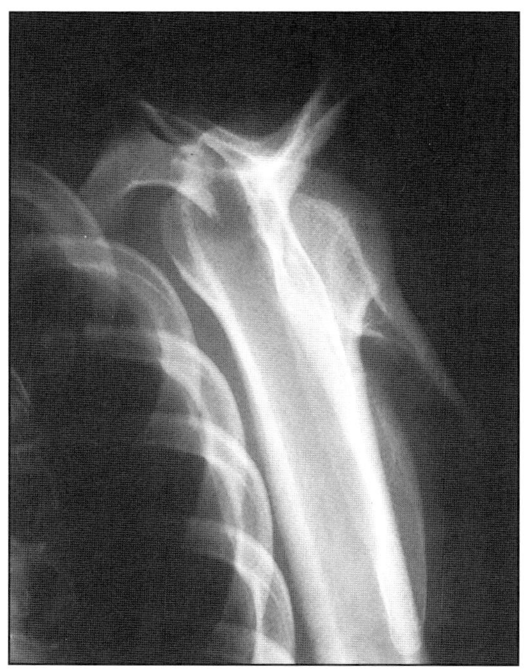

FIGURE 4-10. A man aged 22 years sustained a direct blow to the shoulder from a football block. Scapular Y view reveals a displaced fracture of the scapula body and avulsion of the coracoid at its base.

abducted. If this view is routine, a radiology technologist periodically will be in the undesirable situation of moving an unstable fracture before it is known to exist. Other patients with shoulder trauma with or without a fracture will adamantly refuse to move their shoulder for this view. In such a situation, if the patient can stand, a flat film cassette may be placed on top of the shoulder parallel to the floor, and an x-ray tube on a crane may be placed at floor level pointing toward the ceiling. The patient leans backward over the x-ray tube while holding the cassette with the uninjured hand. If the patient is severely injured or is otherwise necessarily supine, the film cassette is placed in the same position on top of the shoulder perpendicular to the table or cart and the x-ray tube is positioned at approximately knee level aimed parallel to the floor and cephalad at the axilla.

Every anatomic structure is best seen on a particular view. The AP view shows the humeral head and neck, the distal clavicle, the glenoid, the acromion, and the acromioclavicular joint (Figures 4-1 and 4-8). The axillary view visualizes the humeral head and neck, the glenoid, the scapula neck, the acromion, and the clavicle (Figure 4-9). With the Y view, the scapula body is seen in profile and the acromion and coracoid are seen in lateral projection (Figure 4-10). A 45° posterior oblique view, called the Grashey view, demonstrates the humeral head, surgical and anatomic necks, greater tuberosity, the joint space in profile, the glenoid rim, the scapular neck, the coracoid, and the acromion (Figure 4-11). An apical oblique view has an appearance similar to that of the Grashey view in that it is obtained with the same patient position; however, the x-ray tube is angled 45° caudal instead of parallel to the floor as with the Grashey view. We routinely obtain both an AP view and a Grashey view with the shoulder in external rotation. Additional views are obtained according to clinical findings and findings on these first two radiographs. We use the Grashey view because it provides the clinician with the ability to see the articular surfaces of the joint, the desire to no longer miss more than 50% of posterior dislocations [11•], and the ease with which it can be obtained even in a severely multiple injured patient. In such a supine patient, without moving the arm a cassette is placed posterior to the shoulder with its lateral margin elevated to angle it 45° to the table or cart and the x-ray tube is angled 45° medial to lateral.

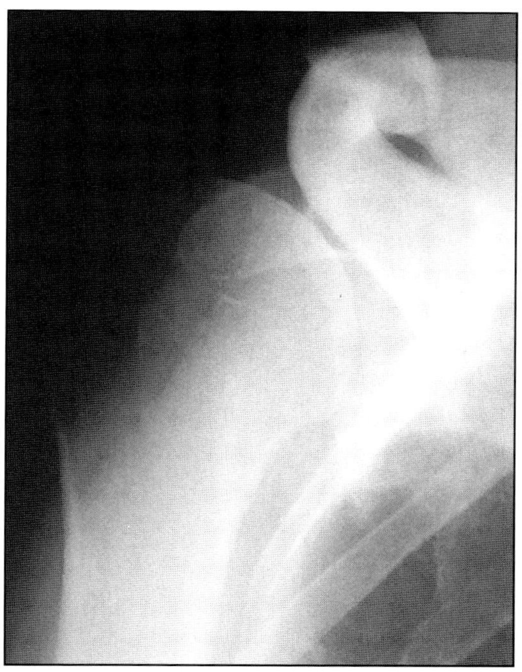

Figure 4-11. Posterior 45° oblique (Grashey) view of the shoulder shows overlap of the glenoid rim and the articular surface of the humeral head from a posterior shoulder dislocation in this man aged 23 years. In a normal shoulder, the two opposing articular surfaces would be separated 3 or 4 mm and parallel with this view.

Plain radiographic examination of the sternoclavicular joints (as in Figure 4-1) has limited value because of overlapping structures and inability to obtain views oriented 90° to one another. CT is the study of choice to evaluate this joint for fracture or dislocation (Figure 4-12). It not only images the sternoclavicular joint but also the underlying airway and vascular structures in the event of a dislocation [12].

The clavicle is not well visualized with AP views because of superimposition on the scapula and ribs. Cephalad angulation of the x-ray beam is needed. Cephalad angulation of 15° frees the distal two thirds of the clavicle from superimposition and as much as 40° may be necessary to throw the proximal clavicle free from the ribs and spine (Figure 4-13). Because of the serpentine shape of the clavicle, some middle and distal third fractures are not visible on AP views but are only seen on cephalic angled views.

The acromioclavicular (AC) joint is seen on AP, axillary, and posterior oblique views of the shoulder as already described (in Figures 4-1, 4-8, 4-9, and 4-11). Stress views are often needed to evaluate the joint for separation. Weights between 10 and 15 lb are strapped to the patient's wrists or forearms for the stress views. Holding the weights in the hands is inadequate because this may cause muscle contraction and reduction of a dislocation.

Scapular fractures tend to be obvious if effort is expended to examine the standard chest or shoulder radiographs. The high incidence of missed scapular fracture occurs because attention is diverted to more pressing, often life-threatening, problems [13]. Obviously, the ultimate prognosis of the patient depends on the associated trauma, not on an overlooked scapular fracture. Routinely, the scapula is imaged using an AP view of the shoulder and a tangential scapular Y view (Figure 4-10). The latter sights tangentially along the body of the bone, showing the scapular spine, the coracoid, and the scapula body in profile. The AP view of the shoulder visualizes the acromion, the glenoid fossa, and the neck of the scapula clear of the ribs. Most of its body is visible but is overlapped by ribs (as in Figure 4-13). Abducting the shoulder 90° rotates the lateral margin and tip of the bone free from the ribs. A Grashey view of the shoulder shows the glenoid fossa, part

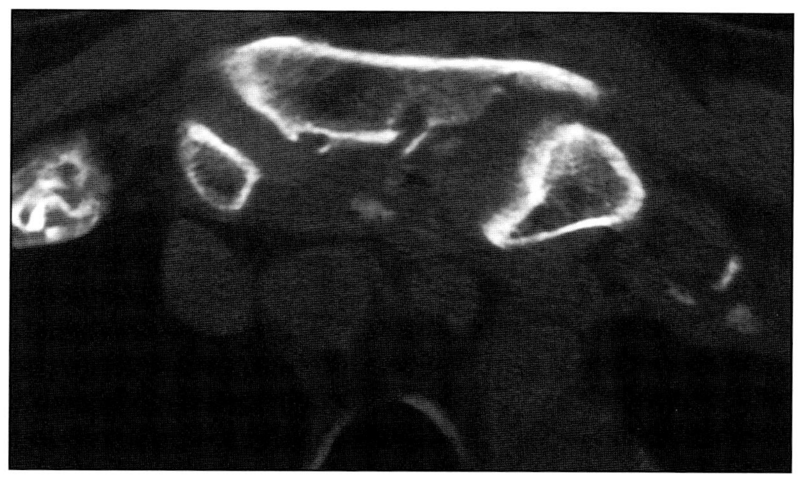

Figure 4-12. A man aged 85 years with a fracture-posterior dislocation of the left sternoclavicular joint demonstrated with computed tomography, the definitive study for evaluating trauma to this joint.

of the acromion, the coracoid, and the scapula neck (as in Figure 4-11). A shoulder axillary view demonstrates the glenoid fossa, the coracoid, and the glenoid neck (as in Figure 4-9).

Anteroposterior and lateral views constitute the standard radiographic examination of the humerus. The films should be long enough to include the shoulder joint and the elbow joint.

SKELETAL SCINTIGRAPHY

Radionuclide bone scanning is used when a plain radiographic study is normal but the patient's symptoms persist in suggesting a fracture. Bone scintigraphy has shown a high sensitivity for detecting occult fractures [14•]. It is also the study of choice when searching for stress fractures [15], because the plain radiographic study is usually normal for 10 days or more after the onset of symptoms and is less expensive than an MRI study. Stress fractures are uncommon in the upper extremity but are seen in association with tennis and other racquet sports, weight lifting, football, gymnastics, and sports involving throwing, such as baseball. Nuclide bone scans are very sensitive but suffer from lack of specificity. A three-phase scan may improve the specificity [15,16].

Connolly *et al.* [17•] advocate use of pinhole collimator magnification for diagnosing injuries to the small bones of the hands and wrists in pediatric patients. The pinhole collimator allows discrimination of abnormalities adjacent to areas with high nuclide activity, such as epiphyseal growth plates. Its use is advocated when images obtained with a high-resolution collimator do not allow confident interpretation of a fracture. The downside of this technique is the approximately twofold time increase necessary to obtain the images when compared with images obtained with a high-resolution, parallel hole collimator.

COMPUTED TOMOGRAPHY

Computed tomography has limited value for fracture detection in the upper extremity. It is used to determine the relationship of the bone fragments for treatment planning of complex fractures or fracture dislocations that are common to the shoulder, the elbow, and the wrist. If difficulty exists in moving the patient for routine radiographs because of multiple injuries, a CT study can be obtained by moving the patient only once. CT arthrography (Figure 4-14) is used in the shoulder and elbow to determine whether a bone fragment adjacent to the joint is within the joint. Small fracture fragments in the wrist may be seen with plain radi-

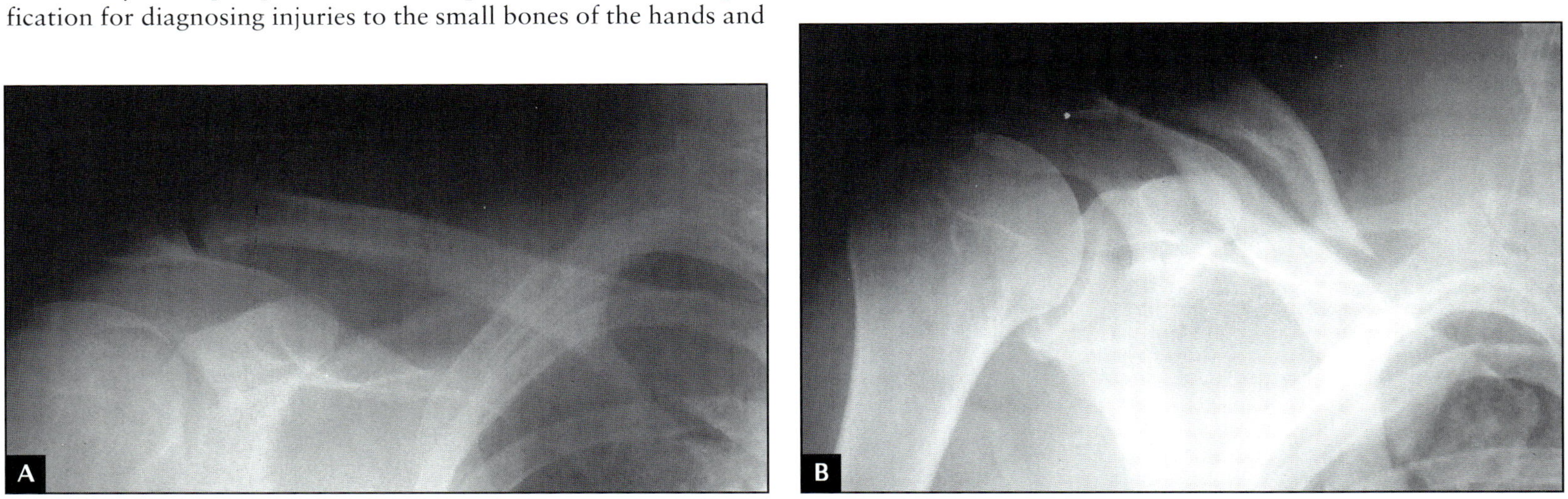

FIGURE 4-13. Displaced clavicle fracture only seen with severe cephalad angulation in a man aged 39 years following a fall. **A**, No fracture is visible with the x-ray beam angulated 10° cephalad. **B**, The fracture was only seen on this rib film where the cephalad angulation exceeded 40°.

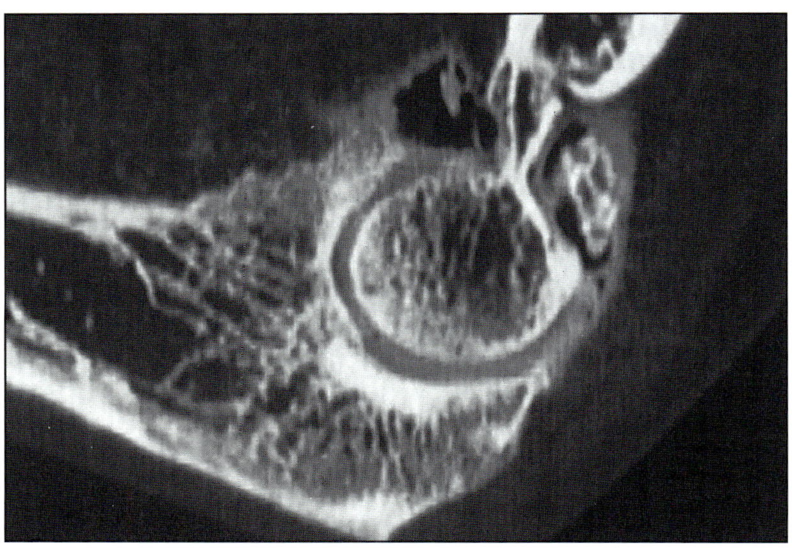

FIGURE 4-14. Multiple avulsion fracture fragments in the elbow of a man aged 35 years with locking, clicking, and a feeling of something loose within his joint following a fall several months earlier. A sagittal computed tomography reconstructed view demonstrates air and contrast from a double-contrast arthrogram outlining parts of two loose bodies in the olecranon fossa.

ographs but CT may be needed if their site of origin must be determined (Figure 4-15) and is often of use in evaluating carpometacarpal fracture-dislocations. Obscure fracture of the glenoid rim, coracoid, acromion, and the sternoclavicular joints may be elucidated with a CT examination. Impaction fractures of the humeral head following anterior dislocation (Hill-Sachs fracture) or posterior dislocation are well seen (Figure 4-16). CT is also valuable in assessing fracture healing as discussed later.

Although CT machines have three-dimensional reconstruction ability, two-dimensional reconstructions are routinely performed and used (*see* Figures 4-4 and 4-14). A three-dimensional reconstruction provides a surface view of the bone containing the fracture that allows the bone to be rotated around any of its three axes for viewing. Because only the external surface of the bone is visible with this technique, the fracture can be seen only where it interrupts the cortical surface of the bone. This is at times useful for preoperative evaluation when many bone fragments are present, but most of the time two-dimensional coronal and sagittal images (as in Figures 4-3 and 4-14) reconstructed from axial images are used to evaluate fractures. They provide information about the course of the fracture through the bone that cannot be seen with the three-dimensional reconstructions. There is current investigation of three-dimensional reconstructed images that allow the clinician to look inside three-dimensional reconstructions (*eg*, in the colon) but it is unclear what effect, if any, this will have on fracture investigation. The Neer [18] classification is in general use to classify shoulder fractures but numerous recent reports have indicated the lack of interobserver agreement using this classification system. Bernstein *et al.* [19•] evaluated the use of CT scans in addition to plain radiographs to see whether CT information improved interobserver agreement in classifying shoulder fractures using this classification. They found that use of axial CT scans caused a slight increase in intraobserver reliability for classification but no increase in interobserver reproducibility. I suspect that further improvement might be expected if coronal and sagittal reconstruction images were also employed to classify the fractures.

MAGNETIC RESONANCE IMAGING

The role of MRI evaluation of fractures falls to detecting occult fractures (Figure 4-17) [2,14,20], diagnosing stress fractures

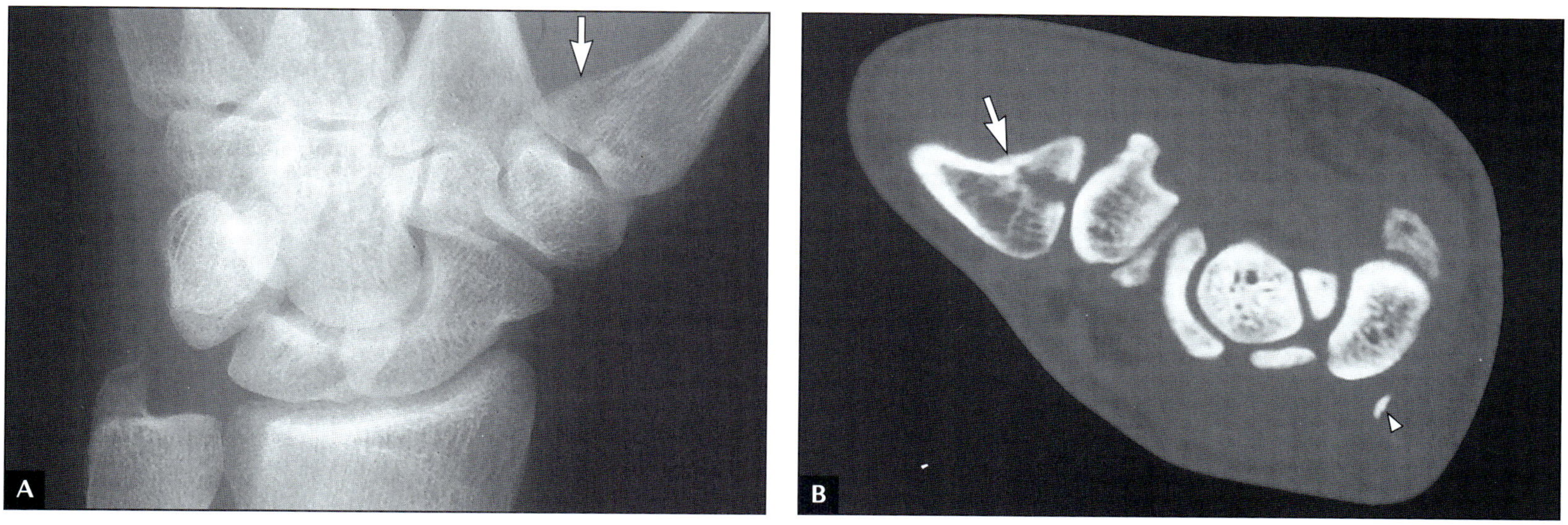

FIGURE 4-15. Fractures of the triquetrum and first metacarpal base resulting from a motorcycle accident in a man aged 27 years were present but not initially detected on the plain radiographic study. A computed tomography (CT) study was done for further evaluation. **A**, Oblique view of the wrist demonstrates an oblique fracture of the first metacarpal base (*arrow*) that was initially missed. **B**, Axial CT view of the wrist shows the triquetral fracture (*arrowhead*) dorsally and the first metacarpal fracture (*arrow*).

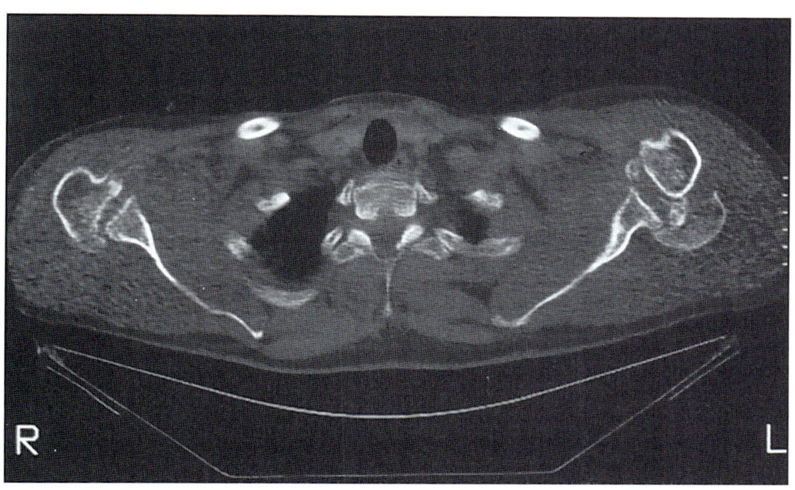

FIGURE 4-16. Computed tomography (CT) scan of both shoulders demonstrates bilateral posterior dislocation of the shoulder joints secondary to a seizure in a man aged 44 years. In the right shoulder, a long vertical impaction fracture of the humeral head is present on the glenoid rim that causes the trough sign [11•] on plain radiographs. In the left shoulder, at least a three-part fracture can be seen from this single image. CT allows the clinician to sort out the relationship of the fracture fragments to one another.

from overuse or osteoporosis [21•], identifying bone marrow edema in an injured area [22•], evaluating physeal injuries in the immature skeleton [4,23], and determining the viability of fracture fragments (Figures 4-18 and 4-19), which is especially applicable to healing scaphoid fractures [1•]. The primary value of MRI for evaluating trauma, however, is to detect injuries to soft tissues: ligaments, tendons, cartilage, and muscle [3•]. It does this better than any other imaging modality, but that discussion falls outside the scope of this chapter. Many technical factors, such as the type of coil used, the size of the field of view, the magnetic field strength and homogeneity, and patient motion are important to obtaining diagnostic images but are also beyond the scope of this chapter.

Hand and Wrist

In patients with a wrist fracture, Spence *et al.* [24] found a combination of undetected fractures (Figure 4-17), fracture extensions, and soft tissue injuries with MRI that were not seen with plain radiographs. Similar findings have also been reported from arthroscopic studies. They suspect that these undetected findings account for the continuing morbidity following restoration of osseous alignment of wrist fractures in some patients.

MRI detected occult fractures in the distal radius or in various carpal bones within hours of an injury when plain radiographs were normal or equivocal for fracture [20,25]. Radionuclide bone scans may not become positive for days following a fracture, according to the findings of Matin [26], although this finding is

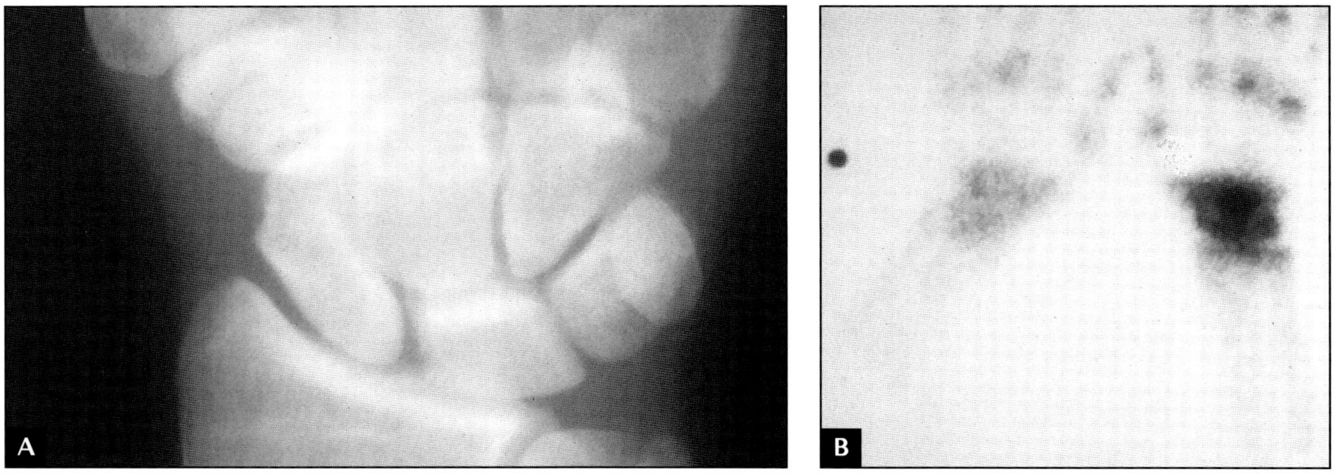

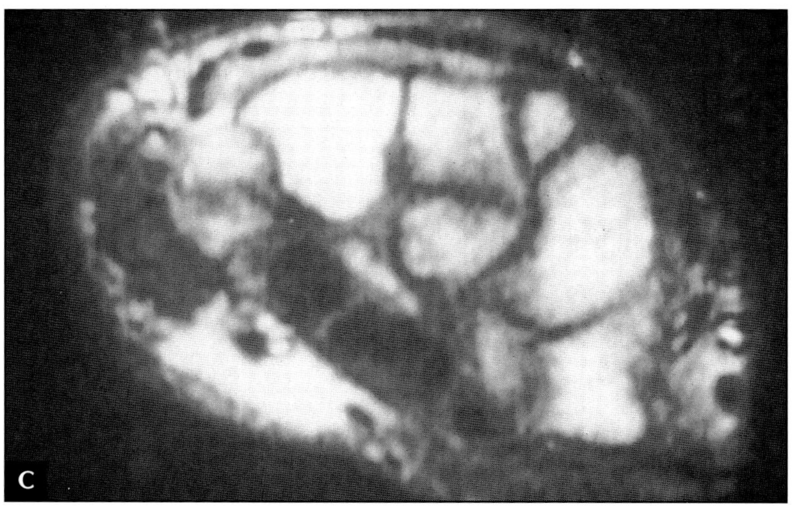

Figure 4-17. An occult fracture of the capitate sustained from a fall onto an outstretched hand. **A**, Plain film posteroanterior view of the wrist fails to show an abnormality. **B**, Because of persistent pain, a nuclide bone scan was obtained that shows increased activity throughout the carpus. **C**, A T1-weighted (TR/TE, 600/15) magnetic resonance image demonstrates the source of pain, a coronal fracture of the capitate. (*Courtesy of* Robert Gould, Chicago, IL.)

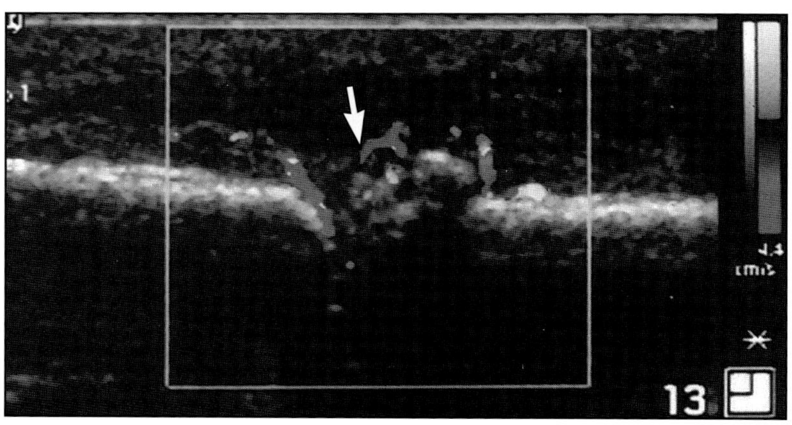

Figure 4-18. Color Doppler superimposed on a gray-scale ultrasound image of a healing comminuted midshaft fracture of the tibia. A comminuted fracture fragment (*arrow*) is seen. The bright horizontal line is the cortex of the tibia. In this fracture site, arterial and venous blood are red and blue on the original image but are gray here and show blood flow to and from the fracture site, indicating that fracture healing is progressing satisfactorily. (*Courtesy of* Joseph Introcaso, Chicago, IL.)

disputed by Holder [16]. MRI has a higher sensitivity and specificity than scintigraphy for detecting occult scaphoid wrist fractures [14•]; I have found this to be true in other bones as well.

Shoulder

Rangger *et al.* [27•] recently published the first report of histologic examination of bone bruises. They found microfractures of cancellous bone, hemorrhage into the fatty marrow, and edema in five patients. Between intact bone trabeculae, they found fatty marrow necrosis, fragmented bony trabeculae, and hyaline cartilage. Histologic findings in this study merely confirm what has been suspected for a long time based on the MRI findings of bone bruises and bone contusions.

Rand *et al.* [22•] found that MRI studies using short tau inversion recovery (STIR) sequences with fat suppression were more sensitive than T1/T2-weighted images for detecting occult fractures and bone bruises in the shoulder (Figure 4-8). Bone bruises have no manifestations on plain radiographs. They are part of a continuum of MRI-detected manifestations of trauma. This continuum has frank fractures at one end and bone marrow edema from bone bruises at the opposite end with injuries less severe than a visible fracture on plain radiographic studies in between. Inversion recovery images with fat suppression are exquisitely sensitive to detecting edema in bone marrow or in soft tissues and their use is essential throughout the musculoskeletal system.

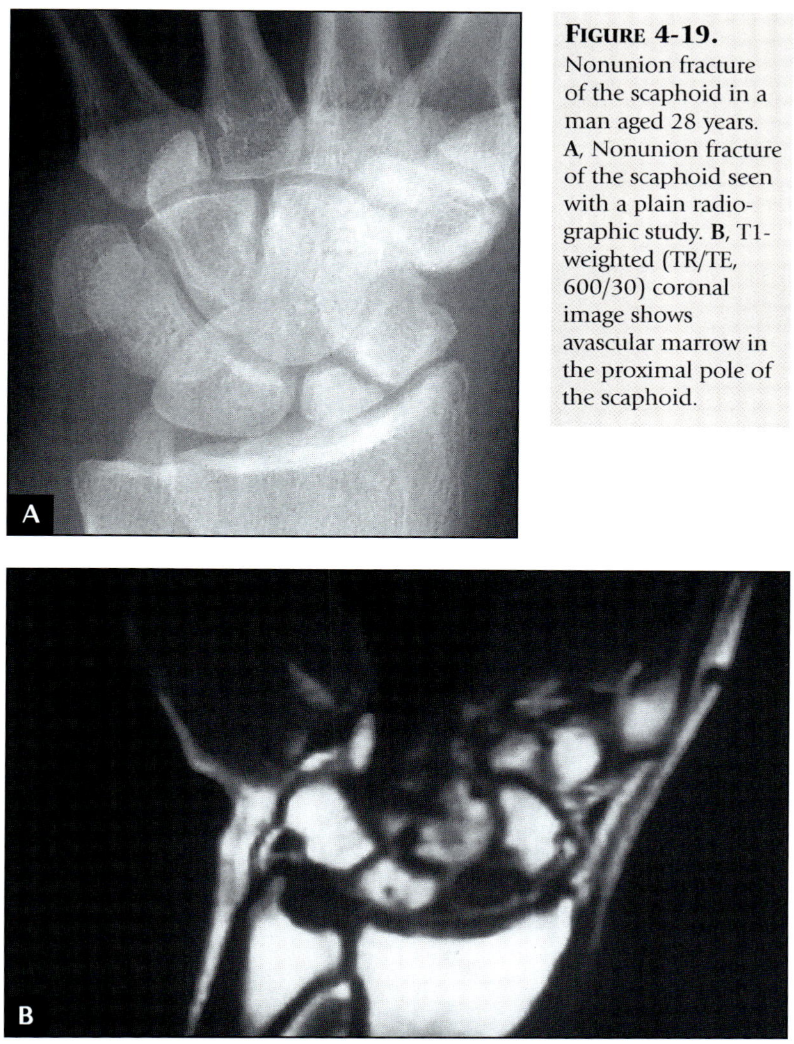

Figure 4-19. Nonunion fracture of the scaphoid in a man aged 28 years. **A**, Nonunion fracture of the scaphoid seen with a plain radiographic study. **B**, T1-weighted (TR/TE, 600/30) coronal image shows avascular marrow in the proximal pole of the scaphoid.

Multiple recent reports [28•] discuss occult fractures of the greater tuberosity demonstrated by MRI in patients with a clinical presentation suspicious for rotator cuff injury following trauma to the shoulder. Plain radiographic studies were interpreted as normal in all patients. MRI showed bone marrow edema and a fracture line in the greater tuberosity to explain the continued shoulder pain in these patients (Figure 4-8).

ULTRASONOGRAPHY

Ultrasound is used to evaluate soft tissue abnormalities in the upper extremity quickly and inexpensively, but it has no currently defined role in detection or evaluation of fractures. Real-time ultrasound can be used to evaluate Hill-Sachs lesions accurately in patients with recurrent shoulder dislocation [29]. This may be a quick, inexpensive way to confirm a clinical suspicion in a patient with suspected recurrent dislocation especially if evaluation of other soft tissue structures (*eg*, rotator cuff) is coincidentally desired. With ultrasound, it is possible to see whether the Hill-Sachs articular defect reaches the glenoid cavity during movement of the shoulder and whether it hinders humeral head motion. Evaluating fracture healing using ultrasound has been shown to be accurate in small numbers of patients to date [30]. Color or power Doppler can be superimposed on a grayscale ultrasound image to show the vascularity of a fracture site (Figure 4-20). A normal healing fracture has increased blood flow to and from the fracture site, whereas increased blood flow is absent with a nonunion. CT, MRI, scintigraphy, or plain radiography studies used to evaluate fractures are performed by technical staff, whereas ultrasound examination of fractures is characteristically performed by a physician. The ultrasound studies are operator dependent and very labor intensive for the physician. Most radiology departments have insufficient personnel and expertise to perform these studies routinely.

FRACTURE HEALING

Imaging is used to determine whether new bone or calcified callus actually bridge a fracture site. Plain radiographs may show an

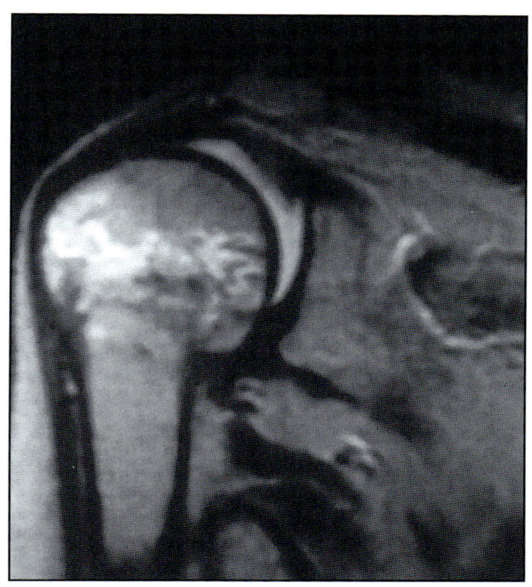

Figure 4-20. Surgical neck fracture in a man aged 50 years. A plain radiograph, not shown, demonstrated a one-part surgical neck fracture. Examination by magnetic resonance imaging with T2-weighted spin-echo image (TR/TE, 2200/80) shows a surgical neck fracture and a joint effusion but also changes of osteonecrosis of the humeral head, which were unexpected.

obvious bone bridge across an uncomplicated fracture, but many fractures are comminuted or spiral and plain radiographic studies may be inconclusive for healing until a relatively large mass of bone bridges them. Bones with peculiar shapes or axes (*eg*, the scaphoid) are also difficult to evaluate with plain films. Newer CT scanners with rapid reconstruction ability in sagittal and coronal planes are uniquely suited to evaluate healing in these more complicated fractures. Views in one plane may be inconclusive, whereas a second or third plane usually provides the needed information (Figures 4-21 and 4-22). In addition, smaller struts of bone across a fracture can be detected in complicated fractures than is possible with plain radiographs. If no bony bridge is seen in three separate planes with CT, certainty is much greater that bone healing is incomplete than through reliance on an image from a single plane.

The most frequent use of CT for fracture healing evaluation in my practice is to evaluate the scaphoid bone. However, the same protocol is used to evaluate fractures of the forearm, elbow, arm, and shoulder. I use a helical CT scanner employing a pitch of 1.0 or less, overlap of 50% or more, as small a field of view as is practicable, and axial scans aligned along the long axis of the scaphoid or transversely for other bones. Reconstructed images are then generated in the coronal and sagittal planes. Thick body areas such as the shoulder are imaged using 140 kV instead of the more common 120 kV used in the extremities to reduce artifacts

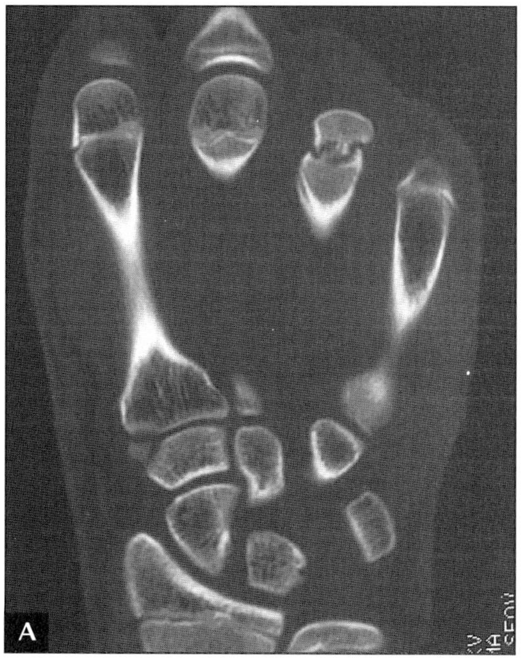

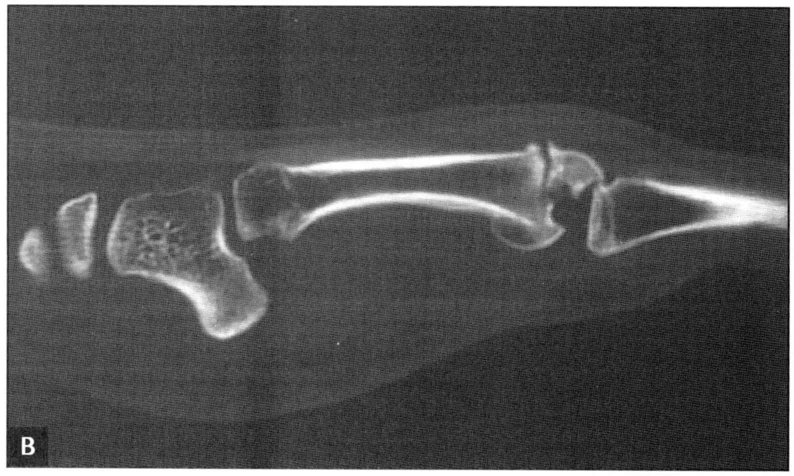

FIGURE 4-21. Nonunion Salter 3 fracture of the fourth metacarpal head in a boy aged 14 years. **A**, Coronal reconstructed image shows abnormal irregularity and widening of the epiphyseal plate. **B**, Sagittal reconstructed image demonstrates volar displacement of the epiphyseal fracture fragment, sclerosis of the fracture surfaces, and an abnormal epiphyseal plate.

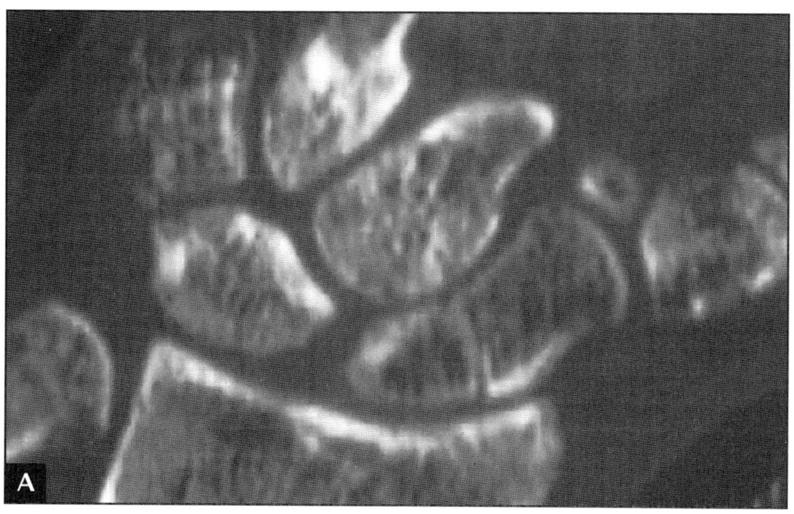

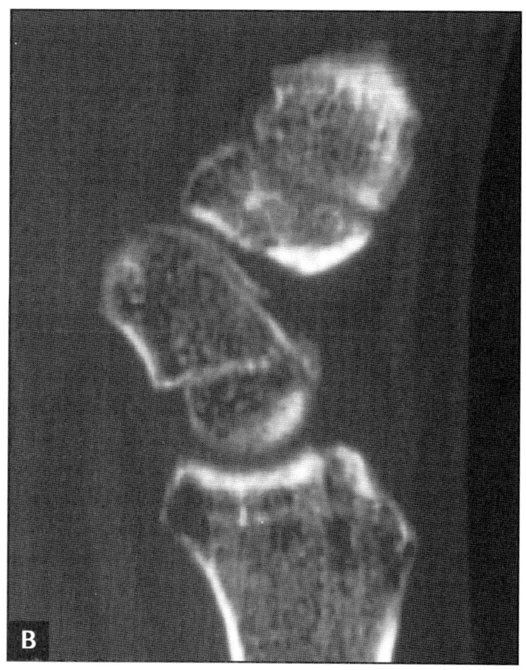

FIGURE 4-22. A man aged 24 years with a questionable nonunion fracture of the scaphoid wrist sustained 4 months earlier. The quality of the reconstructed images is sufficient for them to be relied on to make clinical decisions for this and other patients. **A**, Coronal reconstructed computed tomography (CT) image suggests nonunion of the fracture. **B**, Sagittal reconstructed CT image demonstrates an impacted, displaced fracture with bone bridging across the fracture line seen most convincingly at the volar cortical margin. Axial and other coronal images (*not shown*) demonstrate the same findings of bone bridging as seen here.

on reconstructed images. Pitch has to do with the speed at which the area being scanned moves through the x-ray beam while the scan is being obtained. The higher the number, the faster the area moves, and thus the faster the scan is completed. Slower scans produce better detail so that smaller abnormalities are visible but also diminish the length of area that can be scanned at any given time. The 50% overlap allows reconstruction of images that are almost indistinguishable from the original axial images (as in Figures 4-21 and 4-22). Typical reconstruction images generated from axial images obtained with a pitch larger than 1.0 and overlap of less than 50% have jagged edges or step-off deformities in the images, which makes it difficult to identify small struts of bone bridging a fracture. The bone bridge must be larger before it can be detected with certainty under such circumstances. Before scanners with rapid reconstruction ability were available, we routinely evaluated scaphoid healing using direct CT scans. The patient was repositioned for three separate scans, one for each plane when possible.

Computed tomography imaging to evaluate healing in the scaphoid, other carpal bones, the elbow, metacarpals, the feet, and ankles has changed the care of our patients. The hand surgeons at my institution rely on CT to determine their treatment during healing, especially for scaphoid fractures but also for other small bone fractures, and for healing of carpal fusions. They will perform bone grafting for early nonunions 2 to 3 months earlier than they did when they used conventional tomography to evaluate healing. Shah and Jones [31•] found that Herbert screw fixation success rates in 50 scaphoid nonunion fractures fell off as the duration of nonunion before treatment increased. Early identification of nonunions with CT imaging diminishes the amount of time needed to determine the presence of a nonunion and hopefully improves the success rate of rigid fixation and bone grafting.

MRI studies have predictive value for bone healing. Morgan *et al.* [1•] preoperatively evaluated scaphoid nonunion fractures with MRI prior to internal fixation with a Herbert screw and bone grafting. Intraoperative bone biopsy showed viable marrow in scaphoid fracture fragments with normal marrow signal intensity on preoperative MRI and nonviable bone marrow in fracture fragments with absent marrow signal intensity on preoperative MRI. Scaphoid bones with viable bone marrow on preoperative MRI healed on average within 5 months but those with abnormal marrow signal on MRI but normal bone trabecular pattern on plain films healed with a protracted average time of 10.5 months (Figure 4-18). Patients with abnormal bone marrow signal in the proximal pole on preoperative MRI and abnormal bone trabecular pattern on plain films had not healed at 24 months postoperatively. Patients with normal bone marrow signal on MRI and abnormal cystic changes in the proximal pole bone trabecular pattern on plain films healed in an average time of less than 5 months. MRI can be useful to estimate projected healing time and to select patients who will benefit from and eliminate those who will not benefit from bone grafting.

CONCLUSIONS

Plain radiographic studies are adequate for most fracture detection, treatment, and healing evaluation. A few fractures will be occult to plain film detection and require scintigraphy or MRI for detection. CT with reconstruction views is necessary for healing evaluation to identify either early bone bridging the fracture line or early evidence of nonunion. Stress fractures are identified early with scintigraphy or MRI. Subtle physeal injuries may need scintigraphy or MRI for detection and MRI to detect early epiphyseal closure adjacent to a healed fracture. Marrow edema and marrow viability only can be evaluated by MRI. Digital radiography and PAC systems are soon to be ubiquitous, thus making image transfer almost instantaneous and image manipulation routine. Although ultrasound has no current place in the United States for fracture evaluation, it is used elsewhere in the world for this purpose.

REFERENCES AND RECOMMENDED READING

Recently published papers of particular interest have been highlighted as:
- • Of interest
- •• Of outstanding interest

1.• Morgan WJ, Breen TF, Coumas JM, *et al.*: Role of magnetic resonance imaging in assessing factors affecting healing in scaphoid nonunions. *Clin Orthop* 1997, 336:240–246.

This article reviews estimating bone healing time based on appearance of the bone marrow using MRI.

2. Rogers LF: Occult is a matter of definition. *Am J Roentgenol* 1999, 172:283.

3.• Herzog RJ: Magnetic resonance imaging of the shoulder. *J Bone Joint Surg Am* 1997, 79:934–953.

This is a general review covering MRI shoulder imaging in detail.

4. Jaramillo D, Hoffer FA, Shapiro F, *et al.*: MR imaging of fractures of the growth plate. *Am J Roentgenol* 1990, 155:1261–1265.

5.• Williamson B Jr: The electronic transformation of radiology. *Radiology* 1998, 209:606–608.

This paper provides an overview of sweeping changes coming in the field of imaging.

6.• Murphey MD: Computed radiography in musculoskeletal imaging. *Semin Roentgenol* 1997, 32:64–76.

This article reviews the advantages of CR for musculoskeletal studies.

7.• Erickson SJ: High-resolution imaging of the musculoskeletal system. *Radiology* 1998, 205:593–618.

This is a review of ultrasound, CT, and MRI advances in technology that allow high-resolution image detail in musculoskeletal structures.

8.• Bhalla S, Higgs PE, Gilula LA: Utility of the radial-deviated, thumb-abducted lateral radiographic view for the diagnosis of hamate hook fractures: case report. *Radiology* 1998, 209:203–207.

This paper gives a very useful new view of the hamate hook.

9. Greenspan A, Norman A: The radial head, capitellum view: useful technique in elbow trauma. *Am J Roentgenol* 1982, 138:186–188.

10.• Irshad F, Shaw NJ, Gregory RJH: Reliability of fat-pad sign in radial head/neck fractures of the elbow. *Injury* 1997, 28:433–435.

It is surprising that this study was not done long ago.

11.• Cisternino SJ, Rogers LF, Stufflebaum BC, Kruglik GD: The trough line: a radiographic sign of posterior shoulder dislocation. *Am J Roentgenol* 1978, 130:951–957.

This is a good discussion of plain film imaging of posterior dislocation of the shoulder.

12. Destouet JM, Gilula LA, Murphy WA, *et al*: Computed tomography of the sternoclavicular joint and sternum. *Radiology* 1981, 138:123–128.

13. Imatani RJ: Fractures of the scapula: a review of 53 fractures. *J Trauma* 1975, 15:473–478.

14.• Fowler C, Sullivan B, Williams LA, *et al.*: A comparison of bone scintigraphy and MRI in the early diagnosis of the occult scaphoid waist fracture. *Skeletal Radiol* 1998, 27:683–687.

According to this article, MRI is more sensitive than scintigraphy for early diagnosis of occult scaphoid waist fracture.

15. Patel M: Upper extremity radionuclide bone imaging: shoulder, arm, elbow, and forearm. *Semin Nucl Med* 1998, 28:3–13.

16. Holder LE: Bone scintigraphy in skeletal trauma. *Radiol Clin North Am* 1993, 31:739–780.

17.• Connolly LP, Treves ST, Connolly SA, *et al.*: Pediatric skeletal scintigraphy: application of pinhole magnification. *Radiographics* 1998, 18:341–351.

This paper describes a useful technique in pediatric patients of using pinhole collimation for bone scans; however, the technique is not needed routinely.

18. Neer CS II: Displaced proximal humeral fractures, part I: classification and evaluation. *J Bone Joint Surg* 1970, 52A:1077–1089.

19.• Bernstein J, Adler LM, Blank JE, *et al.*: Evaluation of the Neer system of classification of proximal humeral fractures with computerized tomographic scans and plain radiographs. *J Bone Joint Surg Am* 1996, 78:1371–1375.

This paper reviews an ongoing controversy about the reproducibility of classifying shoulder fractures using the Neer [18] classification.

20. Breitenseher MJ, Metz VM, Gilula LA, *et al.*: Radiographically occult scaphoid fractures: value of MR imaging in detection. *Radiology* 1997, 203:245–250.

21.• Ohashi K, Brandser EA, El-Khoury GY: Role of MR imaging in acute injuries to the appendicular skeleton. *Radiol Clin North Am* 1997, 35:591–613.

This is a comprehensive review of MRI in the extremities.

22.• Rand T, Trattnig S, Haller J, *et al.*: MR imaging in shoulder trauma: value of STIR image. *Acta Radiologica* 1998, 39:273–275.

This article discusses the importance of STIR images.

23. Rogers LF, Poznanski AK: Imaging of epiphyseal injuries. *Radiology* 1994, 191:297–308.

24. Spence LD, Savenor AS, Nwachuku I, *et al.*: MRI of fractures of the distal radius: comparison with conventional radiographs. *Skeletal Radiol* 1998, 27:244–249.

25. Hunter JC, Escobedo EM, Wilson AJ, *et al.*: MR imaging of clinically suspected scaphoid fractures. *Am J Roentgenol* 1997, 168:1287–1293.

26. Matin P: The appearance of bone scans following fractures, including immediate and long-term studies. *J Nucl Med* 1979, 20:1227–1231.

27.• Rangger C, Kathrein A, Freund MC, *et al.*: Bone bruise of the knee. *Acta Orthop Scand* 1998, 69:291–294.

This article describes an important pathologic-MRI correlation in five patients.

28.• Zanetti M, Weishaupt D, Bernhard J, *et al.*: MR imaging for traumatic tears of the rotator cuff: high prevalence of greater tuberosity fractures and subscapularis tendon tears. *Am J Roentgenol* 1999, 172:463–467.

This paper provides useful clinical information concerning unsuspected shoulder pathology.

29. Pancione L, Gatti G, Mecozzi B: Diagnosis of Hill-Sachs lesion of the shoulder: comparison between ultrasonography and arthro-CT. *Acta Radiologica* 1997, 38:523–526.

30. Moed BR, Watson JT, Goldschmidt P, van Holsbeeck M: Ultrasound for the early diagnosis of fracture healing after interlocking nailing of the tibia without reaming. Clin Orthop 1995, 310:137–144.

31.• Shah J, Jones WA: Factors affecting the outcome in 50 cases of scaphoid nonunion treated with Herbert screw fixation. *J Hand Surg* 1998, 23B:680–685.

This article emphasizes the importance of treating scaphoid nonunion fractures as early as possible.

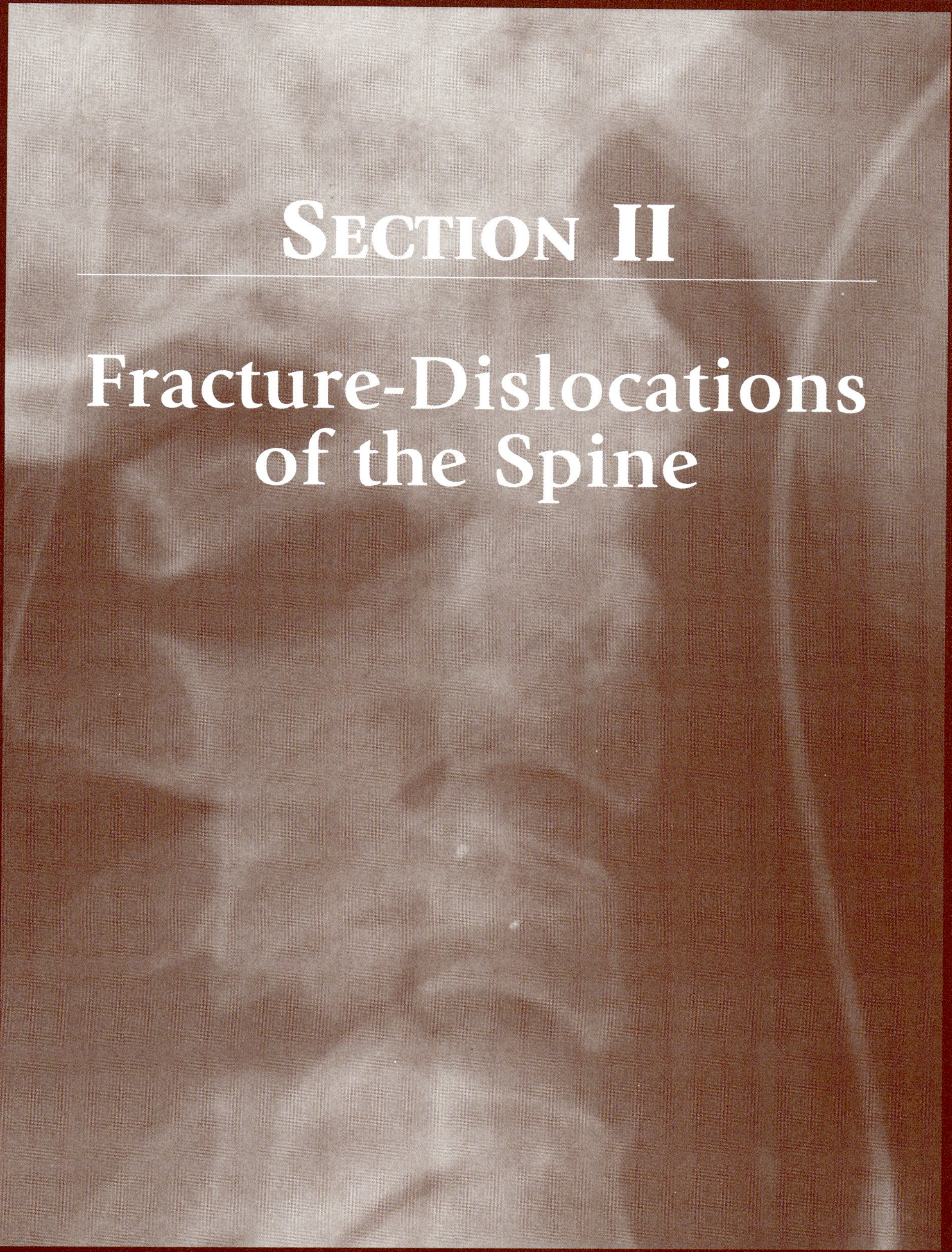

SECTION II

Fracture-Dislocations of the Spine

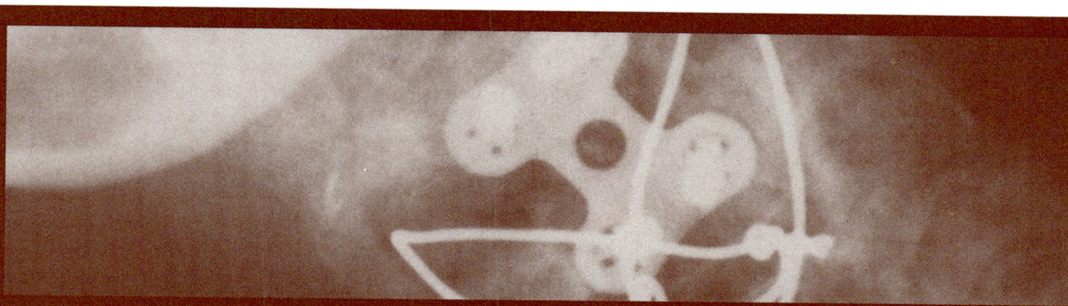

5

Cervical Spine Fractures

Robert F. McLain

Cervical spine injuries range from minor strain and sprain to life-threatening fracture dislocation and spinal cord damage. In any trauma situation, the treating physician's primary concern is to identify cervical spine injuries and to act accordingly to preserve neurologic function and restore stability. Certain aspects to the history and physical examination should heighten suspicion of a cervical injury [1], including high-speed motor vehicle collision or fall from height; facial lacerations or fractures; head injury; transient weakness or numbness at the time of injury; neck pain, stiffness, or apprehension; or persistent neurologic deficits.

Evaluation in the emergency department must include assessment of all cervical motor groups and dermatomes, a careful examination of the head, neck, and shoulder girdles, an evaluation of cord function, and appropriate and properly done screening radiographs of the cervical spine from occiput to T1 [2]. Even if no apparent injury can be identified on examination and screening radiographs, spinal precautions should be maintained in any patient who cannot provide an accurate report of symptoms or cooperate with the examination, including patients who are inebriated, intoxicated, or head injured; unconscious or obtunded; severely injured and in need of rapid resuscitation or surgical care; or distracted by other, more painful injuries. These patients should be protected until a more thorough examination and a coherent history can be obtained, or until a magnetic resonance imaging (MRI) scan can be obtained to rule out soft tissue injuries [3].

After a cervical fracture has been identified, treatment must be prioritized. The cervical spine is initially immobilized in a brace until complete assessment of other injuries is concluded and until emergency surgical procedures are completed. The patient is intubated while awake and cooperative or through fiberoptic control. A complete assessment of the fracture is then completed, including appropriate radiographs, computed tomography (CT) scans, and MRI studies. The fracture is then characterized, classified, and a surgical plan is prepared.

CLASSIFICATION OF INJURIES

SUBLUXATION AND DISLOCATION

Soft tissue injuries of the cervical spine range from trivial to massive and life threatening. Most soft tissue injuries are best characterized as sprains and strains, which consist of minor tears of the posterior ligamentous structures that precipitate muscle pain and spasm. When multiple posterior restraints are damaged, the facet joints may begin to go into subluxation, and when all posterior elements and at least one anterior restraint are disrupted, the spine becomes grossly unstable.

C1–C2 Subluxation

Atlantoaxial instability occurs when the transverse and apical ligaments of the C1–C2 articulation have been disrupted. These ligaments control the relationship between the ring of C1 and the dens. When they are disrupted, the ring of C1 and the dens tend to drift apart, which results in an increased atlantodens interval (ADI) that may increase during flexion and reduce during extension. The normal ADI is up to 3 to 4 mm, and an ADI of 7 mm or more is clearly abnormal (Figure 5-1). These ligamentous injuries do not heal well, and chronic and progressive instability is common. If the instability is allowed to progress unchecked, spinal cord compression results in global weakness, respiratory depression, and eventually death.

Subaxial Subluxation

Subaxial instability occurs when chronic degenerative processes or acute traumatic forces attenuate and disrupt the soft tissue restraints of the posterior cervical column. Normal wear-and-tear changes can lead to sagittal subluxations of up to 3.0 mm between adjacent vertebrae. Subluxations greater than 3.5 mm, either at rest or on flexion-extension radiographs, indicate more significant injury to the posterior restraints [4]. Similarly, increased angulation from one vertebra to the next may signal instability. If the sagittal angulation between adjacent vertebrae exceeds the angulation between surrounding segments by 11°, the injured segment should be considered unstable (Figure 5-2). If instability is severe and remains untreated, sagittal angulation and translation may progress until one or both facets dislocate, often producing root or spinal cord injury.

FRACTURE OF THE ANTERIOR ELEMENTS

The cervical spine is a three-column structure designed to resist excessive compressive, distractive, and torsional forces at the same time it allows flexion, extension, and rotation in those same planes. The anterior column consists of the anterior two thirds of the vertebral body, the anterior longitudinal ligament (ALL), and the anterior portions of the intervertebral disks. The middle column includes the posterior body and disk, the posterior longitudinal ligament (PLL), and the lateral masses and ligaments. The posterior elements include the facets and facet capsules, the laminae and spinous processes, and the ligamentum flavum, interspinous, and supraspinous ligaments.

Compression fractures specifically injure the anterior column. Compression of the vertebral endplate and trabecular bone results in sagittal angulation and loss of vertebral height. Because the middle and posterior columns are unaffected, these injuries are usually

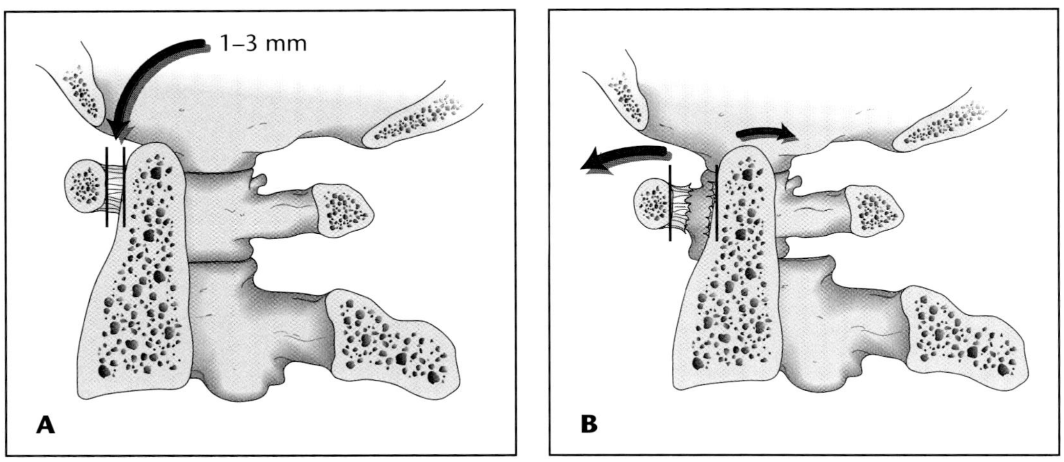

FIGURE 5-1. A and B, Atlantodens interval (ADI). Normal ADI is less than 4 mm. An ADI above 7 mm suggests gross instability.

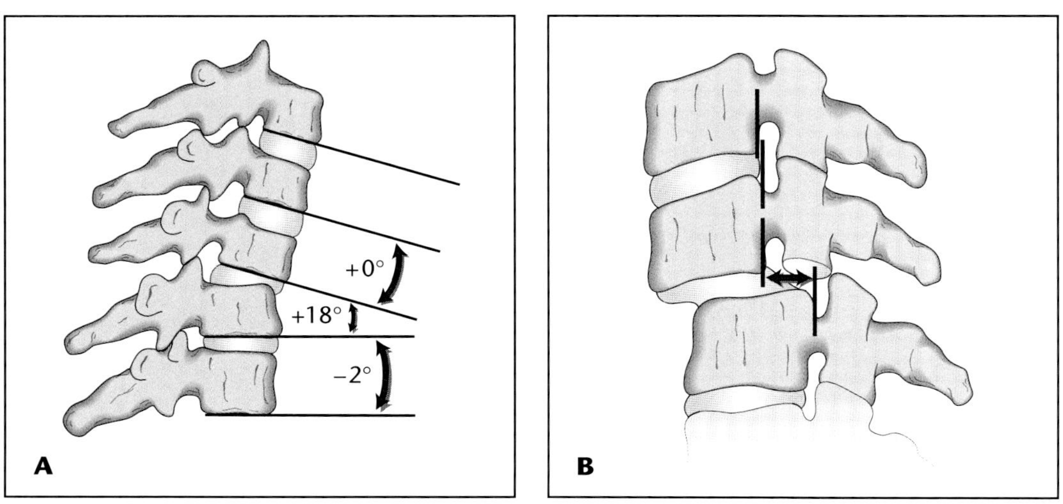

FIGURE 5-2. Cervical instability. Segmental kyphosis that is 11 ° greater than adjacent segments (A) and anterior–posterior translation greater than 3.5 mm (B) are both signs of significant instability.

stable. Burst fractures disrupt both the anterior and middle columns and are more frequently unstable. The posterior column may also be fractured. Fractures that involve all three columns should be considered unstable. Similarly, any fracture associated with a neurologic injury is considered unstable, whether the injury was caused by subluxation or by displacement of fracture fragments into the canal.

Fracture of the Posterior Elements

Stable fractures of the posterior elements include spinous process fractures and some fractures of the laminae. Spinous process fractures may be caused by a direct blow to the process or by an avulsion of the process by its attached musculature (*eg*, clay-shoveler's fracture). Isolated laminar fractures usually result from direct trauma, but a search should be made for associated injuries to the anterior and middle column to avoid overlooking a more serious three-column injury. Facet fractures and dislocations are usually associated with ligamentous injuries and may result in significant rotational instability. Displaced facet fractures may cause nerve root injuries.

Fracture of the Lateral Masses

Lateral mass fractures may occur as an isolated fracture in lateral flexion injuries, or in association with soft tissue trauma in rotational injuries. Lateral mass fractures may cause nerve root injury and may be associated with trauma to the vertebral artery. These injuries are more common in the upper cervical spine.

CRITERIA FOR INSTABILITY AND SURGICAL INDICATIONS

It is difficult to provide a concise, simple definition for "instability" that accounts for all the variables of spinal trauma. White *et al.* [4] have defined clinical instability as the loss of the ability of the spinal elements to maintain alignments and associations between vertebral segments under physiologic loads. Inability of the spinal column to maintain normal relationships results in injury or irritation of the neural structures or in structural changes during loading that result in deformity alone or with pain. Radiographic and clinical criteria for instability have been defined (Table 5-1).

Surgical indications may be absolute or relative. Absolute indications include progressive neurologic deficit, unreduced facet dislocation, and three-column fracture-dislocations. Relative indications include decompression of injured nerve roots above the level of a complete cord injury, stabilization of fractures in spinal cord injured patients, stabilization of two- and three-column fractures in spinally intact patients, and treatment of intractable pain in a patient with an otherwise stable lesion.

TABLE 5-1. RADIOGRAPHIC AND CLINICAL CRITERIA OF INSTABILITY

Greater than 3.5 mm sagittal translation (on 72-in lateral radiograph)
Greater than 11° sagittal angulation in excess of adjacent segments
Three-column fracture or soft tissue disruption
Any neurologic injury
Persistent or unremitting neck pain

Adapted from White *et al.* [4].

SUBLUXATION AND DISLOCATION

C1–C2 Subluxation

Acute disruptions may be treated in a halo brace, with the understanding that a significant number of these cases will not heal and will require subsequent surgery. Treatment of long-term or widely displaced injuries should include closed reduction in traction and C1–C2 spinal fusion. The patient should be placed in halo traction with the neck in slight extension to reduce the subluxation, followed by posterior fixation of C1 and C2 with sublaminar wires (Figure 5-3). Transarticular screws may be placed across the lateral masses at C1–C2 as an alternative to sublaminar wiring. In more protracted cases, the subluxation may not reduce on extension. When no cord compression is found, the injury can be fused in place using sublaminar wires. If there is any evidence of myelopathy, a C1 laminectomy may be necessary, followed by a more extensive fusion from the occiput to C2. Lateral mass screws are more difficult to place in unreduced subluxations.

Subaxial Subluxation

Subluxation results when the posterior ligaments and restraints are stretched or disrupted. Minor subluxations (*ie*, with 2 to 4 mm of translation) are treated in a brace, but evidence of progressive instability must be watched for carefully. In addition, the patient must understand that residual instability and neck pain can be seen after brace treatment and that some patients will still require surgery. When subluxation is associated with signs of mechanical instability, surgical treatment is more often necessary. Most patients benefit from treatment with postural reduction and posterior fusion, with either interspinous wiring or lateral mass plating to stabilize the injury. Interspinous wiring is preferred, if the spinous processes are intact, because it is simple, effective, and carries little operative risk. Lateral mass plating is far more technically demanding, putting the vertebral arteries and nerve roots at some risk with each screw placement, but it provides excellent stability when the spinous processes have been fractured or surgically removed.

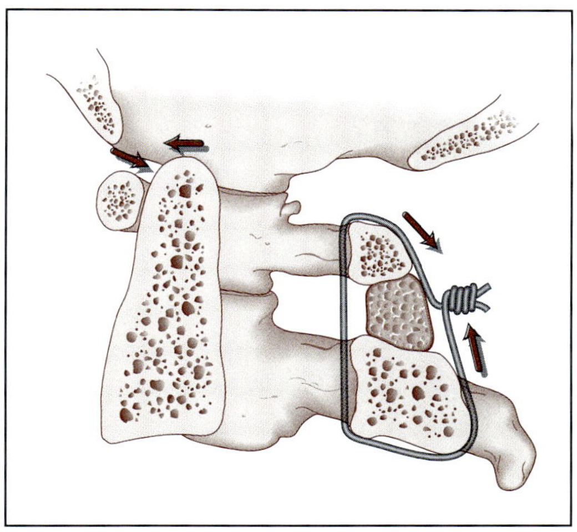

Figure 5-3. Atlantoaxial instability. Posterior sublaminar wiring restores alignment and facilitates fusion.

Unilateral Facet Dislocation

Facet dislocation occurs when the capsular tissues of the facet joint are torn and the interspinous ligaments stretched or disrupted. It is most often seen after motor vehicle accidents or falls from height. The posterior longitudinal ligament is often intact and under tension, which makes closed reduction difficult. The anteroposterior radiograph demonstrates a subtle shift of the spinous processes at the level of injury, with the cranial processes shifted toward the side of the injury. Lateral and oblique radiographs confirm the diagnosis, with the oblique view showing the actual perched facet (Figure 5-4).

Closed reduction of the unilateral facet dislocation should be attempted by applying tongs and traction and gradually increasing the traction force up to 60 to 70 lb. Before attempting a closed reduction, an MRI scan should be obtained of any patient with intact cord function and a unilateral dislocation. This will identify the rare patient with an extruded herniation that might cause cord compression when the deformity is reduced. When such a herniation is present, an anterior approach and diskectomy are recommended before reduction is attempted. If the dislocation does not reduce in traction, surgical treatment is required. In these cases, a posterior approach is used to expose the injured level and to remove just enough of the jumped facet to allow manual reduction under moderate traction. The spine should be stabilized with interspinous wires and autograft bone. If the spinous process is damaged at the site of injury, facet wiring can be used to restore rotational and sagittal stability (Figure 5-5).

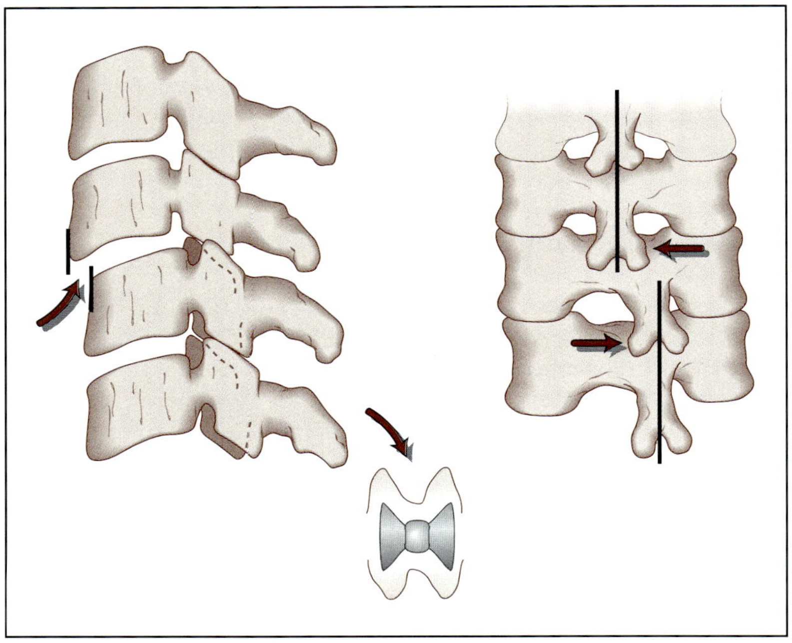

Figure 5-4. Unilateral facet dislocation. Lateral radiograph shows small, unreducible translation at level of injury and "bowtie" sign; facets below the injury are seen in an oblique view because of rotation. An anteroposterior radiograph would reveal a shift in the spinous processes at the level of injury.

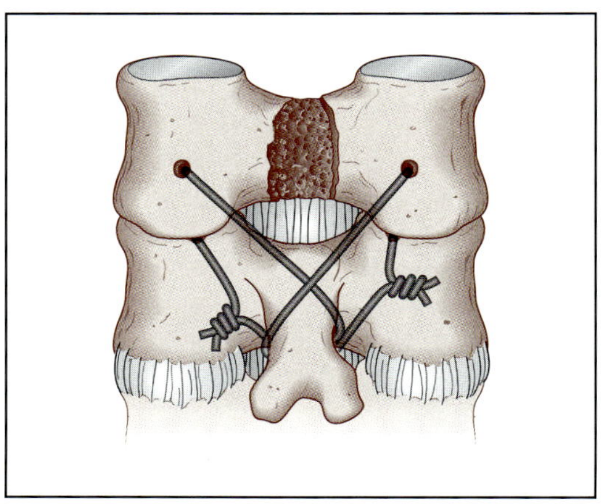

Figure 5-5. Facet wiring is used when the superior spinous process has been fractured or removed.

Bilateral Facet Dislocation

This dislocation is easier to diagnose because vertebral malalignment is readily apparent and associated trauma is usually more severe. Motor vehicle accidents are the usual cause, and spinal cord injury is often seen. With both facets dislocated, the upper vertebra is displaced well forward on the lower vertebra and a marked kyphosis is usually present. Because this injury cannot occur unless the posterior longitudinal ligament and posterior annulus are completely disrupted, the injury is very unstable. This means the dislocation is more easily reduced by traction, but also that it can easily recur unless the spine is stabilized.

In cases of complete spinal cord injury, surgery is indicated to stabilize the spine and allow early rehabilitation. Closed reduction is carried out at the time of admission, but surgery may be delayed until a suitable operative team can be assembled. Urgent treatment will not improve neurologic recovery. Similarly, when no neurologic injury is found, surgery can be delayed until a more suitable time can be arranged.

In cases of incomplete injury with persistent dislocation, urgent operative reduction should be carried out to decompress the cord. Similarly, any patient with progressive neurologic signs deserves rapid evaluation and decompression. An emergency MRI scan will rule out a soft-tissue or disk lesion proximal to the dislocation and help to evaluate the nerve roots at the level of injury. Urgent surgery to decompress the nerve roots is warranted in the quadriplegic patient—every root level salvaged has a major impact on long-term function. Posterior stabilization is carried out in the same way as that for unilateral dislocations. Two additional techniques for posterior stabilization are illustrated in Figure 5-6.

Fracture of the Anterior Elements

Odontoid Fracture

Fractures of the odontoid behave clinically in the same way as atlantoaxial ligamentous injuries. When healing does not occur, progressive instability results in gradual occlusion of the spinal canal, with cord compression at a level incompatible with a normal life. Depending on the type of fracture, patients are more or less likely to need surgery to achieve fracture healing (Figure 5-7) [5]. Type I injuries are usually stable and typically respond well to nonoperative treatment. They are also uncommon. Type II injuries are the most common and the most likely to require surgery. These injuries occur through the base of the odontoid, through a segment that has more cortical bone than cancellous. Nonunions are common. Any amount of angulation and displacement reduces the area of bleeding healthy bone in contact at the fracture. Type III injuries occur through the vertebral body of C2, just below the odontoid base. Nonunions are less common here.

The common treatment for both Type II and Type III fractures is posterior sublaminar wiring. In young patients with a reducible Type II injury, odontoid screw fixation should be considered. Although technically demanding, this procedure preserves the sagittal and rotational motion of the C1–C2 articulation (Figure 5-8).

Compression Fracture

Compression fractures involve only the anterior column of the spine and are rarely unstable. Lateral radiographs show compression of the superior endplate of the injured vertebra, with an occasional fracture

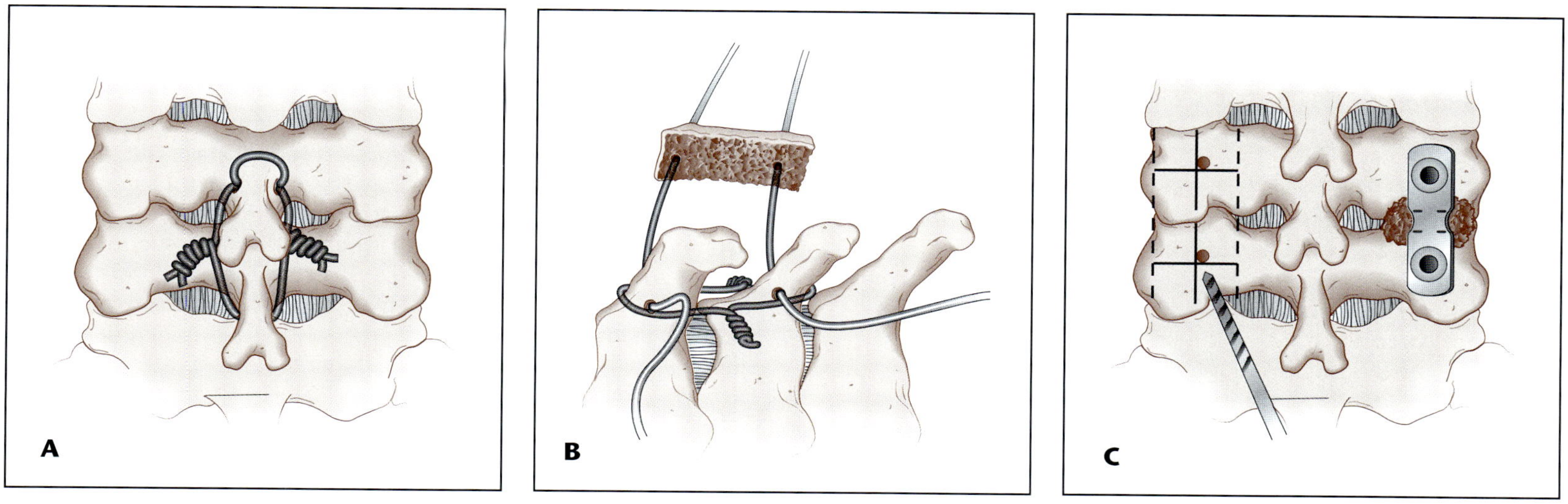

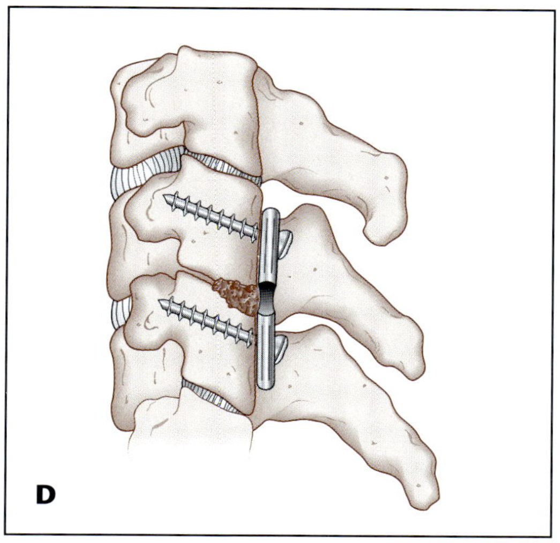

Figure 5-6. **A**, Interspinous wiring for bilateral facet dislocation. This technique uses standard monofilament wire to tie adjacent spinous processes together, locking the facet joints and restricting motion. **B**, To complete interspinous wiring, two smaller wires are passed side-to-side through the spinous processes and two strips of bone graft. As additional wires are tightened, the spinous processes are sandwiched firmly between the grafts, adding stability and speeding the fusion process. **C**, When the spinous process are small, weak, or fractured, a lateral mass plate and screws can be applied. The screw starting point is just above and medial to the midpoint of the lateral mass. The pilot hole is angled eranially by 25° and laterally by 15°. **D**, The plate is applied over the facet joint, which is scraped and packed with bone.

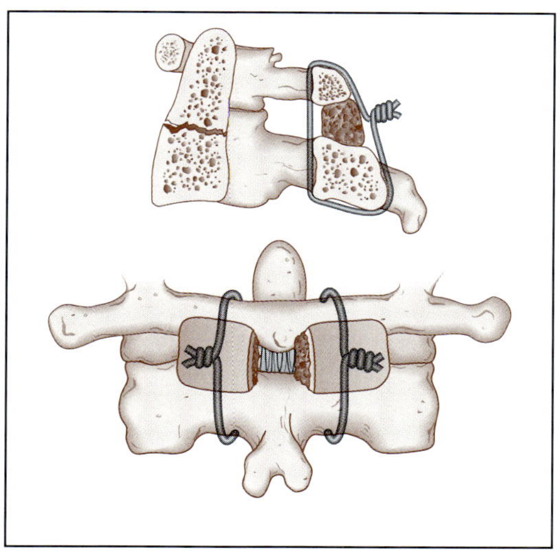

Figure 5-7. Brooks fusion for odontoid fracture.

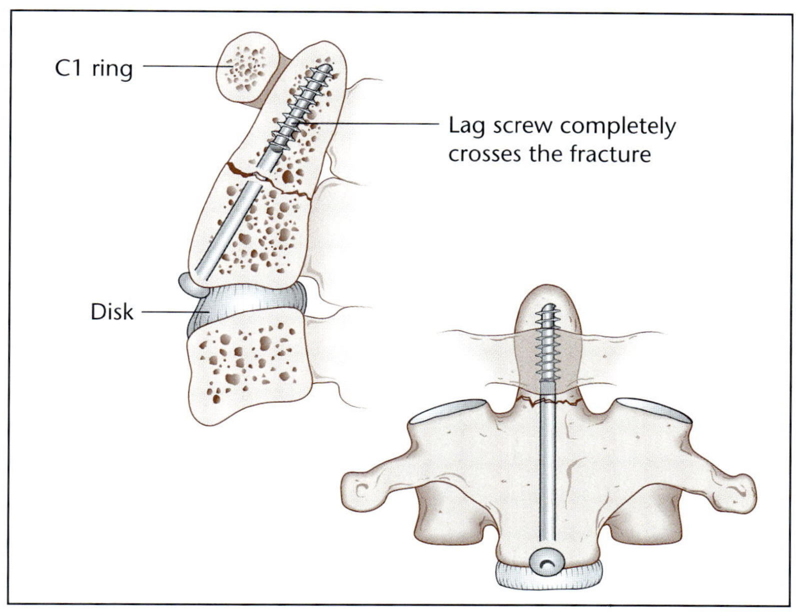

Figure 5-8. Lateral and anteroposterior views of Type II odontoid fracture after anterior odontoid screw fixation.

of the anterior rim. More severe injuries demonstrate fracture of the anterior cortex and mild-to-moderate kyphosis. These injuries are well treated in a brace or collar.

Burst Fracture

Often unstable, these injuries are usually treated in a halo brace or with surgery. The proper approach depends on the presence of neurologic injury, the patient's overall status, and whether the injury disrupts two or three spinal columns. Neurologically intact patients with moderate injuries to the anterior and middle columns of the spine can be treated in a halo vest with reliably good results. Patients with complete cord lesions do not tolerate bracing well and should be stabilized surgically.

If the patient is neurologically intact or has an incomplete lesion, choose an anterior approach to reconstruct the spinal column and decompress the canal. Vertebrectomy, strut graft reconstruction, and plating are enough to stabilize most two-column injuries. The bulk of the vertebral body and both adjacent disks are removed through an anterior approach. Any retropulsed fragments are carefully extracted from the spinal canal. After the resulting defect has been filled with either autograft iliac crest or an allograft fibular strut, a plate and screws are applied to span the adjacent vertebral bodies (Figure 5-9). If the posterior elements have also been disrupted, the anterior construct is either supplemented with a halo and vest or the patient is turned and a posterior triple-wire procedure is performed to ensure success. Failure to recognize a three-column injury can lead to major complications. Combined anterior–posterior fixation eliminates the common causes of failure by restoring the tension-band effect that both anterior plating and posterior wiring need to work against to be most stable [6]. Although the combined approach is more time consuming, the patient can be mobilized rapidly, with confidence that the neural elements will be well protected (Figure 5-10) [7•].

Tear-Drop Fracture

The tear-drop fracture is a subtle and easily overlooked injury [8]. Whereas some compression fractures will cause a small fragment of the anterior vertebral rim to fracture and displace, the true tear-drop fracture is a very unstable *hyperextension* injury, in which that same fragment is produced as an *avulsion*. This injury is uncommon but is sagittally and rotationally unstable in a brace and should be stabilized through anterior interbody fusion and plating. This will restore the anterior tension band and protect the neural elements from injury [9].

Fracture–Dislocation

The difference, mechanically or prognostically, between a severe burst fracture and a fracture–dislocation is a matter of degrees [6]. These injuries result from high-energy trauma, are associated with a high incidence of cord injury, and are usually unstable. To dislocate the vertebral column, all three mechanical columns must be disrupted, either by rupturing the soft tissue restraints or by fracturing the bones. Although alignment is relatively easy to restore, these injuries often displace as soon as physiologic loads are introduced [10]. Surgical treatment is indicated to restore mechanical stability and allow early rehabilitation; decompress the spinal cord

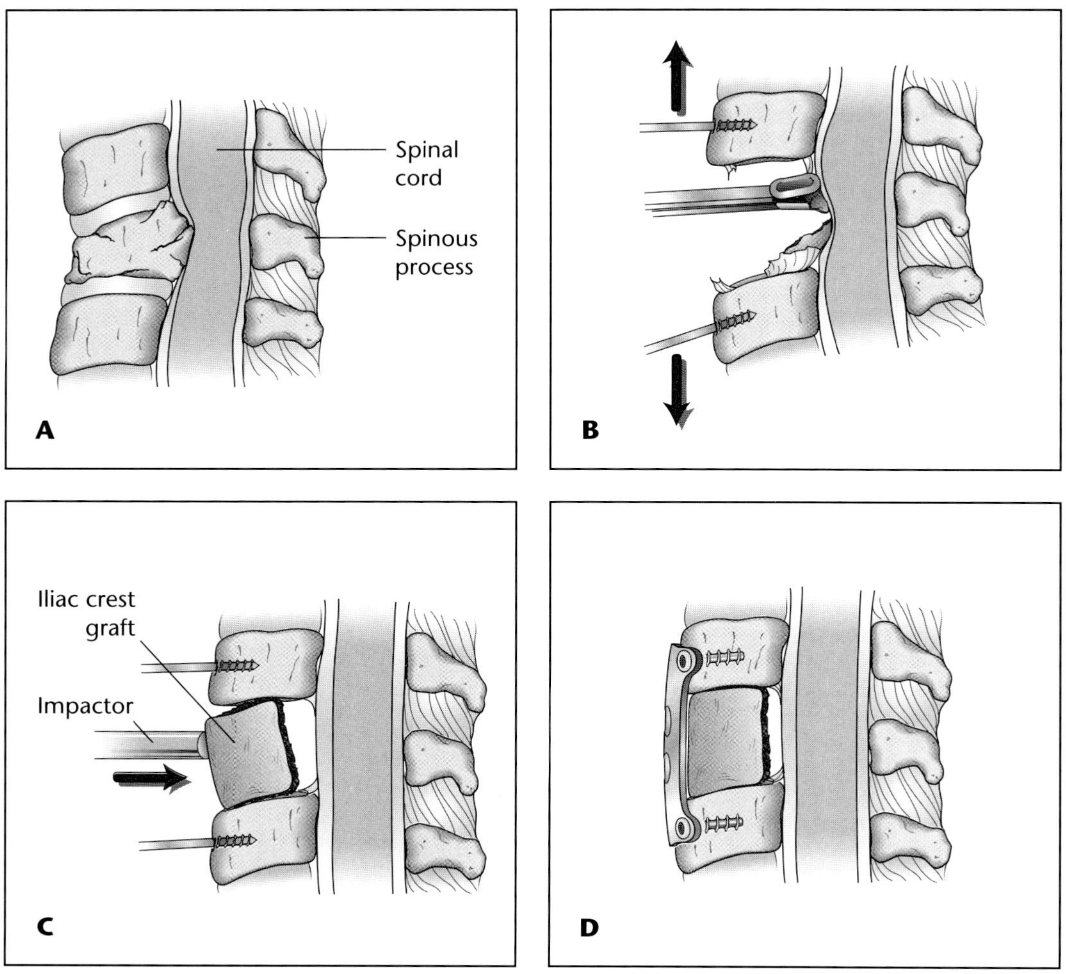

Figure 5-9. A–D, Subaxial burst fracture with cord compression. After removing the fractured vertebra and decompressing the cord, an iliac crest bone graft is harvested and contoured to fill the space and restore normal alignment. The endplates are contoured to hold the graft in place; the plate ensures that it does not move.

and protect it from further injury; and decompress and protect functioning nerve roots.

The head is initially protected with sandbags or rolls, then placed in light traction when the patient is stable. No more than 5 lb of traction should be applied initially and a lateral radiograph should be checked immediately to be sure that the spinal column is not being distracted. Additional weight is applied until the alignment is restored and the dislocation reduced. During this time, necessary imaging studies should be obtained and reviewed and a definitive treatment plan formulated.

For many patients, anterior reconstruction and vertebral plating augmented by halo immobilization are sufficient to restore stability and protect the neural elements [11,12]. In more severe or multilevel injuries, or in patients who cannot tolerate the brace, a combined anterior and posterior reconstruction provides immediate stability and circumferential spinal cord decompression. Posterior plating or wiring alone may not be sufficient to protect the neural elements at the injured level, even when used with a halo.

FRACTURE OF THE POSTERIOR ELEMENTS

Spinous Process Fracture

These injuries are usually stable and easily treated with a soft brace and analgesics. The biggest concern is overlooking a more serious soft tissue injury associated with a benign-looking spinous process fracture. Radiographs must be examined carefully to ensure that the facets are not in subluxation at the level of the injury, that no rotational or translational abnormality is present, and that there is no prevertebral swelling or hematoma. If the injury mechanism is low energy, an MRI scan is not needed and the patient may be placed in a light collar and treated symptomatically. The lateral radiographs in a patient with persistent or progressive symptoms should be repeated if necessary; however, late instability can develop in patients with entirely normal injury radiographs. It is easiest to see this on flexion–extension lateral radiographs obtained 1 to 2 weeks after injury.

Lamina Fracture

As with spinous process fractures, lamina fractures tend to be of two kinds—either isolated injuries that are mechanically stable and easily treated or injuries associated with other, more serious disruptions that render the spinal column unstable. The isolated injuries can be treated symptomatically with reliably good results. The injuries associated with other disruptions must be treated according to the more serious injury. The treatment plan must take into account the presence of laminar fractures, however, because interspinous and facet wiring techniques are usually not possible.

Atlantoaxial Spondylolisthesis

In traumatic spondylolisthesis of the axis ("hangman's fracture"), loads carried anteriorly through the C1–C2 vertebral bodies are transmitted posteriorly to the facets of C2 and C3. As these loads are transmitted axially, the narrow arch of C2 may overload and fail. This produces a unique cervical injury that is a true spondylolisthesis—the anterior elements of C2 are attached to the cranial spine and the posterior elements stay with the caudal spine (Figure 5-11). Fortunately, the displacement tends to widen the neural canal, so that even in unstable fractures, spinal cord injury is not common. Low-grade injuries have minor-to-moderate displacement of the fracture site and can be treated in a four-poster brace or halo. If displacement is more severe, a period of halo traction should be tried before the patient is placed in the halo. For those injuries that cannot be reduced by traction, or if the C2–C3 facet joint is dislocated, open reduction and facet wiring are indicated followed by halo immobilization for 12 weeks.

Facet Fractures

Facet fractures usually occur in higher-energy injuries—motor vehicle collisions, sports trauma—and are similar in mechanism to the unilateral facet dislocations. However, because the facet is fractured, the injury may reduce spontaneously and therefore be somewhat more difficult to spot. Similarly, realignment in a brace or traction is not as difficult as in a fixed dislocation. If the fracture is not displaced, and no neurologic injury is found, the patient can be well treated in a two-poster cervical brace or collar. For

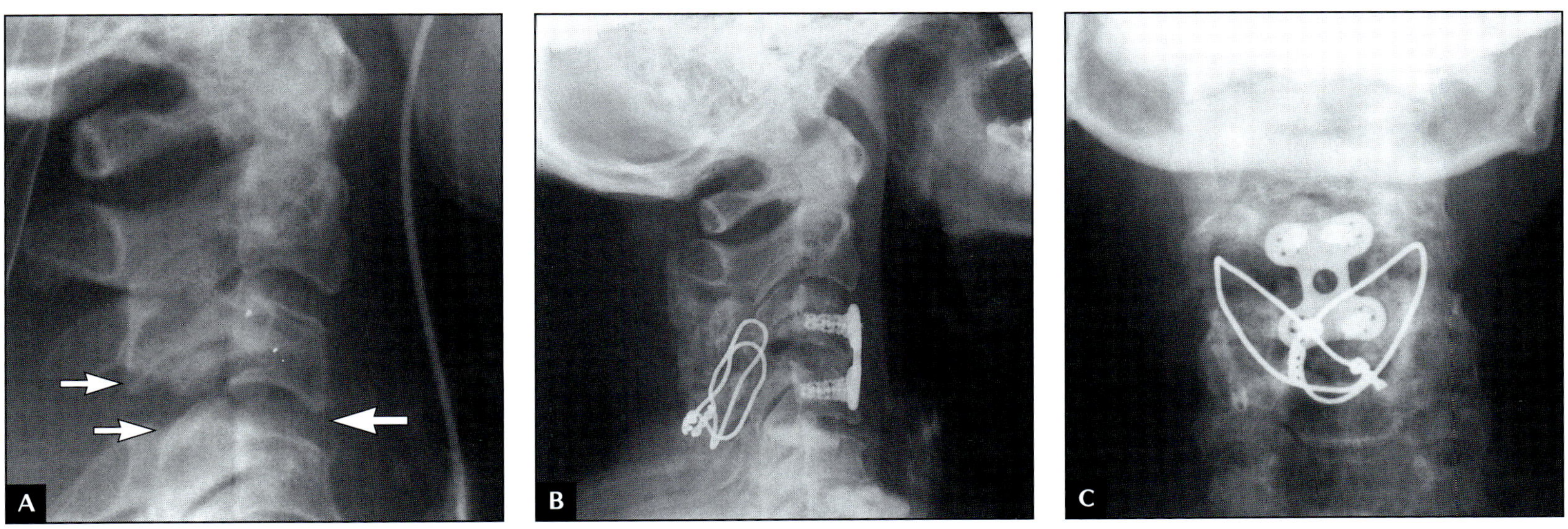

Figure 5-10. Cervical dislocation after motor vehicle accident. A, Alignment is well restored and displacement at the disk is subtle (*large arrow*). The gap between the facet joints is large (*small arrows*). A–C, All structures were seen as disrupted on magnetic resonance imaging scan. Combined anterior and posterior plating restored stability and protected cord and nerve roots. (*From* McLain and Benson [7•]; with permission.)

more severe injuries, or in cases of nerve root injury, a halo may provide more definitive immobilization.

Displaced facet fractures are often rotationally unstable and may remain so after nonoperative treatment. If the fragment is pushed into the neural foramen, severe or persistent nerve root symptoms may be present. In these cases, the most appropriate treatment is a posterior approach with reduction of the fracture and internal fixation. If the entire lateral mass or pillar is fractured, the fixation must be extended to the next vertebral level, because neither lateral mass screws or wire fixation will adequately immobilize the injured segment [13•].

FRACTURES OF THE LATERAL MASSES

Lateral mass fractures usually respond to immobilization and bracing. Displaced injuries may require open reduction and internal fixation to combat rotational instability. Even when the fracture is minimally displaced, facet arthropathy may dispose the patient to pain and dysfunction in the future, and this risk is probably even greater in badly reduced or intra-articular injuries. As long as the patient is aware of this risk, a wait-and-see attitude is reasonable; if significant pain symptoms do develop over time, a single-level posterior fusion can be performed *after the fracture has healed*, thus avoiding the need to extend the fusion to the adjacent levels.

SPINAL CORD AND ROOT INJURY

Evaluation

After a neurologic injury has been recognized, a careful evaluation must be performed to characterize the injury and establish a prognosis and treatment plan. The examining physician must distinguish among complete and incomplete injuries, root and spinal cord trauma, stable and progressive lesions, and isolated and multilevel or multifactorial injuries. It may not be possible to determine whether an injury is complete at the time of admission; intact and partial injuries are as they appear, but spinal cord shock may mask some incomplete cord injuries, thus making it impossible to initially distinguish them from complete cord trauma. After spinal cord shock has resolved (24 to 72 hours), accurate diagnosis is possible.

Diagnosis

Cervical injuries often produce mixed lesions, combining spinal cord and nerve root injuries that have different prognostic implications. Because root lesions can have such a profound impact on long-term function, it is important to identify nerve root compression at or above the level of cord injury and treat it aggressively. The physician must carefully map the dermatomal and motor patterns of injury and look for evidence of residual function—hemiparesis, sacral sparing, and patchy residual sensation. When spinal cord shock has resolved, heralded by the return of the bulbocavernosus reflex, a careful survey will again reveal evidence of complete cord injury or of residual neural function or incomplete root injury. Surgical decompression is indicated if any persistent compression associated with an incomplete cord injury or with nerve root deficit is present.

An MRI scan can provide clues to likely outcome. Complete cord transection, extensive intramedullary hemorrhage, and edema are poor prognostic signs for functional recovery. Specific nerve root lesions can be identified at the level of cord trauma and the potential for decompression assessed. CT provides superior imaging of bony elements and may be helpful in planning stabilization or reconstruction. Electromyograms (EMGs), nerve conduction studies, and bone scans have no role in acute cervical trauma.

Treatment

Initial treatment of spinal cord injury aims at salvaging any injured but still viable cord tissue and at protecting any uninjured but at-risk tissues from further injury. Principles of treatment include indirect decompression of the spinal cord (*eg*, realigning the spinal column, reducing facet dislocations); protection of residual function (*eg*, stabilizing the neck, fiberoptic intubation); and reduction of the injuries' impact on the neural elements (*eg*, aggressive hemodynamic resuscitation, maintenance of adequate perfusion pressures, high dose steroids).

Use of steroids remains controversial. Previous clinical studies have shown equivocal results in terms of neural improvement but an unequivocal increase in complications, such as infection and

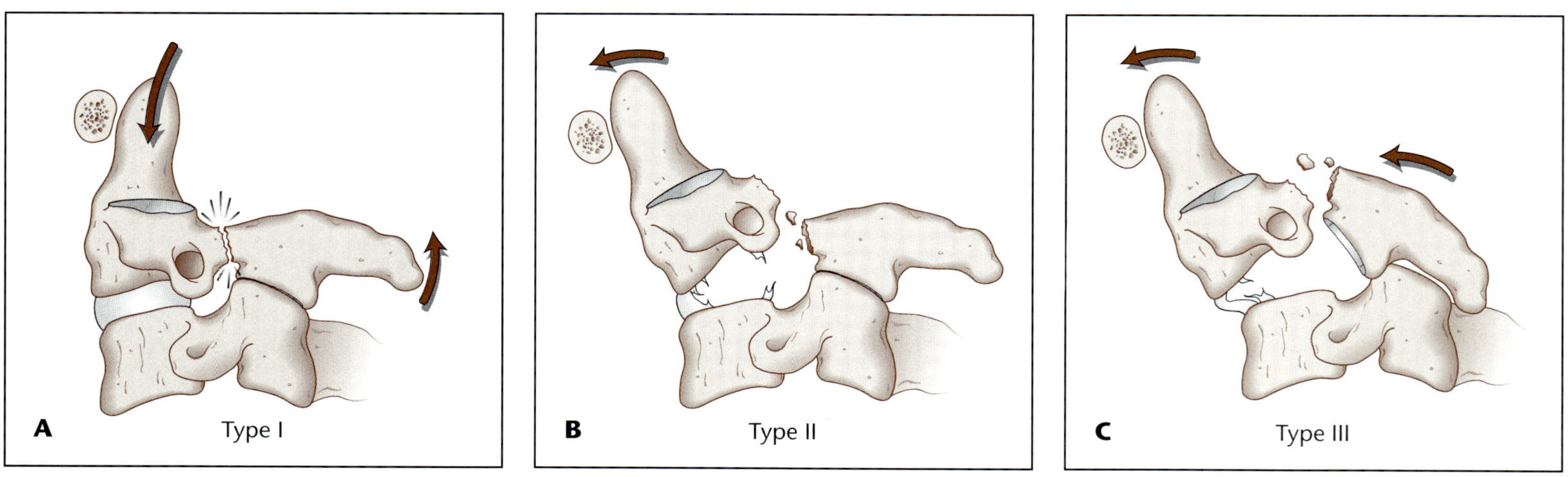

Figure 5-11. A–C, Atlantoaxial spondylolisthesis. Type I injuries are minimally displaced and well treated in a brace or halo. Type II injuries require traction to restore alignment, but heal well in a halo once alignment is regained. Type III injuries cannot often be reduced closed. Open reduction of the dislocated facet is required, followed by wire fixation of the facets.

gastrointestinal hemorrhage. Still, the randomized, prospective trial published by the National Acute Spinal Cord Injury Study [14] did show a small but significant improvement in recovery in patients treated with high-dose steroids immediately after injury. For acute spinal cord injury, the current recommendation is to initiate steroid protocol in incomplete lesions, giving the first dose within 6 hours of injury, using methylprednisolone in an initial bolus of 30 mg/kg and infusion at 5.4 mg/kg/h for 23 hours. Steroid therapy should then be terminated.

Longer courses of steroid medications have shown no additional benefit and are associated with a much greater incidence of serious complications. Results with methylprednisolone have been marginal at best, with the average patient showing less than a single grade of additional improvement. For severe cord deficit with residual compression by either bone or soft tissue, anterior decompression and circumferential stabilization still offer the best and most rapid opportunity for recovery [15].

CONCLUSIONS

Cervical spine fractures and dislocations are among the most dreaded injuries encountered in the emergency department or athletic arena. To avoid precipitating catastrophic iatrogenic injury, simple principles must be learned and followed. The neck must be protected at all times during initial resuscitation, assessment, and examination. Screening radiographs must show the C7–T1 junction clearly and be of good quality. Mechanism of injury, history of neurologic symptoms, and evidence of cranial or facial trauma must be incorporated into direct evaluation of the neck. The cervical spine cannot be "cleared" in a comatose or intoxicated patient. Whenever the cervical spine cannot be definitively "cleared," spinal precautions must be maintained until it can. The neck should never be manipulated in a patient with a suspected neck injury.

After an injury has been identified, the patient can be protected and evaluated in a methodical and complete manner, revealing the mechanical characteristics of the injury, the nature of any neural trauma, and the potential instability of the injury. Such evaluation allows the surgeon to plan the safest and most rational approach, operative or nonoperative, to any cervical injury.

REFERENCES AND RECOMMENDED READING

Recently published papers of particular interest have been highlighted as:
- • Of interest
- •• Of outstanding interest

1. Bohlman HH: Acute fractures and dislocations of the cervical spine. *J Bone Joint Surg* 1979, 61A:1119–1142.
2. Reid DC, Henderson R, Saboe L, Miller JDR: Etiology and clinical course of missed spine fractures. *J Trauma* 1987, 27:980–986.
3. el-Khoury GY, Kathol MH, Daniel WW: Imaging of acute injuries of the cervical spine: value of plain radiography, CT, and MR imaging. *Am J Roentgenol* 1995, 164:43–50.
4. White AA, Southwick WO, Panjabi MM: Clinical instability of the lower cervical spine: a review of past and current concepts. *Spine* 1970, 1:15–270.
5. Clark CR, White AA: Fractures of the dens: a multicenter study. *J Bone Joint Surg* 1985, 67A:1340–1348.
6. McLain RF, Aretakis A, Moseley TA, *et al.*: Subaxial cervical dissociation: anatomic and biomechanical principles of stabilization. *Spine* 1994, 19:653–659.

7•. McLain RF, Benson DR: Missed cervical dissociation: recognizing and avoiding potential disaster. *J Emerg Med* 1998, 16:179–183.

This case report and review outlines the emergency room treatment of unrecognized cervical trauma, emphasizing the proper precautions for cervical stability during major resuscitation and emergency surgery. The authors outline key elements of the history and physical examination that may alert the physician to cervical trauma.

8. Cabanela ME, Ebersold MJ: Anterior plate stabilization for bursting tear-drop fractures of the cervical spine. *Spine* 1988, 13:888–891.
9. Capen DA, Garland DE, Waters RL: Surgical stabilization of the cervical spine. *Clin Orthop* 1985, 196:229–237.
10. Cybulski GR, Douglas RA, Meyer PR, Rovin RA: Complications in three-column cervical spine injuries requiring anterior-posterior stabilization. *Spine* 1992, 17:253–256.
11. Aebi M, Zuber K, Marchesi D: Treatment of cervical injuries with anterior plating. *Spine* 1991, 16:38–45.
12. Suh PB, Kostuik JP, Esses SI: Anterior cervical plate fixation with the titanium hollow screw system. *Spine* 1990, 15:1079–1081.

13.• Steinmann JC, Anderson PA: Subaxial cervical spine fractures with internal fixation: the posterior approach. *Sem Spine Surg* 1996, 8:35–48.

The authors provide a broad overview of current techniques of cervical stabilization following subaxial trauma. Surgical approaches and stabilization techniques are reviewed in detail.

14. Bracken MB, Shepard MJ, Collins WF: A randomized, controlled trial of methylprednisolone in acute spinal cord injury: results of the Second National Acute Spinal Cord Injury Study. *N Engl J Med* 1990, 322:1405–1411.
15. McAfee PC, Bohlman HH: One stage anterior cervical decompression and posterior stabilization with circumferential arthrodesis. *J Bone Joint Surg* 1989, 71A:78–88.

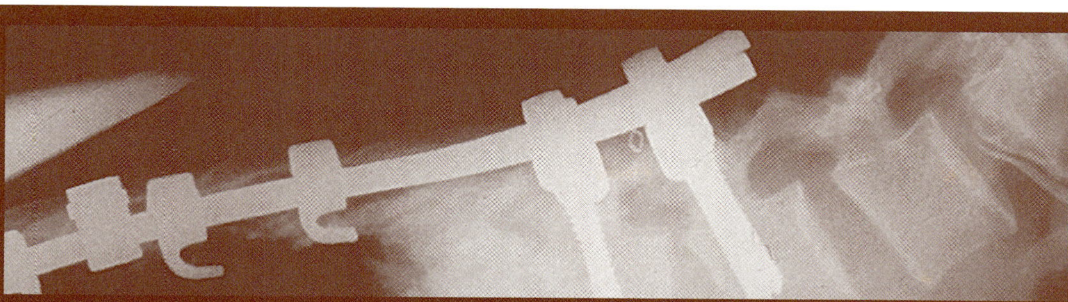

6

Thoracolumbar Fractures and Fracture-Dislocations

Munish C. Gupta
Daniel R. Benson

Thoracolumbar fractures are common and can range from low-energy compression fractures seen in elderly patients that result from minor falls to high-energy fracture-dislocations secondary to motor vehicle accidents. In recent years, the awareness of spine injuries has increased through education, which has made a significant impact on emergency treatment in the field through the use of spinal precautions in preventing further damage to the spinal column and neural elements. However, after a complete spinal cord injury has occurred, it has not been possible to restore neurologic function in any way. The goals for treating patients with thoracolumbar fractures are to preserve and protect function by restoring stability of the spinal column. A secondary goal is to decrease the incidence of late pain or deformity. A spinal cord injury may be only one aspect of a polytraumatized patient. Just as in other patients with multiple trauma, using internal fixation for a spine fracture might be necessary to mobilize the patient and decrease overall morbidity.

PATIENT EVALUATION

Patient evaluation should include a history of the mechanism of injury. Certain mechanisms, such as a seat belt–related or flexion-distraction injury may alert the clinician to the possibility of associated abdominal injuries. The mechanism also may influence the radiologic work-up to include a magnetic resonance image (MRI) to evaluate for ligamentous injury more fully, in addition to the use of plain radiographs and a computed tomography (CT) scan. A complete neurologic examination is essential in treating the injury to the spinal column as well as the neural elements in establishing a baseline for monitoring the neurologic deficit for any further deterioration. For example, an incomplete neurologic deficit in a patient who has a burst fracture is treated with decompression of the canal more readily than in a patient who is intact with a similar bony injury. Radiologic evaluation should include evaluation of the entire spine because of the significant incidence of other spine fractures. After plain anteroposterior (AP) and lateral radiographs have been obtained, CT has been found to be useful for delineating bony injury. MRI has been helpful in instances in which a mismatch is found in the neurologic deficit present and injury seen and in certain mechanisms of injury, which thus suggests ligamentous injury, such as in a flexion-distraction type. After initial patient examination and radiographic evaluation, spinal precautions must be observed to prevent further injury. Steroids should be given as soon as possible to treat the neurologic injury. Finally, spinal injuries should be treated in a definitive manner with coordinated treatment of other injuries as well.

CONCEPT OF STABILITY AND CLASSIFICATION

Holdsworth [1] described mechanisms and classifications for thoracolumbar fractures. He emphasized ligamentous disruption that contributed to instability. He also divided the spine into two columns: anterior and posterior. The anterior column included the anterior longitudinal ligament, vertebral body, intervertebral disk, and posterior longitudinal ligament. The posterior column included the rest of the posterior elements, including the pedicle and all the ligaments. He maintained that a burst fracture did not have any significant posterior ligamentous damage and was thus a stable injury. With the advent of the CT scan, injury to the vertebral body, especially the retropulsed fragments of bone into the canal and the sagittal split of the vertebral body, could be studied. Denis [2] described the middle column as the posterior half of the vertebral body and the annulus, as well as the posterior longitudinal ligament. In his description, the posterior column originally described by Holdsworth [1] remained the same. The anterior column, however, was divided into the anterior and the middle columns. The anterior column comprises the anterior half of the body, the anterior longitudinal ligament, and the anterior half of the disk. Denis pointed out that the middle column was important and that its disruption could create an unstable fracture pattern. James *et al.* [3] did not fully agree with this notion and mentioned that disruption of the posterior elements was more an indication of instability in burst fractures requiring treatment.

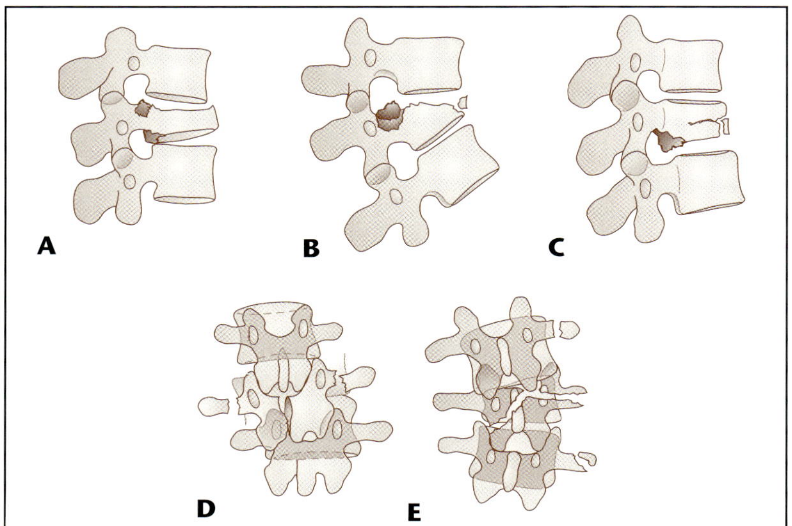

FIGURE 6-1. Classification of burst fractures. Type A has a retropulsed fragment superiorly and inferiorly. Type B, a common pattern, has a superior fragment only. Type C has an inferior retropulsed fragment. Type D has a rotational component and Type E has a distraction component with accompanying posterior element disruption. Both anteroposterior and lateral radiographs are used for this classification. (*Adapted from* Denis [2].)

TABLE 6-1. CATEGORIES OF FRACTURE TYPES

A: **Compression**, including compression fractures and burst fractures
B: Anterior and posterior element injuries with **distraction**, including seat belt–type injuries combined with other flexion distraction injuries
C: Anterior and posterior element injuries with **rotation**

Denis [2] provided a classification of thoracolumbar fractures in which he distinguished between compression fractures and burst fractures. He then further subclassified burst fractures into five types noted from A to E depending on where the retropulsed fragment originated from—superiorly, inferiorly, or both in the middle column (Figure 6-1). In addition, he separated the fractures if any rotation or lateral flexion was seen on the AP radiograph. This subclassification alerts us that retropulsed fragments should be addressed superiorly and inferiorly when decompressing the canal in order to do so fully from one vertebral body superiorly to the other, including the disk spaces. The element of rotation and lateral compression adds to the instability with posterior element disruption. He also classified seat belt–type injuries into a category by themselves in addition to being a mechanism for fracture-dislocation. The fracture-dislocation category includes mechanisms of shear as well as flexion-rotation leading to fracture-dislocation. Gertzbein [4] has described a comprehensive classification of thoracolumbar fractures. Three large categories of fracture types are described in this classification, as shown in Table 6-1.

These three different categories, A, B, and C, are then further subdivided in terms of specific fracture patterns and mechanisms. This classification is more complete, yet it is not widely used possibly because of all the different subgroups it contains. Dall and Stauffer [5] have used angulation and have described four different types (*eg*, I to IV) of fractures in terms of angulation greater or less than 15°. They also distinguish the maximum compromise of the canal occurring at the level of the ligamentum flavum or the pedicles. They found that if significant angulation was present, the chance of neurologic recovery increased to 90%, regardless of the severity of the partial paralysis or the treatment method. Conversely, however, with less than 15° of kyphosis, the chance of neurologic recovery was less than 50% (Figure 6-2) [5]. Kim *et al.* [6] have shown similar findings in which the presence of posterior element disruption correlated with greater improvement in neurologic recovery. This effect may be due to increased space available for neural elements after disruption of posterior structures when retropulsed fragments are pushing anteriorly. The three columns as described by Denis [2] are more commonly used to describe injuries of the thoracolumbar spine (Table 6-2). The thoracolumbar fractures can be subdivided further into four main groups: compression fractures, burst fractures, flexion-distraction injuries, and fracture-dislocation. These groups do not include minor fractures, such as fractures of the transverse processes, pars interarticularis, isolated spinous process, or articular process fractures. The

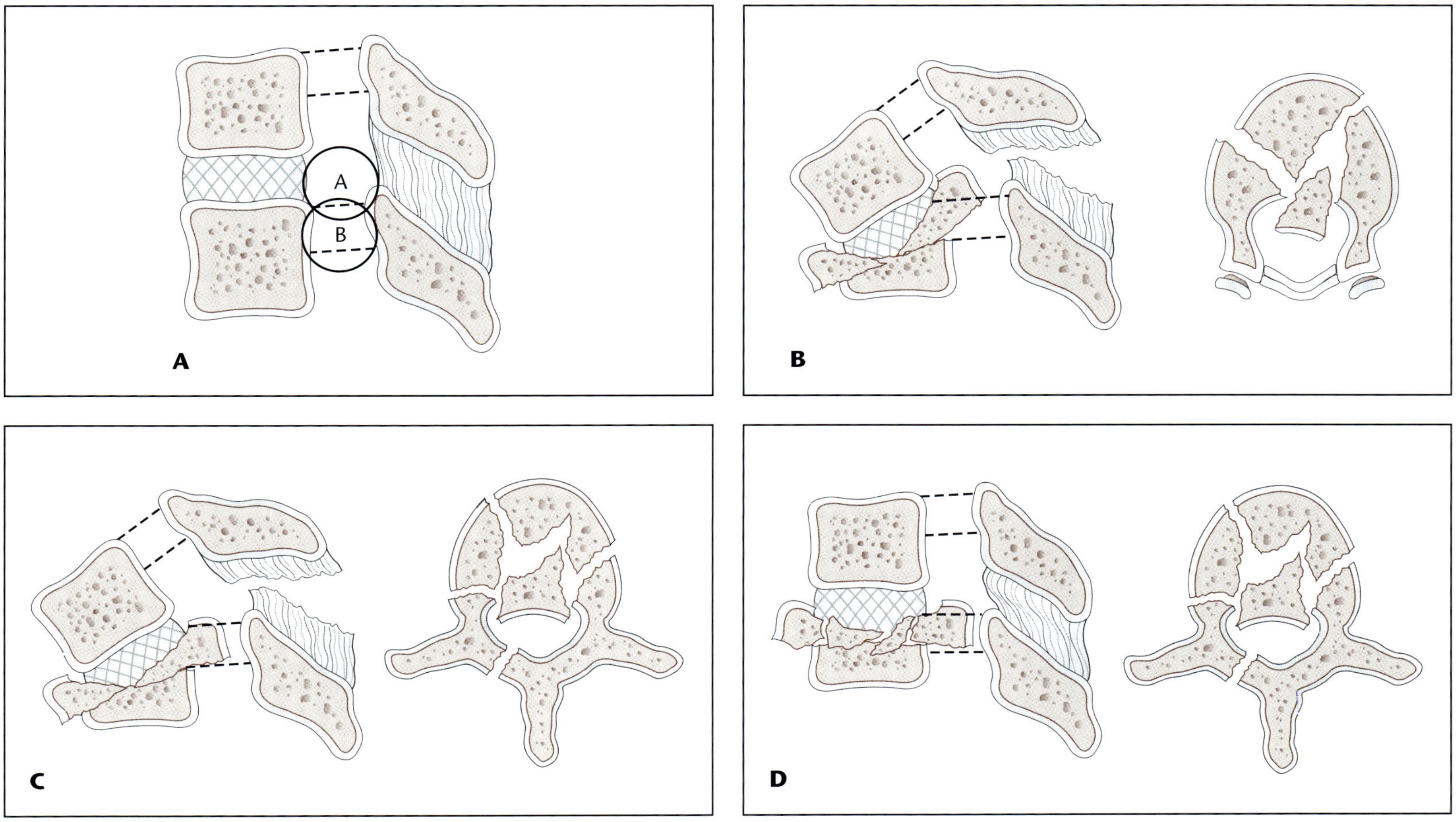

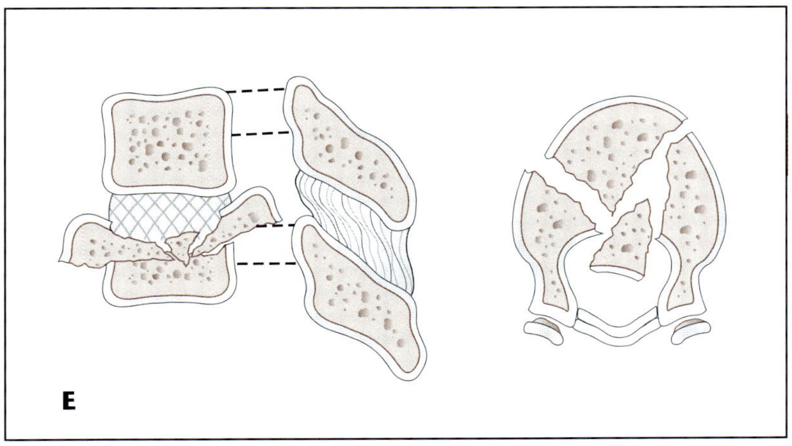

FIGURE 6-2. A, The maximum canal compromise at the midsagittal section varies with location of the fragment and angulation. Types I through IV are described with location of the fragment at the level of the ligamentum flavum (*A*) or pedicle (*B*) and angulation greater than 15° or at or below 15°. **B**, Type I has greater than 15° kyphosis at the level of the disk. **C**, Type II has greater than 15° kyphosis at the level of the pedicle. **D**, Type III has 15° or less kyphosis with maximum bony canal compromise. **E**, Type IV has 15° or less kyphosis at the level of the ligamentum flavum. (*Adapted from* Dall and Stauffer [5].)

TABLE 6-2. BASIC MODES OF FAILURE OF THE THREE COLUMNS IN THE FOUR MAJOR TYPES OF SPINAL INJURIES*

	Column		
Type of Fracture	Anterior	Middle	Posterior
Compression	Compression	None	None or distraction (severe)
Burst	Compression	Compression	None
Seat belt	None or compression	Distraction	Distraction
Fracture-dislocation	Compression rotation shear	Distraction rotation shear	Distraction rotation shear

*In seat belt–type injuries, the component of compression failure of the anterior column is either absent or minimal and takes place in the anterior part of the vertebral body (collapse of about 10% to 20% of the anterior height).

Adapted from Denis [2].

treatment of these minor fractures requires no activity restrictions or brace other than for symptomatic relief (Table 6-3) [7,8].

DIAGNOSIS AND TREATMENT

Compression Fractures

By definition, compression fractures involve the disruption of the anterior column from a flexion force. No disruption occurs in the middle column. These fractures are usually not associated with any neurologic deficit. Treatment includes immobilization in a brace for 3 months. Multiple compression fractures creating kyphosis greater than 30° and loss of height greater than 40% of the vertebral body may signify posterior ligamentous damage and require posterior instrumentation and fusion.

The osteoporotic compression fracture is pathologic and found primarily in elderly postmenopausal women. The osteopenia associated with osteoporosis can be visualized on radiographs. These patients should have a full diagnostic work-up to exclude any other cause of a pathologic fracture, such as tumor or osteomalacia. This work-up may include basic blood tests, bone scans, MRI, and possibly biopsy. These fractures resemble compression fractures with the anterior column compression in the thoracic spine but they can also seem to involve some of the middle column in the lumbar spine where the entire body can be compressed more readily with a flexion force. These patients should be treated with a brace until their symptoms are relieved. Medications such as analgesics and calcitonin are helpful in addition to bracing. New percutaneous techniques, such as

TABLE 6-3. CLASSIFICATION OF THORACIC AND LUMBAR FRACTURES

- A. Vertebral body compression
  - 1. Impaction fracture
    - 1. Endplate infraction
    - 2. Vertebral body collapse
    - 3. Wedge impaction
  - 2. Split fracture
    - 1. Sagittal split
    - 2. Coronal split
    - 3. Pincer fracture
  - 3. Burst fracture
    - 1. Partial burst
    - 2. Burst-split
    - 3. Complete burst
- B. Anterior and posterior element injury
  - 1. Posterior disruption, predominantly ligamentous
    - 1. With transverse disruption of the disk
    - 2. With compression of the vertebral body
  - 2. Posterior disruption, including the arch
    - 1. With transverse disruption through the vertebral body
    - 2. With transverse disruption through the disk
    - 3. With compression of the vertebral body
  - 3. Anterior disruption
    - 1. With hyperextension subluxation of the facet joint
    - 2. Hyperextension spondylolysis
    - 3. With posterior facet dislocation
- C. Anterior and posterior element injury with rotation
  - 1. Vertebral body compression with rotation
    - 1. Impaction
    - 2. Split
    - 3. Burst
  - 2. Distraction with rotation
    - 1. Posterior disruption predominantly
    - 2. Posterior disruption including the arch
  - 3. Rotational shear
    - 1. Slice fracture of the vertebral body
    - 2. Oblique fracture of the vertebral body

Adapted from Wiesel and Boden [7]; with permission.

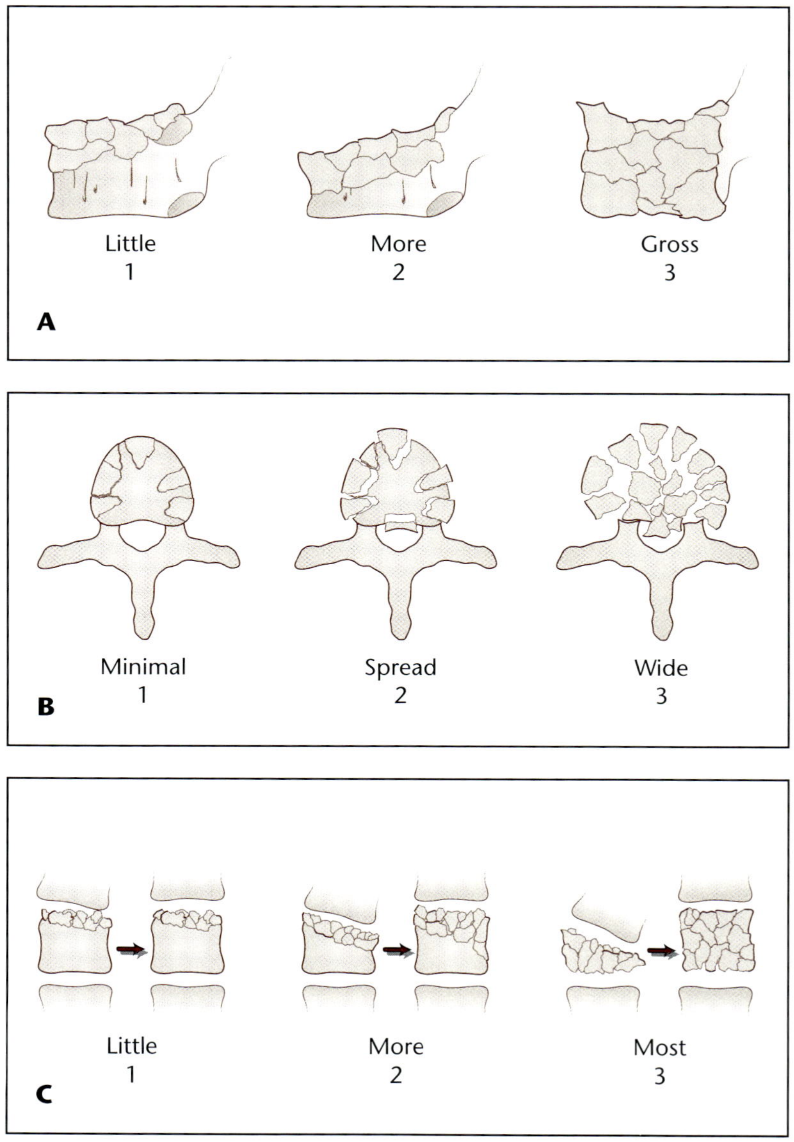

Figure 6-3. Load-sharing classification by assessment of comminution by computed tomography (CT). **A**, In the sagittal plane: little (less than 30% comminution), more (30% to 60% comminution), and gross (more than 60% comminution). **B**, In the axial plane (apposition of fragments): little (minimal), spread (at least 2-mm displacement of less than 50% of the body), and wide (at least 2-mm displacement of more than 50% of the body). **C**, Kyphosis correction on lateral plain radiographs: little (3° or less), more (4° to 9°), and most (10° or more). (*Adapted from* McCormack *et al.* [8].)

vertebralplasty, have been recently described. These techniques restore the height of the vertebral body and place methylmethacrylate in the vertebral body to provide instant stability and subsequent pain relief. Long-term results of this technique are not yet available.

Burst Fractures

Burst fractures constitute some of the most challenging treatment dilemmas associated with thoracolumbar fractures. The burst fracture involves at least the anterior and middle columns. This injury is produced by an axial load with or without the flexion, rotation, and lateral bending components as described by Denis [2]. The posterior column may be disrupted with associated laminar fractures and ligamentous injury. The amount of compression of the vertebral body on plain radiographs and retropulsion of bone seen on CT scans can be useful in selecting the appropriate treatment. McCormack *et al.* [8] showed that comminution of the vertebral body, the spread of the fragments combined with percentage of the fragmented vertebral body, and the amount of correction of angulation needed to restore the vertebral body height can help in selecting those fractures that need anterior column reconstruction but would otherwise have received only less-successful short-segment posterior instrumentation (Figure 6-3).

The presence of a neurologic deficit also plays a key role in selecting the appropriate treatment option. Patients who have a neurologic deficit may or may not have a significant canal compromise with bony elements. This is because the injury to the spinal cord at the instant of maximum deformation of the canal and the velocity of impact of bone hitting the spinal cord can produce an injury that is not fully appreciated at the time the radiographs or CT scans are taken. Trends have been reported by several authors associating greater canal compromise with neurologic injury [6,9]. Decompressing the neural elements can be accomplished indirectly with distraction, a posterolateral transpedicular technique, or a formal anterior intra- or extracavity approach [10–15]. Esses *et al.* [16] compared the two methods of decompression and found that an anterior approach was more efficient in decompressing the canal than a posterior approach. This has been disputed by other surgeons who use primarily posterior instrumentation and achieve canal decompression by fracture reduction and stabilization, infrequently requiring a formal anterior decompression (Figure 6-4) [14]. The technique of decompression is finally left up to the surgeon's training and whether the patient can tolerate the approach, especially anteriorly.

The degrees of angulation measured on the radiograph in a patient lying supine with a thoracolumbar fracture do not truly reflect the angulation the patient will have when sitting or standing. Some increase in angulation is also found in patients treated nonoperatively with a brace [17]. Patients seem to tolerate kyphosis more in the thoracic spine (up to 30°) than in the thoracolumbar spine (up to 20°) [18]. Some controversy still remains about whether the degree of kyphosis is related to the amount of pain at follow-up. The lower the fracture is in the lumbar spine, the lower the chance that the remaining lumbar spine can fully compensate for the kyphosis with hyperextension, which thus increases the chance of low-back pain.

Patients with an incomplete neurologic deficit need to have a decompression of the neural elements with subsequent stabilization and fusion. The anterior approach provides a more direct visualization of the canal and has been shown to be more effective in decompressing the canal (Figure 6-5) [16]. The advantages of the anterior approach are twofold: direct decompression of all offending fracture fragments from the spinal canal and structural support of the anterior column. The disadvantages are increased morbidity when combined with a posterior approach, especially with significant posterior element or ligamentous disruption, and inability to reduce to any significant subluxation when it is present. Anterior decompression can be combined with anterior instrumentation or be supplemented posteriorly [19–25]. Posterolateral transpedicular decompression has been shown to be effective in patients with neurologic deficits [10,14,25]. Advantages of the posterior-only approach include limiting the morbidity to just one approach but has disadvantages of indirect decompression of the canal and less-than-ideal reconstitution of the anterior column. These advantages and disadvantages influence decision making in addition to the training bias of the surgeon and the available support services and facilities.

A patient without a neurologic deficit presenting with a burst fracture with less than 50% compression of the vertebral body, less than 50% canal compromise, and kyphosis less than 20° can be treated in a cast or brace for 3 months. Patients with more than 50% canal compromise have been shown to have a greater chance of developing a neurologic deficit [9]. In terms of complete nonoperative treatment described in the past, prolonged bed rest in today's world is difficult. The treatment should include a hyperextension cast or a well-fitted thoracolumbosacral orthosis after the ileus has resolved. The patient is then braced and monitored with serial radiographs for an average of 3 months.

With greater than 50% vertebral body compression, greater than 50% canal compromise, and more than 20° kyphosis with posterior column disruption, the clinician should consider stabilization and fusion. The need to restore the stability of the spinal column anteriorly after reduction of the burst fracture needs to be determined using criteria such as those described by McCormack *et al.* [8]. Loss of correction and hardware failure has been reported by multiple authors using pedicle screw fixation just one level above and below the level of injury [8,26–29]. Anterior instrumentation and strut grafting can be used in combination not only to restore the body height, thus fortifying the anterior column, but also by limiting the number of segments fused [19,22,23]. The anterior instrumentation should be used cautiously in cases of marked posterior column disruption. Posterior instrumentation with augmentation of the anterior column by transpedicular grafting is another option [26,30,31]. Anterior strut grafting and posterior instrumentation appear to offer the most stable construct and have been reported to give a predictable good result for severe burst fractures with three-column injury (Figure 6-5) [12,32].

The technique of anterior decompression involves a retroperitoneal approach either through the thoracoabdominal approach at the thoracolumbar junction from T10 to L1 or a flank incision for lower lumbar burst fractures. After the fractured vertebral body is dissected out, a complete diskectomy above and below the fracture is performed by doing an annulotomy and then removing the disk using a combination of rongeurs and curets. At this time, an osteotome can be used to debulk most of the fractured body. A curet or bur is used to thin the vertebral body down to the posterior wall. After exposing the vertebral body with a Cobb elevator back to the pedicle and foramen, the posterior wall of the vertebral body is removed by using upside-down curets and pushing the fragments away from the canal. If epidural bleeding is encountered, gel foam and thrombin are helpful in addition to bipolar cautery. After the decompression is performed from pedicle to pedicle and at the end of the vertebral body superiorly and inferiorly, the iliac crest strut can be harvested and placed. Kyphosis can be corrected with a distractor and by pushing at the apex of the kyphosis from the back. The strut graft is impacted in place. Additional bone graft from the vertebral body can be placed anterior to the strut graft for aiding in fusion. At this point, either anterior instrumentation can be placed or the patient can be placed in prone position for posterior instrumentation. Two levels above and below the fractured vertebra need to be instrumented when a combination of hooks, screws, and rods is used. Superiorly, supralaminar hooks can be used and appear to be stronger than transverse process hooks. Two levels of pedicle screws can be used inferiorly. It has been shown that adding another hook significantly reduces the stress on the screw immediately below the fracture level [33]. Some surgeons prefer to place screws above and can obtain short-segment fixation saving levels. The obvious advantage of short-segment fixation is preservation of lumbar motion segments. Anterior instrumentation, such as the Kaneda device and other plates, provides short-segment fixation, but these devices cannot be used with posterior disruption. In such cases, posterior instrumentation needs to supplement the anterior strut grafting. Whether the posterior instrumentation can be short segmented one level above or below, or needs to include two levels above and below, becomes more of an issue in the midlumbar fractures (Figure 6-6). Gurwitz *et al.* [34] have shown that the anterior strut improves the rigidity of the posterior construct when compared with posterior construct alone in short segment constructs. In midlumbar fractures, adding an anterior strut can provide greater stability but this must be balanced with the additional morbidity associated with an anterior approach.

The lower lumbar burst fractures with neurologic deficit can be approached anteriorly at L4 but may be more amenable to posterior decompression, especially at L5 with supplementation from posterior

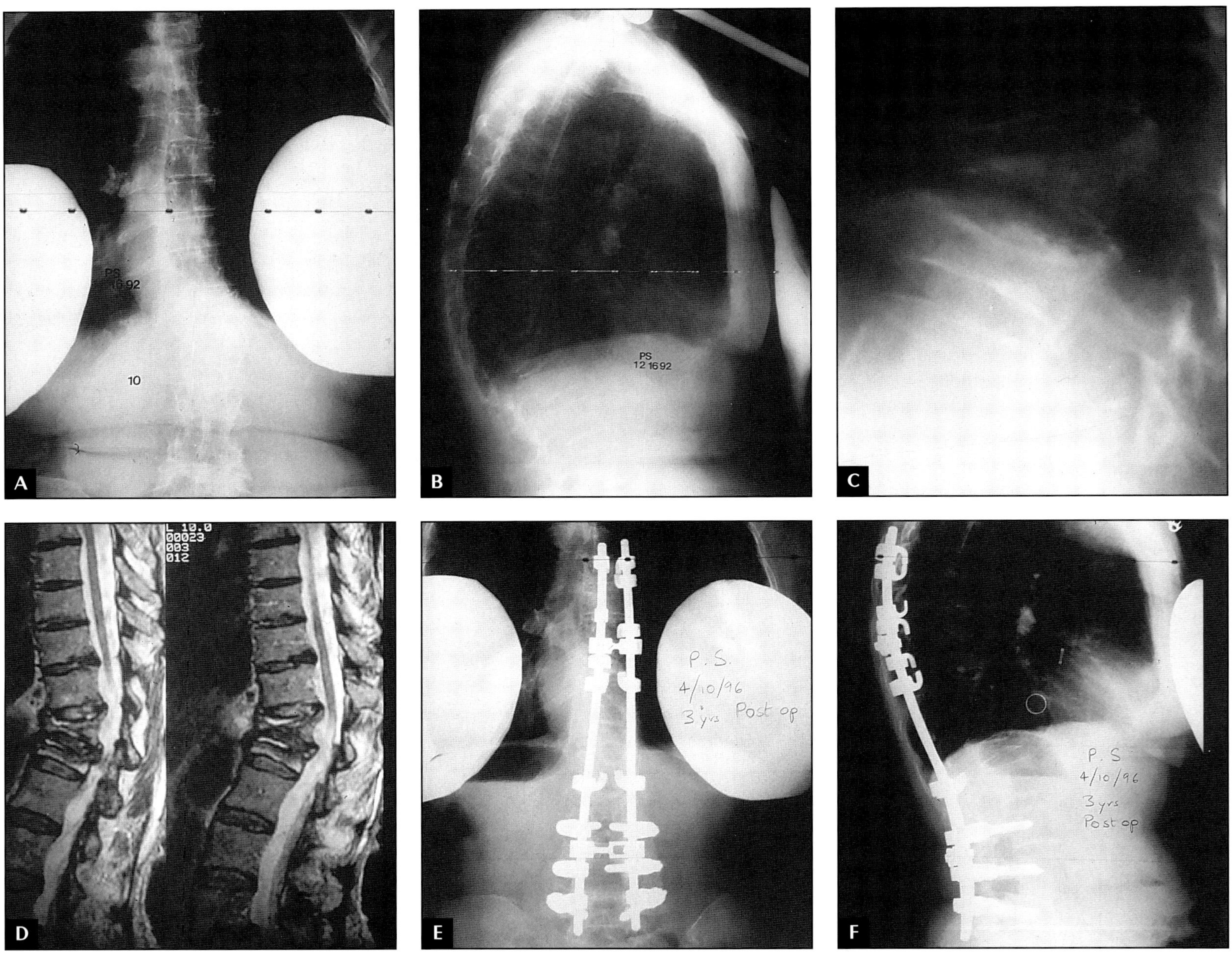

FIGURE 6-4. A–F, Radiographic views from a woman aged 65 years with T12 and L1 compression fractures. Patient was unresponsive to nonoperative measures. She had severe pain over the thoracolumbar region and spinal stenosis from degenerative spondylolisthesis at L4-5. She underwent posterior spinal fusion, instrumentation, and decompression at L4-5 and had resolution of back pain with a solid fusion at 3 years postoperatively.

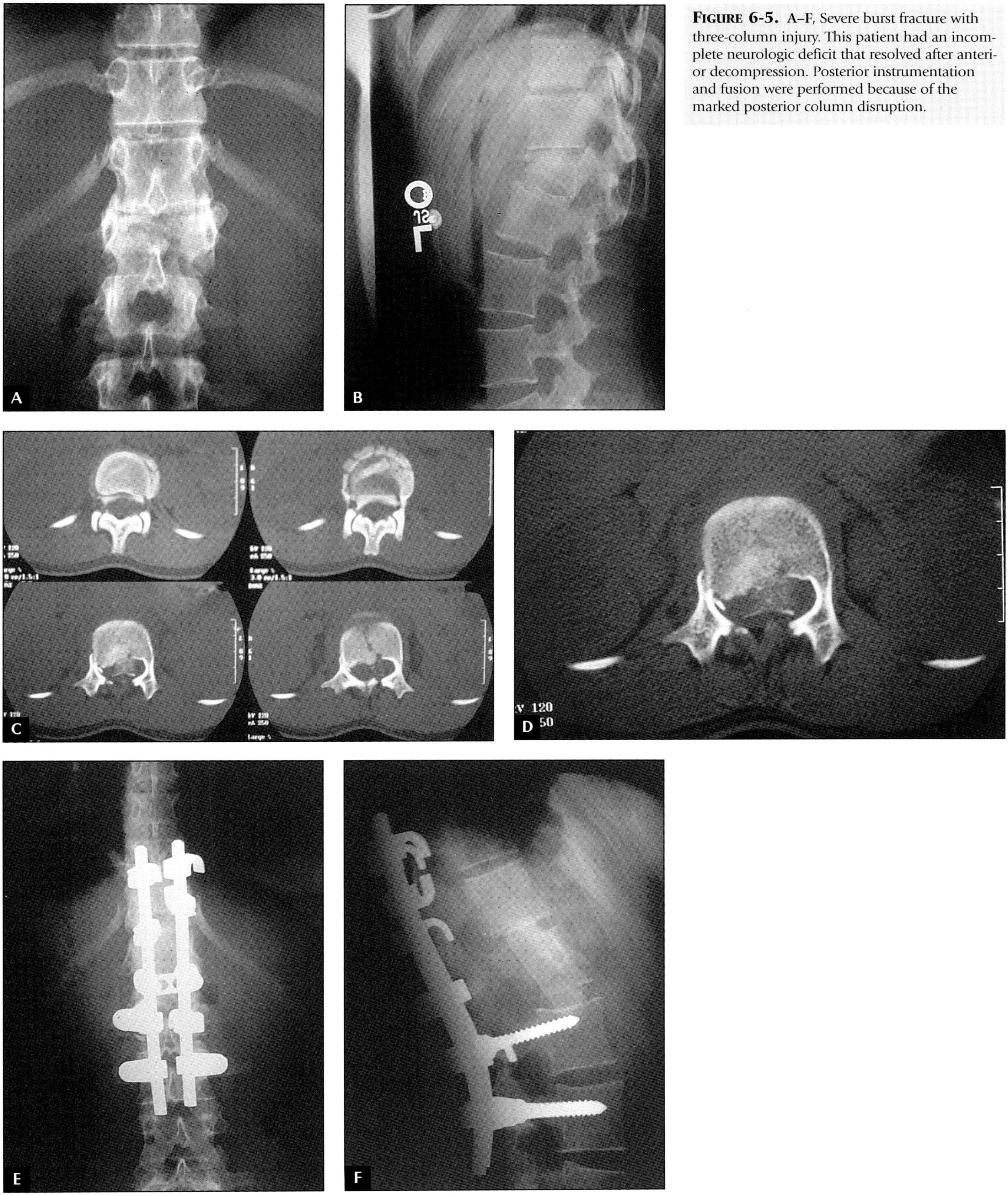

FIGURE 6-5. A–F, Severe burst fracture with three-column injury. This patient had an incomplete neurologic deficit that resolved after anterior decompression. Posterior instrumentation and fusion were performed because of the marked posterior column disruption.

pedicle instrumentation and fusion. Severe burst fracture in the lower lumbar spine can be associated with vertical fractures of the lamina and spinous process. This vertical fracture is associated with dural laceration and entrapment, which need to be decompressed posteriorly [35,36]. Lower lumbar burst fractures without neurologic deficit have been treated successfully with nonoperative care of bed rest and brace treatment with thoracolumbosacral orthosis and a pantaloon extension [17,37]. The lower lumbar burst fractures do not tend to collapse or angulate as much as fracture in the thoracolumbar junction [17]. Long-term results of lower lumbar burst fractures treated with long instrumentation provide greater loss of lordosis and have higher incidence of pain as reported by An *et al.* [38].

Flexion-Distraction Injuries

Flexion-distraction injuries can be of three types: purely osseus, mixed osseus and ligamentous, and purely ligamentous. These injuries usually do not have neurologic deficits but can have a disk herniation, thus giving rise to a deficit. An MRI is helpful in fully delineating the ligamentous damage or presence of a disk herniation leading to a neurologic deficit. On CT scan, the axial images of the involved segments frequently show an empty facet and can show the bony injury through the pedicles or inferior part of the body on a sagittal reconstruction. The pure osseus injury originally described as a Chance fracture can be successfully treated with

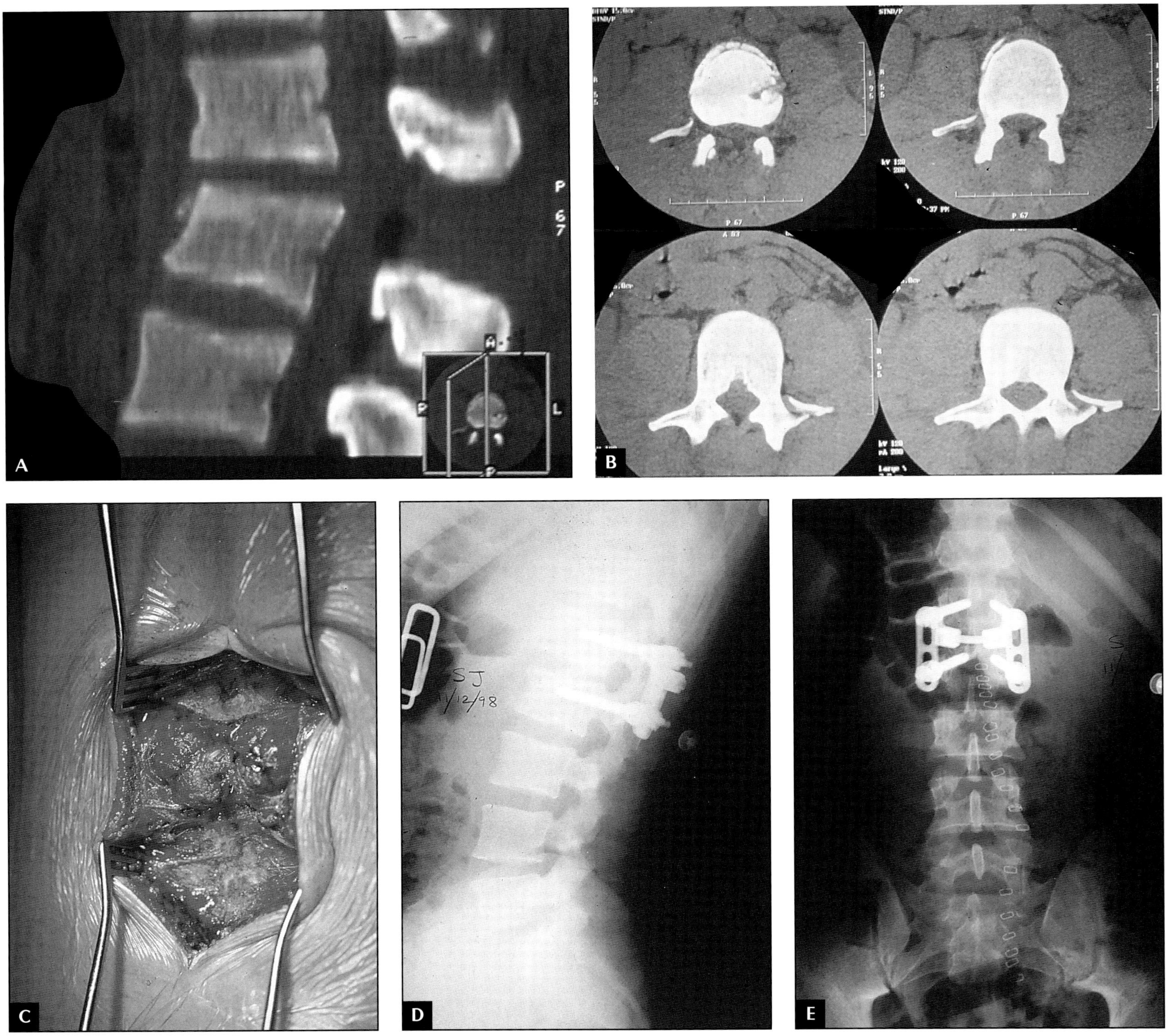

Figure 6-6. A–E, This patient was involved in an airplane crash and suffered a flexion-distraction injury because of the seat belt. Marked disruption of the fascia with muscle herniation is present. Short-segment compression and posterior instrumentation were performed.

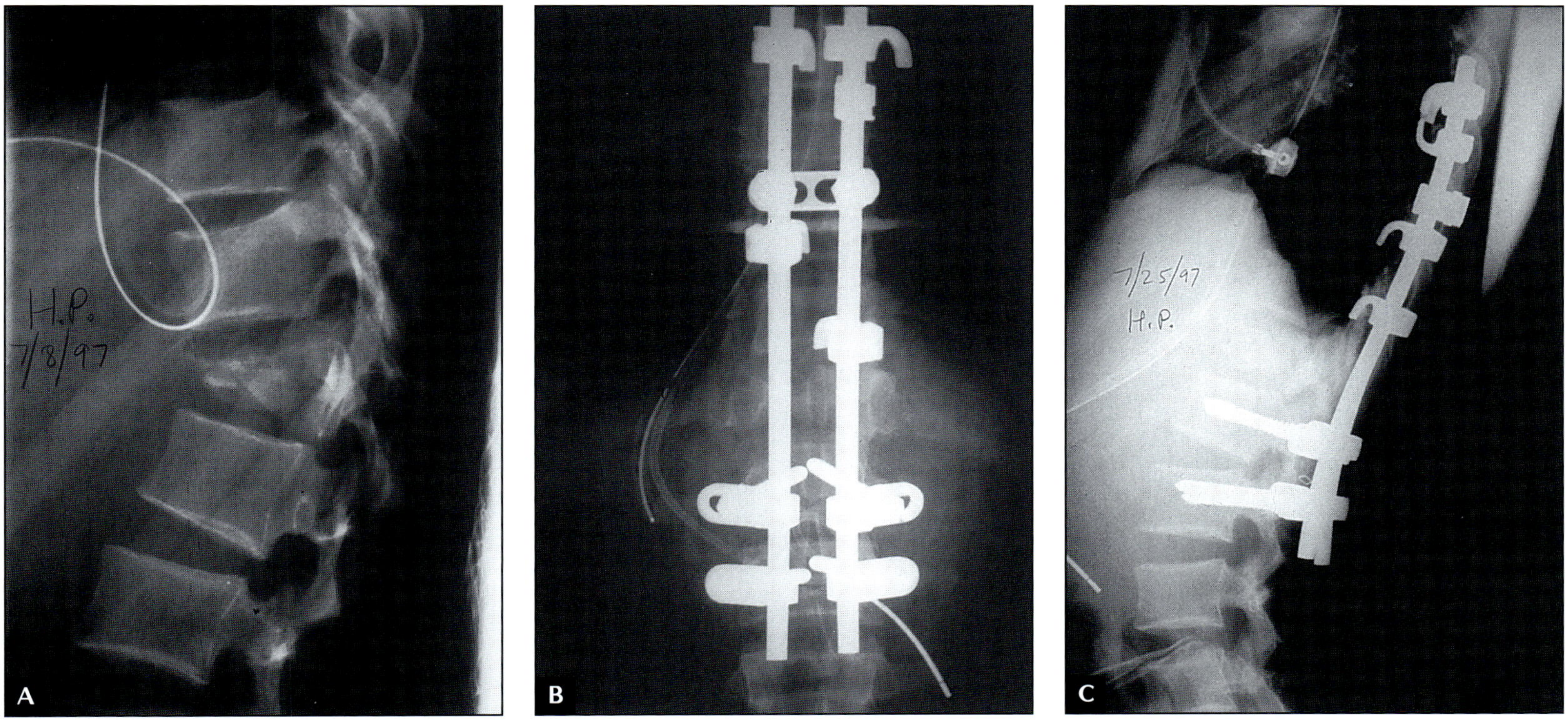

FIGURE 6-7. A–C, This fracture-dislocation was reduced with posterior segmented instrumentation.

nonoperative measures, such as a cast or a brace, for 3 months. The mixed ligamentous injury must be assessed individually as to the amount of ligamentous damage and percentage of bony apposition that could be obtained if treated nonoperatively. These injuries can be treated successfully with short-segment compression instrumentation. If the axis of rotation in a flexion-distraction injury is in the posterior portion of the vertebral body, compression of the vertebral body is possible. Purely ligamentous injuries should be treated with short-segment compression instrumentation (Figure 6-6).

FRACTURE-DISLOCATIONS

Fracture-dislocations of the spine occur with mechanisms of flexion rotation, shear, and flexion-distraction [2]. These injuries are highly unstable and usually accompanied by neurologic deficit. In the thoracic spine, fractures can be seen at multiple levels and can be fully evaluated using a CT scan. The translation present on AP and lateral radiographs are pathognomonic for fracture-dislocation. The goal in these injuries is to stabilize the spine with multiple levels of fixation above and below the area of the injury and combine it with early rehabilitation to decrease overall morbidity and mortality from this injury. In cases with an incomplete deficit, especially in the thoracolumbar region, a posterior alignment procedure with instrumentation should be performed first, followed by an anterior decompression if necessary. In the thoracic spine, hook and rod systems with segmental fixation should be used at multiple segments above and below to provide stability (Figure 6-7). In the thoracolumbar region, hooks can be used in the thoracic spine and screws in the lumbar spine to provide stability. The reduction of these fracture-dislocations has to be individualized to the mechanism of the fracture. Placing the patient prone on the four-poster frame usually helps to align the spine somewhat. Final reduction of the spine can be achieved by first placing the proximal fixation and then using cantilever mechanism, especially for the flexion-rotation injury to reduce the kyphosis by bringing the rod to the screws that are placed in the lumbar spine.

CONCLUSIONS

Thoracolumbar fractures can be treated effectively with the newer anterior instrumentation and posterior segmental spinal instrumentation systems. When possible, short-segment instrumentation should be used to save motion segments. The success of nonoperative treatments of certain fractures should not be forgotten in the enthusiasm of using new instrumentation and techniques. The next step in thoracolumbar fracture treatment would be to achieve the ability to enhance neural recovery from potentially devastating spinal cord injuries.

REFERENCES AND RECOMMENDED READING

Recently published papers of particular interest have been highlighted as:

- • Of interest
- •• Of outstanding interest

1. Holdsworth F: Fractures, dislocations, and fracture-dislocations of the spine. *J Bone Joint Surg Am* 1970, 52:1534–1551.
2. Denis F: The three column spine and its significance in the classification of acute thoracolumbar spine injuries. *Spine* 1983, 8:817–831.
3. James K, Wenger K, Schlegel J, Dunn H: Biomechanical evaluation of the stability of thoracolumbar burst fractures. *Spine* 1994, 19:1731–1740.
4. Gertzbein S: Thoracolumbar trauma: a new classification of thoracic and lumbar injuries. *Semin Spine Surg* 1995, 7:70–90.

5. Dall B, Stauffer E: Neurologic injury and recovery patterns in the burst fracture at the T12 or L1 motion segment. *Clin Orthop* 1988, 233:171–176.
6. Kim N, Lee H, Chun I: Neurologic injury and recovery in patients with burst fracture of the thoracolumbar spine. *Spine* 1999, 24:290–294.
7. Weisel SW, Boden SD: Classification of thoracic and lumbar fractures. In *Spine Surgery: Thoracolumbar Trauma*. Edited by Hanley EN Jr. Philadelphia: WB Saunders; 1995:73.
8. McCormack T, Karaikovic E, Gaines R: The load sharing classification of spine fractures. *Spine* 1994, 19:1741–1744.
9. Trafton P, Boyd C: Computed tomography of thoracic and lumbar spine injuries. *J Trauma* 1984, 24:506–515.
10. Garfin S, Mowery C, Guerra J, *et al.*: Confirmation of the posterolateral technique to decompress and fuse thoracolumbar spine burst fractures. *Spine* 1985, 10:218–223.
11. Whitesides T, Shah S: On the management of unstable fractures of the thoracolumbar spine: rationale for use of anterior decompression and fusion and posterior stabilization. *Spine* 1976, 1:99–107.
12. Dimar J, Wilde P, Glassman S, *et al.*: Thoracolumbar burst fractures treated with combined anterior and posterior surgery. *Am J Orthop* 1996:159–165.
13. Bohlman H, Eismont F: Surgical techniques of anterior decompression and fusion for spinal cord injuries. *Clin Orthop* 1981, 154:57–67.
14. Sjostrom L, Karlstrom G, Pech P, *et al.* Indirect spinal canal decompression in burst fractures treated with pedicle screw instrumentation. *Spine* 1996, 21:113–123.
15. DeWald L: Burst fractures of the thoracic and lumbar spine. *Clin Orthop* 1984, 189:150–161.
16. Esses S, Botsford D, Kostuik J: Evaluation of surgical treatment for burst fractures. *Spine* 1990, 15:667–673.
17. Mumford J, Weinstein J, Spratt K, *et al.* Thoracolumbar burst fractures. *Spine* 1993, 18:955–970.
18. Grimes P, Vaccaro A, Garfin S: Treatment complications of thoracolumbar spine trauma. *Semin Spine* 1995, 7:141–151.
19. Ghanayem A, Zdeblick TA: Anterior instrumentation in the management of thoracolumbar burst fractures. *Clin Orthop* 1997, 335:89–100.
20. Dunn H: Anterior stabilization of thoracolumbar injuries. *Clin Orthop* 1984, 189:116–124.
21. Okuyama K, Abe E, Chiba M, *et al.*: Outcome of anterior decompression and stabilization for thoracolumbar unstable burst fractures in the absence of neurologic deficits. *Spine* 1996, 21:620–625.
22. Kaneda K, Abumi K, Fujiya M: Burst fractures with neurologic deficits of the thoracolumbar-lumbar spine: Results of anterior decompression and stabilization with anterior instrumentation. *Spine* 1984, 9:788–795.
23. Kostuik J: Anterior fixation for burst fractures of the thoracic and lumbar spine with or without neurological involvement. *Spine* 1988, 13:286–293.
24. Kostuik J: Anterior spinal cord decompression for lesions of the thoracic and lumbar spine, techniques, new methods of internal fixation results. *Spine* 1983, 8:512–531.
25. Kirkpatrick J, Wilber R, Likavec M, *et al.*: Anterior stabilization of thoracolumbar burst fractures using the Kandea device: a preliminary report. *Orthopedics* 1995, 18:673–678.
26. Daniaux H, Seykora P, Genelin A, *et al.*: Application of posterior plating and modifications in thoracolumbar spine injuries. *Spine* 1991, 16:S125–133.
27. McLain R, Sparling E, Benson D: Early failure of short-segment pedicle instrumentation of thoracolumbar fractures. *J Bone Joint Surg Am* 1993, 75:162–167.
28. Louis C, Gauthier V, Louis R: Posterior approach with Louis plates for fractures of the thoracolumbar and lumbar spine with and without neurologic deficits. *Spine* 1998, 23:2030–2039.
29. Carl A, Tromanhauser S, Roger D: Pedicle screw instrumentation for thoracolumbar burst fractures and fracture-dislocation. *Spine* 1992, 17:S317–S324.
30. Ebelke D, Asher M, Neff J,*et al.*: Survivorship analysis of VSP spine instrumentation in the treatment of thoracolumbar and lumbar burst fractures. *Spine* 1991, 16:S428–S432.
31. Dick W, Kluger P, Magerl F, *et al.*: A new device for internal fixation of thoracolumbar and lumbar spine fractures: the "Fixateur Interne." *Paraplegia* 1985, 23:228–232.
32. Schnee C, Ansell L: Selection criteria and outcome of operative approaches for thoracolumbar burst fractures with and without neurological deficit. *J Neurosurg* 1997, 86:48–55.
33. Yerby S, Ehteshami J, McLain R: Offset laminar hooks decrease bending moments of pedicle screws during in situ contouring. *Spine* 1997, 22:379–381.
34. Gurwitz G, Dawson J, McNamara M, *et al.*: Biomechanical analysis of three surgical approaches for lumbar burst fractures using short-segment instrumentation. *Spine* 1993, 18:977–982.
35. Pickett J, Blumenkopf: Dural lacerations and thoracolumbar fractures. *J Spinal Disorders* 1989, 2:99–103.
36. Denis F, Burkus J: Diagnosis and treatment of cauda equina entrapment in the vertical lamina fracture of lumbar burst fractures. *Spine* 1991, 16:S433–439.
37. Chan D, Seng N, Kann K: Nonoperative treatment in burst fractures of the lumbar spine (L2–L5) without neurologic deficits. *Spine* 1993, 18:320–325.
38. An H, Simpson J, Ebraheim N, *et al.*: Low lumbar burst fractures: comparison between conservative and surgical treatments. *Orthopedics* 1992, 15:367–376.

SECTION III

Fractures of the Pelvis and Acetabulum

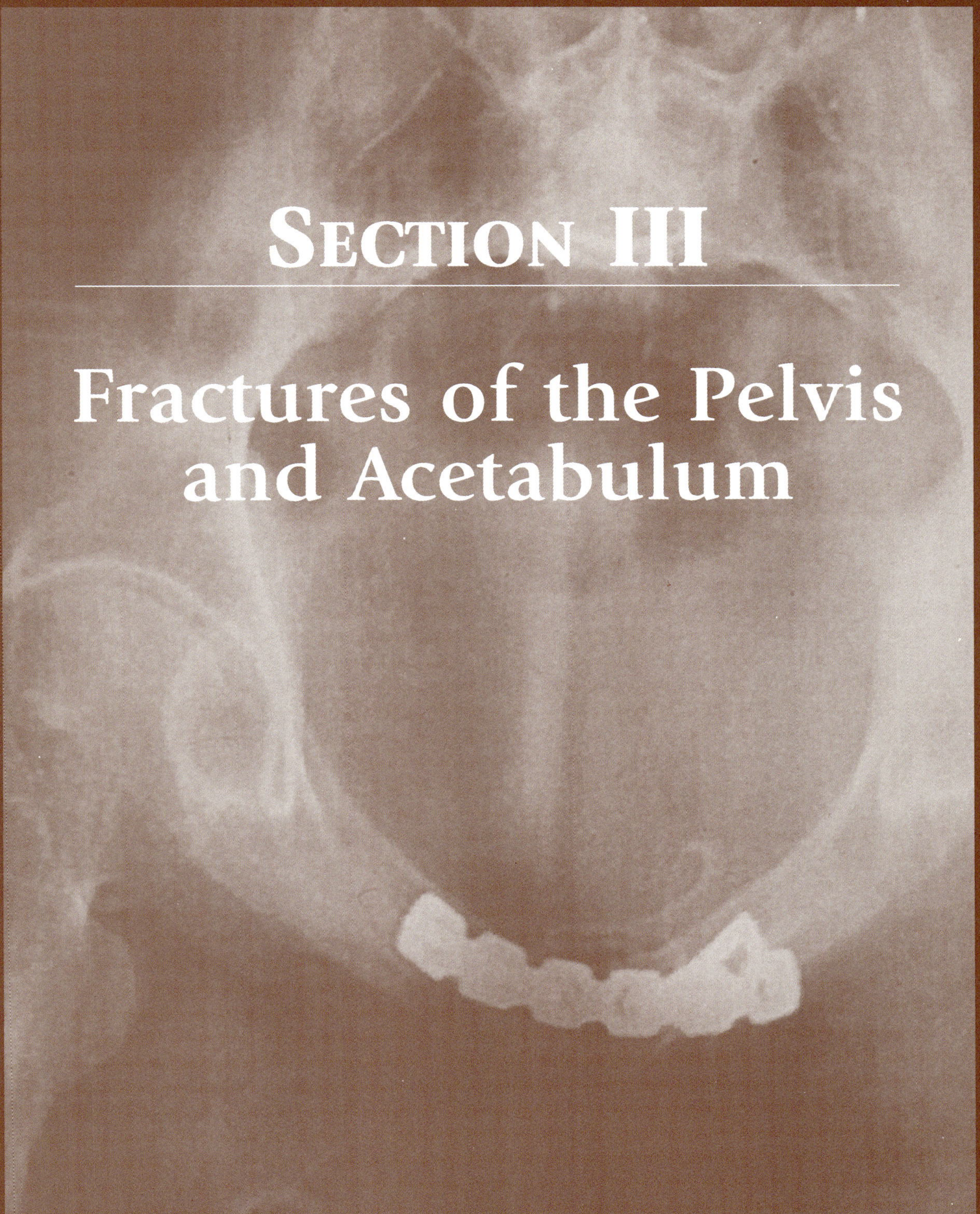

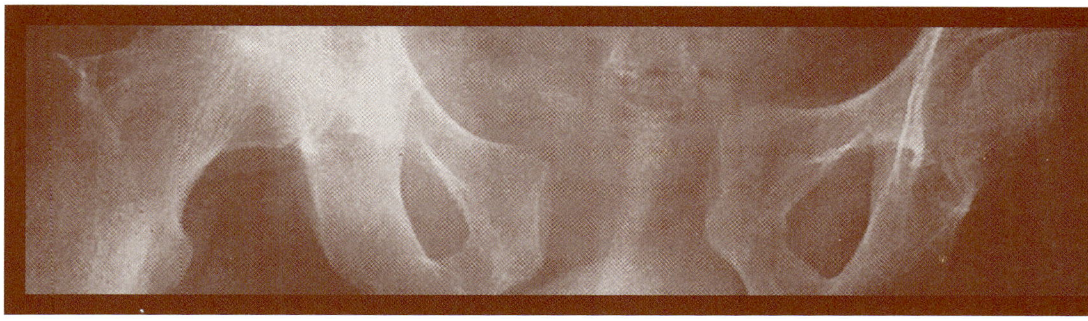

7

Current Diagnosis and Management of Pelvic Ring Fractures

Kenneth A. Egol
James F. Kellam

DIAGNOSIS

Mechanism of Injury

As with most types of fractures, the history of the injury leads the treating physician down certain algorithmic paths. The kinetic energy associated with the injury is the first point of concern. Is the patient a young person involved in a high-speed motorcycle crash or is the patient a frail, elderly person who fell from standing height on the sidewalk? Clearly, the low-energy pelvic fracture suffered by the elderly patient has different implications in the acute phase compared with the high-energy pelvic disruption.

In the high-energy blunt polytrauma patient, mechanism of injury has significant prognostic implications for morbidity and mortality [1,2]. Patients who are involved in motor vehicle crashes are more likely to sustain a lateral compression-type fracture (inherently more stable fracture patterns) with a mortality of between 6.6% and 13.4%. These patients are likely to die from associated head or abdominal trauma [1,2]. Motorcyclists or pedestrians who are struck by motor vehicles are more likely to sustain unstable types of pelvic fractures. The mortality rate in these patients ranges from 20% to 26% with the cause of death related to hemorrhage associated with pelvic vascular injuries [1,2]. Falls from a height are more likely to produce a vertically unstable fracture pattern, with mortality rates from 0% to 25% also related to pelvic and visceral injuries [1,2].

Physical Examination

Physical examination of the high-energy blunt polytrauma victim differs little from that made in the elderly to assess their low-energy fracture pattern. The resuscitation phase of treatment, if needed, occurs simultaneously with the diagnostic phase. Examination of pelvic stability involves inspection and palpation. The flank is inspected for signs of contusion or hematoma indicative of significant retroperitoneal bleeding. Scrotal hematoma indicates severe anterior injury with disruption of the genitourinary floor [3]. Deformity is assessed by measurement of leg length discrepancy and rotational deformity. Open wounds are important because they may indicate an open fracture. Following inspection, palpation of the area of injury is carried out to determine soft tissue disruption, bony gap, and hematoma. All male patients should have a rectal examination to assess the prostate and female patients ought undergo a pelvic speculum examination [3–6].

Applying internal and external rotational forces to the iliac crests to determine whether the pelvis opens or closes assesses rotational instability of the pelvis. A senior member of the trauma team should perform this maneuver. If gross instability is demonstrated, no further manipulation of the pelvis should be attempted to avoid disrupting any pelvic clots that may have formed. If the examination cannot be performed in the trauma department, an examination under anesthesia is advisable [7]. Neurologic examination of the extremities is mandatory to determine whether the lumbosacral plexus has been injured.

Classification

Although a detailed classification of pelvic ring injuries is beyond the scope of this chapter, it is necessary to discuss the comprehensive classification in order to understand management principles. According to Tile [8] (Figure 7-1), Type A fractures preserve the bony and ligamentous integrity of the posterior pelvic complex and the pelvic floor. These include avulsion fractures, iliac wing fractures, and transverse sacral fractures (Figure 7-2). Because these iliac fractures do not involve the posterior weight-bearing arch of the pelvis, they are stable and thus require only symptomatic care. The transverse sacral injury may need reduction and sacral root decompression if the fracture displacement appears to be such that the sacral roots are being clinically compromised.

Type B fractures are incomplete disruptions of the posterior pelvic complex. These fractures include internal (lateral compression) and external rotational injuries (open book) to the hemipelvis. Depending on the magnitude and direction of force, these injuries exhibit a range of rotational instability (Figure 7-2).

Type C fractures encompass those fractures that exhibit rotational as well as translational instability. These fractures are associated with complete bony or ligamentous disruption of the posterior pelvic complex and the pelvic floor. These fractures generally require operative stabilization. Denis [9] has further classified the sacral fractures associated with a pelvic ring injury [10,11]. Zone 1 includes fractures through the sacral ala. They have an incidence of neural injury up to 24%, usually involving the fifth lumbar root. Zone II fractures are through the foraminal region of the sacrum. There is a higher incidence of neurologic injury with these fractures than Zone I. Zone III fractures traverse the interforaminal area and include the transverse fracture. They have the highest incidence of neurologic injury [10,12].

It must be remembered that this subclassification of sacral fracture is part of the overall pelvic injury. Treatment decision will be determined by the fracture and injury personality as outlined in the comprehensive classification.

Radiographic Assessment

Radiographic evaluation of the pelvis is critical in making the diagnosis. Before definitive fixation decisions can be made, a complete radiographic assessment of the pelvis is done. A single anteroposterior (AP) pelvic radiograph, commonly obtained during the initial resuscitation phase, is used in most trauma centers to determine the presence or absence of pelvic ring stability. If displacement has occurred posteriorly, major bleeding should be suspected and resuscitation continued [8]. Further understanding of the injury is obtained from inlet and outlet views of the pelvis as well as a computed tomography (CT) scan to completely define the injury pattern and displacement [4,8].

The AP radiograph is taken with the patient supine and the x-ray beam directed from midpelvis to the floor. Anterior ring fractures are obvious on this view; however, posterior injuries are often more subtle. Signs of potential pelvic instability include bilateral pelvic injuries, avulsion fractures of the L5 transverse processes or the ischial spine, and vertical pubic rami fractures [8].

The inlet view is taken with the patient supine and the x-ray beam angled 60° caudally, perpendicular to the pelvic brim. This view demonstrates AP displacement, as well as rotational deformity, very nicely [4,6,8,13]. Furthermore, sacral crush fractures seen as interruption of the arcuate line are visible as well [4]. The outlet view is taken with the patient supine and the x-ray beam directed 45° cranially. This radiographic view is useful in determining vertical migration of the hemipelvis. In addition, fractures horizontal or vertical through the sacral foramina are visualized. Oblique radiographs of the sacroiliac joint may be obtained; however, the advent of CT has replaced these views. In addition, CT has enhanced assessment and diagnosis of posterior pelvic ring injuries. Two- and three-dimensional reconstruction has

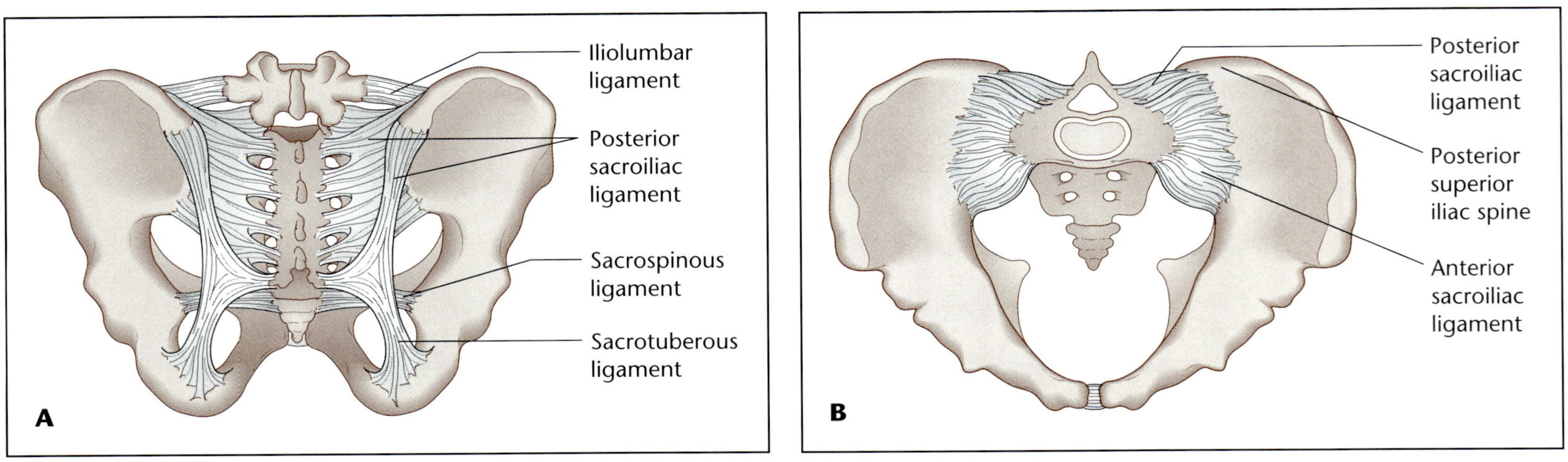

Figure 7-1. A, Strong ligamentous support of the posterior pelvis. B, Anterior and posterior sacroiliac ligaments.

greatly improved visualization and understanding of the displaced posterior pelvic ring; in particular, it has improved visualization of the injury to the sacrum or sacroiliac joints as either impacted and stable or displaced and unstable.

MANAGEMENT

Indications for Stabilization

Absolute indications for acute stabilization of pelvic fractures include acute hemorrhagic blood loss in association with rotational or translational instability of the pelvic ring and open pelvic fractures into the perineum. A relative indication for pelvic stabilization in the acute phase includes the multiply injured patient with associated fractures. In this case, external fixation of the pelvis may help control pain, aid in mobilization, and facilitate nursing care. Absolute indications for delayed stabilization of the pelvic ring include displacement of the symphysis greater than 2.5 to 3.0 cm; displaced sacroiliac dislocations and fracture dislocations; severe rotational deformity resulting in the inability to reach neutral limb position; and translational injury with a resultant leg length discrepancy of greater than 2 cm. Relative indications for delayed stabilization include a locked symphysis pubis, impingement of sacral nerves, tilt fractures, and a sacral fracture with a gap of greater than 5 mm (*ie,* with a potential for nonunion [4,6,8,13–17].

Generally, sacral fractures associated with pelvic ring injuries are treated as part of the pelvic ring injury. The displaced transverse sacral fracture with neurologic injury usually requires reduction, decompression, and stabilization to improve the chance of neurologic recovery [10,11].

Hemodynamically Unstable Patient

General assessment of the hemodynamically unstable patient with a presumed pelvic fracture starts with the resuscitative effort following the standard Advanced Trauma Life Support Program protocol (Figure 7-3). Key to management of the pelvic injury in these patients is determination of pelvic fracture pattern

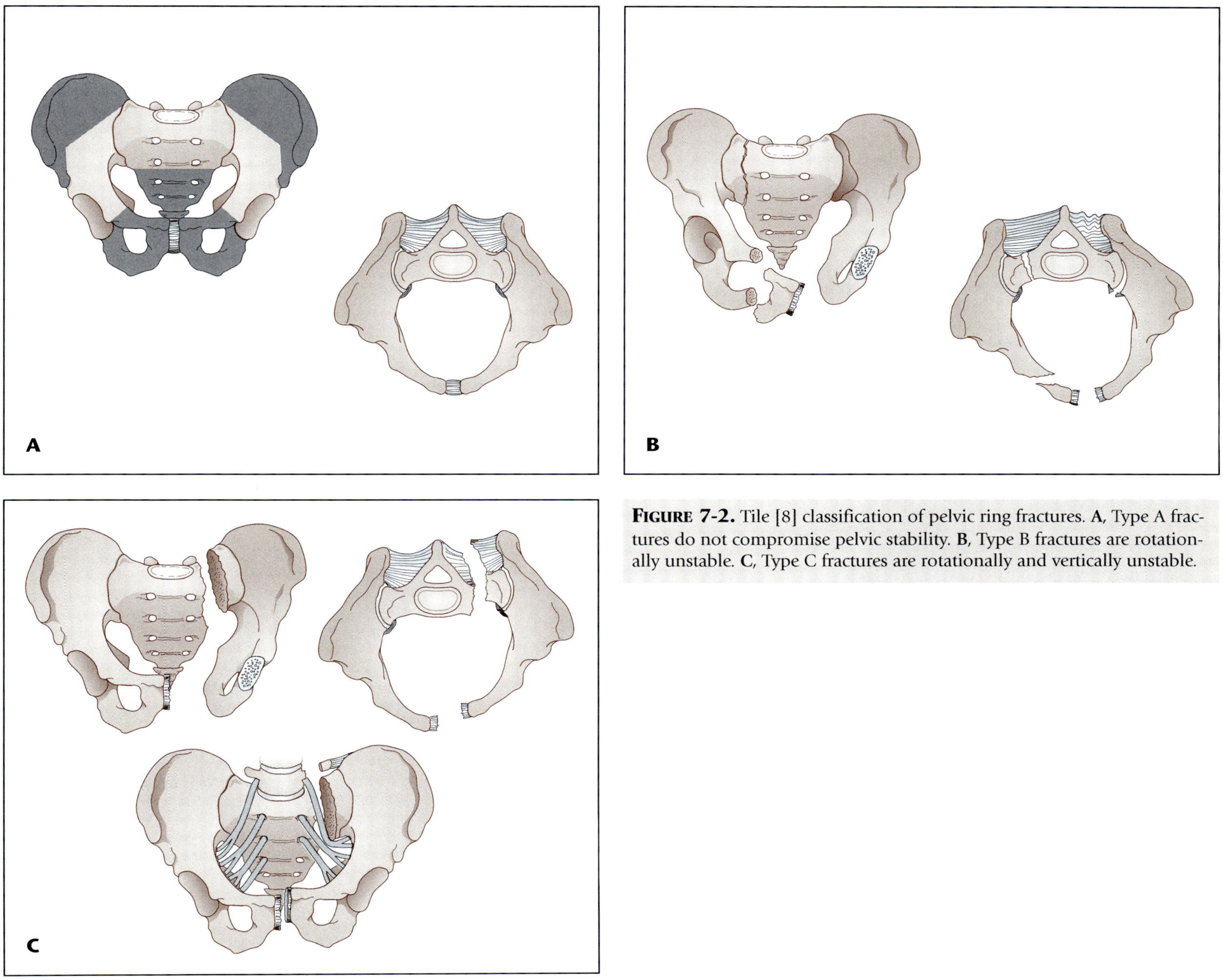

Figure 7-2. Tile [8] classification of pelvic ring fractures. **A,** Type A fractures do not compromise pelvic stability. **B,** Type B fractures are rotationally unstable. **C,** Type C fractures are rotationally and vertically unstable.

instability and its contribution to the overall status of the patient. After airway and breathing have been stabilized, care of the circulatory system is mandatory. If the patient is in decompensated hypovolemic shock, the source of bleeding must be found and corrected. Five potential sites of blood loss exist in the polytrauma patient: the chest, the abdomen, the retroperitoneum, the extremity in the case of a long bone fracture, and onto the floor in the case of any open wounds. Continued hemodynamic instability in the face of a rotationally or completely unstable pelvic fracture requires determination of the presence of intra-abdominal bleeding. If positive for blood, a laparotomy and stabilization of the pelvis on an emergency basis is required to control the bleeding. If negative, then noninvasive pelvic stabilization and arteriography are performed on an urgent basis [4,12,18,19].

Several options exist for rapid stabilization of the pelvis in the emergency department. The pneumatic antishock garment is an inflatable device that is placed over the lower extremities and abdomen and works by increasing peripheral resistance. This device cannot be used on a long-term basis (*ie*, more than 2 hours) because of concern about compartment syndromes in the legs. Another simple modality is the vacuum beanbag. The beanbag is placed around the pelvis to close down an externally rotated pelvis and thus decrease pelvic volume. This technique is an excellent temporary stabilizer that allows for patient transport from the emergency department to the CT scanner and to the operating room (Figure 7-4). If no other alternative is available, a sheet wrapped circumferentially around the patient can accomplish something of the same result [5]. A more invasive and technically challenging way to control the pelvis is application of the pelvic resuscitative clamp [16]. The C-clamp device is applied to the posterior pelvis at the level of the sacroiliac joints and achieves a reduction of the displaced posterior pelvis. These clamps require some expertise in application. The standard method for controlling the unstable hemipelvis in the hemodynamically unstable patient is application of an anterior external fixator. Usually, this is performed in the operating room within 20 to 30 minutes of arrival; however, it can be applied in the emergency department if proper facilities and equipment are available. These techniques are more effective if longitudinal traction is applied prior to their application. This is best done through skeletal traction with a tibial or femoral traction pin and 20 to 30 lb of weight (Figure 7-5).

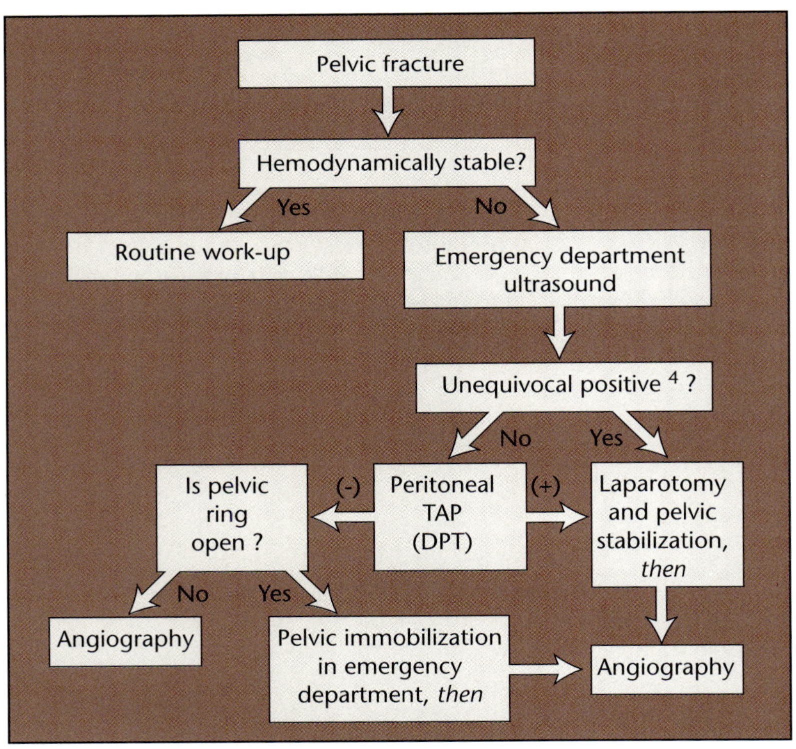

Figure 7-3. Algorithm for emergency department management of patients with a suspected pelvic injury.

Further decision making is guided by the patient's response to resuscitation [19]. If hemodynamic stability is not obtained with placement of the external fixator, angiography is indicated to determine the source of the bleeding and coil any potential bleeders. If angiography is readily available around the clock, angiography before external fixation may be considered. With the patient stabilized, reassessment with regards to definitive management is made (Figure 7-4).

Hemodynamically Stable Patient—Unstable Fracture Pattern

If the patient with a pelvic ring disruption is hemodynamically stable on arrival or following resuscitation and acute stabilization, reassessment of the pelvic injury must be undertaken. History, physical examination, and a complete radiographic assessment including CT scan are required to fully establish fracture pattern stability. The timing of stabilization is determined when the fracture is fully defined, the patient is physiologically stable, and the appropriate equipment and facilities are available.

In the rotationally unstable open-book pelvic fracture, treatment options include reduction and treatment with the external fixator or open reduction and internal fixation with plates and screws. The key to external fixation of the pelvis is secure placement of the pins into the iliac crest. In the procedure, two or three 5-mm (diameter) pins should be used, each spaced 1 cm apart to increase stability. The pins should be placed between the inner and outer tables of the pelvis in the thick anterior half of the pelvis. Following fluoroscopic verification of pin placement, the frame can be constructed. The hemipelvis is reduced manually and the frame tightened. Inlet and outlet fluoroscopic images confirm the reduction (Figure 7-4).

Open reduction and internal fixation of the symphysis is accomplished through a Pfannansteil incision (Figure 7-4). Before surgery, a Foley catheter is placed to decompress the bladder. After exposure is complete, a reduction clamp is used to reduce the disruption. Choice of fixation with a stable posterior injury is either a 2- or 4-hole plate across the reduced symphysis. If the posterior complex is disrupted and requires stabilization, similar plates may be used across the symphysis. The size of plate should match the patient's pelvis (either a 3.5-mm or 4.5-mm plate and appropriately sized screws). However, if posterior instability will not be addressed and the only fixation will be anterior, some authors recommend two plates at 90° from each other (Figure 7-4).

Fixation of the posterior pelvic complex can be achieved anteriorly, posteriorly, or through percutaneous means. Advantages of the anterior approach include excellent visualization of the sacroiliac joint for reduction (Figure 7-6). The disadvantage is risk to the L5 nerve root and potential malrotation in the reduction. The advantage of the posterior approach is the ease of exposure of the iliac wing or sacroiliac joint. The disadvantage is the need to place the fixation into the sacral ala under image control with anterior neurovascular structures at risk. The anterior approach is not indicated for sacral fractures or in cases where a colostomy or suprapubic catheter might cause a high risk for infection. Because of the potential soft tissue complications with the posterior approach through crushed tissue, the concept of percutaneous placement of iliosacral screws is an excellent option. This technique is suitable for sacroiliac dislocations and sacral fractures. The screw must start on the outer table of the iliac wing and cross the sacroiliac joint into the S1 body. A thorough understanding of the bony and neurovascular anatomy is needed to perform the procedure safely (Figure 7-7). An adequate reduction must also be obtained, either closed or open [4–7,15,17]. Sacral fractures are stabilized with either percutaneous or open iliosacral screws. Plate stabilization of sacral fractures is performed using a 4.5-mm reconstruction plate contoured to fit across the dorsal aspect of the sacral lamina and down the outer aspect of the posterior iliac tubercles (Figure 7-8). The use

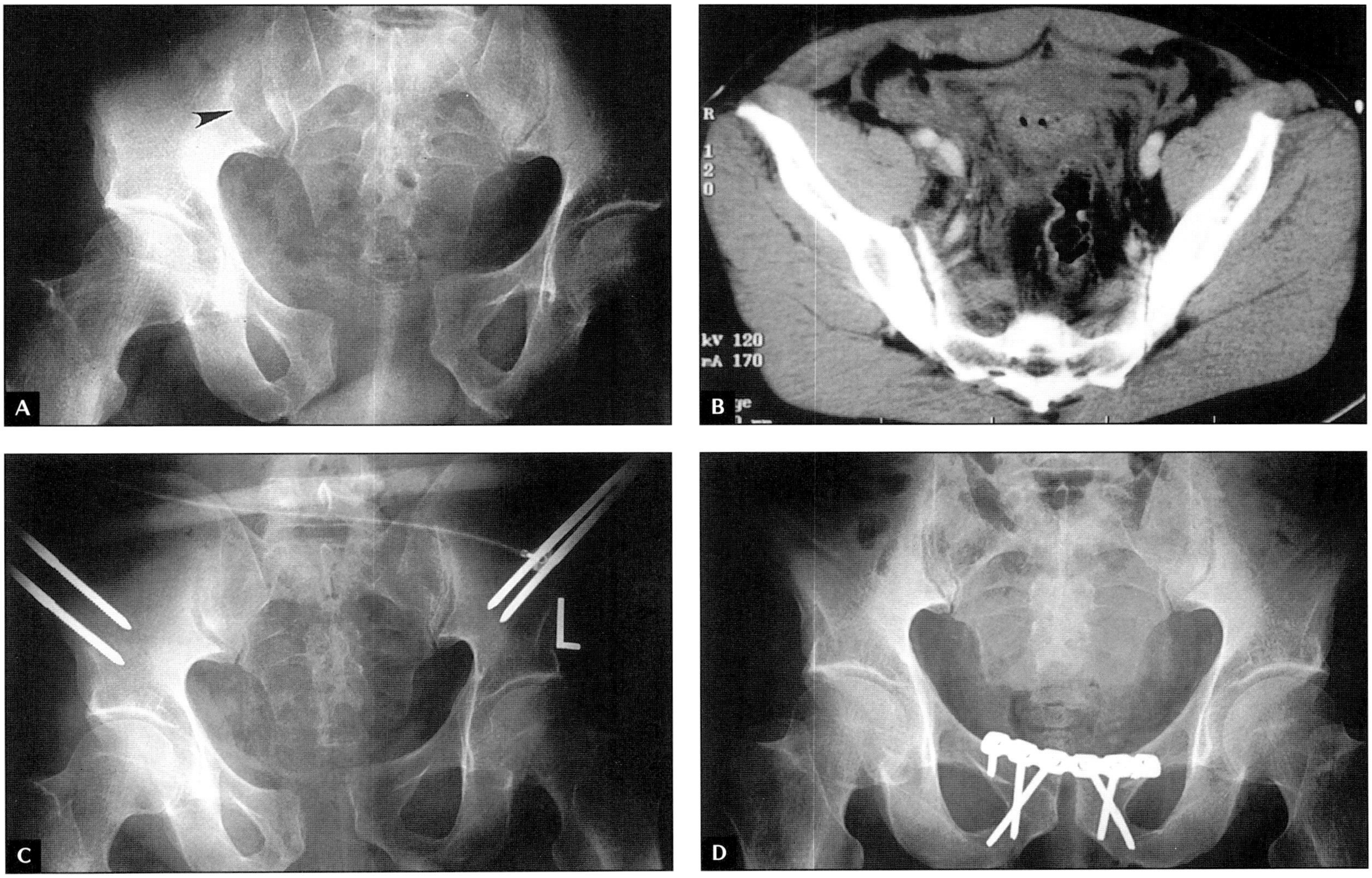

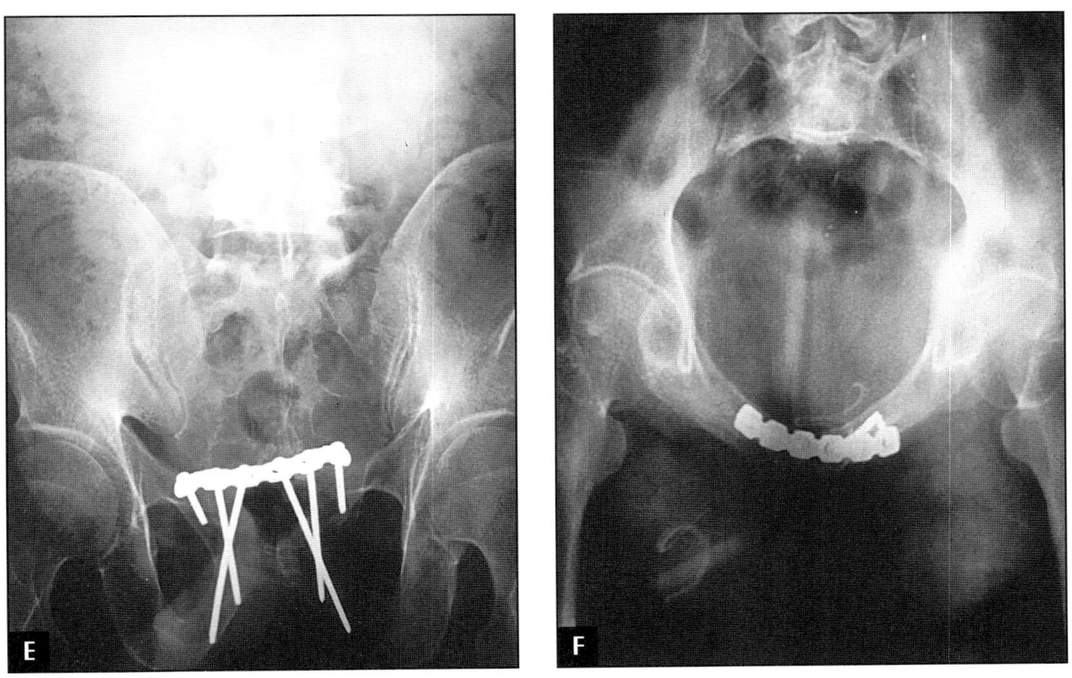

FIGURE 7-4. Radiographs of a man aged 42 years who was involved in a motorcycle accident. The patient was hemodynamically unstable. **A**, Anteroposterior radiograph demonstrating an open book injury with a displaced sacroiliac joint on the right (*arrowhead*). The patient was immediately placed in a circumferential beanbag and became stable. **B**, Computed tomography scan demonstrating the pelvis closed down in the back with the beanbag in place. **C**, A temporary external fixator was placed following a negative angiogram. **D–F**, When the patient's condition improved, he was taken for definitive symphyseal fixation.

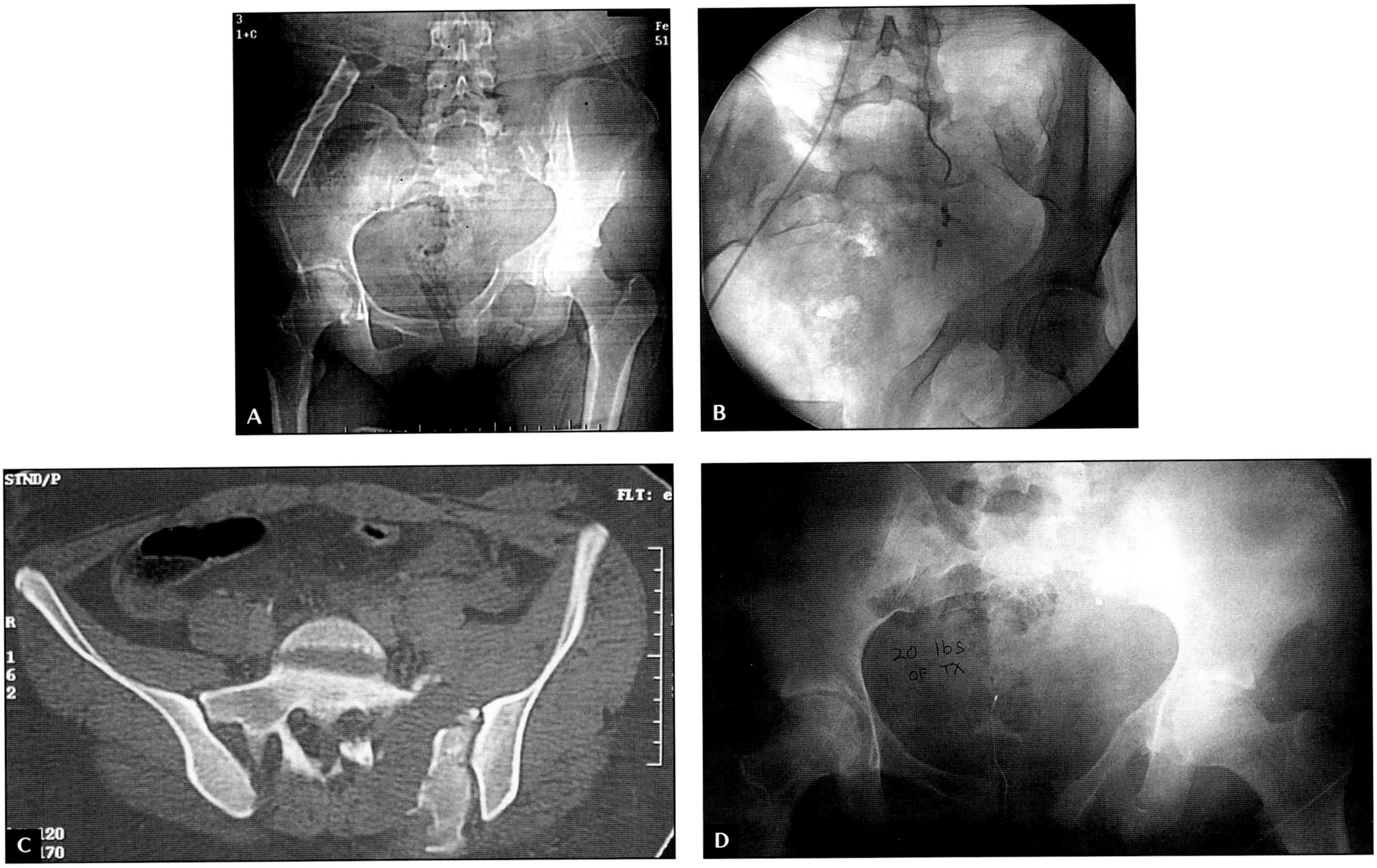

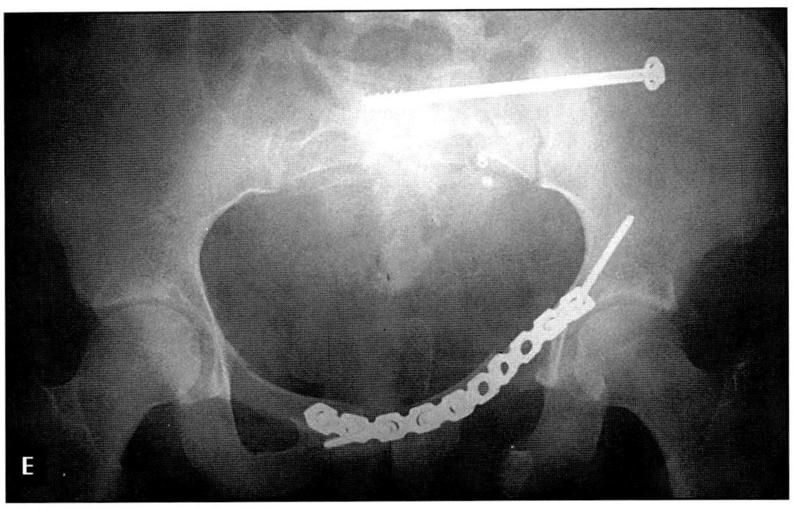

FIGURE 7-5. Hemodynamically unstable woman aged 18 years who was involved in a motor vehicle accident. Anteroposterior radiograph (**A**) demonstrates a vertically unstable fracture pattern. The patient was taken to angiography, where she was found to have an injured internal iliac artery. The arterial injury was coiled (**B**). Computed tomography scan (**C**) shows the extent of the posterior injury. The patient was immediately placed in skeletal traction, which helped to reduce the fracture (**D**). When the patient's condition stabilized, she was fixed definitively with a plate anteriorly and a percutaneous iliosacral screw posteriorly.

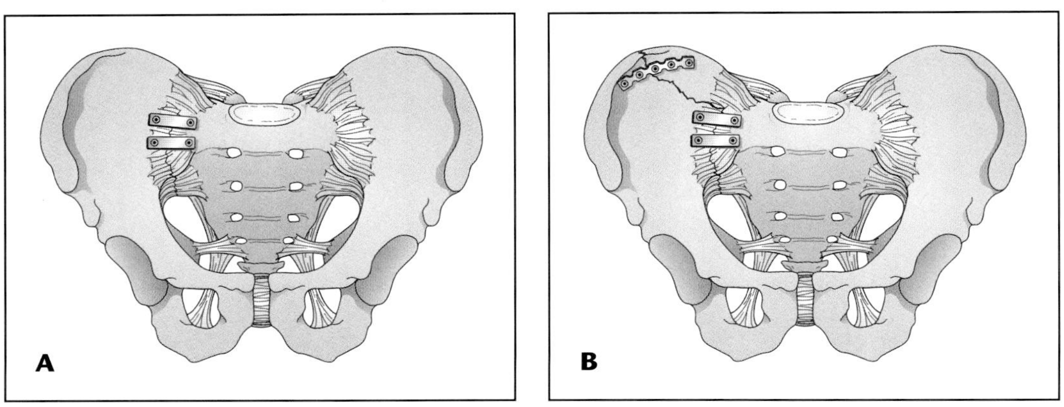

FIGURE 7-6. **A**, Plate fixation of a disrupted sacroiliac joint. **B**, Supplemental fixation of the iliac wing in a crescent fracture.

of iliosacral bars demands that one hemipelvis is stable to support the construct (Figure 7-9) [20]. Displaced transverse sacral fractures require reduction, decompression of the sacral roots, and stabilization. The stabilization is difficult and must be individualized. Plates and connection to the lumbar spine are often necessary. No one specific method of treatment exists. The surgeon

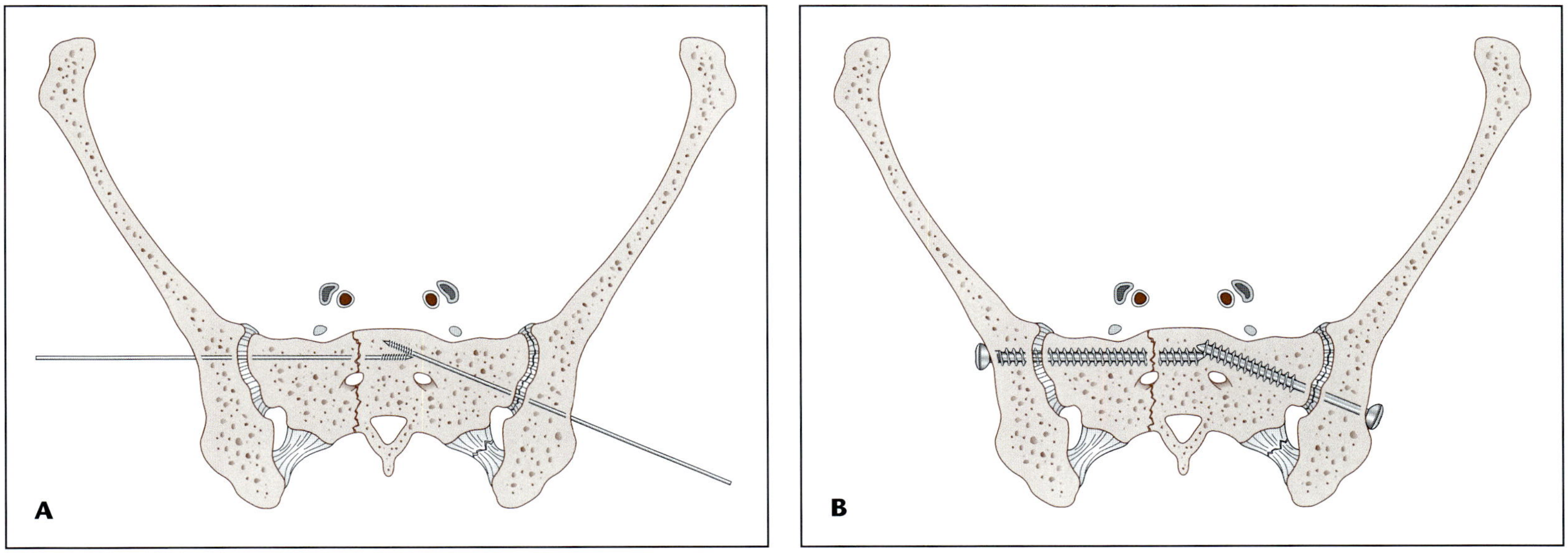

FIGURE 7-7. Proper placement of iliosacral screws for either a sacroiliac joint disruption or a sacral fracture. Note the proximity of neurovascular structures anterior to the sacrum.

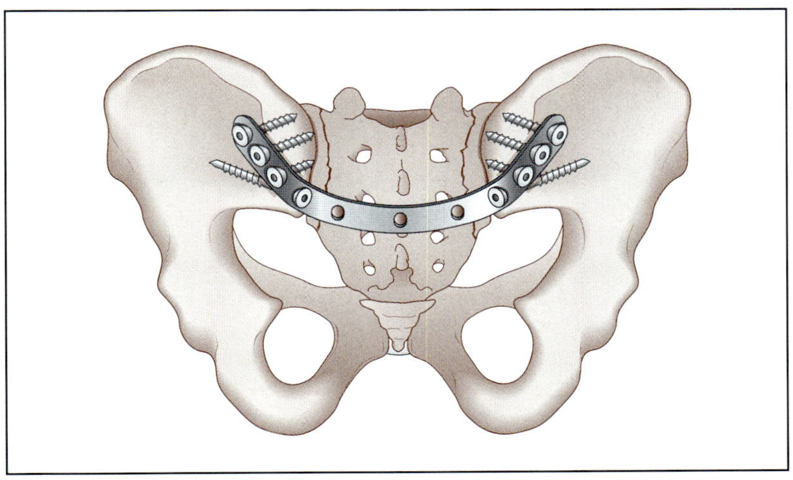

FIGURE 7-8. Proper placement of a contoured reconstruction plate along the posterior aspect of the pelvis to act as a tension band.

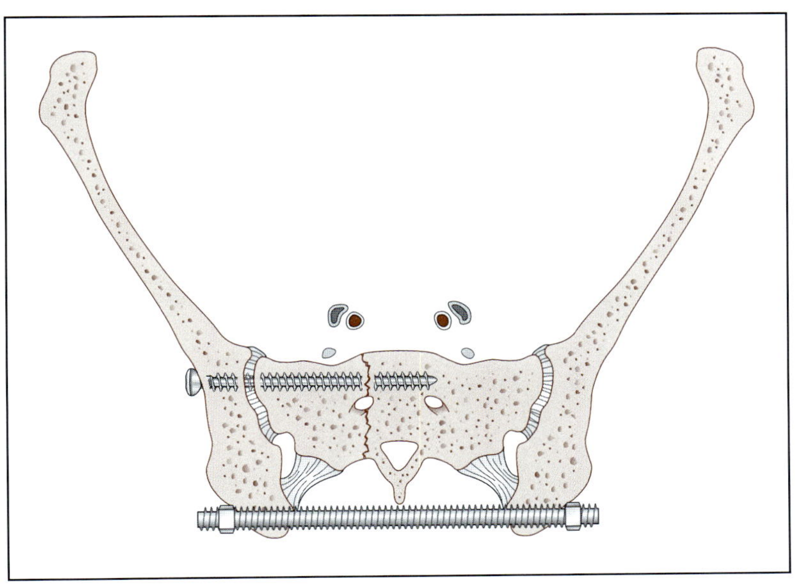

FIGURE 7-9. Use of transiliac bars to supplement fixation of the hemipelvis.

treating these injuries operatively must be able to individualize treatment options depending on the fracture, the soft tissue injury, and the patient's condition.

Postoperative management follows general guidelines. Patients are mobilized over the first 2 to 3 days postoperatively. Weight bearing is allowed on the uninvolved side, whereas only 30-lb touchdown weight bearing is allowed on the side with the posterior disruption. This regimen is continued for 6 to 8 weeks, at which time weight bearing is advanced as tolerated. If a bilateral posterior injury is present, patients are kept non–weight bearing and mobilized bed to chair only for 6 to 8 weeks.

Hemodynamically Stable Patient–Stable Fracture Pattern

Stable pelvic fractures include all Tile [8] Type A fractures, including avulsion fractures seen around the pelvis in children and adolescents and the majority of lateral compression fractures. These are most common in the elderly population as the result of simple falls and usually are diagnosed as fractures of the pubic rami. In general, these injuries are treated symptomatically with gentle mobilization, protected weight bearing, and strengthening when pain has subsided. Most such patients have a good prognosis with regard to long term function and pain relief [21].

CONCLUSIONS

The diagnosis and management of pelvic ring injuries differ depending on the mechanism and acuity of the presentation. The acute management of a high-energy injury is aimed at the recognition of bleeding associated with the pelvic fracture and its subsequent control. The definitive management requires an in-depth understanding of the surgical anatomy and techniques to operatively stabilize the fracture. Accurate diagnosis leads to appropriate decision making and thus improved patient outcome.

REFERENCES AND RECOMMENDED READING

Recently published papers of particular interest have been highlighted as:
- • Of interest
- •• Of outstanding interest

1. Burgess AR, Eastridge BJ, Young JWR, *et al.*: Pelvic ring disruptions: Effective classification system and treatment protocol. *J Trauma* 1990, 30:848–856.
2. Dalal AA, Burgess AR, Siegel JH, *et al.*: Pelvic fracture in multiple trauma: classification by mechanism is key to pattern of organ injury, resuscitative requirements and outcome. *J Trauma* 1989, 29:981–1002.
3. Olsen SA, Pollack AN: Assessment of pelvic ring stability after injury. *Clin Orthop* 1996, 329:15–27.
4. Kellam JF, Browner BD: Fractures of the pelvic ring. In *Skeletal Trauma: Fractures, Dislocations, Ligamentous Injuries* edn 2. Edited by Browner BD, Jupiter JB, Levine AM, *et al.* Philadelphia: WB Saunders; 1998:1117–1179.
5. Routt ML, Simonian PT, Swiontkowski MF: Stabilization of pelvic ring disruptions. *Orthop Clin* 1997, 28:369–388.
6. Wolinsky PR: Assessment and management of pelvic fracture in the hemodynamically unstable patient. *Orthop Clin* 1997, 28:321–329.
7. Kellam JF, McMurtry RY, Paley D, *et al.*: The unstable pelvic fracture: operative treatment. *Orthop Clin* 1987:18:25–41.
8. Tile M: Management. In *Fractures of the Pelvis and Acetabulum* edn 2. Edited by Tile M. Baltimore: Williams & Wilkins; 1995:102–134.
9. Denis F, Davis S, Comfort T: Sacral fractures: an important problem. *Clin Orthop* 1988, 227:61–65.
10. Kellam JF: Sacral fractures. In *Fractures of the Pelvis and Acetabulum* edn 2. Edited by Tile M. Baltimore: Williams & Wilkins; 1995:200–209.
11. Kellam JF, Browner BD: Fractures of the pelvic ring. In *Skeletal Trauma: Fractures, Dislocations, Ligamentous Injuries* edn 2. Edited by Browner BD, Jupiter JB, Levine AM, *et al.* Philadelphia: WB Saunders; 1998:1117–1179.
12. Nerlich M, Maghsudi M: Algorithms for early management of pelvic fractures. *Injury* 1996, 27(suppl):29–37.
13. Tile M: Pelvic ring fractures: should they be fixed? *J Bone Joint Surg Br* 1988, 70:1–12.
14. Jones AL, Powell JN, Kellam JF, *et al.*: Open pelvic fractures: A multicenter retrospective analysis. *Orthop Clin* 1997, 28:345–350.
15. Kellam JF, McLaren A, Tile M: Internal fixation. In *Fractures of the Pelvis and Acetabulum* edn 2. Edited by Tile M. Baltimore: Williams & Wilkins; 1995:150–199.
16. Latenser BA, Gentillello LM, Tarver AA, *et al.*: Improved outcome with early fixation of skeletally unstable pelvic fractures. *J Trauma* 1991, 31:28–31.
17. Matta JM, Saucedo T: Internal fixation of pelvic ring fractures. *Clin Orthop* 1989, 242:83–97.
18. Goldstein A, Phillips F, Sclafani SJA: Early open reduction and internal fixation of the disrupted pelvic ring. *J Trauma* 1986, 26:325–333.
19. Gruen GS, Leit ME, Gruen RJ, *et al.*: The acute management of hemodynamically unstable multiple trauma patients with pelvic ring fractures. *J Trauma* 1994, 36:706–713.
20. Buckle R, Browner BD, Morandi M: A new fixation device for emergent reduction and stabilization of displaced pelvic fractures associated with massive hemorrhage. *J Orthop Trauma* 1993, 7:177–178.
21. Koval KJ, Aharonoff GB, Schwartz MC, *et al.*: Pubic rami fracture: a benign pelvic injury? *J Orthop Trauma* 1997, 11:7–9.

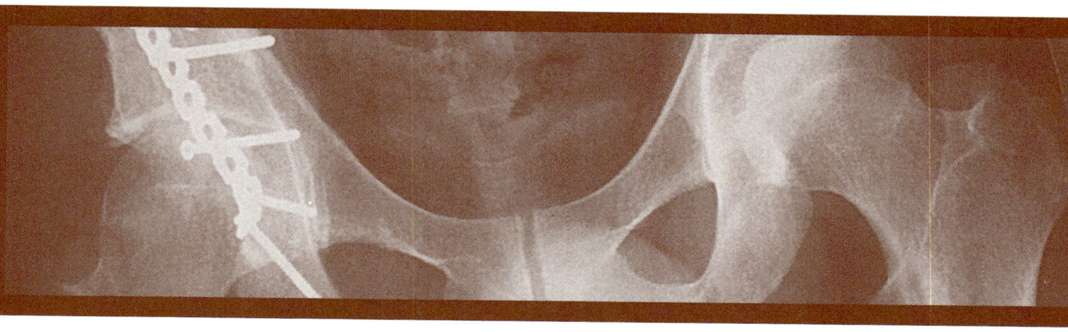

8

Fractures of the Acetabulum

H. David Moehring

Displaced fractures of the acetabulum are best treated by open reduction and internal fixation. The goals of acetabulum surgery are to allow early mobilization of the patient by providing stability and relief of pain initially and ultimately to prevent posttraumatic arthritis and loss of function. The former is more predictable than the latter. Acetabular fractures frequently occur in young and middle-aged adults as a result of a motor vehicle accident, fall from a height, or similar high-energy trauma. Relative contraindications to surgery are few, provided the patient is physiologically fit [1]. Nonoperative treatment, consisting of balanced skeletal traction alone or with a period of restricted weight bearing, is indicated for patients with nondisplaced or stable fracture patterns. Surgical treatment of acetabulum fractures poses significant technical challenges and is characterized by a steep learning curve. Nevertheless, the requisite skills can be acquired by the dedicated surgeon. Level one trauma centers and university hospitals provide the optimal environment and necessary resources to treat patients with complex musculoskeletal trauma.

DIAGNOSIS

Rapid screening examination of the spine, pelvis, and extremities is performed coincident with resuscitation and treatment of life-threatening injuries if they coexist. Careful neurologic examination should be performed and gross deformities of the extremities reduced and splinted prior to obtaining radiographs. The pelvis is examined for evidence of instability and rectal, vaginal, and urethral evaluation is performed with any evidence of bleeding from these areas or an open perineal wound. Following completion of physical examination, radiographs are reviewed. Standard evaluation requires anteroposterior (AP) and 45° oblique (Judet) radiographs, as already discussed. The appropriate selection of the surgical approach can be made on the basis of the AP and oblique radiographs. A computed tomography (CT) scan can add valuable information regarding unsuspected sacral fractures, bone fragments in the joint, and marginal impaction and is also helpful in planning optimal screw orientation and starting points.

CLASSIFICATION

Judet *et al.* [2] developed an anatomic classification of fractures in 1964. Letournel [3] refined this classification into five so-called "simple" patterns, involving either a single column or wall of the acetabulum, or transverse fractures, which bisect both columns of the acetabulum. Letournel [3] further subdivided transverse fractures into transtectal, juxtatectal, and infratectal types to define more specifically those fracture lines crossing the superior acetabular articular surface, the cotyloid fossa, and inferior region of the joint, respectively. In addition, five associated patterns were defined in general, adding another level of complexity to the simple patterns. This original classification was again modified by the AO group to fit their ABC classification. This classification is shown in Figure 8-1 [4]. Basically, classifications indicate gradations of severity and as such can provide information regarding treatment and prognosis. They are also a form of discipline that helps the clinician understand the three-dimensional anatomy and evaluate functional outcomes in a standardized fashion.

TREATMENT

Nonoperative treatment can be entertained for nondisplaced fractures, minimally displaced stable fractures, or those that involve only small portions of the articular weight-bearing surface. This includes certain low transverse or T-type fractures as well as low anterior column–high superior ramus fractures. In addition, certain displaced fractures of both columns in high-risk patients can be treated nonoperatively if they resolve to a so-called "secondary congruence." In this situation, the acetabular columns and articular segments are spread apart, but generally they move together and group themselves around the femoral head. This is in contradistinction to displacement of one column or major segment, leaving the other intact, so that the femoral head subluxes and abnormal contact stresses cause rapid joint degeneration and chondrolysis.

Selection of the appropriate surgical approach is fundamental to successful treatment of the fractured acetabulum (Figure 8-2) [4]. Although no singular surgical approach is ideal for all fractures of

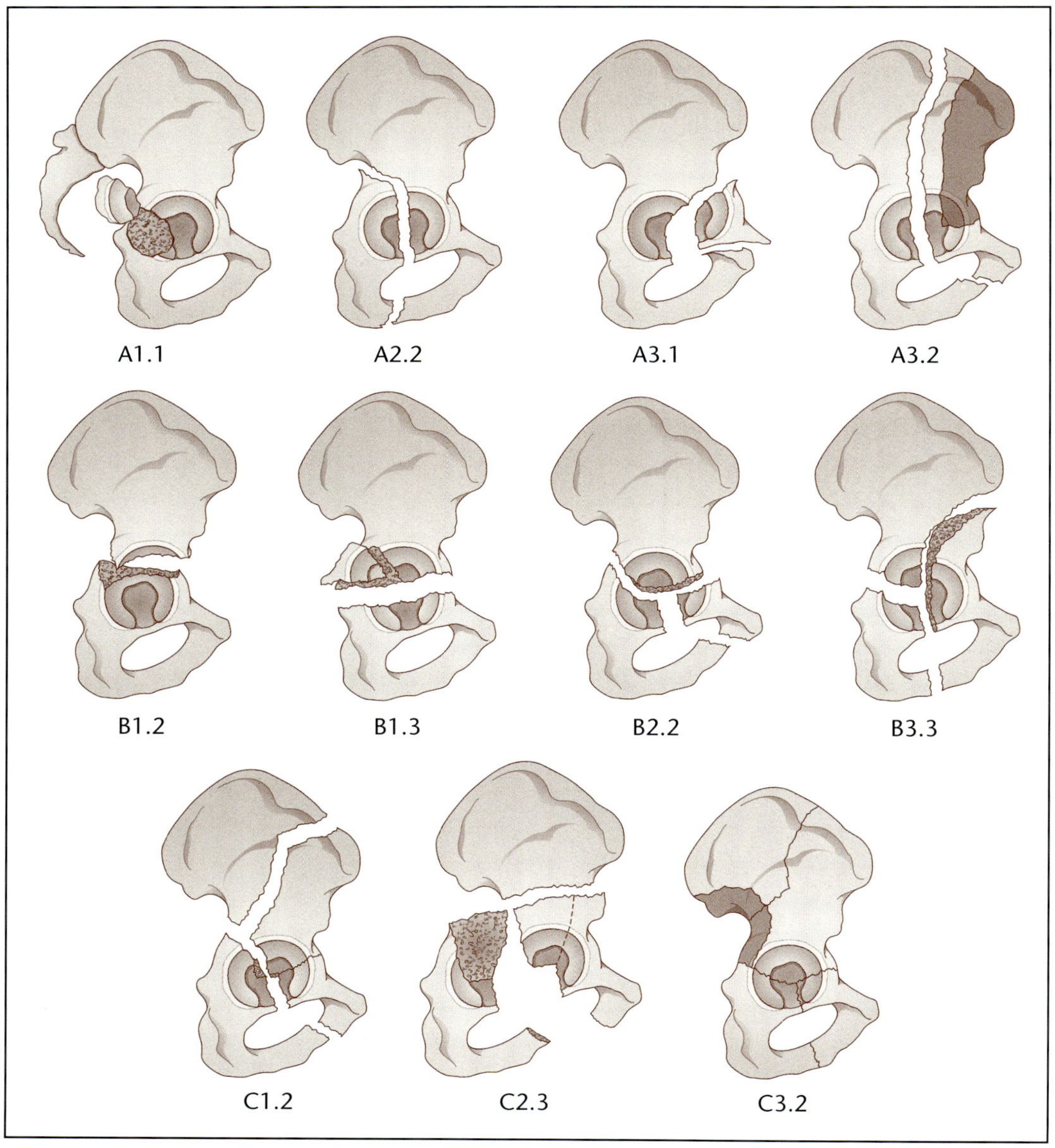

FIGURE 8-1. AO classification of acetabulum fractures. This classification has been modified to fit the groups A, B, and C of the AO classification. (*Adapted from* Müller *et al.* [4].)

the acetabulum, most patients can be treated with a single surgical approach. Nearly all acetabulum fractures can be treated through either a posterior (Kocher-Langenbeck) or anterior (ilioinguinal) approach or occasionally both in combination. The Kocher-Langenbeck approach addresses the posterior column and wall, giving limited access to the anterior column through the greater sciatic notch. The ilioinguinal approach primarily exposes the anterior column and internal aspect of the innominate bone. The posterior column and the quadrilateral surface can be approached along the internal aspect of the pelvic brim in the second window of this approach. The ilioinguinal approach is associated with the most rapid recovery and lowest rate of complications and therefore should be used whenever a fracture can be reduced by this approach. Heterotopic ossification and nerve injury are virtually nonexistent with this approach. The scar is cosmetically pleasing and the patient's postoperative progress is relatively rapid [5]. The extended iliofemoral, the straight lateral, and the triradiate approaches are used for complex or subacute fractures, which present late and are associated with early callus formation [6]. These surgical approaches are well described in standard texts. The indications, patient positioning, and salient features of each are summarized in Table 8-1.

REDUCTION AND FIXATION

Reduction techniques are shown in Figures 8-3 through 8-9 [4]. When the patient's leg is draped and free, an additional assistant is necessary to apply traction. A percutaneous Schantz pin inserted in the greater tuberosity for lateral traction is useful (Figure 8-4). The femoral distractor is useful in exposing the acetabulum in posterior approaches with an intact iliac wing. Alternatively, a fracture table may be used (Figure 8-3). Examples of characteristic fracture patterns and methods of fixation are shown in Figures 8-10 through 8-18.

ADJUNCTIVE TECHNIQUES

Flip Trochanteric Osteotomy

The so-called digastric slide involves a partial osteotomy of the greater trochanter, maintaining the attachments of the gluteus medius and minimus proximally and some attachments to the vastus lateralis distally (Figure 8-13) [7]. The osteotomized greater trochanteric medallion is then flipped or turned 90°, much as the patella is everted in knee surgery, providing increased exposure of the retroacetabular region. This procedure is not usually necessary, but it may be helpful when dealing with a very large posterior column/wall fragment that would require excessive retraction of the gluteus medius and perhaps jeopardize the superior gluteal neurovascular bundle (Figure 8-12). It also may aid in exposure of certain T-type fractures from the posterior approach. Given that the blood supply from the osteotomized fragment is preserved, it heals rapidly when replaced with screws or sutures, and it produces lower risk for postoperative pulloff.

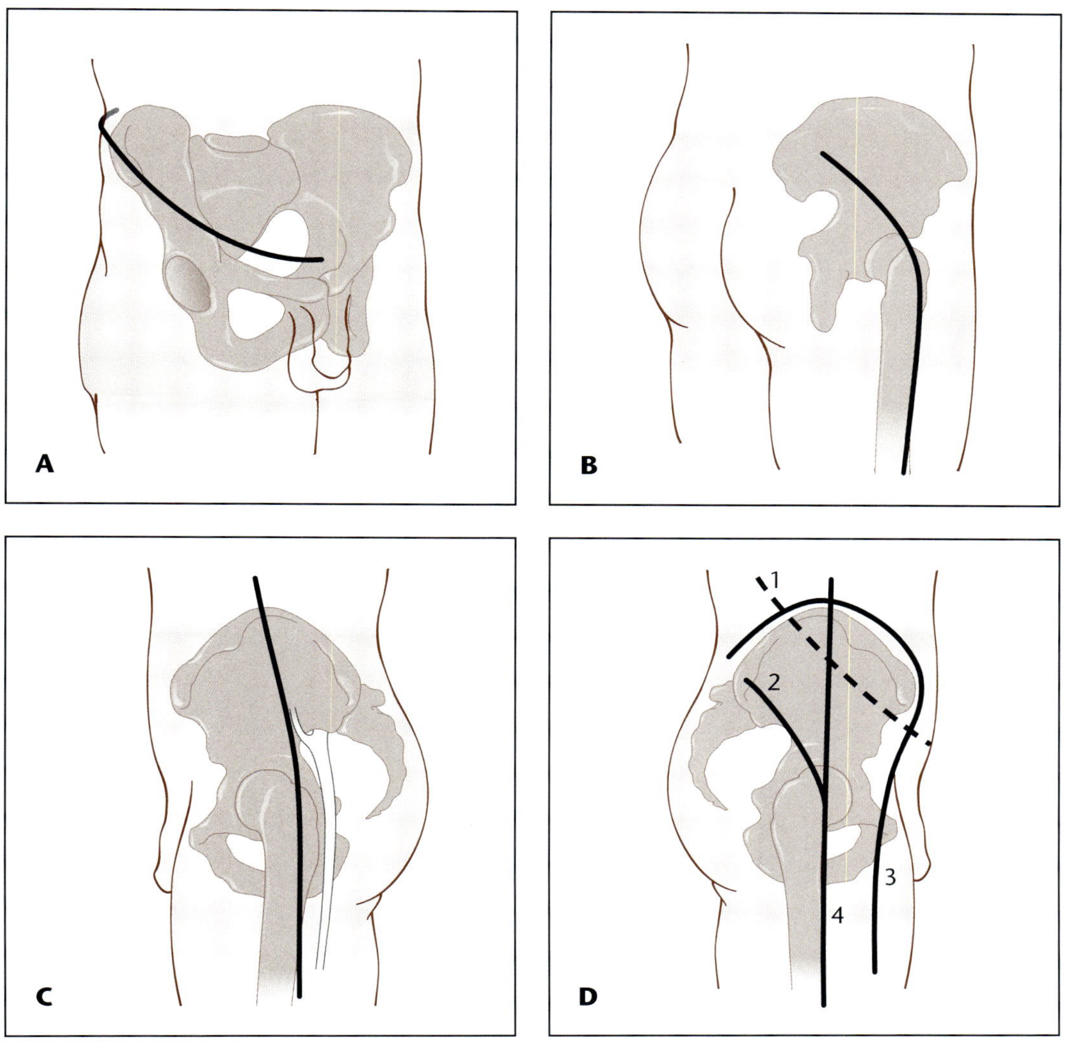

Figure 8-2. Four common surgical approaches to the acetabulum. **A**, Ilioinguinal; **B**, Kocher-Langenbeck; **C**, straight lateral; **D**, 1) Ilioinguinal, 2) Kocher-Langenbeck, 3) *extended iliofemoral*, and 4) straight lateral. (*Adapted from* Müller *et al.* [4].)

PERCUTANEOUS SCREWS

Not infrequently, the ability to place a screw percutaneously through the skin and soft tissue adjacent to standard surgical incision enables the surgeon to secure fixation without necessitating an additional incision. Occasionally, percutaneous fixation alone is useful in undisplaced or minimally displaced fractures, which are at jeopardy for displacement [8]. A case can be made for this if other findings include contralateral injuries, soft-tissue compromise, or the fracture pattern suggests the potential for displacement (Figure 8-13). The image intensifier is essential to insert these screws safely and in correct orientation. The anterior column screw is placed with the patient in the supine position and basically is located as has been described above. Its direction is lateral to medial and directed posteriorly and distally to enter the superior pubic ramus, which is a narrow window, or exit the anterior column through the superior portion of the quadrilateral plate. The later is a safer position for the 6.5- or 7.0-mm cannulated screws. The 3.5-mm screw is used if the ramus is selected. The clinician must use the image intensifier to monitor the direction of the screws to avoid penetrating the joint or possibly damaging the neurovascular bundle. The combination of outlet obturator oblique and inlet iliac-oblique views are useful in correct screw placement. The anterior column screw can also be placed in retrograde fashion from the pubic tubercle up the superior ramus across the fracture site. This requires a small incision to select the appropriate starting point on the symphysis pubis.

Retrograde posterior column screws are inserted in the ischial tuberosity (Figure 8-13). The entire gluteal area in this region should be thoroughly draped to avoid contamination from the rectal area. With the hip flexed and the patient in the decubitus position, the ischial tuberosity can be palpated and a cannulated guide pin inserted slightly laterally to ensure that the sciatic nerve is not injured. The direction of this screw is determined by the starting point, which is somewhat hard to control. It is best to enlarge the opening in the tuberosity with a 3.2-mm (or larger) drill to allow more leeway for guide-pin insertion. The posterior column should be essentially nondisplaced or reducible. After drilling the cortex of the ischial tuberosity, an appropriate-length cannulated screw is selected and inserted under C-arm control. As with an antegrade

TABLE 8-1. INDICATIONS, PATIENT POSITIONING, AND SALIENT FEATURES OF VARIOUS SURGICAL APPROACHES

Approach	Patient Position	Indications	Salient Features
Kocher-Langenbeck	Lateral, or prone if fracture table is used	Posterior fracture dislocations that require reduction of the posterior wall or column, T-shaped fractures, and transverse patterns. (AO types A 1 to 3; B1 and B2, and C2) In conjunction with the ilioinguinal exposure if necessary for the latter two fracture patterns, or complex both column fractures	Exposes posterior wall, column, and sciatic notch, quadrilateral plate by palpation, and acetabulum by distracting the femoral head or wall fracture.
Ilioinguinal	Supine or "floppy lateral"	Anterior column-wall fractures Anterior column and posterior hemitransverse fractures, both column fractures Occasionally, difficult T-type or transverse fracture patterns. (AO types A3, B3, and C1,2)	Anterior column, wall, and superior public ramus. Quadrilateral plate through second window, and posterior column and acetabulum indirectly.
Combined anterior (ilioinguinal) and posterior (Kocher-Langenbeck)	Floppy lateral	Complex both column, transverse, or certain T-type fractures and whenever necessitated by inability to obtain anatomic reduction through a single approach (AO types B2; C1, C2, and C3)	
Extended ileofemoral	Lateral	Complex both column fracture patterns in which the posterior column is extensively comminuted or extends distally into the ischium Fractures presenting late with early healing and callus formation or fractures that extend into the posterior illium and sacroiliac joint. (AO types B1, B2, C1, C2, and C3)	Primarily exposes lateral aspect of innominant bone, but gives the best simultaneous exposure to both columns. However, access to anterior column and pubic ramus is limited and a plate along the pelvic brim to the pubis cannot be used effectively. A commanding exposure is obtained, but with greater morbidity, more wound problems, and a higher incidence of heterotopic ossification. In addition, residual abductor weakness is frequent and can compromise results even if the joint is anatomically reduced.
Straight lateral	Lateral	Complex posterior column fractures, transverse and posterior wall fractures, certain T-shaped fractures. (AO types B1, B2, C1, and C2)	Exposures obtained include posterior column and the distal half of the iliac wing, acetabular roof, and limited access to the anterior column Disadvantages include limited access to the anterior column, heterotopic ossification and potential abductor weakness

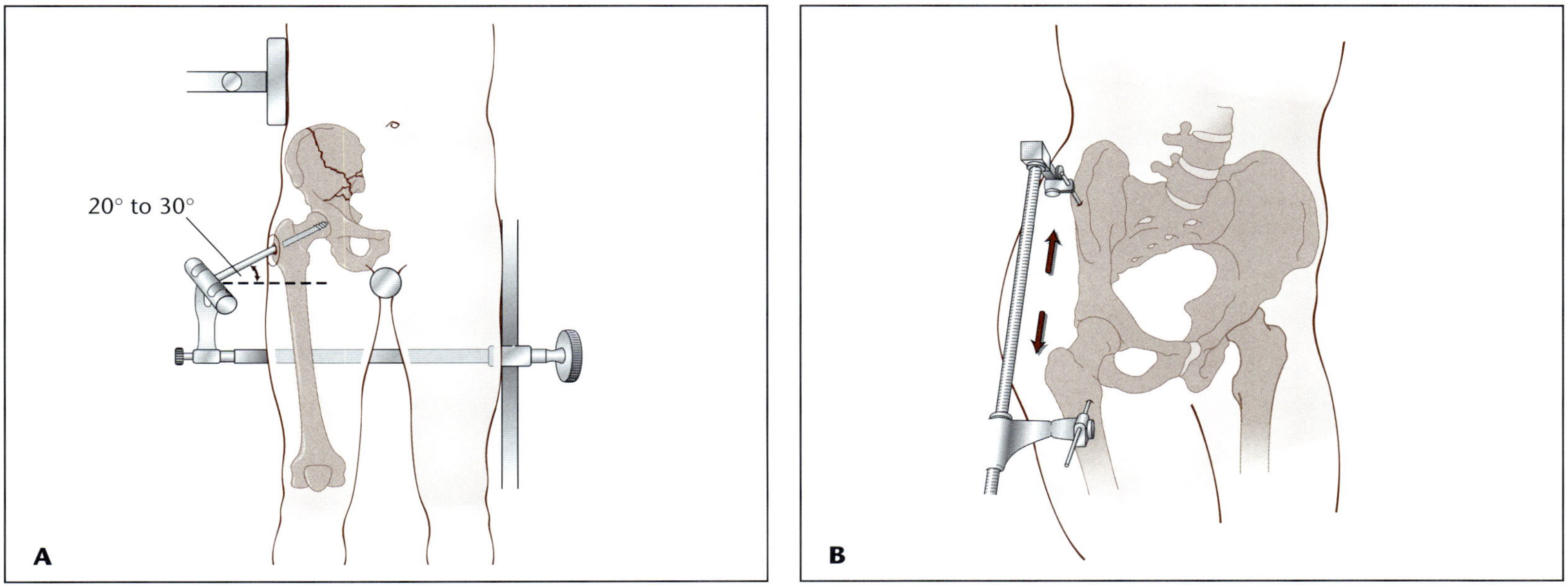

FIGURE 8-3. A, Fracture table provides lateral and longitudinal traction but requires prolonged anesthesia and set-up time. Careful monitoring is needed to prevent sciatic nerve palsy. **B**, Femoral distractor is useful for pulling femoral head out of acetabulum and improving visualization of fracture. Not useful with ileoinguinal approach. (*Adapted from* Müller *et al.* [4].)

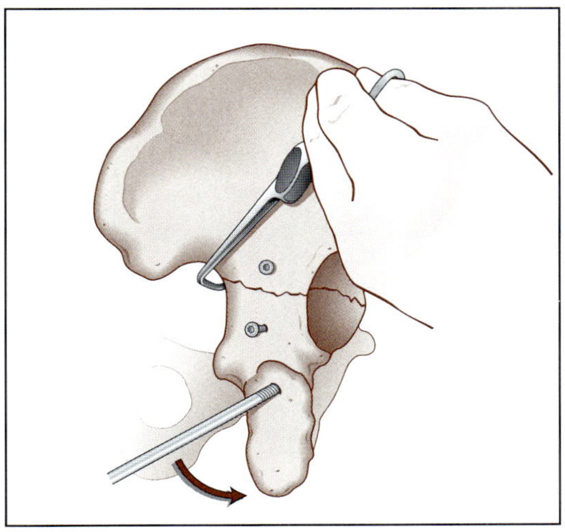

FIGURE 8-4. Reduction of the posterior column of a tranverse acetabular fracture. Schantz pin in the ischial tuberosity and a hook in the sciatic notch help to derotate the posterior column.

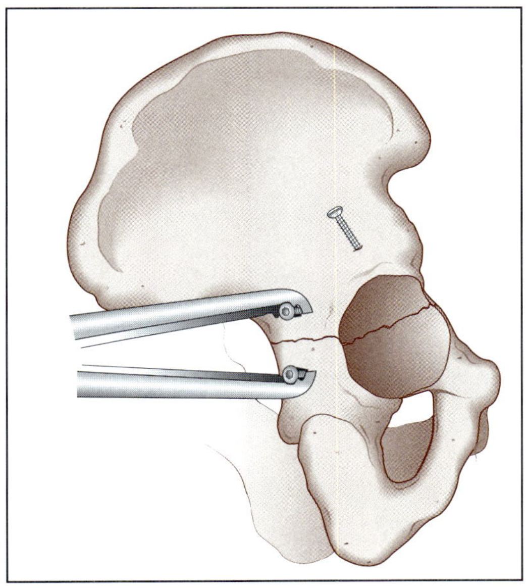

FIGURE 8-5. Use of pelvic reduction forceps to secure reduction of posterior column.

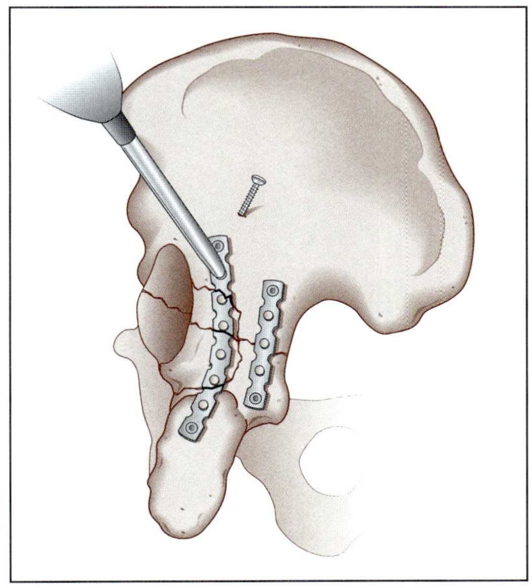

FIGURE 8-6. Fixation of transverse and posterior wall acetabular fracture using dual reconstruction plates and anterior column cannulated screw.

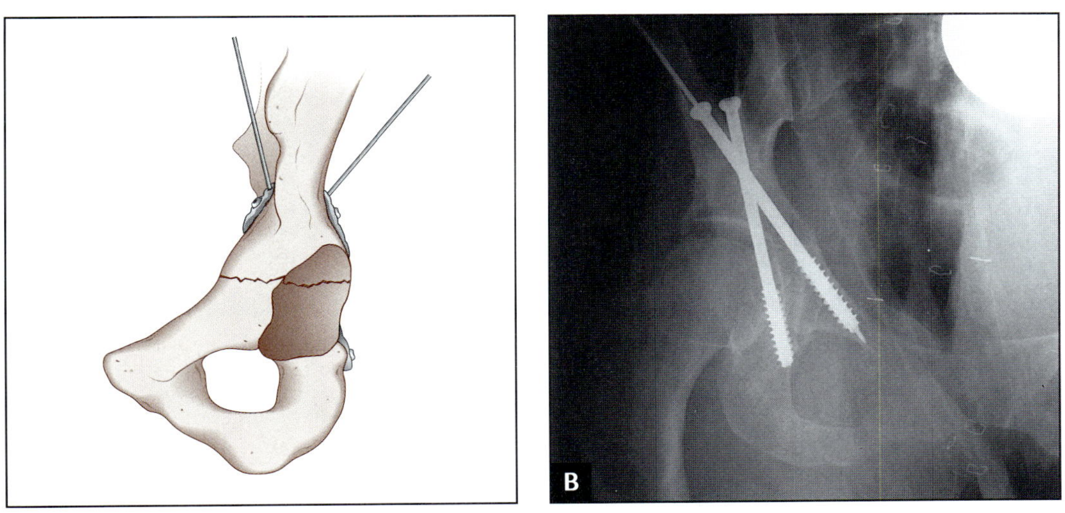

FIGURE 8-7. A, Direction of cannulated screw guide pins, or regular 3.5-mm screws for fixation of the anterior and posterior columns. **B**, Intraoperative radiograph illustrating direction of anterior and posterior column screws for treatment of transverse acetabular fracture.

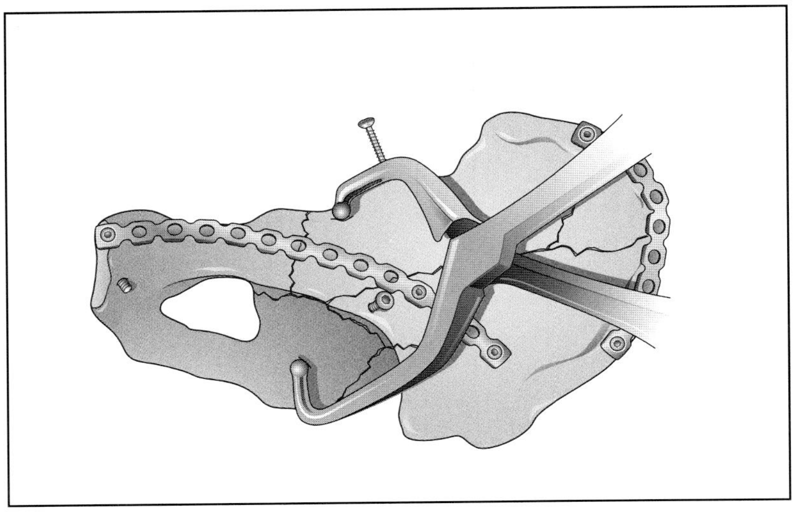

FIGURE 8-8. Reduction of posterior column through the "second window" of an ilioinguinal approach. Note the direction of anterior screw above angled pelvic reduction forceps as well as the direction of the posterior column screw, just anterior to the intersection of the reduction forceps and the posterior plate. Additional posterior column screws can be placed carefully through the reconstruction plate into the posterior column.

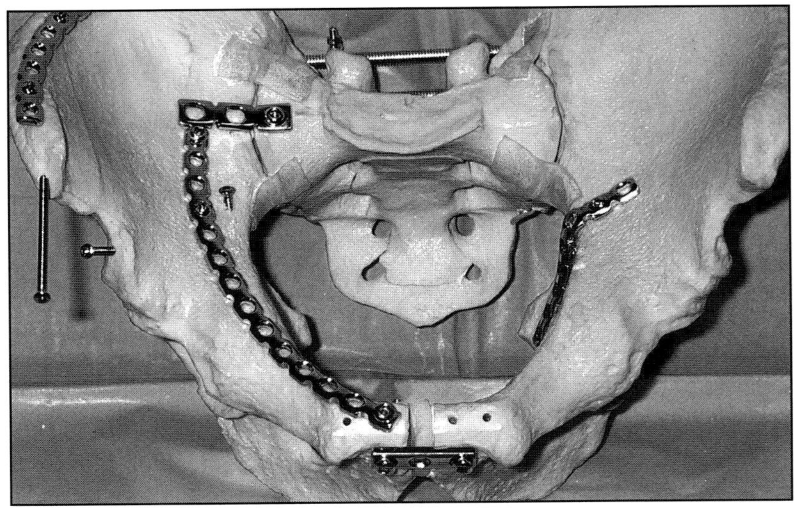

FIGURE 8-9. Types of pelvic-acetabular fixation. Generally, stabilization of pelvis, including the anterior sacroiliac or iliosacral screw and pubic plating, should precede fixation of an acetabular fracture. Posterior column screws can be seen paralleling the quadrilateral plate medial to the pelvic reconstruction plate, above the pelvic brim. Note the quadrilateral plate–posterior column buttress plate on right.

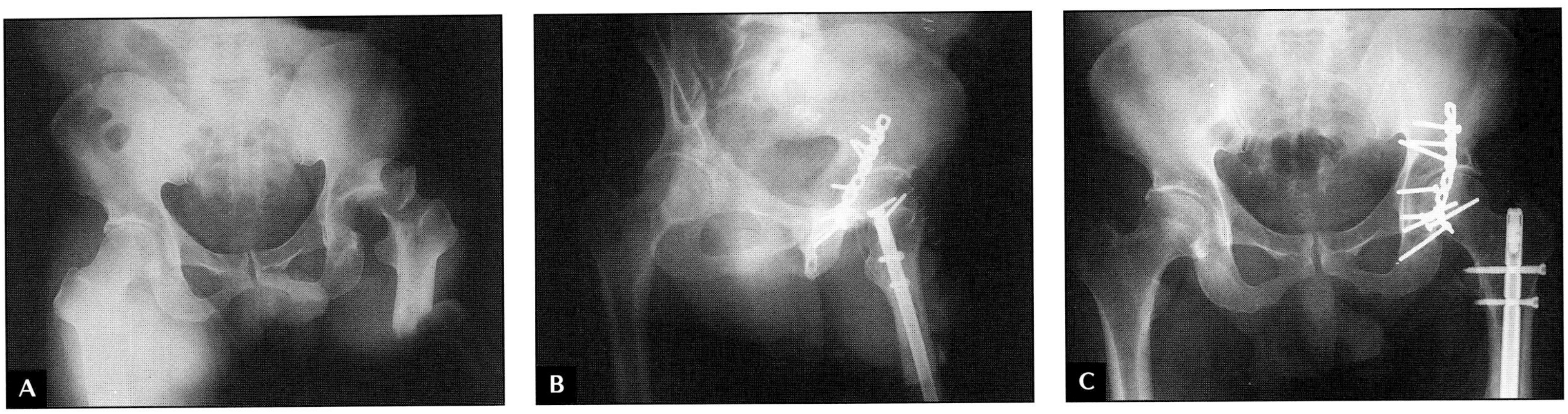

FIGURE 8-10. A, Unusually severe injury including dislocation of hip joint, fractured femoral head, fractured posterior wall acetabulum, and subtrochanteric fracture of the femur. **B**, Immediate postoperative view after stabilization of all fractures and reduction of hip joint. **C**, Three-year follow-up showing maintenance of joint space and healing of subtrochanteric, acetabular, and femoral head fractures, associated with good functional result.

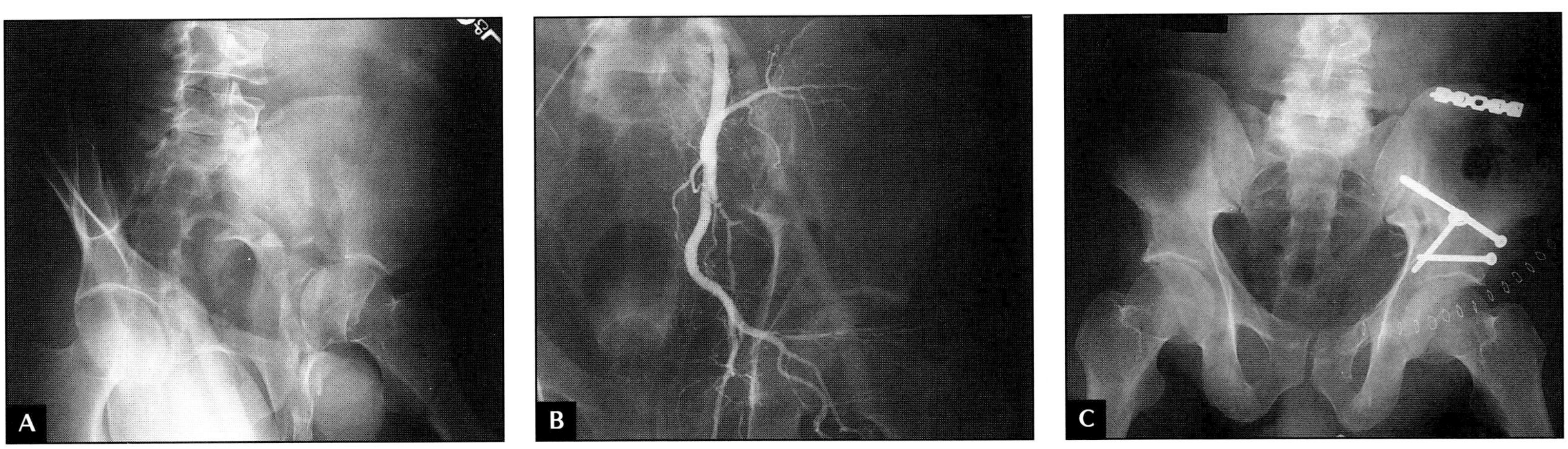

FIGURE 8-11. A, Marked displacement of iliac wing and acetabular fracture associated with polytrauma and hemorrhagic shock. **B**, Most bleeding from acetabular fractures is venous or bony in origin. However, with wide displacement, arterial avulsion can occur. Note arteriogram showing cut-off of superior gluteal artery. Embolization by the radiologist can be helpful in these instances. **C**, Postoperative film showing anatomic reduction of joint through an ilioinguinal approach, using lag-screw fixation. Patient died as a result of adult respiratory distress syndrome and multiple organ failure 10 days postoperatively.

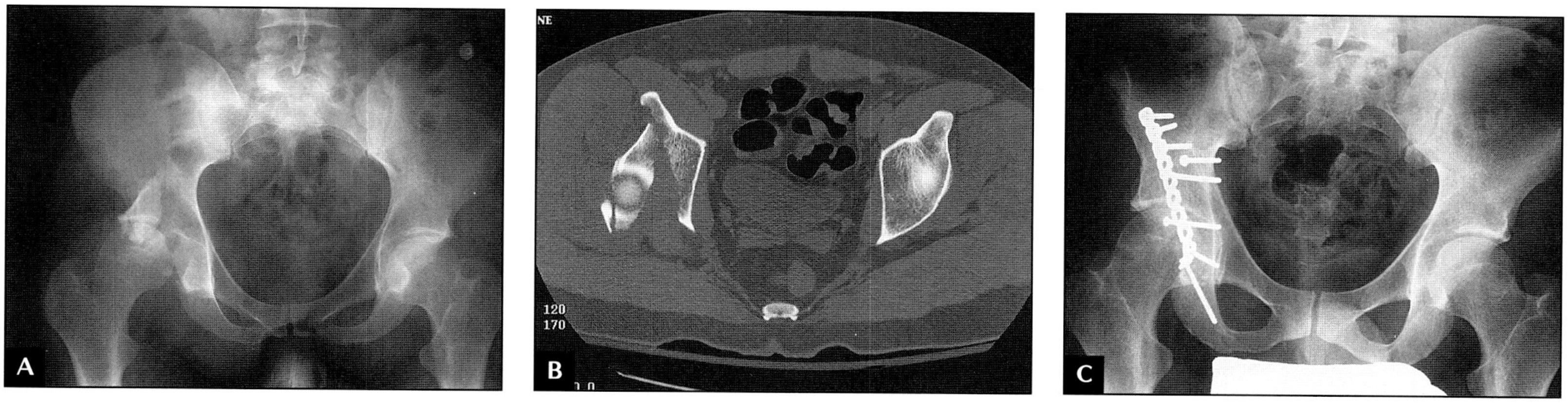

FIGURE 8-12. A, Large posterior column–wall acetabular fracture. B, Fracture extends to anterior/inferior iliac spine and includes dome of acetabulum over dislocated femoral head. C, Anatomic reduction and fixation using a Kocher-Langenbeck approach with the "flip" trochanteric osteotomy because of proximal extension. Superior gluteal neurovascular bundle can be stretched if plate extends too far proximally above the joint.

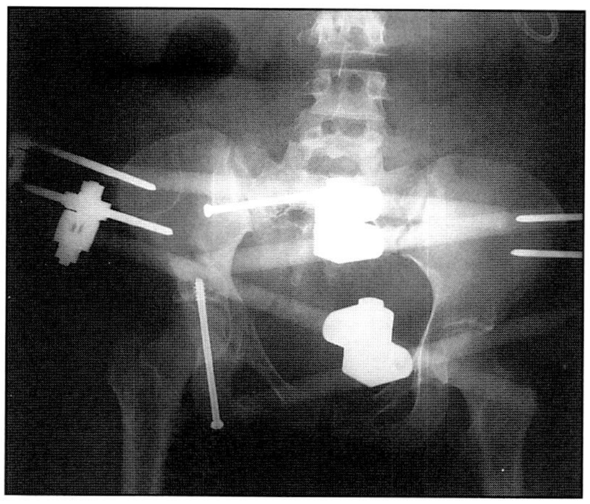

FIGURE 8-13. Polytrauma victim with widely open pelvic disruption. Stabilization was provided by pelvic external fixator and percutaneous iliosacral and retrograde posterior column acetabular screws.

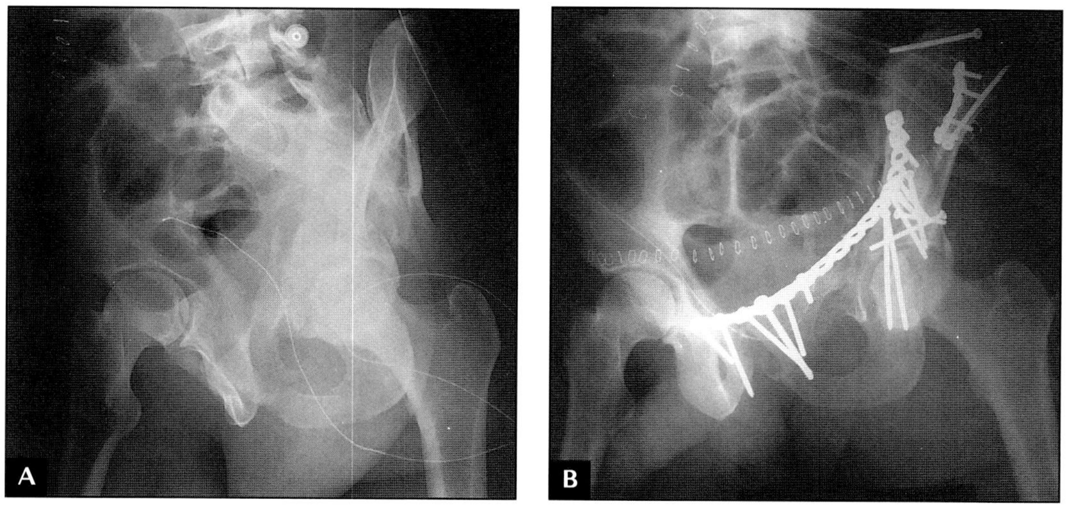

FIGURE 8-14. A, Typical fracture of both columns with large spur sign. B, Ilioinguinal approach with extension of plate to contralateral nonfractured pubis. Note long posterior column screws.

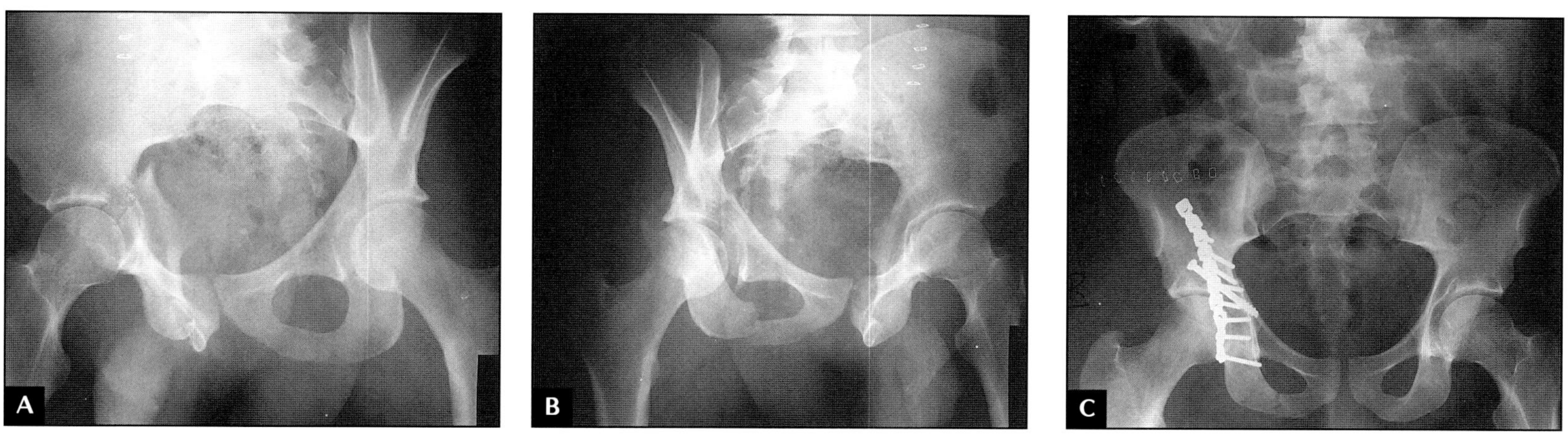

FIGURE 8-15. A, Iliac oblique radiograph showing apparent transverse acetabular fracture. B, Obturator oblique view clearly illustrates fracture extending into obturator foramen with displaced inferior pubic ramus, indicating a T-type fracture pattern. C, Representative postoperative anteroposterior view showing anatomic reduction and fixation through a posterior approach.

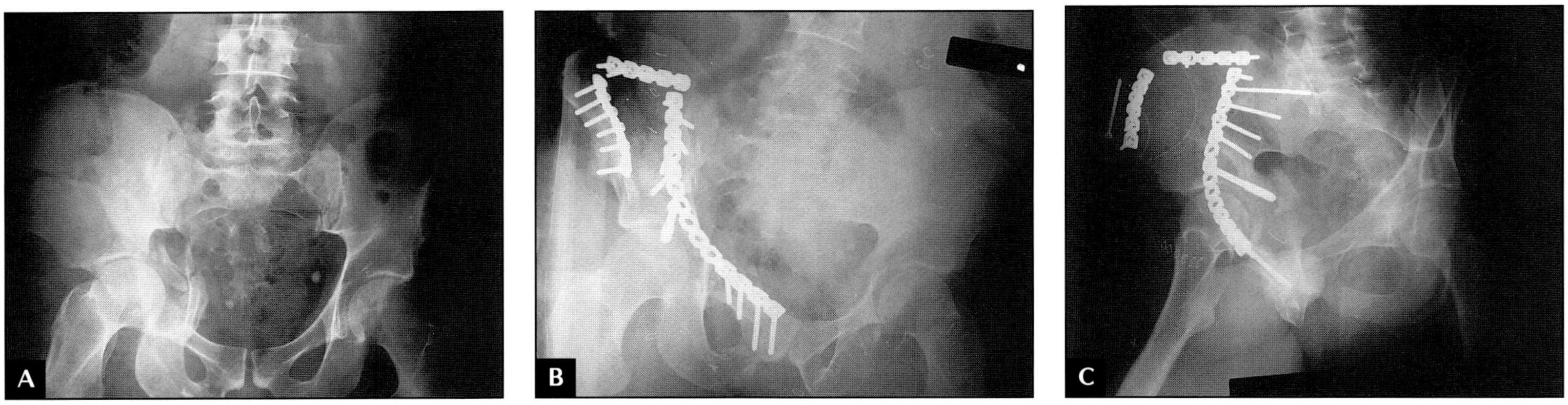

FIGURE 8-16. A, Comminuted acetabular fracture of both columns. B, Anatomic reduction and internal fixation through an ilioinguinal approach.

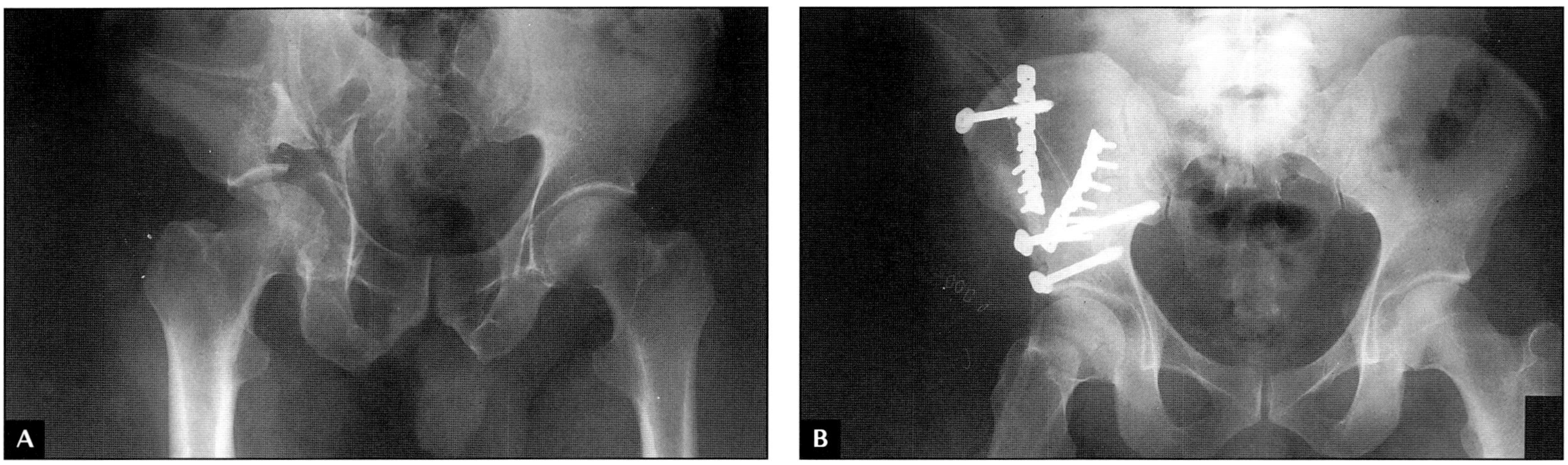

FIGURE 8-17. A, Comminuted anterior column fracture with associated posterior hemitransverse extending proximally into the sciatic notch. B, Reduction in iliolingual approach. The inferior lag screw captures the high posterior-column fragment.

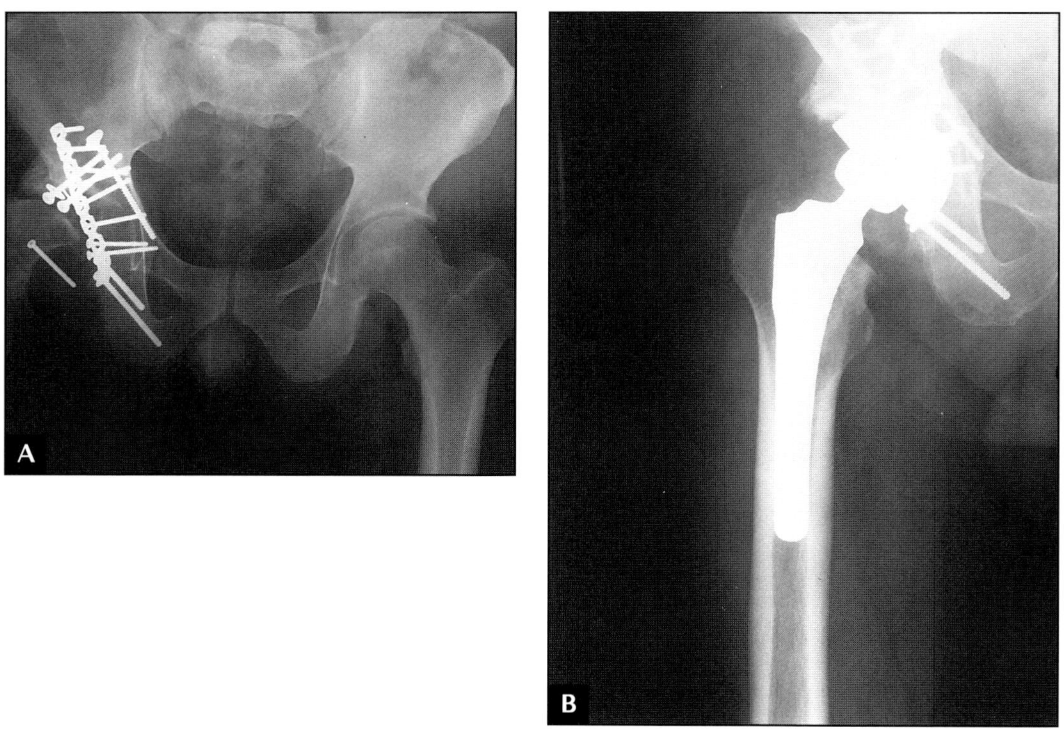

FIGURE 8-18. A, Four-year postoperative view of posterior wall and transverse acetabular fracture. Posterior wall has undergone avascular necrosis, chondrolysis, and mechanical wearing away of the femoral head. This is frequently mistaken for avascular necrosis of femoral head. B, Salvage by a total hip arthroplasty. Primary total hip arthroplasty can be considered in acetabular fractures associated with severe damage to the femoral head.

posterior column screw inserted from an ilioinguinal approach, the screw will appear superimposed on the AP and obturator oblique views but should be seen out of the joint on an iliac oblique view. If the screw can be demonstrated to be out of the joint on any view, it is nonarticular.

POSTOPERATIVE CARE

Drains are retained for 24 to 48 hours until collection levels have decreased. Intravenous antibiotics are continued for 72 hours or until the soft tissue is benign. When the Kocher-Langenbeck or any of the extended approaches are used, heterotopic ossification prophylaxis is indicated with 75-mg indomethacin daily for 14 days or postoperative radiation of 7-Gy dosage [9–12]. This is not necessary when the ilioinguinal approach is used. All patients should receive some form of prophylaxis against deep venous thrombosis (DVT) [13,14]. Sequential compression devices and subcutaneous heparin, followed by low-dose coumadin, is an excellent regimen. Anticoagulation should be continued for at least 3 and preferably 6 weeks or beyond in patients at risk. The latter include advanced age, male gender, and previous DVT. Vena caval filters may also be indicated in this group [14]. Patients should be mobilized from bed to chair as soon as they are comfortable and begin physical therapy at day one or two. Full weight bearing is not allowed for at least 8 to 10 weeks. Range-of-motion and muscle-strengthening exercises are graduated and encouraged. For patients who have had the straight lateral or extended iliofemoral approach, an abduction orthosis is worn for a minimum of 6 weeks.

PREVENTION OF COMPLICATIONS AND CAVEATS

Complications cannot be eliminated entirely, but they can be greatly reduced by careful and safe operative techniques. When using the ilioinguinal approach, look carefully for aberrant vessels between the obturator and inferior epigastric vessels or external iliac vessels (corona mortis) [15]. These should be ligated or coagulated to prevent troublesome bleeding. Reconstruct the inguinal canal or make sure that it is intact at the time of closure to prevent possible development of hernia. Appropriate drainage of wounds should prevent hematoma formation; however, if it occurs, prompt return of the patient to the operating room and evacuation of the hematoma may be indicated.

Dissect carefully and directly on bone in the region of the ischial tuberosity and spine because the sciatic nerve is in direct proximity to these structures [16]. Retractors placed in the sciatic notch do not usually cause a problem, provided the hip is extended and the knee flexed. Retractors in the lesser sciatic notch or on the tuberosity need to be placed carefully and not left in place for a prolonged time. Remember to avoid excessive traction and release it periodically when the fracture table is used. All patients should have a screening duplex ultrasound to rule out DVT, because it is not uncommon, especially in patients who have been transferred from an outside facility on a delayed basis. Most pulmonary complications can be prevented or reduced by mobilization of the patient and the use of an aggressive incentive spirometry regimen. Most hemorrhage is venous or bony in origin; however, markedly displaced fractures involving the sciatic notch and associated with clinical signs of bleeding require an arteriogram and embolization of bleeding sources, especially if they involve the superior gluteal vessels (Figure 8-11). Anticipate increased blood loss in these cases despite embolization as mobilization of the fracture through the notch may reactivate bleeding.

Be sure that the hollow drill and cannulated screw guide pins are new and have not been burred. If resistance is found when drilling over a guide pin, stop and insert another guide pin and remove the bent or burred pin. It is helpful to predrill a pilot hole to prevent bending of the cannulated guide pins. If they are sawed off by the drill, they can be difficult or impossible to remove.

Use a postoperative CT to confirm that suspicious hardware is out of the joint if necessary, but avoid the routine postoperative use of this study because a great deal of radiation to the patients' gonadal area occurs. Many experienced surgeons find the incidence of iatrogenic nerve palsies so low that it does not justify the routine use of somatosensory evoked potential nerve monitoring during surgery [11]. Nevertheless, this modality can be helpful when used during a posterior approach to the acetabulum and might prompt the removal of traction or change the position of a retractor should signals go down. A significant incidence of false positives and false negatives is associated with this study. Its use with the ilioinguinal approach is less helpful, because injury to the sciatic nerve is quite rare.

PROGNOSIS

Even the most trivial of acetabular fractures are serious injuries, for which a biologic price is likely to be exacted at some point in time [17]. Reported results vary and are probably overly optimistic representing the unavoidable bias of the surgeon [1,9,18,19]. Letournel [3] reported nearly 80% good and excellent results following acetabular surgery. Matta [5] also reported approximately 70% good results in his series. Other authors have reported less favorable results [20]. To date, few good midterm or long-term functional outcome studies have appeared. It is likely that "results from the patients' side" will reveal varying degrees of disability in a significant number of patients. Although patients cannot be given a guarantee that they will avoid future arthritis, accurate and careful open reduction and internal fixation certainly optimizes their chances.

REFERENCES AND RECOMMENDED READING

Recently published papers of particular interest have been highlighted as:
- • Of interest
- •• Of outstanding interest

1. Helfet DL, Borrelli J Jr, Dipasuale T, *et al.*: Stabilization of acetabular fractures in elderly patients. *J Bone Joint Surg Am* 1992, 74:753–765.
2. Judet R, Judet J, Letournel E: Fractures of the acetabulum: classification and surgical approaches for open reduction. *J Bone Joint Surg Am* 1964, 46:1615–1638.
3. Letournel E: The results of acetabular fractures treated surgically: twenty-one years' experience. In *The Hip: Proceedings of the Seventh Open Scientific Meeting of the Hip Society.* St. Louis: Mosby; 1979:42–85.

4. Müller ME, Allgöwer M, Schneider R, Willenegger H: Acetabulum. *Manual of Internal Fixation: Techniques Recommended by the Ao-Asif Group* edn 3. New York: Springer Verlag; 1991:501–513.
5. Matta JM: Operative treatment of acetabular fractures through the ilioinguinal approach: a ten-year perspective. *Clin Orthop Rel Res* 1994, 305:10–19.
6. Johnson EE, Matta JM, Mast MW, *et al.*: Delayed reconstruction of acetabular fractures 21–120 days following injury. *Clin Orthop Rel Res* 1994, 305:20–31.
7. Sienbenbrock KA, Gautier J, Ziran BH, *et al.*: Trochanteric flip osteotomy or cranial extension and muscle protection in acetabulum fracture fixation using a Kocher-Langenbeck approach. *J Orthop Trauma* 1998, 12:387–391.
8. Starr AJ, Reinert CM, Jones AL: Percutaneous fixation of the columns of the acetabulum: a new technique. *J Orthop Trauma* 1998, 12:51–58.
9. Kaempffe FA, Bone LB, Border JR: Open reduction and internal fixation of acetabular fractures: heterotopic ossification and other complications of treatment. *J Orthop Trauma* 1991, 5:439–445.
10. Moed BR, Maxey JW: The effect of indomethacin on heterotopic ossification following acetabular fracture surgery. *J Orthop Trauma* 1993, 7:33–38.
11. Middenbrooks ES, Sims SH, Kellam JF *et al.*: Incidence of sciatic nerve injury in operatively treated acetabular fractures without somatosensory evoked potential monitoring. *J Orthop Trauma* 1997, 12:327–329.
12. Moed BR, Letournel E: Low-dose irradiation and indomethacin prevent heterotropic ossification after acetabular fracture injury. *J Bone Joint Surg Br* 1994, 76:895–900.
13. Fishmann AF, Greeno RA, Brooks LR, *et al.*: Prevention of deep vein thrombosis and pulmonary embolism in acetabular and pelvic fracture surgery. *Clin Orthop Ref Res* 1994, 305:122–138.
14. Montgomery KD, Potter HG, Helfit DL: Detection and management of proximal deep venous thrombosis in patients with acute acetabular fractures: a follow-up report. *J Orthop Trauma* 1997, 11:333–336.
15. Teague D, Graney DO, Routt ML: Retropubic vascular hazards of the ilioinguinal exposure: a cadaveric and clinical study. Presented at the Orthopaedic Trauma Association annual meeting, Los Angeles, California, September, 1994.
16. Fassler PR, Swiontkowski MF, Kilroy AW, *et al.*: Injury f the sciatic nerve associated with acetabular fracture. *J Bone Joint Surg Am* 1993, 75:1157–1166.
17. Borrelli J Jr, Torzill PA, Grigiene R, *et al.*: Effect of impact loading on articular cartilage: development of an intraarticular fracture model. *J Orthop Trauma* 1997, 11:319–326.
18. Brumback RJ, Holt ES, McBride MS, *et al.*: Acetabular depression fracture accompanying posterior fracture dislocation of the hip. *J Orthop Trauma* 1990, 4:42–48.
19. Mayo KA: Open reduction and internal fixation of fractures of the acetabulum: results in 163 fractures. *Clin Orthop Rel Res* 1994, 305:31–38.
20. Wright R, Barrett K, Christie MJ, *et al.*: Acetabular fractures: long-term follow-up of open reduction and internal fixation. *J Orthop Trauma* 1994, 8:397–403.

SECTION IV

Fractures of the Hip and Femur

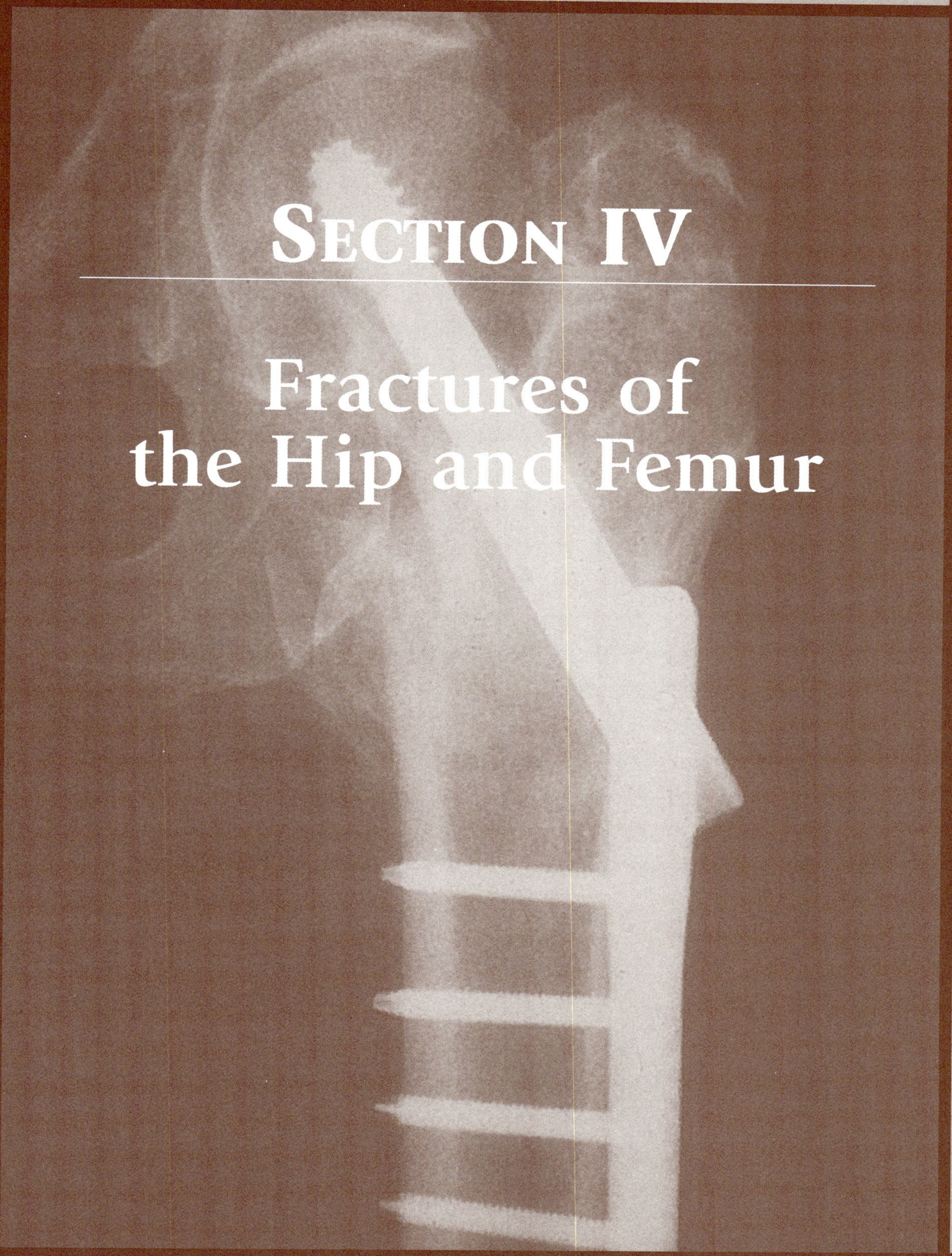

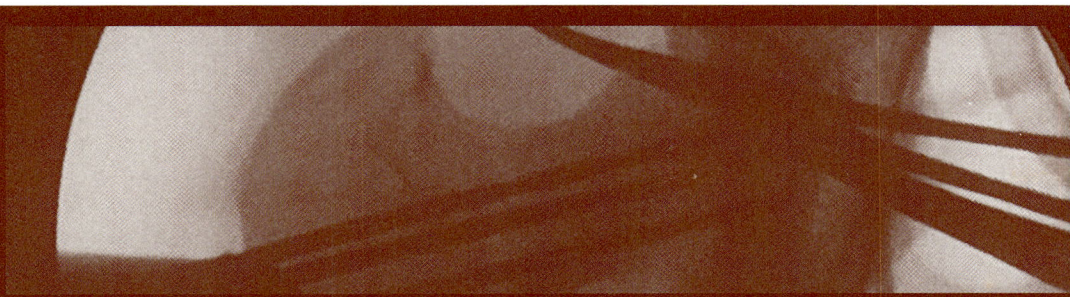

9

Femoral Neck Fractures

David C. Teague
Marc F. Swiontkowski

Femoral neck fracture commonly occurs in two disparate patient populations. Most patients are elderly individuals who sustain low-energy fractures from falls while standing or walking. Fewer than 5% of femoral neck fractures occur in high-energy trauma patients younger than 50 years of age. These fractures typically result from vehicular trauma or falls from significant height. Decidedly different management algorithms are used for these two injury types. This chapter details current standards of management for these two patient populations and explores current debates within the field.

ANATOMY

The adult femoral neck shaft angle measures approximately 130° in both men and women. Femoral neck anteversion typically measures 10° in both genders. A detailed understanding of the vascular supply of the femoral head supports a rational approach to certain aspects of surgical management of femoral neck fractures [1]. Most of the femoral head receives its blood supply from the lateral epiphyseal artery, the terminal branch of the medial femoral circumflex artery of the profunda femoris system (Figure 9-1) [2]. The inferior metaphyseal artery—that is, the terminal branch of the ascending portion of the lateral femoral circumflex artery—provides the only significant anterior blood supply. This vessel enters the mid-portion of the anterior hip capsule and supplies mostly anterior and inferior metaphyseal bone. The final component of the femoral head blood supply is a branch of the obturator arterial system, which enters the head through the ligamentum teres and branches out through the medial epiphyseal artery. In effect, the only vessels that absolutely require protection during a surgical approach to the hip are the lateral epiphyseal vessels contained within the retinacular reflection at the posterior-superior femoral neck.

PATHOPHYSIOLOGY

Femoral neck fracture significantly damages the blood supply to the femoral head; increasing displacement correlates with severity of damage to the lateral epiphyseal arterial system [3]. Although osteocyte loss from uncrushed trabeculae proximal to a femoral neck fracture requires 3 weeks to reach completion, irreversible cellular changes occur after 12 hours of ischemia. Dynamic blood flow studies in an animal model confirm a 60% decrease in femoral head blood flow following a minimally displaced femoral neck fracture despite an anatomic reduction [4]. Femoral head osteonecrosis results when this blood supply fails to reconstitute adequately.

Despite the certain injury to the femoral head vascularity that occurs coincident with femoral neck fracture, at least two surgical interventions positively influence outcome. First, optimal reduction of the femoral neck fracture lowers the rate of femoral head avascular necrosis [5]. As demonstrated by Claffey [6], even complete, displaced femoral neck fractures can occur without disruption of the lateral epiphyseal arterial system. In the displaced state, these intact vessels likely have poor flow due to kinking and direct pressure from fracture fragments in the same way that a malaligned fractured lower leg might exhibit distal pulselessness even with intact vessels until the limb has been reduced and splinted. Reduction of the femoral neck fracture may reestablish flow through unkinked vessels or at least lead to more rapid arterial recanalization.

The second surgical maneuver directly under the surgeon's control is performing an anterior capsulotomy. Severely displaced femoral neck fractures disrupt the posterior hip capsule [7], especially in high-energy injuries. If the displacement measures less than half the diameter of the neck, however, the capsule may remain intact. A significant intracapsular hematoma can accumulate in this situation, and the resulting pressure elevation may occlude the capsular venous drainage system or even halt arteriolar flow in the retinaculum reflection of the superior femoral neck. Numerous studies document an adverse effect on femoral head blood flow secondary to increased intracapsular pressure [8–10]. Because intracapsular pressures exceeding local arteriolar pressures are common, anterior capsulotomy probably plays a salutary role in minimizing femoral head ischemia [11].

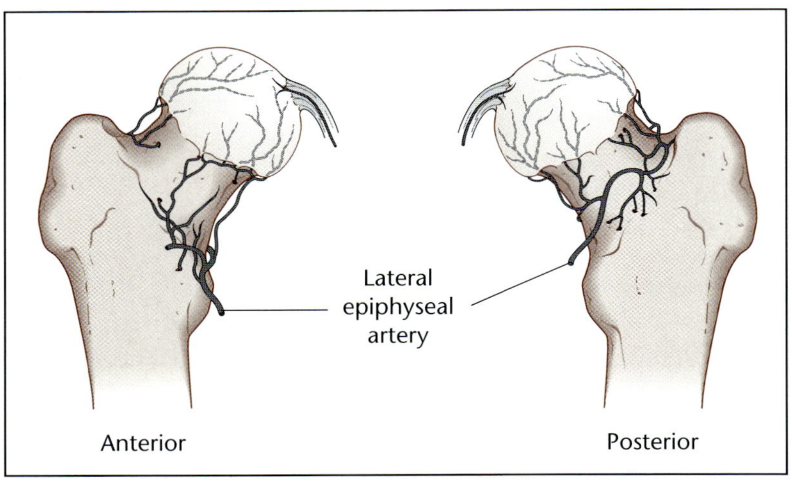

FIGURE 9-1. The lateral epiphyseal artery provides the majority of the femoral head blood supply in more than 90% of adults. The area of insertion of the anterior capsule contributes little to the femoral head arterial supply. (*Adapted from* Browner *et al.* [2].)

SURGICAL MANAGEMENT

Open Reduction

Most surgeons prefer to use a fracture table to assist with obtaining and maintaining reduced position of the fragments. For displaced fractures, a gentle closed reduction often substantially improves the position. The maneuver involves traction with the hip extended to restore length followed by internal rotation until the neck axis aligns with the femoral head. Multiple forceful reduction attempts should not be undertaken. The operative capsulotomy affords a visual check of the reduction and allows adjustment of the position, obviating the need for multiple closed reduction attempts.

For nondisplaced fractures, release of the capsular hematoma may mitigate excessive pressures producing vascular tamponade. This capsular tamponade appears to be the most plausible explanation for posttraumatic avascular necrosis following nondisplaced and impacted valgus fractures. For these injuries, reduction requires neither manipulation nor visualization. A limited capsulotomy under fluoroscopic guidance avoids the additional dissection necessary for open reduction yet provides the physiologic benefit of release of the capsular hematoma.

For displaced fractures, the Watson-Jones incision provides adequate access both to the proximal lateral femur and the anterior capsule and femoral neck [12]. The incision is centered over the greater trochanter. A straight lateral incision through the fascia lata exposes the vastus lateralis distally. Proximally, the interval between the gluteus medius and the tensor fascia muscles requires development. Blunt dissection in this interval proceeds down to the anterior hip capsule. Elevation of the vastus lateralis origin from the intertrochanteric ridge exposes the capsular insertion at this level. Distally, the vastus lateralis may be elevated anteriorly or split in line depending on the size of the patient and the surgeon's preference. Anterior hip capsulotomy performed in line with the femoral neck releases any intracapsular hematoma and provides digital and visual access to the fracture site. At the intertrochanteric ridge, 1-cm superior and inferior extensions of the capsulotomy result in a T-capsular incision that is tagged to assist with retraction and visualization. A bone hook placed about the greater trochanter permits lateral traction to the femoral shaft and allows disimpaction of the fracture site. Next, the limb is externally rotated by adjusting the fracture table. The femoral neck fragment attached to the shaft typically lies anterior to the femoral head fragment. Often, a blunt curved instrument placed between the fracture surfaces allows reduction of this offset as lateral traction is released. The reduction must be precise and confirmed with good-quality biplanar fluoroscopic images. Clinical outcome depends significantly on the quality of the reduction; angulation more than 20° on the lateral film produces a high incidence of failure [5].

Provisional reduction is maintained with a pointed reduction clamp or a 2-mm Kirschner wire placed centrally through the femoral neck in both fluoroscopic planes. After anatomic reduction has been confirmed, the cannulated screw system provides the most efficient means for stabilization (Figure 9-2). Three parallel cancellous screws placed in an inverted triangular configuration along the appropriate femoral neck axis adequately stabilize these fracture patterns, and additional screws do not afford increased strength to the construct [13–15]. Density of the bone is the most critical component with regard to fracture stability, and the implantation of a fourth or fifth screw produces no additional mechanical advantage. At least one screw should be placed within

3- to 5-mm of the subchondral bone. When poor bone quality exists, positioning one screw within 3 mm of the inferior femoral neck cortex may promote optimum stability [16]. These screws must achieve compression, so all threads should be in the femoral head fragment only, with no threads bridging the fracture site. If stable anatomic reduction cannot be achieved, a compression hip screw and side plate may be a better implant choice. This device transfers load to the lateral shaft rather than across the fracture. Again, the clinician must note that the quality of the reduction is the most critical aspect of management that remains directly under the surgeon's control.

When inserting multiple screws to fix a femoral neck fracture, attention to the lateral starting points is critical (Figure 9-3) [17]. Implants inserted through the thick lateral cortical bone distal to the point opposite the middle of the lesser trochanter predispose the limb to subtrochanteric fracture. Unfilled distal drill holes and screws placed from too distal a location produce stress concentrations that may lead to catastrophic failure in the early postoperative period even with a low-energy fall or twist. Management of this complication usually requires revision of the fixation to a compression hip screw and side plate sufficiently long to obtain at least four bicortical screws below the subtrochanteric fracture. Leaving one or two of the original screws in place prevents loss of position of an incompletely united femoral neck fracture during the revision surgery.

HEMIARTHROPLASTY

Although many regional variations exist, most surgeons prefer a posterolateral modified Gibson approach for hemiarthroplasty for femoral neck fracture. This approach requires a posterior capsulotomy; flexion and internal rotation provide exposure of the proximal femur. Lateral approaches do not violate the posterior capsule, potentially simplifying rehabilitation. Commonly used intervals include the Watson-Jones, between the tensor and gluteus medius muscles, and the direct lateral of Hardinge, between the anterior and posterior halves of the gluteus medius [1]. The direct lateral approach is associated with an 11% occurrence of permanent superior gluteal nerve palsy and resultant Trendelenburg gait [18]. These two approaches employ an anterior capsulotomy followed by hip flexion and external rotation to deliver the femoral head into the surgical field. A modular cemented unipolar or bipolar prosthesis is typically inserted for elderly patients.

CURRENT DEBATES

CAPSULOTOMY

Many surgeons still prefer closed reduction and percutaneous stabilization for intracapsular femoral neck fractures. Many, if not most, surgeons perform percutaneous stabilization for valgus impacted and nondisplaced intracapsular femoral neck fractures. Besides the obvious advantage of providing reduction under direct vision, we contend that a capsulotomy may be protective of the femoral head blood supply. Intracapsular tamponade can reduce blood flow to the femoral head in fractures with an undisrupted capsule [19,20]. Intracapsular pressure can rise to a level that impedes the venous drainage or arterial supply to the femoral head. The anterior capsulotomy effectively decompresses this tamponade effect and allows anatomic reduction under direct vision. Additionally, optimum reduction of femoral neck fractures results in a lower rate of avascular necrosis of the femoral head [11]. Presumably, timely reduction allows reestablishment of flow through the remaining intact

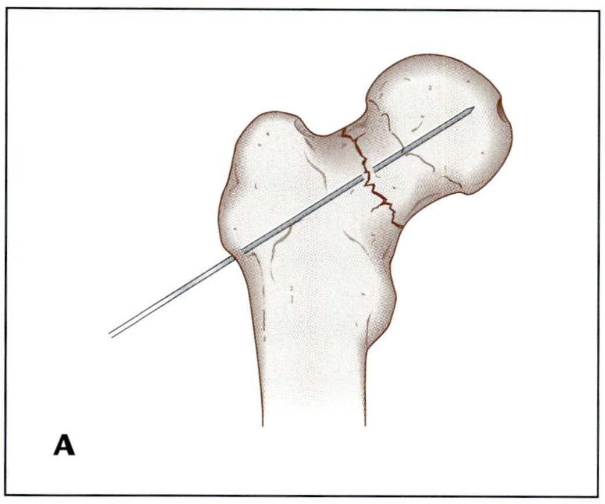

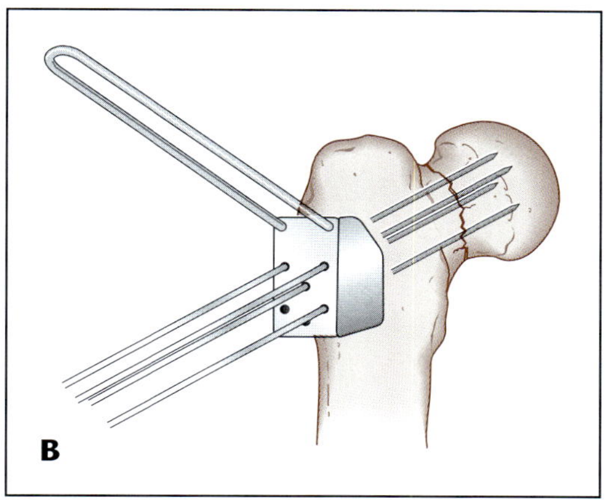

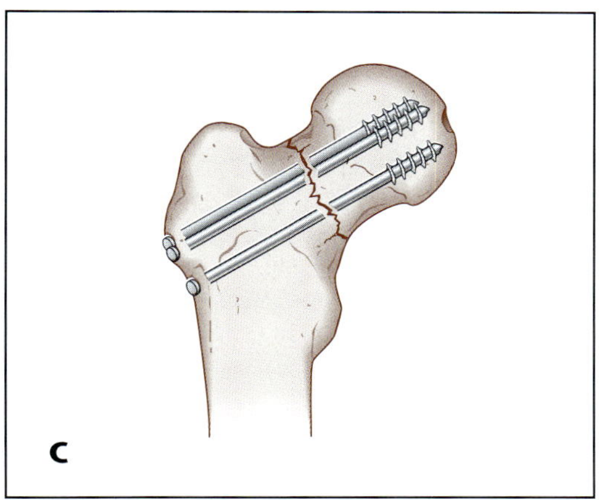

FIGURE 9-2. Cannulated screw fixation. A, The central control guide wire placed along the femoral neck axis provides provisional stabilization of the anatomically reduced fracture. B, Using a parallel drill guide, three guide wires are placed in an inverted triangle pattern. The initial wire may be maintained if its position is acceptable, or removed when a better configuration is obtained. C, Screws are inserted to within approximately 5 mm of subchondral bone. Most screws are self-tapping, but a cannulated drill and tap are necessary in young trauma patients with dense cancellous bone.

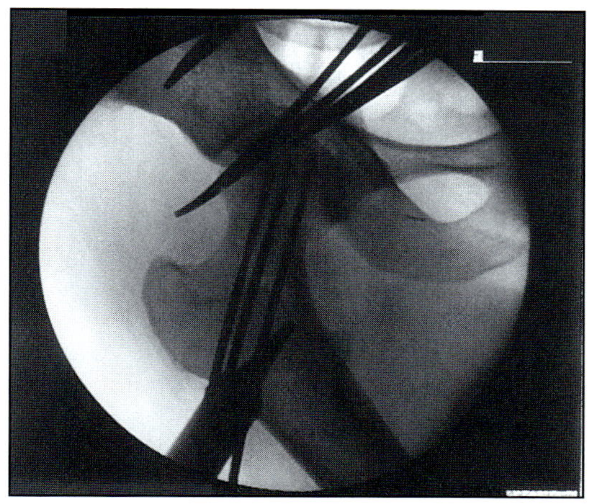

FIGURE 9-3. High-quality fluoroscopic image confirms anatomic reduction and parallel insertion of drill bits in an inverted triangle configuration. As noted, current systems allow use of cannulated drills and screws. Note that final screw position will be proximal to the midpoint of the lesser trochanter. (*From* Swiontkowski [17]; with permission.)

retinacular vessels, and stabilization provides an appropriate mechanical environment for revascularization. Thus, in young, high-energy trauma patients, an anterior capsulotomy should be performed both to release the intracapsular hematoma and to provide visualization of the reduction. The combined effect of this maneuver may reduce the danger of ischemia to the femoral head. In older patients with nondisplaced fractures, a limited capsulotomy may likewise diminish the risk of avascular necrosis.

Timing of Fixation

No series has reported a complete absence of avascular necrosis after internal fixation. Avascular necrosis occurs at a higher rate in younger adults with high-energy injuries. Almost all patients younger than age 50 years who develop this complication require a reconstructive procedure, whereas many older individuals with avascular necrosis tolerate these symptoms without need for a reconstructive procedure [21,22]. Several investigations have indicated that reduction of a displaced femoral neck fracture improves femoral head blood flow [4–6]. Superior displacement of the femoral head by up to one half of the femoral neck diameter can occur without disruption of the lateral epiphyseal artery complex [6]. As previously noted, the reduction likely "unkinks" or straightens these vessels in situations in which the epiphyseal artery complex remains intact. In one series of high-energy femoral neck fractures in patients aged younger than 50 years, the avascular necrosis rate was 20% when femoral neck fractures were reduced and stabilized with compressive internal fixation within 8 hours [11]. This information mandates an emergent reduction of femoral neck fractures in younger patients. Many young patients with this injury present with multisystem trauma. Lifesaving intervention clearly takes precedence in these settings. However, when orthopedic intervention is deemed appropriate, a displaced femoral neck fracture in a young patient should be considered a true emergency. Due to the limited options for treatment of posttraumatic avascular necrosis of the femoral head, the management of these fractures should be superseded only by addressing pelvic ring instability associated with serious bleeding, by débriding contaminated open fractures, and by reducing cervical spine subluxations and dislocations.

Ipsilateral Femoral Neck and Shaft Fractures

The uncommon but not rare ipsilateral femoral neck and shaft fractures present difficult treatment choices. Authors now agree that priority should first be given to the anatomic reduction and stabilization of the femoral neck component of the injury. The severe functional sequelae of failed femoral neck fixation in this typically young patient population mandate aggressive and precise management of the intracapsular injury. Second-generation cephalomedullary nails allow fixation of both the femoral neck fracture and the shaft fracture with a single implant. However, this surgery is technically demanding, even in experienced hands [23]. Numerous authors now detail the efficacy of retrograde femoral nail insertion for femoral shaft fractures [24,25]. This technique compares favorably with antegrade nailing for routine femoral diaphyseal fractures, although certain reservations exist with regard to long-term knee joint function, potential for knee septic arthritis associated with a deep infection about the nail, and possible problems with hardware removal. Nevertheless, the early success of retrograde femoral nailing makes it the recommended technique for stabilizing a femoral diaphyseal fracture below a femoral neck fracture (Figure 9-4). The intracapsular fracture should first be addressed with open reduction and internal fixation with multiple cannulated screws. Screw placement is simplified because no consideration need be given to antegrade nail passage through the piriformis fossa, and the retrograde nail seldom needs to extend proximal to the lesser trochanter. Reaming the diaphyseal fracture minimizes nail insertion pressure, which protects the femoral neck fixation during nail placement.

Hemiarthroplasty Versus Internal Fixation in the Elderly

Most orthopedists agree that the ideal result in elderly patients is a healed femoral neck fracture, thus preserving the patient's native femoral head and avoiding avascular necrosis. Stability of fixation, or the ability to achieve stable internal fixation with compression across the fracture, depends primarily on the density of the bone. Therefore, a certain subset of patients with poor bone quality, limited life span, or chronic disease will be better served with prosthetic replacement. However, we contend that open reduction and internal fixation should be strongly considered for most elderly patients with femoral neck fracture. Obtaining adequate reduction and stable fixation with multiple parallel screw technique decreases the rate of nonunion to 10% or less in most recent series [26]. Avascular necrosis continues to occur in up to 30% of united, initially displaced femoral neck fractures, but may not be sufficiently symptomatic to require additional treatment, especially in elderly patients with lower demands [22,27]. Patients more than 64 years of age who sustain a nondisplaced femoral neck fracture definitely should undergo open reduction and internal fixation [27]. A series of 215 displaced femoral neck fractures in elderly patients treated exclusively with open reduction and internal fixation demonstrated only a 17% reoperation rate [28]. A similar protocol that pro-

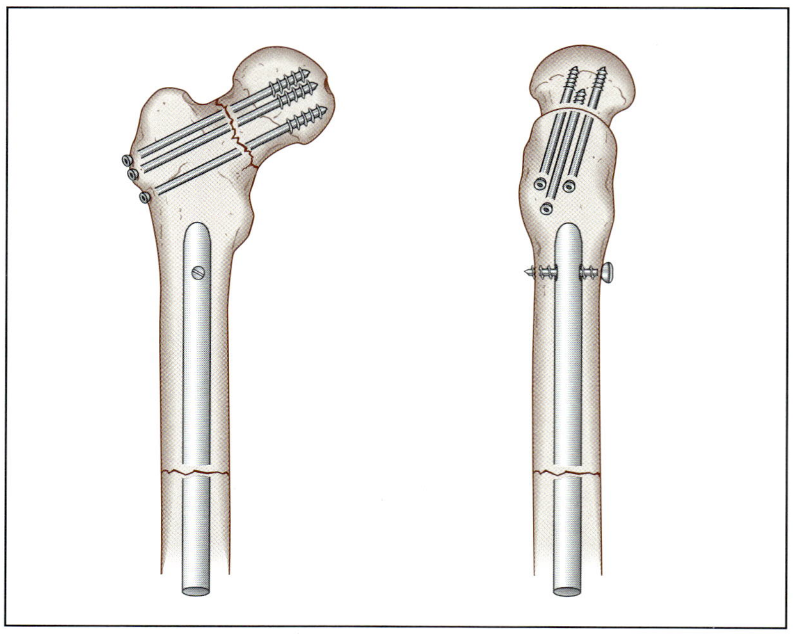

Figure 9-4. Ipsilateral femoral neck and shaft fractures stabilized with cannulated screws and retrograde intramedullary nail. This type of case ought to be performed with the entire leg draped into the field on a fluoroscopy table. The clinician should reduce and fix the femoral neck fracture first under direct vision, then proceed with closed interlocking nailing of the shaft through an intra-articular distal femoral starting point. Most retrograde nails require freehand anterior to posterior proximal locking.

vides for primary hemiarthroplasty in significantly osteopenic patients or those with chronic disease likely could produce an even lower rate of reoperation.

Unipolar Versus Bipolar Devices

First-generation hemiarthroplasty devices provided an alternative to internal fixation for femoral neck fractures but introduced inherent problems, including prosthetic loosening, acetabular erosion, and dislocation. Bipolar prosthetic designs were developed in response to these problems. These bicentric devices were expected to reduce frictional wear between the prosthesis and the acetabular articular cartilage. Two recent series identify no improvement in functional outcomes after femoral neck fractures in patients treated with cemented modular unipolar versus cemented modular bipolar prostheses [29,30]. Patients with bipolar hemiarthroplasty typically have slightly better range of motion at the hip with regard to rotation and abduction and frequently can manage a faster walking speed than patients treated with unipolar devices. Unipolar prostheses cost approximately $700 (U.S.) less than bipolar prostheses. Only 10% of patients with hip fractures at age 75 will still be alive 10 years later. A therapeutic strategy that favors unipolar hemiarthroplasty over bipolar hemiarthroplasty provides a substantial cost savings and is not likely to produce significant functional problems for long-term survivors. A similar analysis recommends hemiarthroplasty over total hip arthroplasty, but some noncontrolled reports suggest that total hip arthroplasty may provide better functional outcome for these elderly patients [31].

Surgical Approach for Hemiarthroplasty

The reported incidence of dislocation after primary prosthetic arthroplasty ranges from 0.3% to 11% [32]. The surgical technique used in most of these series includes a posterior approach and posterior capsulotomy. This approach possibly predisposes the prosthesis to posterior dislocation, particularly in debilitated elderly patients who may have difficulty adhering to hip flexion and internal rotation precautions. Consequently, lateral approaches employing an anterior capsulotomy for proximal femur delivery were thought to be indicated to diminish the dislocation rate. Despite a few early reports that appeared to demonstrate lower complication rates after anterior approaches, recent reports fail to support this advantage and specifically fail to demonstrate differences in medical or surgical complications following anterior or posterior approaches for hemiarthroplasty [27]. Either approach may provide acceptable results, and the choice should be based on the surgeon's experience and preference.

NEW MATERIALS AND TECHNIQUES

Cement Augmentation

A meta-analysis by Lu-Yao *et al.* [33] demonstrated an overall nonunion rate of 33% in displaced femoral neck fractures treated with internal fixation. This complication presents a greater management problem than does development of avascular necrosis, because most patients with nonunion develop severe pain and require a secondary procedure. The major predisposing factor for nonunion is the inadequate strength of severely osteoporotic bone surrounding the compression implants and comminution at the fracture site. These conditions reduce the ability to achieve stable fixation with compression at the fracture site and diminish the bone's load-sharing capacity. It can be demonstrated that the less stable the fracture is at surgery following fixation, the higher the risk will be for healing complications [34]. New high-strength cements, which are biocompatible and susceptible to remodeling and replacement, may prove to be valuable adjuncts in the treatment of femoral neck fractures in patients with poor bone quality. To prove useful, the cement must be injectable and fast setting to fill defects and improve mechanical holding strength in prepared osteoporotic bone. Norian SRS (Norian Corporation, Cupertino, CA) cement, an osteoconductive carbonated apatite with chemical and physical characteristics similar to those of the mineral phase of bone, cures nonexothermically at a physiologic pH [35]. In dynamic biomechanical tests of paired femoral neck fractures fixed with cancellous screws in an inverted triangle configuration, cement-augmented specimens fail at significantly higher loads (170%) than controls [36]. Control fracture constructs with the lowest strength of repair achieve the greatest improvement with cement augmentation, which suggests usefulness especially in patients with advanced osteoporosis. This material is approved by the U.S. Food and Drug Administration for use in distal radius and mandible fractures. European clinical trials remain under way for femoral neck fractures and intertrochanteric fractures.

Femoral Head Drilling

For patients in whom either internal fixation or hemiarthroplasty could potentially be considered, a new technique from Gill *et al.* [26] offers an intraoperative assessment of femoral head vascularity. All patients selected for open reduction had a straight lateral approach with an anterior capsulotomy. The capsulotomy allowed visualization of the fracture site and the femoral head. Acceptable reduction was achieved followed by drilling of the femoral head with a 2.0-mm drill directed from the base of the head fragment into the superior quadrant of the femoral head. Two to four holes were placed. These holes were then examined for the presence or absence of bleeding. Of these patients, 87% had bleeding from the drill holes after reduction, and none developed avascular necrosis. Another 13% of patients had no bleeding from the drill holes after reduction, and all developed avascular necrosis. This technique requires evaluation by other investigators. It may prove prognostically useful and provide assistance with intraoperative decision making regarding internal fixation versus hemiarthroplasty in a given subset of patients.

Our Approach

We favor open reduction and internal fixation for nondisplaced and displaced femoral neck fractures when appropriate. Younger patients who have sustained high-energy injuries receive emergent open reduction with capsulotomy and multiple screw fixation. Instead of a traditional fracture table, we prefer positioning the patient on a fluoroscopy table with the entire extremity and hip prepared and draped into the surgical field (Figure 9-5). A bump under the ipsilateral buttock elevates the operative site and facilitates obtaining lateral fluoroscopic views intraoperatively. This position obviates the need for an unscrubbed assistant. A bicortical Schanz pin placed at the level of the lesser trochanter provides control of the distal fragment and greatly assists with reduction maneuvers. The minimal shortening typically present is easily overcome, and sustained traction is not necessary once reduction is provisionally secured with a clamp or Kirschner wire.

Specific treatment choices for older individuals are based on pertinent factors including age, functional demands, comorbidities,

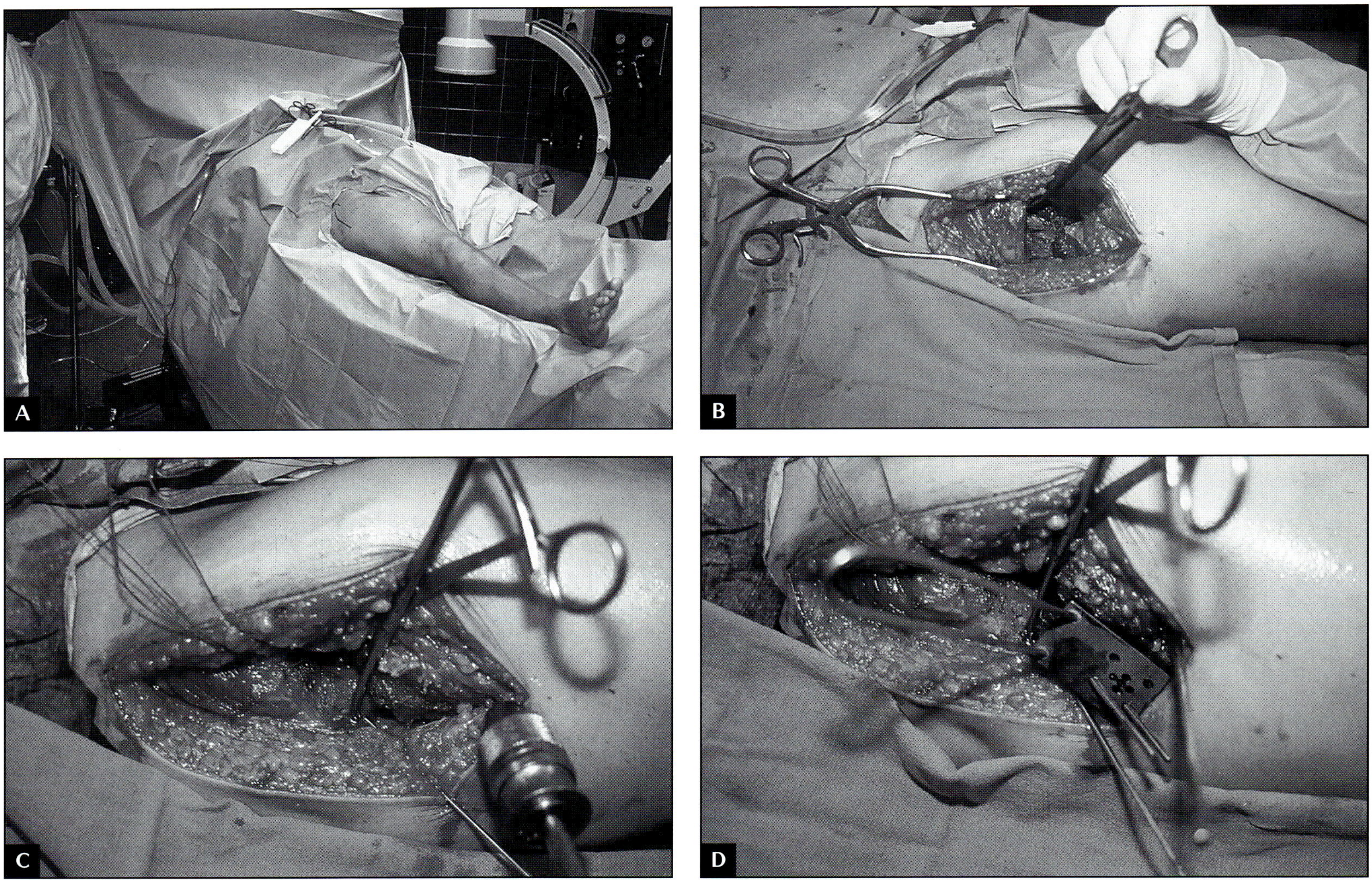

FIGURE 9-5. Open reduction and internal fixation of a high energy femoral neck fracture. **A,** Entire lower extremity prepared for surgery. **B,** Lateral incision centered over greater trochanter, and Watson-Jones interval developed for exposure of anterior capsule. **C,** Tag sutures in reflected capsule and Schanz screw in diaphyseal segment provide visualization of fracture and facilitate reduction, respectively. Pointed forceps maintain anatomic reduction with one point on the medial neck of the proximal fragment made accessible by the capsulotomy and the other on the lateral cortex of the distal fragment. A central guide wire further secures the reduction and provides a reference for the cannulated screw system. **D,** The parallel guide facilitates appropriate placement of cannulated screw guide wires. (*From* Swiontkowski [17]; with permission.)

and bone quality. Activity level and comorbidities, elicited from a careful history, are the most important factors for deciding therapy. Healthy elderly patients with high functional demands and good bone density merit a prompt open reduction, capsulotomy, and multiple screw fixation. Older patients with normal life expectancy but poor bone density or chronic illness typically receive cemented hemiarthroplasty with some consideration given to total hip arthroplasty. Elderly, low-demand patients with characteristically poor bone quality are best served by cemented unipolar hemiarthroplasty following appropriate medical work-up. Preoperative management of correctable medical conditions improves survival, which emphasizes the importance of medical consultation in this subset of patients [37,38].

Finally, we recommend a fundamental commitment to hip fracture prevention. We orthopedists must educate ourselves about the treatment and prevention of osteoporosis [39]. We should consistently advocate a lifestyle for all our patients that includes adequate calcium replacement, 400 to 800 units of vitamin D, appropriate exercise, and cessation of smoking. For our elderly patients, we need to prioritize fall-prevention efforts, including eliminating shag carpets and poor footwear, avoiding benzodiazepines, and encouraging routine exercise and annual visual acuity checks. For at-risk elderly patients, bisphosphonates, hormones, and calcitonin can restore bone mass and decrease the occurrence of fragility fractures. In nursing-home patients, hip-protective devices decrease the incidence of hip fracture [40]. Given that two thirds of the cost of osteoporosis in the United States is due to hip fractures, orthopedic surgeons can significantly improve the economy of medical care and the quality of life of our patients if we focus more of our efforts on these prevention issues [39].

REFERENCES AND RECOMMENDED READING

Recently published papers of particular interest have been highlighted as:
- • Of interest
- •• Of outstanding interest

1. Trueta J, Harrison MHM: The normal vascular anatomy of the femoral head in adult man. *J Bone Joint Surg Br* 1953, 35:442–461.

2. Browner BD, Jupiter JB, Levine AM: *Skeletal Trauma: Fractures, Dislocations, Ligamentous Injuries* edn 2. Philadelphia: WB Saunders; 1997.
3. Catto M: A histological study of avascular necrosis of the femoral head after transcervical fracture. *J Bone Joint Surg Br* 1965, 47:749–776.
4. Swiontkowski MF, Tepic S, Rahn B, *et al.*: The effect of femoral neck fracture on femoral head blood flow. In *Bone Circulation and Bone Necrosis: Fourth International Symposium on Bone Circulation*. New York: Springer Verlag; 1990:150–153.
5. Garden RS: Malreduction and avascular necrosis in subcapital fractures of the femur. *J Bone Joint Surg Br* 1971, 53:183–197.
6. Claffey TJ: Avascular necrosis of the femoral head: an anatomical study. *J Bone Joint Surg Br* 1960, 42:802–809.
7. Drake JK, Meyers, MH: Intracapsular pressure and hemarthrosis following femoral neck fracture. *Clin Orthop* 1984, 182:172–176.
8. Strömqvist LI, Ljung P: Preoperative and postoperative scintimetry after femoral neck fracture. *J Bone Joint Surg Br* 1984, 66:49–54.
9. Swiontkowski MF, Tepic S, Perren SM, *et al.*: Laser Doppler flowmetry for bone blood flow measurement: correlation with microsphere estimates and evaluation of the effect of intracapsular pressure on femoral head blood flow. *J Orthop Res* 1986, 4:362–371.
10. Swiontkowski MF, Tepec S, Rahn BA, *et al.*: The effect of femoral neck fracture on femoral head blood flow. *Orthop Trans* 1987, 11:344–345.
11. Swiontkowski MF, Winquist RA, Hansen ST: Fractures of the femoral neck in patients between the ages of twelve and forty-nine years. *J Bone Joint Surg Am* 1984, 66:837–846.
12. Watson-Jones R: Fractures of the neck of the femur. *Br J Surg* 1936, 23:787–808.
13. Springer ER, Lachiewicz PF, Gilbert JA: Internal fixation of femoral neck fractures: a comparative biomechanical study of Knowles pins and 6.5 mm cancellous screws. *Clin Orthop* 1991, 267:85–92.
14. Swiontkowski MF, Harrington RN, Keller TS, *et al.*: Torsion and bending analysis of internal fixation techniques for femoral neck fractures: the role of implant design and bone density. *J Orthop Res* 1987, 5:433–444.
15. Van Audekercke R, Martens M, Mulier JC, *et al.*: Experimental study on the internal fixation of femoral neck fractures. *Clin Orthop* 1979, 141:203–212.
16. Lindqvist S, Tornkvist H: Quality of reduction and cortical screw support in femoral neck fractures: an analysis of 72 fractures with a new computerized measuring method. *J Orthop Trauma* 1995, 9:215–221.
17. Swiontkowski MF: Femoral neck fractures: open reduction internal fixation. In *Master Techniques in Orthopedic Surgery: Fractures.* Edited by Wiss D. Philadelphia: Lippincott-Raven; 1998: 213–221.
18. Ramesh M, O'Byrne JM, McCarthy N, *et al.*: Damage to the superior gluteal nerve after the Hardinge approach to the hip. *J Bone Joint Surg Br* 1996, 78:903–906.
19. Crawford EJP, Emery RJH, Hansell DM, *et al.*: Capsular distension and intracapsular pressure in subcapital fractures of the femur. *J Bone Joint Surg Br* 1988, 70:195–198.
20. Strömqvist B, Nilsson L., Egund N, *et al.*: Intracapsular pressures in undisplaced fractures of the femoral neck. *J Bone Joint Surg Br* 1988, 70:192–194.
21. Protzman RF, Burkhalter WE: Femoral neck fractures in young adults. *J Bone Joint Surg Am* 1976, 58:689–695.
22. Barnes JT, Brown JT, Garden RS, *et al.*: Subcapital fractures of the femur: a prospective review. *J Bone Joint Surg Br* 1976, 58:2–24.
23. Kang S, McAndrew MP, Johnson KD: The reconstruction locked nail for complex fractures of the proximal femur. *J Orthop Trauma* 1995, 9:453–463.
24. Moed BR,Watson JT, Cramer KE, *et al.*: Unreamed retrograde intramedullary nailing of fractures of the femoral shaft. *J Orthop Trauma* 1998, 12:334–342.
25. Ostrum JT, DiCicco J, Lakatos R, *et al.*: Retrograde intramedullary nailing of femoral diaphyseal fractures.*J Orthop Trauma*1998, 12:464–468.
26. Gill TJ, Sledge JB, Ekkernkamp A, *et al.*: Intraoperative assessment of femoral head vascularity after femoral neck fracture. *J Orthop Trauma* 1998, 12:474–478.
27. Hudson JI, Kenzora JE, Hebel JR, *et al.*: Eight-year outcome associated with clinical options in the management of femoral neck fractures. *Clin Orthop* 1998, 348:59–66.
28. Strömqvist B, Hansson LI, Nilsson, LT, *et al.*: Hook-pin fixation in femoral neck fractures: a two-year follow-up study of 300 cases. *Clin Orthop* 1987, 218:58–62.
29. Cornell CN, Levine D, O'Doherty J, *et al.*: Unipolar versus bipolar hemiarthroplasty for the treatment of femoral neck fractures in the elderly. *Clin Orthop* 1998, 348:67–71.
30. Wathne RA, Koval KJ, Aharonoff GB, *et al.*: Modular unipolar versus bipolar prosthesis: a prospective evaluation of functional outcome after femoral neck fracture. *J Orthop Trauma* 1995, 9:298–302.
31. Broos PL: Hip fractures in elderly people: the surgical treatment in Leuven, Belgium. *Acta Chir Belg* 1994, 3:130–135.
32. Hunter GA: Should we abandon primary prosthetic replacement for fresh displaced fractures of the neck of the femur? *Clin Orthop* 1980, 152:158–161.
33. Lu-Yao GL, Keller RB, Littenberg B, *et al.*: Outcomes after displaced fractures of the femoral neck: a meta-analysis of one hundred and six published reports. *J Bone Joint Surg Am* 1994, 76:15–25.
34. Rehnberg L, Olerud C: Fixation of femoral neck fractures: comparison of the Uppsala and von Bahr screws. *Acta Orthop Scand* 1989, 60:579–584.
35. Goodman SB, Bauer TW, Carter D, *et al.*: Norian SRS cement augmentation in hip fracture treatment. *Clin Orthop* 1998, 348:42–50.
36. Stankewich CJ, Swiontkowski MF, Tencer AF, *et al.*: Augmentation of femoral neck fracture fixation with an injectable calcium-phosphate bone mineral cement. *J Orthop Res* 1996, 14:786–79.
37. Eiskjaer S, Ostgard SE: Risk factors influencing mortality after bipolar hemiarthroplasty in the treatment of fracture of the femoral neck. *Clin Orthop* 1991, 270:295–300.
38. Kenzora JE, McCarthy RE, Lowell JD, *et al.*: Hip fracture mortality: relation to age, treatment, preoperative illness, time of surgery, and complications. *Clin Orthop* 1984, 186:45–56.
39. Lane JM, Nydick M: Osteoporosis: current modes of prevention and treatment. *J Am Acad Orthop Surg* 1999, 7:19–31.
40. Zohman GL, Lieberman JR: Perioperative aspects of hip fracture care: guidelines for intervention that will impact prevalence and outcome. *Am J Orthop* 1995, 1:666–671.

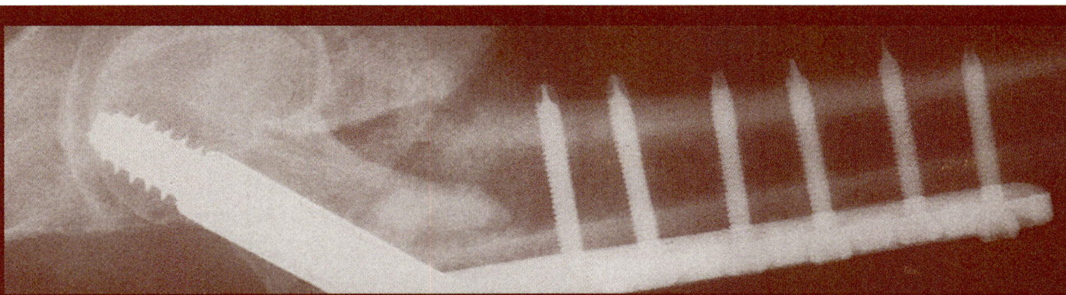

10

Intertrochanteric Hip Fractures

Richard F. Kyle
Thomas J. Ellis

Hip fracture in the elderly is a common and potentially devastating injury. Currently, more than 300,000 fractures occur annually in the United States, and this number is expected to double by the year 2050 [1]. Half of all hip fractures are intertrochanteric fractures. Because this is such a frequent injury, the orthopedic surgeon must understand current treatment principles of intertrochanteric hip fractures.

EPIDEMIOLOGY

The patient with an intertrochanteric hip fracture is generally slightly older and has higher morbidity and mortality than does the patient with femoral neck fractures [2]. The mechanism of injury is generally a fall with both a direct force applied to the greater trochanter as well as a torsional force applied to the shaft of the femur. The pull of the iliopsoas muscle on the lesser trochanter and of the abductor muscles on the greater trochanter also contribute to the fracture pattern [3]. Gait instability and osteoporosis are identified risk factors for hip fractures. In the younger population, high-speed trauma from motor vehicle accidents or falls from a height are the leading causes of hip fractures.

ANATOMY

Intertrochanteric fractures occur in the peritrochanteric area around the insertion of the abductor musculature, a region with a generous blood supply. The bony anatomy of the upper end of the femur is extremely important because it dictates where the surgeon must place his internal fixation devices for maximum purchase in the femoral head. The internal trabecular pattern was first described Ward [4] in 1938 (Figure 10-1). The major trabecular pattern consists of the primary compressive trabeculae and primary tensile trabeculae. These coalesce in the center of the femoral head to give maximum density of the trabecular bone in this area. The primary compressive trabeculae run in line with the weight-bearing forces that act on the hip at approximately 159°. The area between the primary and secondary trabeculae is called Ward's triangle. This space has minimal trabecular bone and provides extremely poor purchase for internal fixation devices. The triangle in the inferior portion of the head between the two primary trabecular patterns also has low-quality trabecular bone and provides poor fixation. The calcar femorale is a vertical plate of bone seen on a lateral view of the upper end of the femur (Figure 10-2). It originates from the posteromedial portion of the femoral shaft next to the lesser trochanter and radiates laterally toward the greater trochanter. It is thickest medially and gradually thins as it passes laterally. This plate of bone provides support in the posterior aspect of the femoral neck and resists posterior rotational forces exerted on the hip during normal activities of rising from the sitting position and stair climbing.

Singh *et al.* [6] devised a classification system for radiographically determining the degree of osteoporosis that depends on the presence or absence of these trabeculae. This has not proven to be a reliable indicator of osteoporosis because of poor interobserver and intraobserver reliability [7]. The surgeon can make an estimate of the degree of osteoporosis based on radiographs by noting the loss of primary and secondary compressive trabeculae. Tensile trabeculae are lost first and reflect moderate osteoporosis. Loss of compressive trabeculae reflects more severe osteoporosis.

BIOMECHANICS OF THE HIP

Forces passing through the hip joint are substantial. The total force at the hip during single-limb stance is approximately three times body weight. It has been shown that, in men, an average hip-joint reaction force of four times body weight occurs immediately after heel strike, with another peak of seven times body weight at toe-off [8]. During patient-care activities in bed and during passive exercises in physical therapy, substantial loading of up to four times body weight occurs [9]. In addition, variations in neck shaft angle (coxa vara or coxa valga) influence the efficiency of the abductor muscles and thereby influence the joint reactive force. Therefore, any internal fixation used to treat intertrochanteric hip fractures will be subjected to considerable stress.

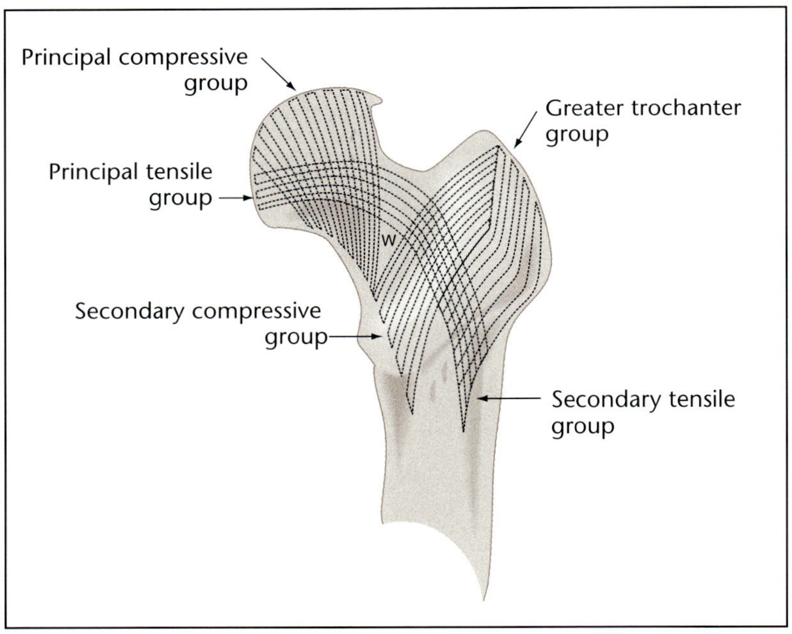

FIGURE 10-1. Internal trabecular pattern of the proximal third of the femur. The primary compressive and tension trabeculae coalesce in the center of the head. W—Ward's triangle. (*Adapted from* Rockwood *et al.* [5].)

With an intertrochanteric hip fracture, significant comminution of the posteromedial wall may occur as well as a fracture of the lesser trochanter. These posteromedial fragments account for much of the stability in the intertrochanteric region, and their comminution results in an unstable fracture. After the large posteromedial buttress is gone and stability has been lost, reestablishment of the medial buttress must be obtained to establish stability. Use of a sliding device can allow the impaction necessary to close the mechanical defect created by the fracture.

To apply these sliding devices correctly, it is essential to understand the mechanics of the devices and the forces that they must withstand. In a 1935 study, Pauwels [10] concluded that the forces acting on the hip in a single-limb stance amount to approximately three times the body weight applied at an angle of 159° to the vertical plane. These results were confirmed by other authors [10,11]. This same force acts on any hip fixation device that is placed across the fracture site.

A sliding device with a screw-plate angle closest to this combined force vector allows optimal ease of sliding and impaction. The closer the nail plate angle is to the resultant force across the hip, the more force is available to assist impaction (Figure 10-3) [12]. Devices with lower angles are subject to lower forces parallel and greater forces perpendicular to the sliding axis; these perpendicular forces act to jam or bend the device, thereby preventing impaction. Technically, however, the surgeon cannot place the sliding device at an angle greater than 150°.

The need to position the hip screw at the highest angle should not overshadow the need to place the screw in the center of the femoral head in both the anteroposterior (AP) and lateral views [13]. The most dense pattern of cancellous bone is located in the center of the femoral head, where primary compression and tension trabeculae coalesce. Clinically, center-head placement of the lag screw is associated with the lowest incidence of failure after open reduction internal fixation of intertrochanteric fractures (Figure 10-4) [14]. Therefore, it is mechanically desirable to place the sliding fixation device at as high an angle as clinically possible and still maintain center-head placement of the fixation device to prevent cutout.

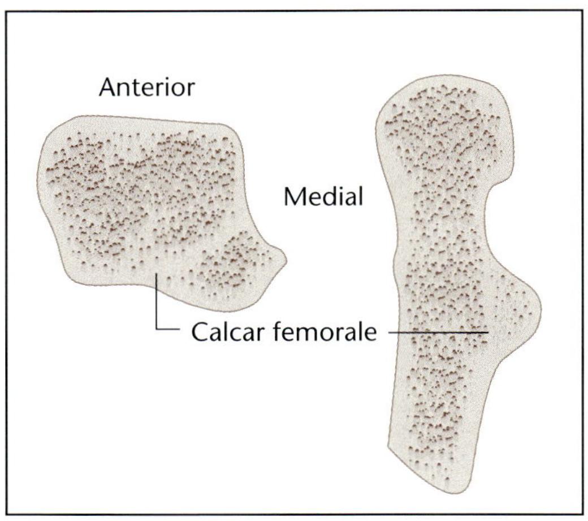

FIGURE 10-2. The calcar femorale is a vertical column of bone seen on a lateral view of the upper end of the femur. (*Adapted from* Rockwood *et al.* [5].)

Mechanical testing has shown that if fracture fragments are allowed to produce an impact, they carry a large portion of the load transmitted across the hip, thereby reducing the stresses on the fixation device and decreasing the chance of failure [15]. Properly placed sliding devices after anatomic reduction allow spontaneous impaction and medial displacement of all intertrochanteric fractures into a stable configuration (Figure 10-5). This allows early mobilization of the patient with weight bearing in most cases.

CLASSIFICATION

A fracture classification system is only of value if it leads to better care of the fracture or permits a more accurate prognosis. In intertrochanteric fractures, the classification should allow the surgeon to predict the stability of the fracture because stability is the key to successful treatment.

Intertrochanteric fractures can be classified as either stable or unstable. In a stable intertrochanteric fracture, the posteromedial buttress remains intact or is minimally comminuted. Collapse of the fracture fragments is minimal, and stability is obtained with reduction and reestablishment of the medial cortical contact. In an unstable intertrochanteric fracture, however, a large segment of the posteromedial wall is comminuted and the hip collapses into varus.

The classification devised by Kyle [16] identifies basic types of intertrochanteric fractures (Figure 10-6). Type I fractures consist of nondisplaced, stable intertrochanteric fractures without comminution (21%). Type II fractures represent stable, minimally comminuted but displaced fractures (33%). These stable fractures are not problem fractures because the bone is basically in a stable configuration once they are fixed. They can be fixed with either dynamic hip screws or with intramedullary hip screws.

Types III and IV fractures are unstable. Type III fractures (24%) have a large posteromedial comminuted area. These fractures are also most appropriately managed with a dynamic hip screw. Type IV fractures (14%) consist of an intertrochanteric fracture with a subtrochanteric component. This is a difficult fracture to treat because of the great force in the subtrochanteric region of the femur [13,17]. These can be managed with a 95° dynamic condylar screw or blade plate, a high-angled hip screw, or a second-generation intramedullary rod.

A newly described fracture is a Type V fracture (8%). This is an intertrochanteric fracture that has significant extension into the femoral neck. This pattern is very unstable and has a 50% failure rate when treated with a dynamic hip screw. In Kyle's [16] experience, the main failure mechanism is excessive collapse, probably because of the extensive comminution extending into the femoral neck. If the fracture is treated with a dynamic hip screw, then the construct should have a short barrel to allow for greater collapse.

Two other fractures patterns are important to mention. The reverse oblique fracture should be fixed with either a 95° blade plate or dynamic condylar screw or with a second-generation intramedullary nail. Successful treatment with an intramedullary nail is difficult because a posterior split in the greater trochanter can occur when reaming the small proximal fragment before placement of the nail. The second fracture is the basicervical femoral neck fracture. This is treated in a manner similar to that used for a stable intertrochanteric fracture. An additional guide pin or screw can be placed above the lag screw as a derotation pin during insertion of the lag screw. However, this does not add to the overall strength of the fixation [18].

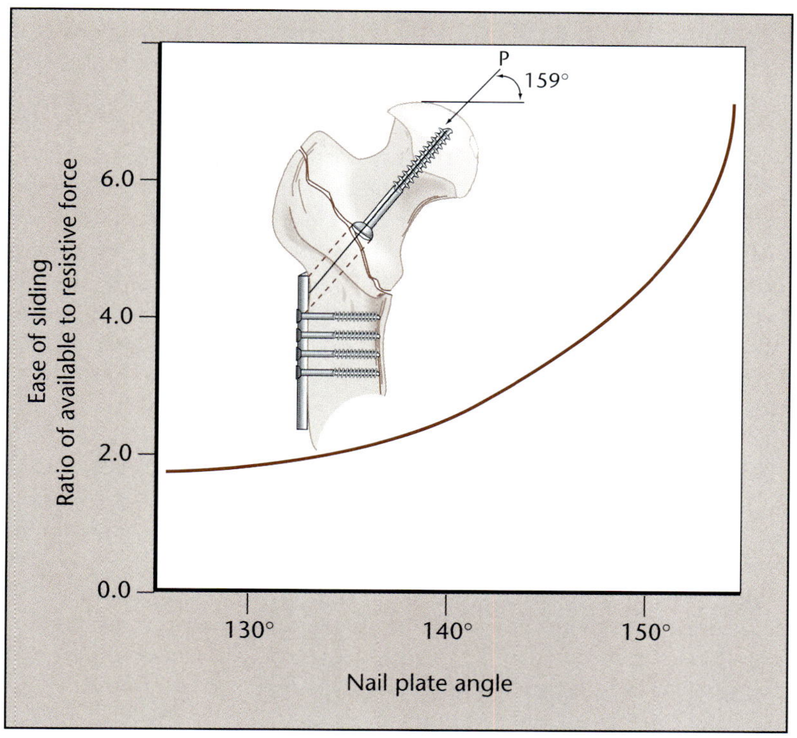

FIGURE 10-3. When ease of sliding is plotted against nail plate angle, the greater the ease of sliding. The closer the nail plate angle is to the resultant force across the hip, the more force is available to assist impaction of the sliding screw.

CLINICAL SIGNS

The patient with a hip fracture has a shortened and externally rotated leg. Any attempt to move the leg causes severe pain, so

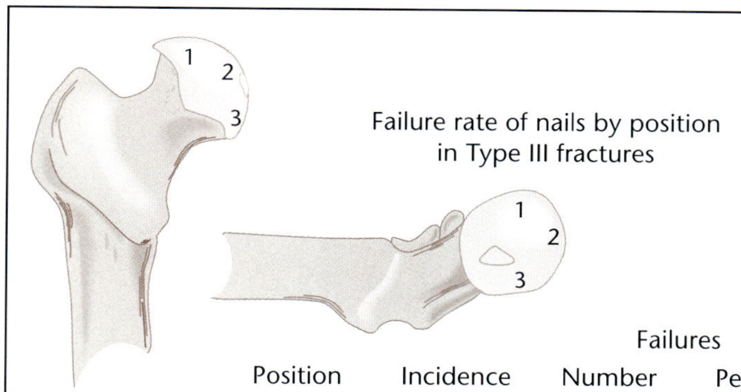

Position	Incidence	Failures Number	Failures Percent
2/2	34	0	0
2/3	22	1	4.5
2/1	4	0	0
1/2	6	2	33
1/3	4	1	25
3/3	4	1	25

FIGURE 10-4. The 2/2 position, or center head placement, gives the lowest failure rate in unstable intertrochanteric fractures.

forced attempts at range of motion should not be performed. In the elderly patient, a preoperative medical evaluation is important. Kenzora *et al.* [19] have shown that stabilization of the patient is essential prior to surgery and timing of surgery is dictated by the patient's medical condition. The old adage that patients are most stable when they come through the emergency department door is simply not true. Generally, patients can be stabilized within 12 to 24 hours.

RADIOGRAPHIC EVALUATION

Standard AP and lateral hip radiographs are obtained for evaluation. On the AP view, a fracture is seen between the greater and lesser trochanters. The larger the lesser trochanter fracture, the more unstable the fracture will be. If no fracture is seen but one is suspected based on results of a clinical examination, a magnetic resonance image (MRI) of the hip should be obtained. If the MRI is negative, it can be assumed that the patient does not have a hip fracture. If the MRI is positive for an intertrochanteric hip fracture, then the treatment plan is less clear and needs to be dictated by the physical examination findings. A patient who has minimal discomfort and is able to perform a straight leg raise can be treated nonoperatively and mobilized as tolerated. If symptoms worsen, then the surgeon should recommend open reduction and internal fixation of the fracture.

SURGICAL TECHNIQUE

Successful treatment of intertrochanteric fractures depends on the stability of the fracture fixation. The ability of the fixation device to obtain firm purchase in the proximal and distal fragments depends on the degree of osteoporosis of the bone fracture pattern and correct use of the fixation device. In severe osteoporosis, the ability of the bone to carry a substantial amount of the load is impaired even when a collapsing device is used. The purchase of the cortical screws through side plates in osteoporotic bone may also be impaired and result in the plate's pulling away from the femoral shaft. Using cerclage wires or methylmethacrylate in the side plate screw holes may minimize this risk.

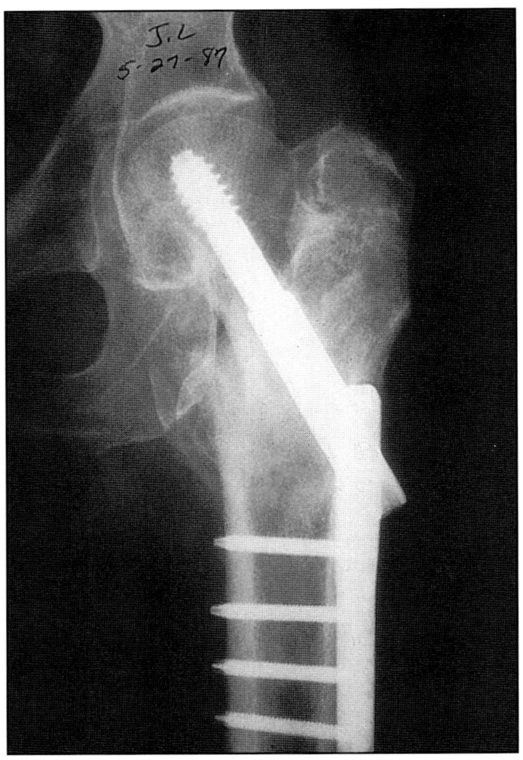

FIGURE 10-5. Sliding devices properly placed after anatomic reduction allow spontaneous impaction and medial displacement of all intertrochanteric fractures to a stable position.

The patient is brought to the operating room and placed supine on a standard fracture table. The unaffected hip is held in a gently flexed, abducted, and externally rotated position to assist in obtaining cross-table lateral radiographs of the affected hip. The fracture is reduced with traction applied to the affected leg; reduction is confirmed with image intensification. The fracture should be reduced in an anatomic or slight valgus position. If this cannot be obtained with traction, then the leg should be slightly abducted to 15° or 20°. A lateral view on the image intensifier should be taken during reduction to evaluate posterior sag of the fracture and to assess the amount of anterior angulation of the femoral neck. If the patient has persistent posterior sag of the shaft, a crutch can be used outside the sterile field to elevate and hold the shaft reduced to the neck. It is important to obtain a good reduction of the fracture in both the AP and lateral planes *before* prepping the hip.

The hip is prepped and draped in the usual sterile manner. An incision is made over the lateral aspect of the thigh, beginning at the flare of the greater trochanter and extended 12 to 15 cm distally. The dissection is carried down though the skin and subcutaneous tissue to the fascia lata, which is split along its posterior extent. This exposes the vastus lateralis, which is retracted superiorly with an Israel retractor and split longitudinally. The lateral aspect of the femoral shaft is exposed with a periosteal elevator; the vastus lateralis and fascia lata are retracted anteriorly with a Bennett retractor. Dissection of the vastus lateralis muscle is limited to 4 to 5 cm around the level of the lesser trochanter.

A ⅛-in guide pin is placed on the anterior aspect of the femoral shaft and neck, with the blunt end projecting toward the midline of the patient. The guide pin should appear in its proper position at a high angle, bordering the medial cortex and appearing to lie within the center of the femoral head on the AP view. This allows visualization with the image intensifier to ensure that the hole drilled in the lateral aspect of the shaft is at the appropriate level.

The lateral aspect of the femoral shaft is perforated at the appropriate level dictated by the anterior ⅛-in guide pin. This is accomplished using a drill that is slightly larger than the selected guide pin. If the femoral head and neck lie posterior in the lateral plane, the drill hole should start slightly anterior on the lateral aspect of the femur. Conversely, if the head and neck lie anterior, the drill hole should be started slightly posterior.

The drill is advanced across the fracture site to the subcapital level of the femoral head. During drill advancement, the position of the drill is checked under image intensification in both the AP and lateral planes to ensure proper position of the drill. This is the single most important step in fixation of intertrochanteric hip fractures. The drill should lie at the highest angle anatomically possible and be positioned in the center of the femoral head in both the AP and lateral projections. The drill is then removed, and the guide pin is passed through the hole made by the drill to the level of subchondral bone (Figure 10-7).

The angle of the side plate is determined by using a variable angled guide. Some surgeons like to use the variable-angled guide to pass the guide pin. Most hip fixation devices come in variable angles in 5° increments. This allows an accurate fit of the plate to the shaft

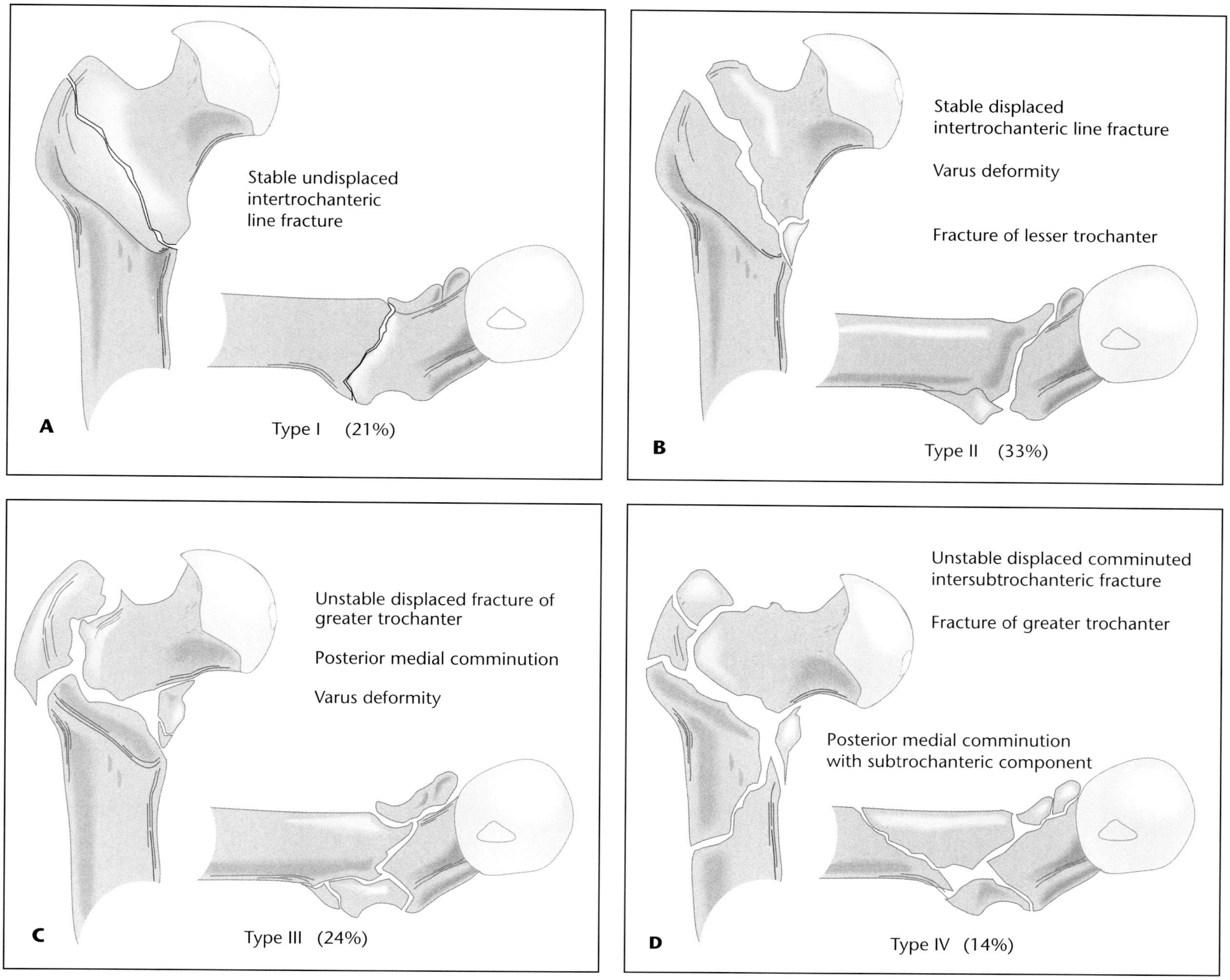

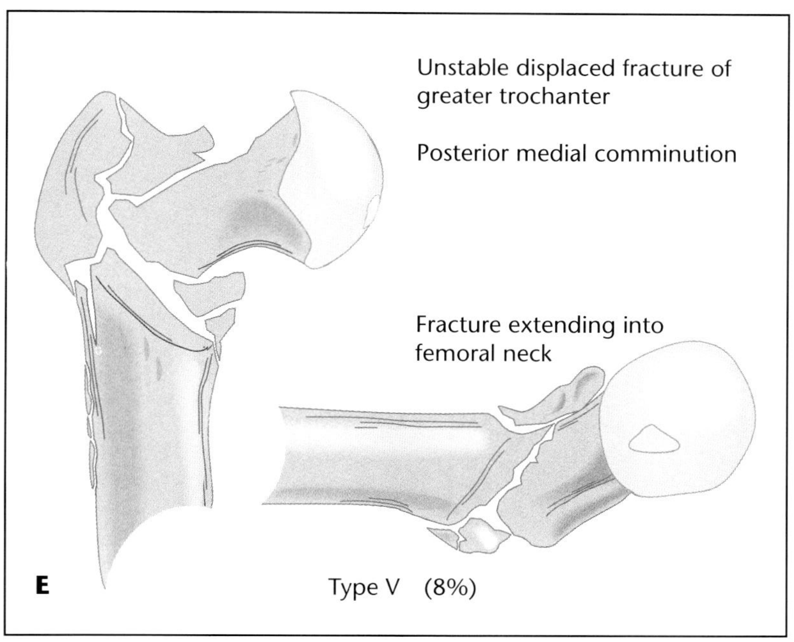

FIGURE 10-6. A–E, Classification of intertrochanteric fractures used at Hennepin County Medical Center. The classification is based on stability. Types III and IV are unstable. Type V is a newly described fracture and has the highest failure rate (*Adapted from* Kyle [16].)

of the femur. The length of the lag screw is determined from the guide pin. A cannulated reamer is then passed over the guide pin and passed to within 10 mm of subchondral bone. Depending on the bone quality, a tap may be inserted across the fracture site into the neck and head fragment within 5 mm of subchondral bone. The screw is then placed over the guide pin and inserted under image intensification to within 5 mm of subchondral bone.

After the screw has been seated, engage the side plate into the lag screw and make sure the plate lies parallel to the shaft. To limit stripping of the vastus lateralis muscle, the side plate is first slid distally underneath the muscle and then engaged to the lag screw. A fixed-angle screw and side plate that do not lie parallel to the shaft after the screw has been inserted may cause a subtrochanteric fracture if the plate is forced down on the shaft. If an inappropriate angle has been selected so that the plate diverges by more than 5° from the shaft, the plate should be removed and the appropriately angled side plate should be selected. The plate is fixed to the lateral aspect with cortical bone screws. In good bone, three cortical screws affixed into the side plate are probably sufficient [20]. However, in patients with osteoporotic bone, additional screws may be needed. If the fracture is comminuted and significant collapse is anticipated, a short barrel on the side plate should be used.

Traction is then released from the affected hip, and the knee is grasped through the sterile drapes to ensure that traction is released and that impaction can occur. Fracture fragments receive an impact either by a direct blow with an impactor or by compression with a compression screw as dictated by the system used. If a compression screw is used, care must be taken not to pull the hip screw out of the head in osteoporotic bone. The hip is rotated freely on the fracture table and a quick view is obtained with the image intensifier to ensure that the screw is within the confines of the femoral head.

The wound is thoroughly irrigated and hemostasis is obtained by electrocautery as needed. The wound is then closed in the usual fashion and a sterile dressing is placed.

POSTOPERATIVE CARE

The patient is allowed to sit as tolerated. If solid fixation was obtained in intertrochanteric fractures of Types I, II, or III, the patient is allowed to work on transfers and gait-training weight bearing as tolerated on the injured extremity. A study by Koval *et al.* [21] found that patients voluntarily limit loading of their injured extremity after open reduction of hip fractures. If the bone is highly osteoporotic or poor fixation is obtained, delayed weight bearing is necessary until fracture callous is evident. In Type IV fractures, the patient should be toe-touch weight bearing until callous formation is present. After callous formation is present, the patient is allowed to increase weight bearing as tolerated. Prophylactic perioperative antibiotics have reduced the incidence of infection to less than 1%. These patients also are at risk for deep venous thrombosis. Early mobilization and either mechanical or chemical deep venous thrombosis prophylaxis are indicated.

PROSTHETIC REPLACEMENT

Primary prosthetic replacement is rarely indicated in an intertrochanteric hip fracture because of the difficulty of the surgery. It may be necessary in patients with severe osteoarthritis or rheumatoid arthritis, or when a tumor has invaded the femoral

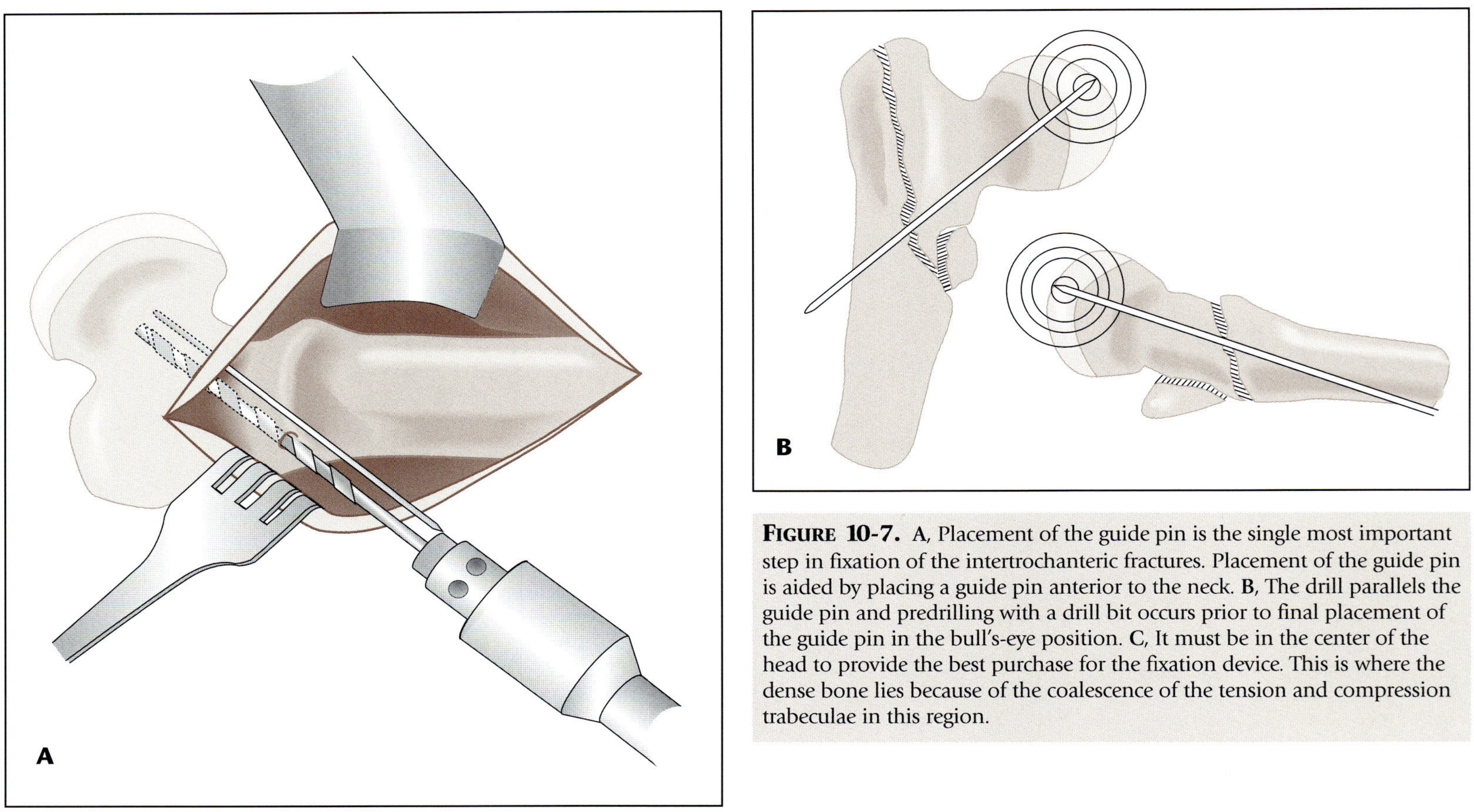

FIGURE 10-7. A, Placement of the guide pin is the single most important step in fixation of the intertrochanteric fractures. Placement of the guide pin is aided by placing a guide pin anterior to the neck. **B**, The drill parallels the guide pin and predrilling with a drill bit occurs prior to final placement of the guide pin in the bull's-eye position. **C**, It must be in the center of the head to provide the best purchase for the fixation device. This is where the dense bone lies because of the coalescence of the tension and compression trabeculae in this region.

head or acetabulum. It may also be indicated in the severely osteoporotic patient with a Type V fracture. Determining the appropriate anteversion and length of the prosthesis is difficult because the normal landmarks are involved in the fracture. It is important to repair the trochanter if possible to maintain competent abductors and decrease the risk of postoperative dislocation.

COMPLICATIONS

Results of intertrochanteric fracture fixation are gratifying. Nonunion occurs in less than 1% of cases [16]. When nonunion does occur, the patient may be treated with repeat internal fixation and bone grafting. If evidence of varus deformity is present, an osteotomy is performed in the intertrochanteric region, and a valgus alignment is created with simultaneous bone grafting of the medial cortex. Avascular necrosis occurs in less than 1% of intertrochanteric hip fractures [16]. If the patient is symptomatic with segmental collapse, then a total hip replacement may be necessary.

Most complications in intertrochanteric fracture treatment are secondary to screw cutout and varus deformity (Figure 10-8). These complications result from poor placement of the fixation device [16]. The incidence of cutout or varus deformity ranges from 6% to 10%. When contemporary devices composed of high-strength stainless steel or titanium are used, fracture of the implant is under 1% [22,23]. If cutout and varus deformity do occur, the surgeon may elect to revise the fixation before destruction of the femoral head and acetabulum. This may be accomplished with another screw placed at a different angle if sufficient bone remains within the femoral head. If sufficient bone is not present within the femoral head, a blade plate is a good alternative. Regardless of the implant used, the fracture should be fixed in slight valgus and in most cases, bone graft should be applied.

REFERENCES AND RECOMMENDED READING

Recently published papers of particular interest have been highlighted as:
- • Of interest
- •• Of outstanding interest

1. Hudson JI, Kenzora JE, Hebel JR, *et al.*: Eight year outcome associated with clinical options in the management of femoral neck fractures. *Clin Orthop* 1998, 348:59–66.
2. Allfram PA: Epidemiologic study of cervical and trochanteric fractures of the femur in an urban population. *Acta Orthop Scand Suppl* 1964, 65:1–109.
3. Inman VT: Functional aspects of the abductor muscles of the hip. *J Bone Joint Surg* 1947, 23:803–810.
4. Ward FO: *Human Anatomy*. London: Renshaw; 1938.
5. Rockwood CA Jr, Green DP, Bucholz RW: *Rockwood and Green's Fractures in Adults,* edn 3, vol 2. Philadelphia: JB Lippincott; 1991.
6. Singh M, Nagrath AR, Maini PS: Changes in the trabecular pattern of the upper end of the femur as an index of osteoporosis. *J Bone Joint Surg Am* 1970, 52:457–467.
7. Gustilo RB, Kyle RF, Hoeltzel DA: An evaluation of the reproducibility of the Singh index system for evaluation of osteoporosis. Presented at 18th Annual Orthopedic and Trauma Seminar, Minneapolis, MN; 1984.
8. Paul JP: *Forces at the Human Hip Joint* [thesis]. Chicago: University of Chicago; 1967.
9. Frankel VH, Burstein AH, Lyge L, *et al.*: The telltale nail: Proceedings of American Association of Orthopaedic Surgeons. *J Bone Joint Surg Am* 1971, 53:1232.
10. Pauwels F: Der Schenkenholsbruck, Mechanisches Problem. Grundlagen des Heilungsvorganges. Prognose und kausale Therapie. *Z Orthop Chir,* 1935.
11. Massie WK: Extracapsular fractures of the hip treated by impaction using a sliding nail-plate fixation. *Clin Orthop* 1962, 22:180–202.
12. Kyle RF, Wright TM, Burstein AH: Biomechanical analysis of the sliding characteristics of the compression hip screws. *J Bone Joint Surg Am* 1979, 61:1308–1314.
13. Kyle RF, Gustilo RB, Premer RF: Analysis of 622 intertrochanteric hip fractures: a retrospective and prospective study. *J Bone Joint Surg Am* 1979, 61:216–221.
14. Baumgaertner MR, Curtin SL, Lindskog DM, *et al.*: The value of tip-apex distance in predicting failure of fixation of peritrochanteric fractures of the hip. *J Bone Joint Surg Am* 1995, 77:1058–1064.
15. Frankel VH: *The Femoral Neck: Function, Fracture Mechanism and Internal Fixation—An Experimental Study*. Springfield, IL: Charles C. Thomas Publishers; 1960.
16. Kyle RF: Intertrochanteric fractures. In *Operative Orthopaedics*. Edited by Chapman MW. Philadelphia: JB Lippincott; 1988:353–359.
17. Wile PB, Panjabi MM, Southwick WO: Treatment of subtrochanteric fractures with a high angle compression hip screw. *Clin Orthop* 1983, 175:72–78.
18. Blair B, Koval KJ, Kummer F, *et al.*: Basicervical fractures of the proximal femur. *Clin Orthop* 1994, 306:256–263.
19. Kenzora JE, McCarthy RE, Lowell JD, *et al.*: Hip fracture mortality: relation to age, treatment, preoperative illness, time of surgery, and complications. *Clin Orthop* 1984, 186:45–56.
20. Yian EH, Banerji I, Matthews LS: Optimal side plate fixation for unstable intertrochanteric hip fractures. *J Orthop Trauma* 1997, 11:254–259.
21. Koval KJ, Sala DA, Kummer FJ, *et al.*: Postoperative weight-bearing after a fracture of the femoral neck or an intertrochanteric fracture. *J Bone Joint Surg Am* 1998; 80:352–356.
22. Dimon JH: The unstable intertrochanteric fracture. *Clin Orthop* 1973, 92:100–107.
23. Naiman PT, Schein AJ, Siffert RS: Medial displacement fixation for severely comminuted intertrochanteric fractures. *Clin Orthop* 1969, 62:151–155.

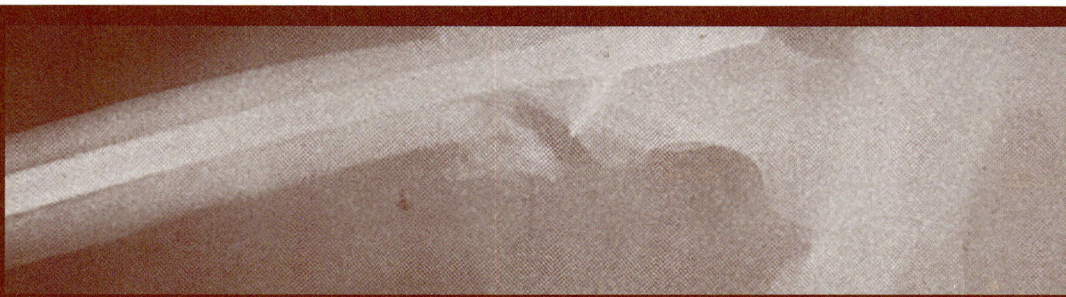

11

Subtrochanteric Fractures of the Femur

Ronald W. Lindsey
Zbigniew Gugala

Subtrochanteric fractures represent a subset of proximal femur fractures associated with a high incidence of complications [1]. Regional specific factors involving the anatomy, biology, and biomechanics may inhibit the surgeon's ability to adequately reduce, stabilize, mobilize, and ultimately heal these fractures. The subtrochanteric fractures literature is difficult to analyze because most clinical studies tend to combine all subtrochanteric fractures, although these fractures can be quite different depending on the type of patient and mechanism of injury [2]. Many clinical reports include various implants or surgical techniques, making distinctions between different treatment methods more obscure [3]. Existing fracture classification systems vary and are not always comprehensive, and pertinent associated factors, such as bone quality or postoperative mobilization, are not always accurately described. This chapter presents a modern approach to subtrochanteric fractures, their analysis, treatment options, and ultimate functional objectives.

SUBTROCHANTERIC REGION

Subtrochanteric fractures occur in a region of the femur that is well identified although not always accurately defined (Figure 11-1). Fielding and Magliato [4] and Fielding [5] described the subtrochanteric portion of the femur as beginning at the upper level of the lesser trochanter and extending distally for 7.5 cm into the femur diaphysis. This definition, however, does not account for the size of the femur. We prefer the designation of Kinast *et al.* [6], who modified this definition to include the area of the proximal femur from the upper border of the lesser trochanter extending a distance three times the height of the lesser trochanter.

EPIDEMIOLOGY

Subtrochanteric fractures comprise between 10% and 35% of all fractures of the proximal femur [5–8]. Patients with this fracture usually present in a bimodal distribution according to age. Most patients are elderly with osteopenic bone and have been injured by relatively minor trauma (*eg,* a fall). The second, smaller group includes younger patients and victims of high-energy insults (*eg,* motor vehicle accidents). In a clinical review of subtrochanteric fractures, Bergman *et al.* [9] found the mean age of patients with low-energy fractures to be approximately 76 years compared with a mean age of 40 years in those with high-energy injuries. This disparity in the mean age and the mechanisms of injury has a significant effect on optimal treatment selection. Elderly patients usually have lower functional demand but poor bone quality in which to achieve fixation. Younger patients tend to have better bone quality, but their fractures are typically more comminuted, their functional expectations are high, and these fractures frequently occur with other injuries.

Bergman *et al.* [9] also recognized two additional subgroups of patients. One group consisted of those with pathologic fractures secondary to metastatic or primary neoplasms or metabolic bone disease. Stable fixation is especially challenging in these patients because healing can be either limited or prolonged. The other group consisted of patients with fractures secondary to nonunion or a failed attempt at previous fixation. Successful salvage of the elderly patient requiring rapid mobilization may consist of hemiarthroplasty [10].

BIOLOGIC AND BIOMECHANICAL CONSIDERATIONS OF SUBTROCHANTERIC FRACTURES

Biologically, the subtrochanteric region of the proximal femur is composed of thick cortical bone as opposed to the cancellous bone found in the intertrochanteric region. The enveloping musculature is well vascularized, but this cortical bone heals at a slower rate than the adjacent metaphysis and is at greater risk for delayed or nonunion. Prolonged healing times are especially prevalent in comminuted fractures, which usually benefit from supplemental bone grafting [11].

Biomechanically, the subtrochanteric region transfers load from the hip onto the shaft of the femur through a relatively small area that is repeatedly subjected to enormous mechanical loads. These stresses, generated by body weight and hip musculature, result from the bending moment and compressive forces at the hip joint. In 1917, Koch [12] calculated the subtrochanteric medial compression load of a 200-lb male during weight bearing to be approximately 1200 lb/in^2, whereas the lateral tensile loads were approximately 1000 lb/in^2. Frankel and Burstein [13] later demonstrated that, even with bed rest, simple activity such as hip flexion and extension created significant loads through this area. Typically, the muscles on the lateral aspect of the proximal femur partially offset the high compressive stresses on the medial cortex. However, this region is loaded eccentrically, and most of the load is resisted by the subtrochanteric posterior medial cortex, which is critical for the stability of this region. Fielding and Magliato [4] emphasized the importance of maintaining or reestablishing medial cortex continuity in minimizing the risk for implant fatigue failure.

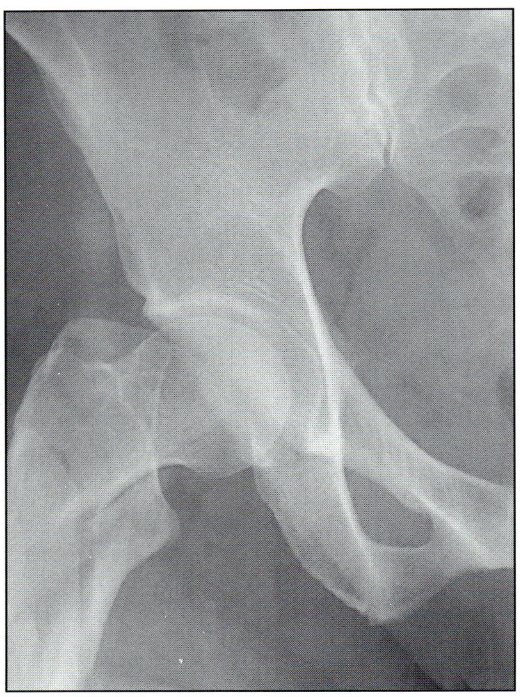

FIGURE 11-1. A comminuted fracture of the right proximal femur that begins at the intertrochanteric region and extends into the subtrochanteric region below the lesser trochanter.

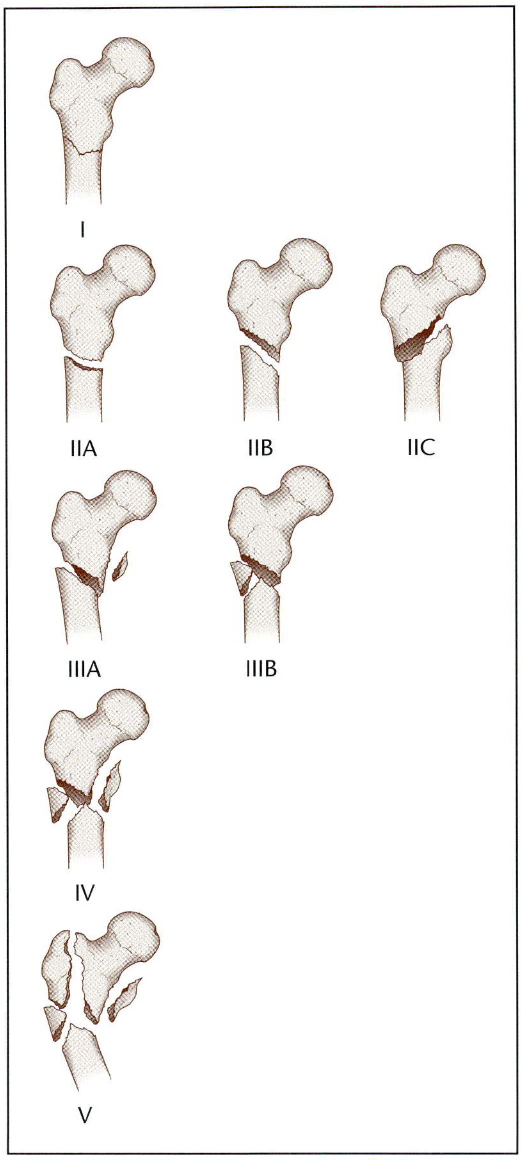

FIGURE 11-2. Seinsheimer [17] classification for subtrochanteric fractures.

Further biomechanical study recognized that, apart from fracture characteristics, limb stability was also affected by the type of fixation employed. The bending moment was noted to be greater on fixation placed further from the line of joint reaction forces (*ie*, plate and screws) compared with the more central intramedullary device [14]. It was later determined that the torsional loads through this region created considerable rotational shear and fatigue, which was reduced by implants with static interlocking [15]. Tencer *et al.* [16] tested various implants and concluded that large intramedullary nails provided the best bending stiffness; torsional stiffness improved to only 40% of the intact femur with plate and screw constructs (although considerably better than the 5% with open slot nails); and slotted nails in single load to failure withstood approximately twice the body weight of screw-and-slide-plate devices.

Finally, proximity of the fracture to the hip joint and the large hip musculature can complicate fracture reduction and stabilization. The iliopsoas attaches to the lesser trochanter and, when intact, places the proximal fragment in flexion and external rotation. The large hip abductors abduct the proximal fragment through its attachment on the greater trochanter. Meanwhile, the distal fragment is both abducted and shortened by the hamstrings and adductors. Fixation of subtrochanteric fractures, which is ultimately limited by the amount and quality of bone proximal to the fracture, must resist these displacement forces. Therefore, the increased time to union, the enormous cyclic loads across the region, and the limited available bone for proximal fixation combine to place subtrochanteric fractures at high risk for fixation failure, delayed union, or nonunion.

CLASSIFICATION

Ideally, a classification system both categorizes injuries and assists in determining optimal treatment or providing insight into the clinical outcome. Many subtrochanteric fracture classification systems are primarily intertrochanteric or shaft fractures descriptions that have been expanded to include the subtrochanteric region. We prefer the Seinsheimer [17] classification, because it is specific for the subtrochanteric region and identifies the principal fracture fragments as well as their location and configuration. Most important, this system allows the clinician to differentiate between stable and unstable fractures easily and to select appropriate fixation. The Seinsheimer classification system is depicted in Figure 11-2 and a Seinsheimer Type IIIA fracture is shown in Figure 11-3. Subtrochanteric fractures are categorized into five basic types, as described in Table 11-1.

DIAGNOSIS

Patients sustaining subtrochanteric fractures usually offer a history of either extremely high- or low-energy trauma. Patients with low-energy trauma are usually elderly; when low-energy trauma occurs in the younger patient, a pathologic basis for the injury should be considered. High-energy fracture patients can be older, but these injuries usually are reported in a younger patient population. In these patients, a thorough emergency trauma evaluation should be performed to rule out the presence of associated injuries.

Patients with subtrochanteric fractures clinically present with severe pain on passive or active motion of the affected limb and are unable to bear weight. The limb posture is usually shortened with the foot externally rotated. Significant thigh swelling and tenderness are present about the hip. Evidence of neurovascular involvement is rarely found except in cases of gunshot injury. Emergency application of either traction or a Thomas splint provides some pain relief and decreases thigh hemorrhage.

IMAGING

Standard anterior posterior and lateral plain radiographs are indicated to permit analysis of the type and extent of the fracture. These radiographs should include images of both hip and knee joints in both views. Additional skeletal radiographs may be considered in polytraumatized patients to exclude other bony injuries. Occasionally, the true geometry of the fracture cannot be established until traction is applied to the limb. In traction, the physi-

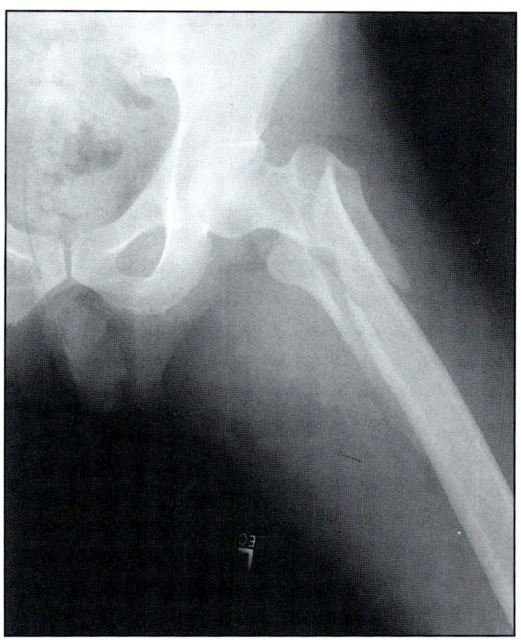

FIGURE 11-3. Frontal view of a Seinsheimer [17] Type IIIA fracture. The femoral head neck is abducted into varus angulation.

TABLE 11-1. CATEGORIZATION OF SUBTROCHANTERIC FRACTURES ACCORDING TO SEINSHEIMER'S CLASSIFICATION

Type I. Nondisplaced or less than 2-mm displacement
Type II. Two-part fractures with greater than 2-mm displacement, subdivided into
IIA. Transverse
IIB. Spiral with the lesser trochanter on the proximal fragment
IIC. Spiral with the lesser trochanter on the distal fragment (reverse obliquity)
Type III. Three-part fracture, subdivided into
IIIA. Spiral fracture with a medial lesser trochanter butterfly fragment
IIIB. Spiral fracture with a lateral cortical butterfly fragment
Type IV. Comminuted fracture with four or more fragments
Type V. Subtrochanteric fractures with intertrochanteric extension.

Data from Seinsheimer [17].

cian can frequently better assess the extent of fracture displacement, its pattern, and the degree of comminution. Additionally, if an intramedullary device is being considered for stabilization, the dimensions of the medullary canal can be determined. The presence of severe osteopenia or lysis in the subtrochanteric region warrants biopsy to determine the source of the pathologic lesion. Extensive comminution may warrant radiographs of the contralateral limb to establish leg length accurately.

DEFINITIVE TREATMENT OPTIONS

Traction

All subtrochanteric fractures should initially be placed in traction. This preliminary stabilization, either through a Buck's boot or skeletal pin, minimizes limb shortening, improves limb alignment, decreases thigh swelling, and provides relief from pain. In the modern era of fracture management, all but the select subtrochanteric fractures warrant surgical stabilization. Traction as definitive therapy was used in the past; authors such as DeLee [18] reported excellent healing with minimal complications. However, most of the clinical experience has been less than favorable with this method [2,19]. Reasonable fracture alignment can be maintained and acceptable rates of union can be achieved with considerable effort. Such affected patients are restricted to bed, and prolonged immobilization is equally hazardous for the elderly and the younger polytraumatized patient. Therefore, we would reserve this treatment for the rare patient who simply cannot be medically cleared for surgery.

If traction is employed, the technique proposed by DeLee *et al.* [2] should be followed. A Steinmann's pin is placed in either the distal femur or the proximal tibia. Approximately 25 lb (12 kg) should be applied initially for the average-size patient; the weight should then be adjusted depending on the amount of distraction required. As previously noted, the proximal fragment is usually in a position of flexion, abduction, and external rotation, and the distal fragment must be positioned accordingly to facilitate reduction. This requires 90-90 alignment (*ie,* 90° of flexion at the hip and at the knee) with distal limb abduction and external rotation. After acceptable alignment has been achieved, periodic radiographs are necessary to ensure that alignment is maintained. After 3 weeks in the 90-90 position, hip and knee flexion is gradually decreased until a neutral position is obtained with care being taken to avoid anterior fracture angulation. At 4 weeks of traction, a cast brace is applied with the hip in 5° of flexion and with the knee in extension. The patient is permitted to bear weight partially during ambulation, progressing quickly onto full weight bearing as tolerated. The cast is removed approximately 12 to 16 weeks after its application.

External Fixation

External fixation (*ie,*unilateral), although rarely promoted as favorable fixation of these fractures, was reported by Dhal and Singh [20] as a simple, minimally invasive treatment alternative in the management of subtrochanteric fractures. Uneventful fracture union was achieved by 6 months in 94% (48 of 51) of patients using external fixation. The authors cited acceptable fracture reduction, preservation of vascularity, and adequate stabilization without late deformity [20]. This technique permits gradual frame destabilization, thus promoting a more "biologic" healing without static stress shielding. As opposed to traction, external fixation patients have some mobilization potential, albeit limited, and therefore are not restricted to bed.

External fixation of subtrochanteric fractures creates a fulcrum at the fracture with the fixator acting as either a tension band or a buttressing cantilever, depending on the stable or unstable nature of the fracture. The principal biomechanical disadvantage of unilateral external fixation is the large bending moment on the pins, which are at risk for loosening, failure, or subsequent fracture malunion, especially in unstable fractures. Therefore, early mobilization must be approached with caution; patients in the Dhal and Singh series [20] were non–weight bearing for 8 weeks, partially weight bearing for another 8 weeks, and then fully weight bearing for 4 weeks with the frame before its removal at a median of 5 months (up to 9 months or more). The cumbersome nature of the fixator, its requirement for restricted mobilization, and its prolonged period of application limit its indications for patients who are either poor surgical candidates or not able to tolerate prolonged traction (*eg,* patients with closed head injuries).

Extramedullary Internal Fixation

Fixed-Angle Plate and Screw Device

Fixed-angle plate and screw devices have been successfully employed in the treatment of various subtrochanteric fractures [4,6,21–23]. In the stable subtrochanteric fracture, these implants allow for adequate direct reduction and sufficient stabilization as the plate is maintained under tension. The 95° fixed-angle blade plate or dynamic condylar screw is especially indicated for Seinsheimer [17] reverse obliquity

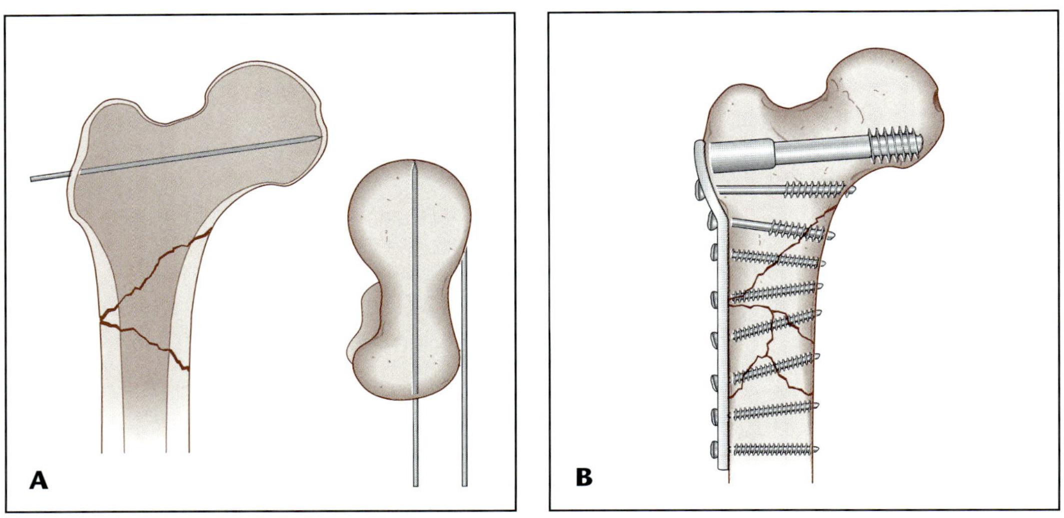

Figure 11-4. Fixed-angle blade plate and condylar screw devices require accurate placement of the blade or screw using image intensification. In the coronal plane, the proximal fixation should extend across the femoral neck into the inferior portion of the femoral head (A). In the sagittal plane, the proximal fixation should be centered in the femoral neck and head (B). After fixation of the side plate to the lateral femoral cortex, additional screws can be placed in the proximal fragment. When feasible, additional screws can also be used to reestablish medial cortical stability.

injuries (Type IIC, IV, or V) to prevent excessive shortening and distal shaft medialization (Figures 11-4 and 11-5).

The principal disadvantage of the fixed-angle plate device is the enormous bending stresses to which the plate is subjected along the lateral aspect of the femur in the unstable comminuted fracture with loss of medial column buttress. An in vitro biomechanical study by Tencer *et al.* [16] demonstrated that combined compression-bending loads to failure in an unstable subtrochanteric model was significantly lower for extramedullary plate devices compared with results using intramedullary implants. In a clinical report by Seinsheimer [17], three of four blade plates used in the fixation of Seinsheimer Type IIIA fractures failed. Hanson and Tullos [21] recommended avoiding weight bearing until some bony healing had occurred, whereas other authors concluded that these devices were not suitable for the unstable subtrochanteric fracture [22,23].

Kinast *et al.* [6] demonstrated that a fixed-angle plate device could be used effectively if fracture healing occurred in a timely fashion. They emphasized that medial-column anatomic reduction and stable interfragmentary compression were less important than limb alignment and minimizing vascular disruption at the fracture site. They advocated indirect surgical reduction techniques in an effort to achieve more rapid bony union and decrease the risk for hardware failure. The side plate should be tensioned so that it slightly overdistracts the medial column and reduces the medial fragments without direct exposure. The fracture is then axially compressed to retain its periosteal attachment (Figure 11-6).

Compression Hip Screw

In recent years, the most popular implant for the management of subtrochanteric hip fractures has been the compression hip screw (CHS) [24–27]. Although the CHS was not specifically designed for subtrochanteric fractures, it has proven to be quite successful, especially in stable fractures (Figure 11-7). The sliding component of the construct, ideal for the high subtrochanteric fracture, creates dynamic stability by the impaction and medial displacement of the shaft [26]. Waddell [27] reported good results in 88% of 24 patients treated with the CHS, and surmised that the single large proximal screw optimized fixation in the proximal fragment. Mullaji *et al.* [25] reported a 91% union rate in 42 elderly patients with subtrochanteric fractures treated with the CHS and concluded that the limited functional capacity of the older patient was more ideally suited for this implant. Patients were mobilized early, but this was restricted to partial weight bearing for 6 to 8 weeks.

The CHS is compromised by the extensive surgical dissection required for its implantation and the inability to ensure fracture stability during the early postoperative phase in the unstable subtrochanteric fracture. Whitelaw *et al.* [28] reported implant-related complications in 16% of patients treated with a CHS for unstable subtrochanteric femur fractures. Device modifications have been made to make the CHS more durable by increasing the side-plate strength. However, the lateral position of the side plate is still subjected to high bending loads, especially when the medial cortex is deficient and remains at risk for fatigue failure, screw cutout, or breakage [26,28]. In stable fractures, weight bearing can commence immediately; in the unstable fracture, activity should be restricted until medial calcar bony reconstitution has occurred.

Intramedullary Internal Fixation

Ender Flexible Nails

Ender condylocephalic flexible nails have been advocated for subtrochanteric fractures as a minimally invasive, biomechanically sound mode of fixation. Kuderna *et al.* [29] reported excellent results using Ender nails in 26 patients with subtrochanteric or combined intertrochanteric/subtrochanteric fractures. In their series, all patients required external cast or brace support but were

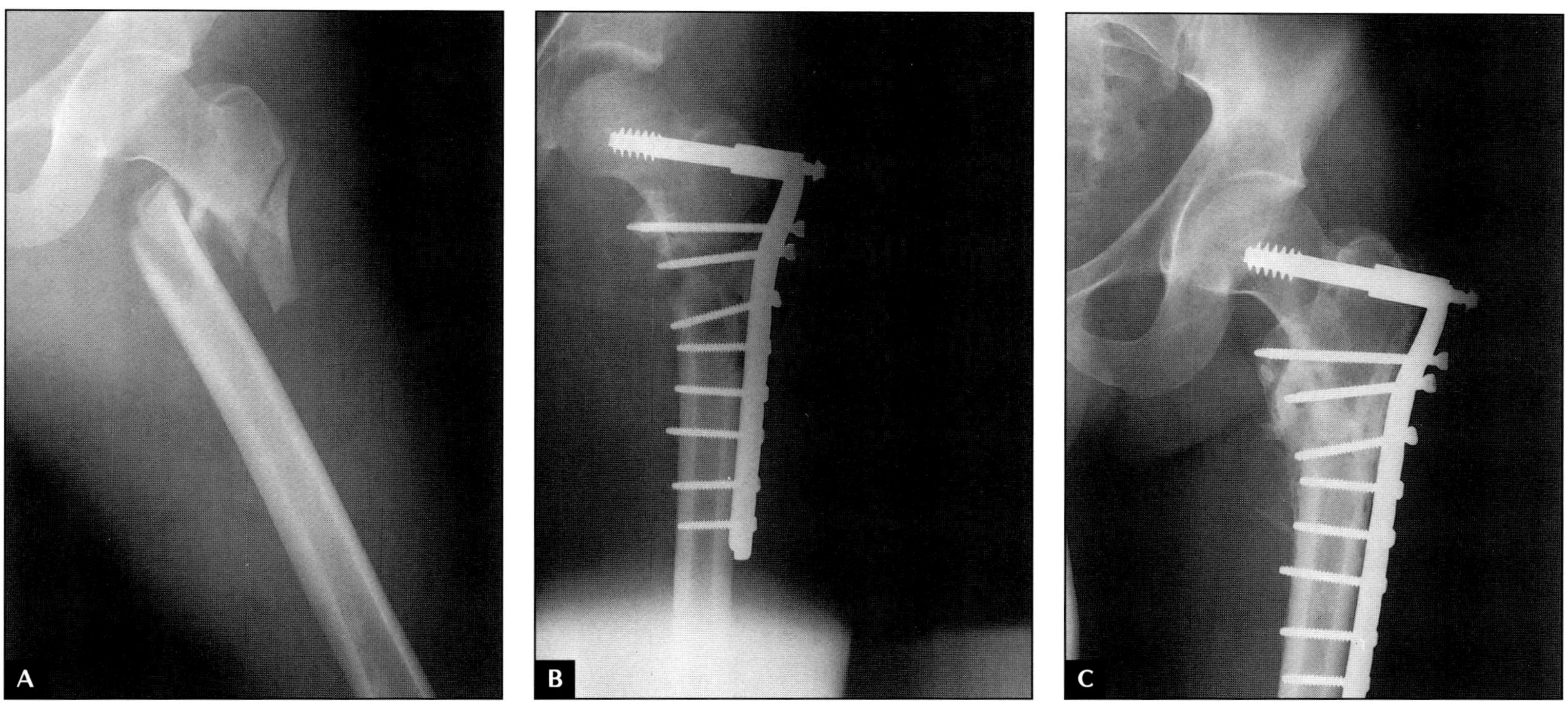

Figure 11-5. A, Frontal view of a Seinsheimer's [17] Type IIC or IIIB fracture. Fracture pattern is a reverse obliquity (at 95° to the normal intertrochanteric line.) This fracture tends to excessively shorten and medially displace the shaft with a conventional sliding hip screw configuration. B, Stable limb alignment and length are better achieved with a 95° dynamic condylar screw and side plate supplemented with bone graft. C, The fracture has consolidated in acceptable alignment after 8 months.

able to bear full weight immediately without loss of alignment or fixation. The principal advantages of this technique include reduced risks for infection, a close, indirect method of reduction, and early ambulation irrespective of the fracture complexity [29]. Despite this encouraging initial experience, Ender nails have quickly lost favor to more modern antegrade interlocking intramedullary devices. Levy *et al.* [30] reported both torsional and axial instability with Ender nails, especially in comminuted, unstable fractures. Closed reduction of the subtrochanteric fracture with retrograde Ender nails was often difficult, necessitating surgical dissection for direct open reduction [26]. Pankovich and Tarabishy [31] concluded that Ender nails were preferably indicated for intertrochanteric fractures and reported the incidence of nail migration with or without subsequent loss of fixation to be most prevalent in subtrochanteric fractures.

Intramedullary Nails

Intramedullary nail fixation of subtrochanteric fractures has had wide appeal because of decreased bending movement on the intramedullary device. When noninterlocked intramedullary nails were employed, the proximal fixation was so tenuous that it warranted almost the routine addition of either other internal fixation, external casting, or both [32]. First-generation interlocking nails generally have had better success with proximal fragment fixation; however, they require an intact lesser trochanter with or without sufficient frank cortical continuity at least in the upper subtrochanteric region [33]. Although these authors noted that intramedullary nail application for these fractures could be challenging, their results were promising.

The technical difficulty of intramedullary nailing of subtrochanteric fractures has been identified by several other authors

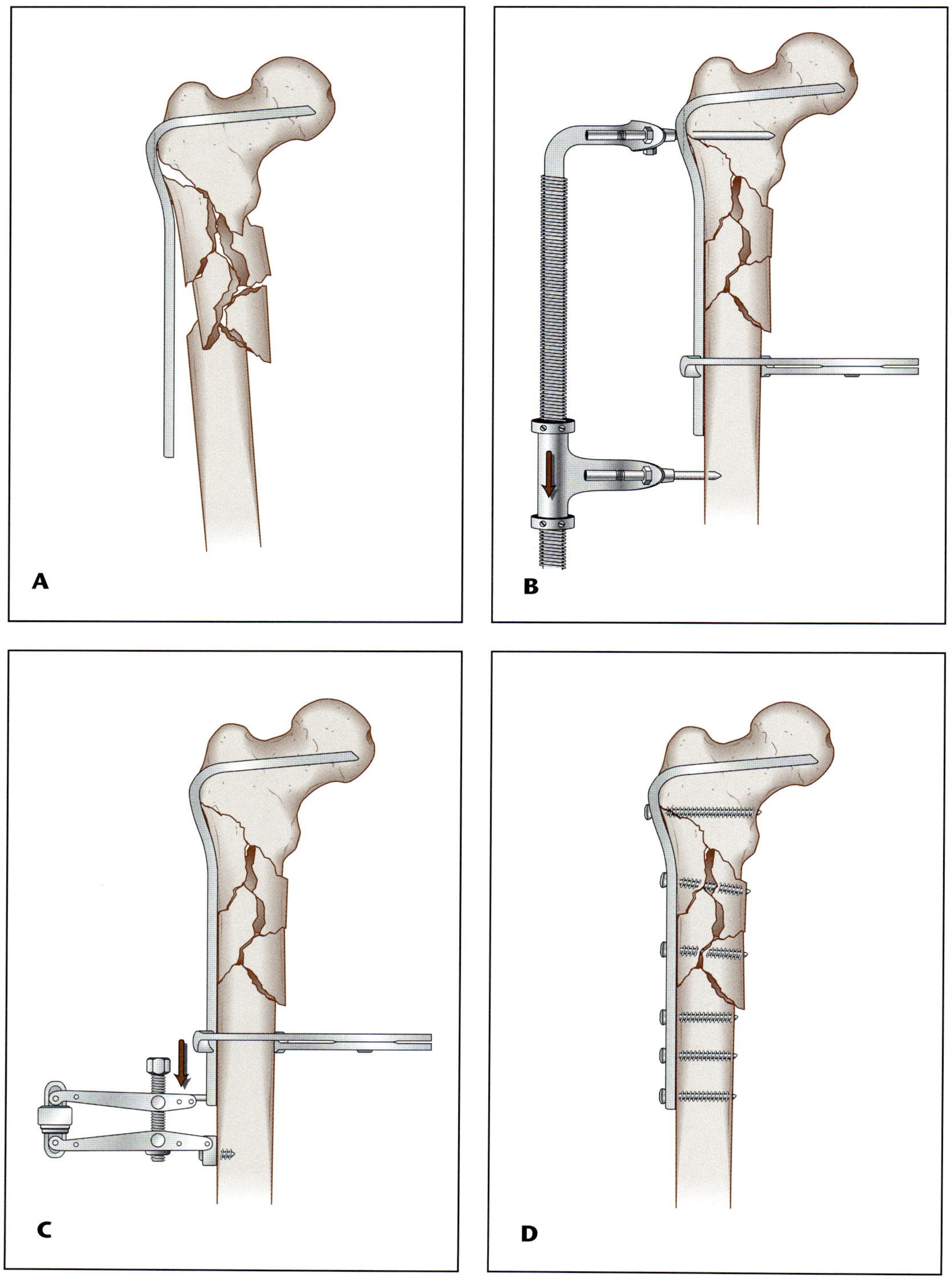

FIGURE 11-6. **A**, The indirect surgical reduction technique advocated by Kinast *et al.* [6] consists of proper placement of the proximal fixation in the inferior aspect of the femoral head at an angle that would correct fracture varus malalignment with eventual reduction of the side plate. **B**, Tensioning of the side plate with a femoral distractor slightly overdistracts the medial column and facilitates medial fragment reduction without surgical exposure. **C**, After the medial comminution has been reduced without direct fracture exposure, the side plate tension is then converted to axial compression to complete the reduction. **D**, Interfragmentary screw fixation of the medial comminution is achieved again without direct surgical exposure or disruption of the periosteum. (*Adapted from* Kinast *et al.* [6].)

[17,26,27]. As previously noted, the flexed and abducted posture of the short proximal fragment make indirect closed reduction and access to the piriformis fossa difficult. Even in the lesser trochanter, where it can be captured by a proximal first-generation interlocking screw, the high subtrochanteric fracture with medial comminution remains at risk for varus malalignment and shortening (Figure 11-8) with early hip activity. Gross proximal fragment instability results if the proximal fracture is more complex and extends into the intertrochanteric region. Distally, rotational and axial instability compromise the effectiveness of nonlocked nails. Although distal fragment forces are better controlled with distal interlocking, slotted nails are less rigid and still permit healing with more residual external rotation.

Evolution of second-generation reconstruction intramedullary nails has improved the success of femoral nailing in the subtrochanteric fracture [34]. In the modified cephalomedullary design, the proximal portion of the reconstruction nail is enlarged and allows for placement of two screws into the femoral head for improved fracture fixation and alignment (Figure 11-9). In vitro biomechanical testing has demonstrated the nail's resilience to bending loads of unstable fracture patterns compared with first-generation intramedullary nails, Ender nails, fixed-angle plate and screw devices [16,35], or short and long intermedullary hip screws [36].

French and Tornetta [37] reported a 100% union rate in 45 subtrochanteric fractures without proximal intertrochanteric extensions that were treated with the reconstruction nail. No cases of implant failures occurred, and excellent hip and knee mobility was regained. However, 61% of patients experienced varus malreduction created by the adducted position of the femur necessary to facilitate nail insertion but not corrected before placement of interlocking screws. The technique also required a prolonged mean operative time of 270 minutes, which the authors attributed to the difficulty of nail insertion and placement of the proximal interlocking screws, as well as the time for surgical set-up. In two patients, the piriformis fossa, which is crucial for the stability of this implant, was fractured during the implantation and prompted the authors to seek an alternate mode of stabilization. Therefore, the major limitations of the reduction nail include its restricted use to select subtrochanteric fractures and the difficulty of placing two screws proximally while maintaining acceptable femoral head and neck reduction.

Zickel Nail

The Zickel nail was the first intramedullary implant designed specifically for treatment of subtrochanteric femur fractures. The objectives of its design were to provide a rigid implant strong enough to resist bending stresses, to eliminate screws to avoid loosening, and to achieve sufficient proximal fixation in the femoral head and neck with a single implant. The result was a solid rectangular rod through which a separate cephalad flange could be placed into the femoral head and fixed. In a clinical series by Villar and Thomas [38], there were no construction failures with Zickel nail compared with a 17% mechanical failure rate with a fixed nail plate. In another report by Bergman *et al.* [9], 131 patients with subtrochanteric fractures were managed with the Zickel device with a satisfactory outcome achieved in 90%. Nonunion occurred in only 5%. The authors' overall experience was highly favorable but most notably in the treatment of unstable fractures. This success was attributed to the excellent load-sharing properties of the device.

The Zickel nail, however, is not recommended for complex subtrochanteric fractures with intertrochanteric extension or comminution because of the risk of varus displacement of the femoral head [7]. The incidence of technical difficulties associated with insertion of a Zickel nail can be significant and include trochanteric fractures, femoral head-neck perforations, and femoral shaft displacement [38,39]. The absence of distal static locking has been implicated in the rotatory instability of the distal fragment [23,26]. Finally, the most disturbing complication has been the risk for

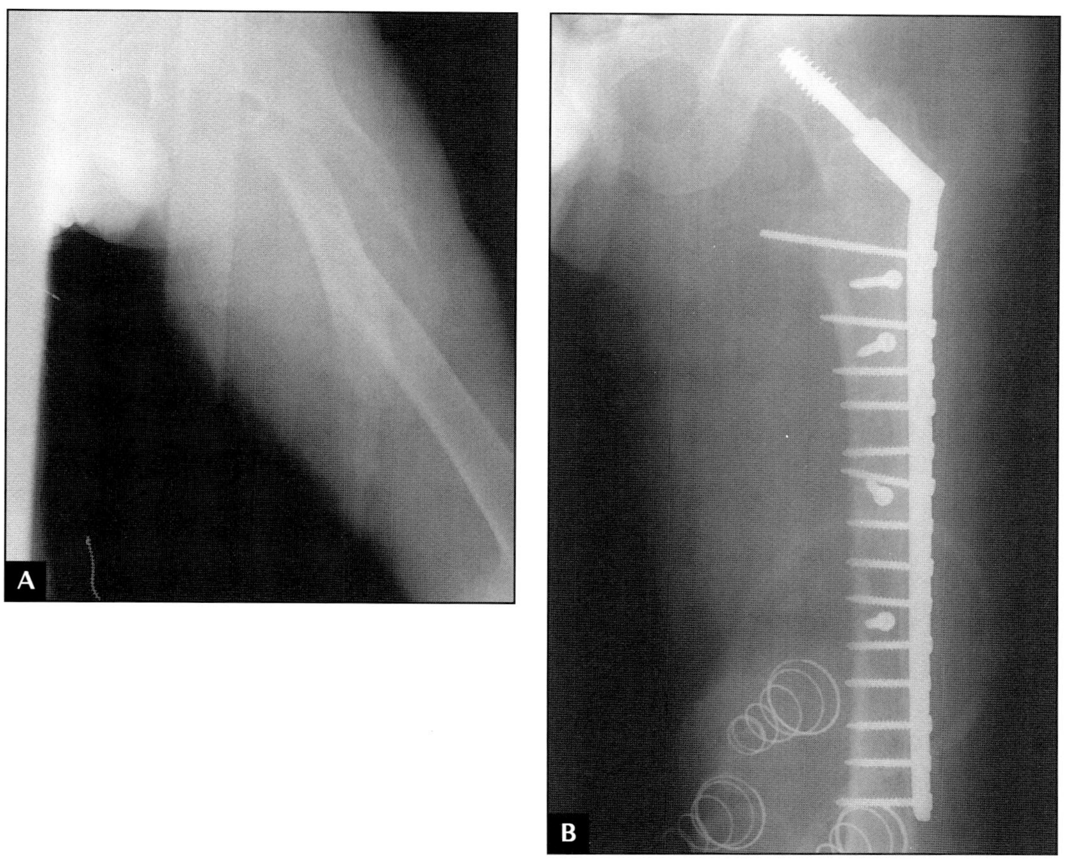

FIGURE 11-7. **A**, Frontal view of a Seinsheimer [17] Type IIIA fracture with a large medial butterfly fragment extending down to the isthmus of the femoral shaft. **B**, The compression hip screw has been used to reduce the fracture and stabilize the previously displaced medial cortical buttress. The diaphyseal extension associated with this type of fracture requires an extremely long side plate (as well as extended surgical dissection) to achieve fixation.

refracture associated with attempts at implant removal [40,41]. These authors cited the implant's size, rigidity, and configuration as the probable cause. Some authors have suggested that the Zickel nail should not be employed in younger patients [41].

Gamma Nail

The Gamma nail, which combines the merits of both intramedullary fixation and sliding screw technology, was designed specifically to address many biomechanical challenges of subtrochanteric fracture management. In an in vitro biomechanical evaluation of the Gamma nail, Rosenblum *et al.* [42] demonstrated a sixfold increase in the area moment of inertia for the Gamma nail compared with that of the sliding hip screw and found a significant increase in resistance to bending. This bending stiffness was noted to cause almost no strain on the medial calcar, regardless of the fracture pattern (Figure 11-10).

Clinical studies have supported the theoretic biomechanical advantages of the implant. Halder [43] reviewed 25 subtrochanteric fractures treated with the Gamma nail; all healed with few complications (one screw cut-out and one distal shaft fracture). Stable fixation was achieved without reduction of the posterior medial comminution. Compared with its use in intertrochanteric fractures, use of the Gamma nail for subtrochanteric fracture was technically more difficult, took longer, required more time for fluoroscopy, and resulted in greater blood loss [43].

Among the positive attributes of the Gamma nail is its ability to tolerate early, unrestricted ambulation. In a prospective clinical review of consecutive subtrochanteric fractures treated with the Gamma nail, Chevalley and Gamba [44] reported that all patients could attempt full weight bearing immediately regardless of the fracture pattern. They surmised that the Gamma nail allowed the surgeon to treat subtrochanteric fractures of varying complexity with a standard, mini-

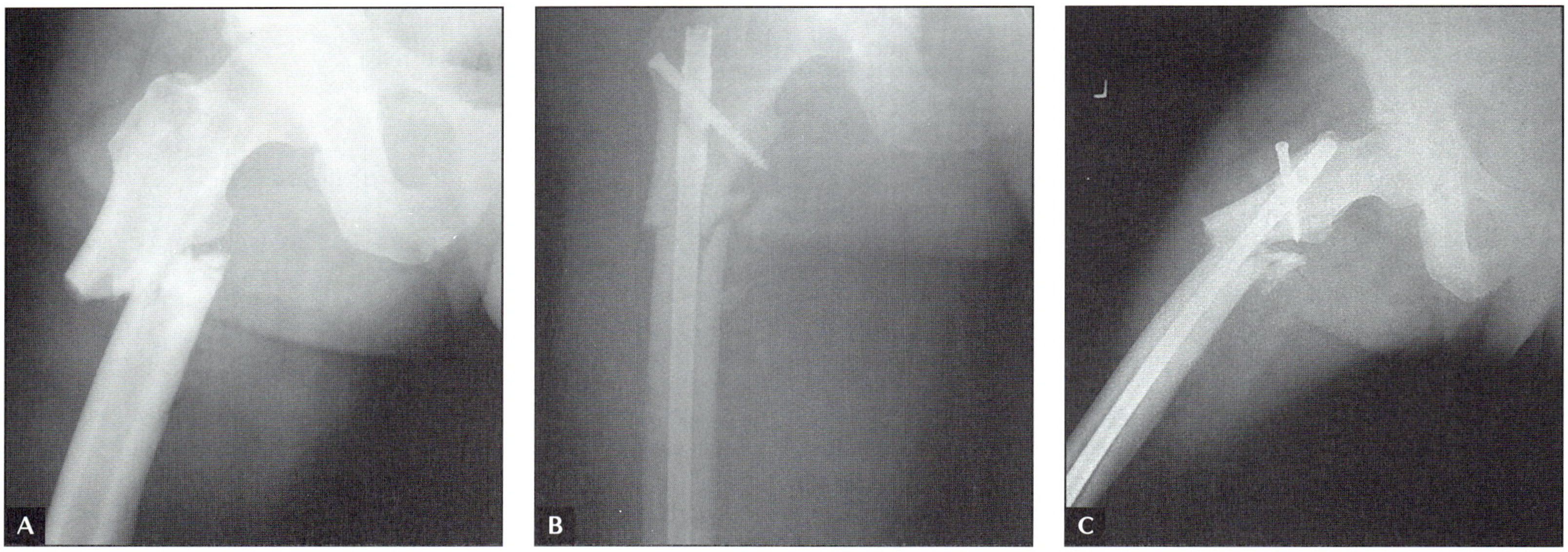

FIGURE 11-8. A, Seinsheimer's [17] Type IIA fracture of the right femur. B, Reduction and fixation using a first-generation interlocking intermedullary nail with proximal screw fixation into the lesser trochanter. C, After early limited weight bearing, the proximal fragment has displaced into varus and external rotation due to marginal proximal fragment fixation.

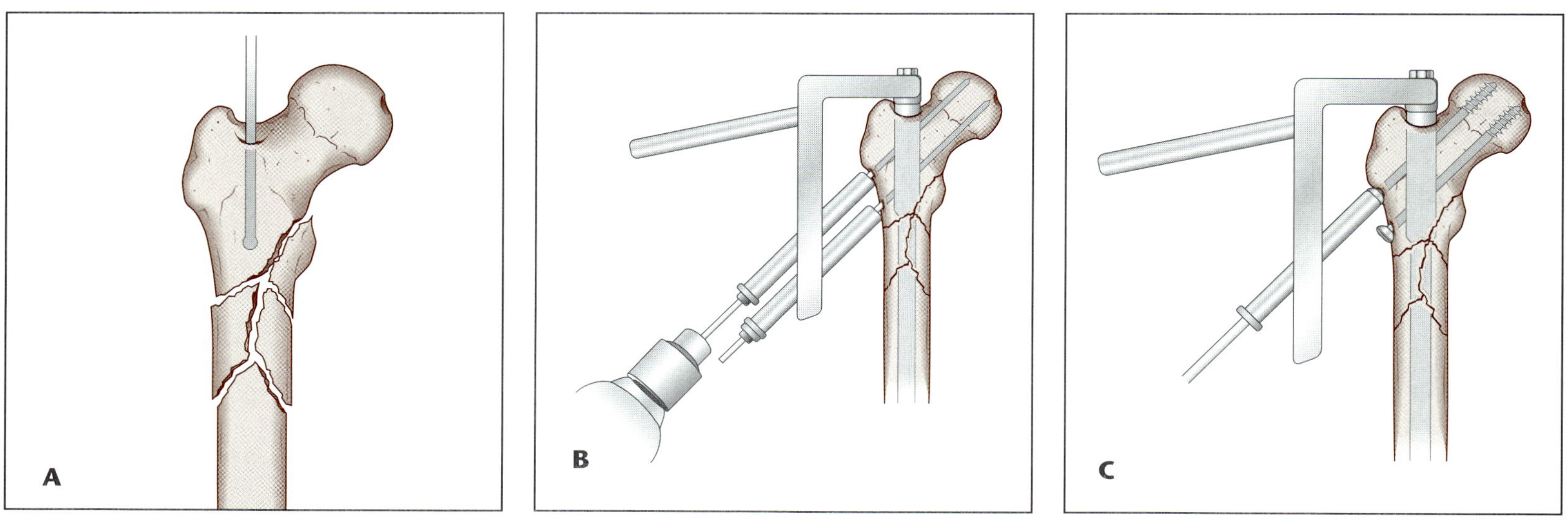

FIGURE 11-9. A, A guide wire is inserted through an intact piriformis fossa followed by standard femoral nail reaming and nail insertion. B, The proximally attached guide is used to insert two parallel 2.4-mm guide pins into the femoral neck and heads. C, The guide pins are then replaced with a caudal 8.0-mm lag screw and a more cephalad 6.4-mm lag screw.

mally invasive technique with consistently good results. The most prevalent complication with the original short Gamma nail was thigh pain in 8 of 45 patients (18%), which was thought to result from stress transfer from the medial calcar to the distal locking screws or the tip of the implant in the proximal femur diaphysis [45].

In another clinical study comparing the CHS with the Gamma nail, Goldhagen *et al.* [45] concluded that use of the Gamma nail was technically more demanding than the CHS. Among the Gamma nail biomechanical advantages cited were the intramedullary position of the implant, its shorter lever arm and decreased bending moment, the sliding screw femoral-head fixation, and the increased stiffness of the nail's design.

A prospective study in elderly patients also demonstrated a shorter convalescence period with earlier full weight bearing in Gamma nail patients compared with those whose implantation used the CHS [44,46]. However, intraoperative complications were again more prevalent. These complications were attributed to the implant's original design, size, configuration, and stiffness, which did not easily accommodate the femur of many smaller patients and resulted in either trochanteric fractures or proximal shaft fractures.

Bone Graft

Regardless of the fixation device or technique employed, the supplemental bone graft can be essential, especially for unstable subtrochanteric fractures with comminuted medial cortical deficiency [11,27,47]. The delicate balance between sufficient bone healing and the high risk of hardware failure dictates a low threshold for bone grafting in these fractures. Clearly, bone graft is an absolute indication in all cases of delayed union or nonunion. Intramedullary reamed devices can indirectly supply bone graft to the more distal fractures; however, proximity of the more proximal fracture site to the wound usually warrants an open procedure with direct graft placement. Procedures that minimize soft tissue dissection, such as indirect reduction techniques, do not devascularize the comminuted bone fragments and for this reason frequently may not require supplemental grafting [6].

Open Subtrochanteric Fractures

Open fractures of the subtrochanteric femur are infrequent and have been reported in fewer than 10% of high-energy fractures [18]. Typically, open subtrochanteric fractures occur secondary to gunshot injury; neurovascular injuries are more prevalent than in closed fractures. Definitive treatment may or may not require local wound débridement, depending on the energy level of the missile. As with closed fractures, gunshot-related injuries are best managed with surgical stabilization. Bone grafting is usually warranted if either comminution or decompression are found in the fracture hematoma. Occasionally, extremely high-energy fractures are best managed with delayed definitive fixation after repeat débridement (Figure 11-11).

AUTHORS' PREFERRED TREATMENT METHOD AND POSSIBLE COMPLICATIONS

We prefer the long Gamma nail for the treatment of subtrochanteric fractures. The complications that haunted the short Gamma nail have been addressed with this new longer design. Clearly, proximal shaft fractures from either distal locking screws or a stiff short nail have been eliminated. By decreasing the lateral bend of the proximal nail from 10° to 7°, the implant has been made more applicable to a wider variety of proximal femur configurations. The distal aspect of the nail is only 11 mm, which eliminates the larger sizes available in the original design and their tendency to fill the canal.

The long Gamma nail involves a single implant and technique that is suitable for all fractures, whether stable or unstable (Figures 11-11 and 11-12). Indicated injuries include fractures with extensions into the greater trochanter, the piriformis fossa, and the femur diaphysis. Axial and torsional instability can be neutralized with distal static locking, whereas the large compression screw component of the construct can be fixed or allowed to collapse with or without controlled

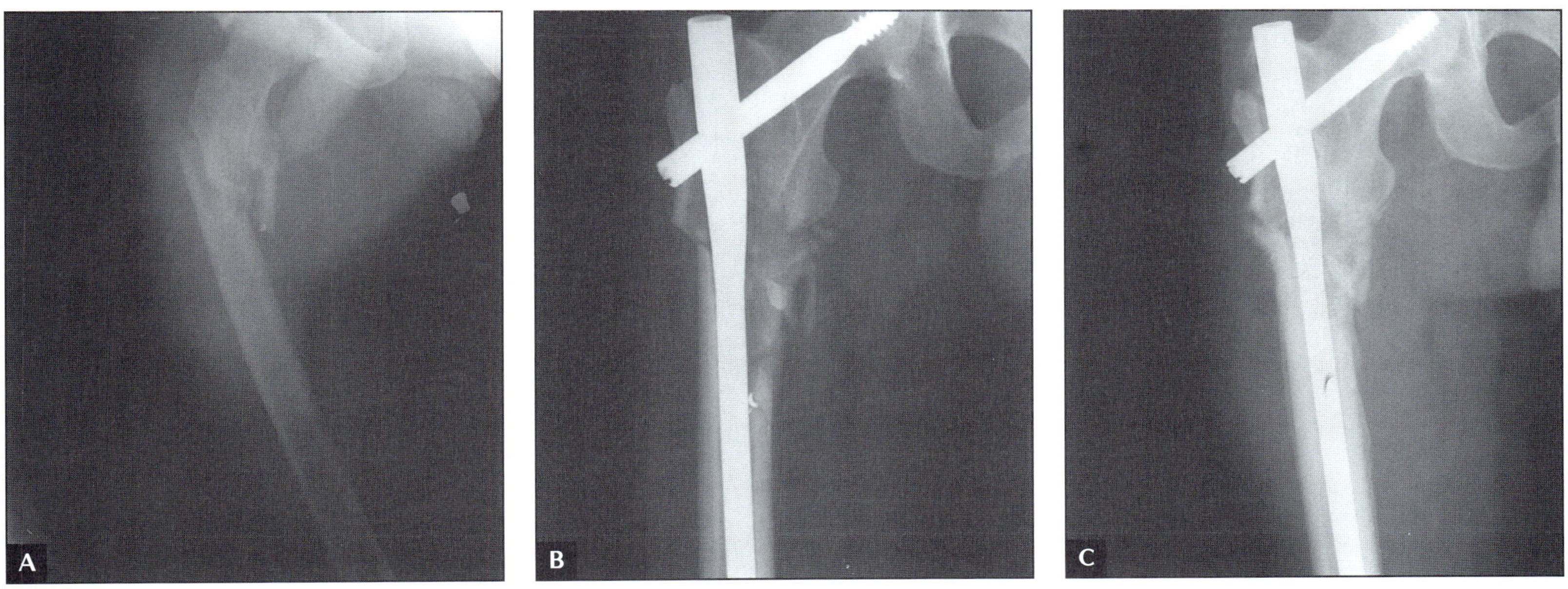

Figure 11-10. A, Seinsheimer [17] Type IIIA subtrochanteric fracture with extensive comminution of the medial cortex. B, Reduction and fixation with the Gamma nail; bone graft was provided solely by the intramedullary reamings. C, Despite immediate unrestricted weight bearing, the fracture and medial comminution are healing without compromise of alignment or fixation.

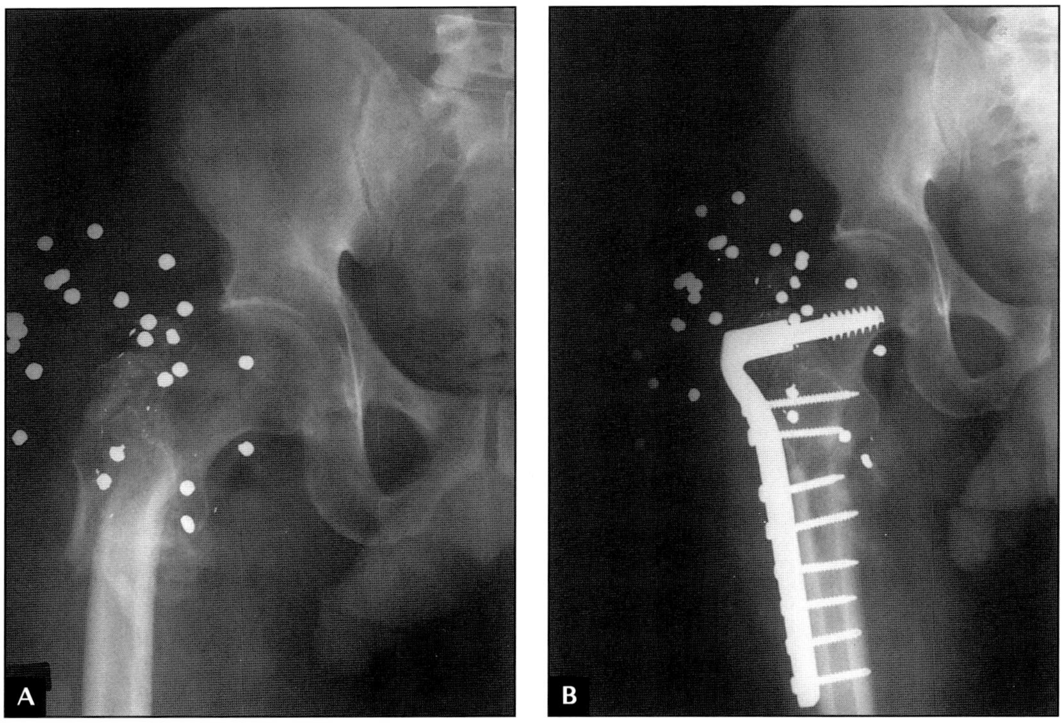

FIGURE 11-11. **A**, Subtrochanteric fracture secondary to shotgun injury (Seinsheimer [17] Type V). **B**, Open reduction and external fixation with a 95° dynamic condylar screw and side plate.

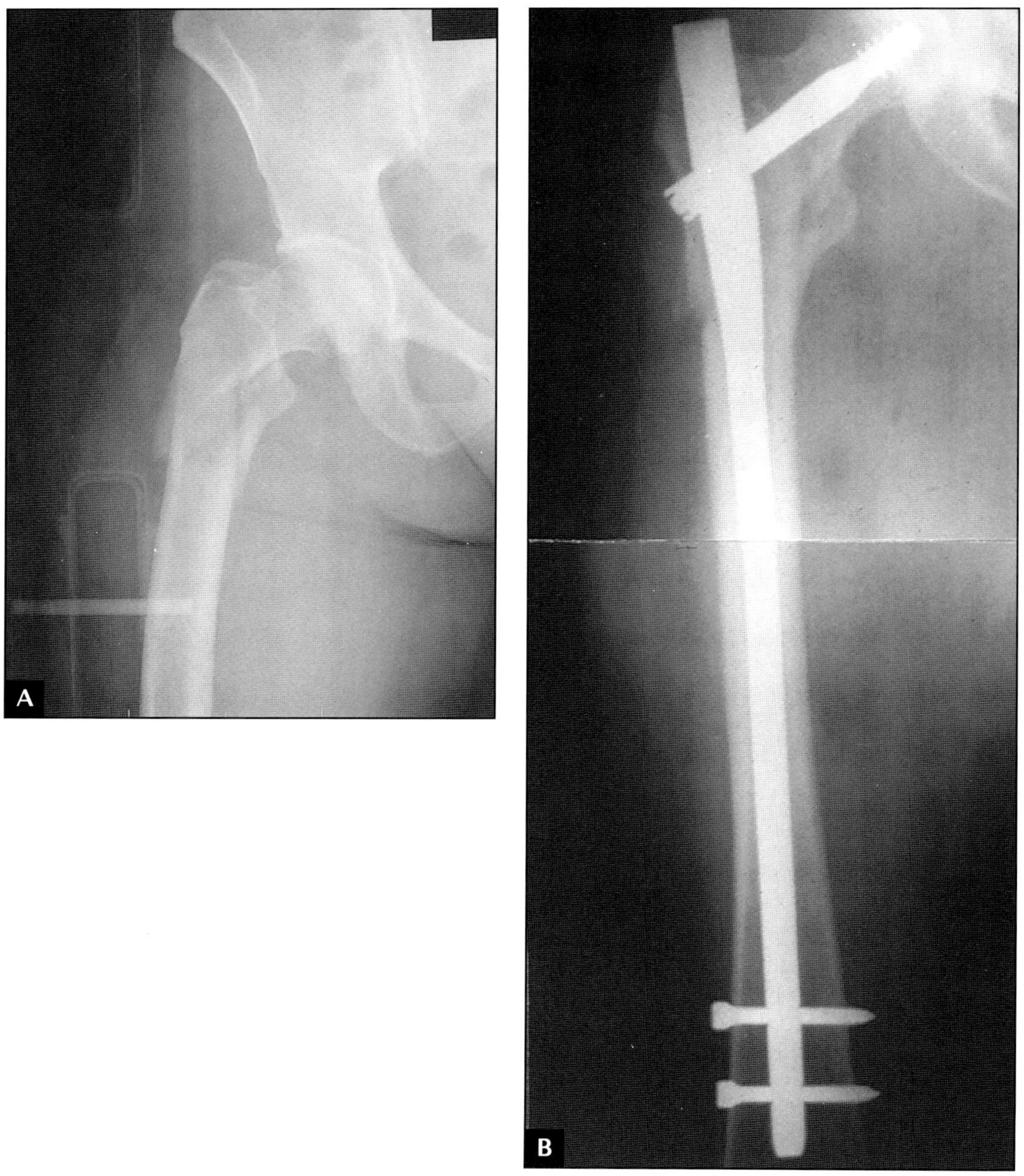

FIGURE 11-12. **A**, Seinsheimer [17] Type IIIA subtrochanteric fracture of the region of the femur. **B**, Long Gamma nail used for reduction and stabilization.

screw rotation. The fixed-angle option makes the long Gamma nail effective for reverse-obliquity fractures of Seinsheimer IIC, IV, or V (Figure 11-13). However, for these select fracture types, we prefer the 95°-angle blade plate or dynamic condylar screw and side plate, except in cases in which the fracture extends into the femur diaphysis.

Coupled with the implant's excellent resistance to bending loads, early minimally controlled weight bearing is a feasible objective in these patients. Biologically, the technique requires limited exposure, indirect reduction, and incorporates all benefits of intramedullary reaming with secondary bone grafting to stimulate fracture healing.

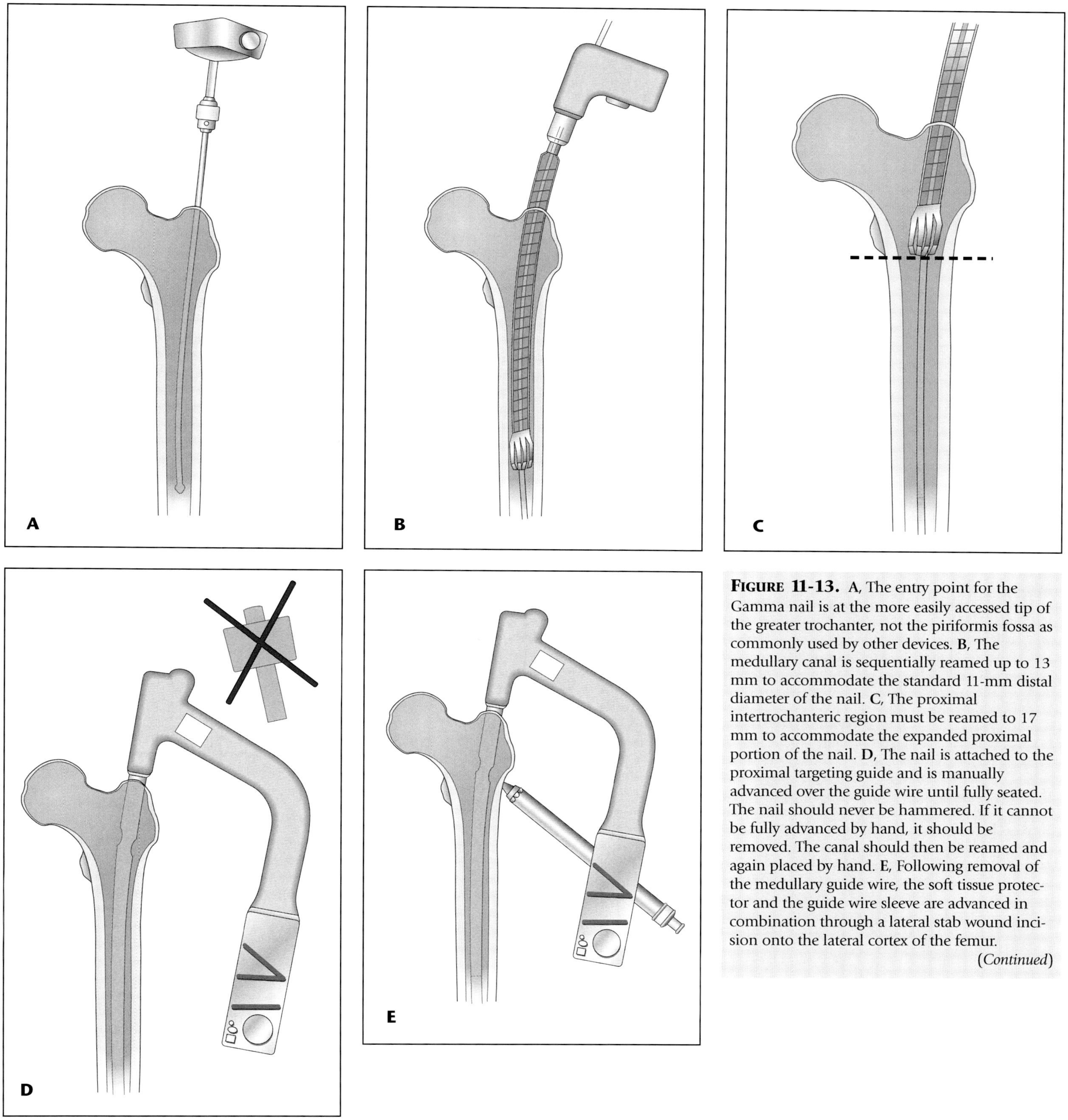

FIGURE 11-13. **A**, The entry point for the Gamma nail is at the more easily accessed tip of the greater trochanter, not the piriformis fossa as commonly used by other devices. **B**, The medullary canal is sequentially reamed up to 13 mm to accommodate the standard 11-mm distal diameter of the nail. **C**, The proximal intertrochanteric region must be reamed to 17 mm to accommodate the expanded proximal portion of the nail. **D**, The nail is attached to the proximal targeting guide and is manually advanced over the guide wire until fully seated. The nail should never be hammered. If it cannot be fully advanced by hand, it should be removed. The canal should then be reamed and again placed by hand. **E**, Following removal of the medullary guide wire, the soft tissue protector and the guide wire sleeve are advanced in combination through a lateral stab wound incision onto the lateral cortex of the femur.
(*Continued*)

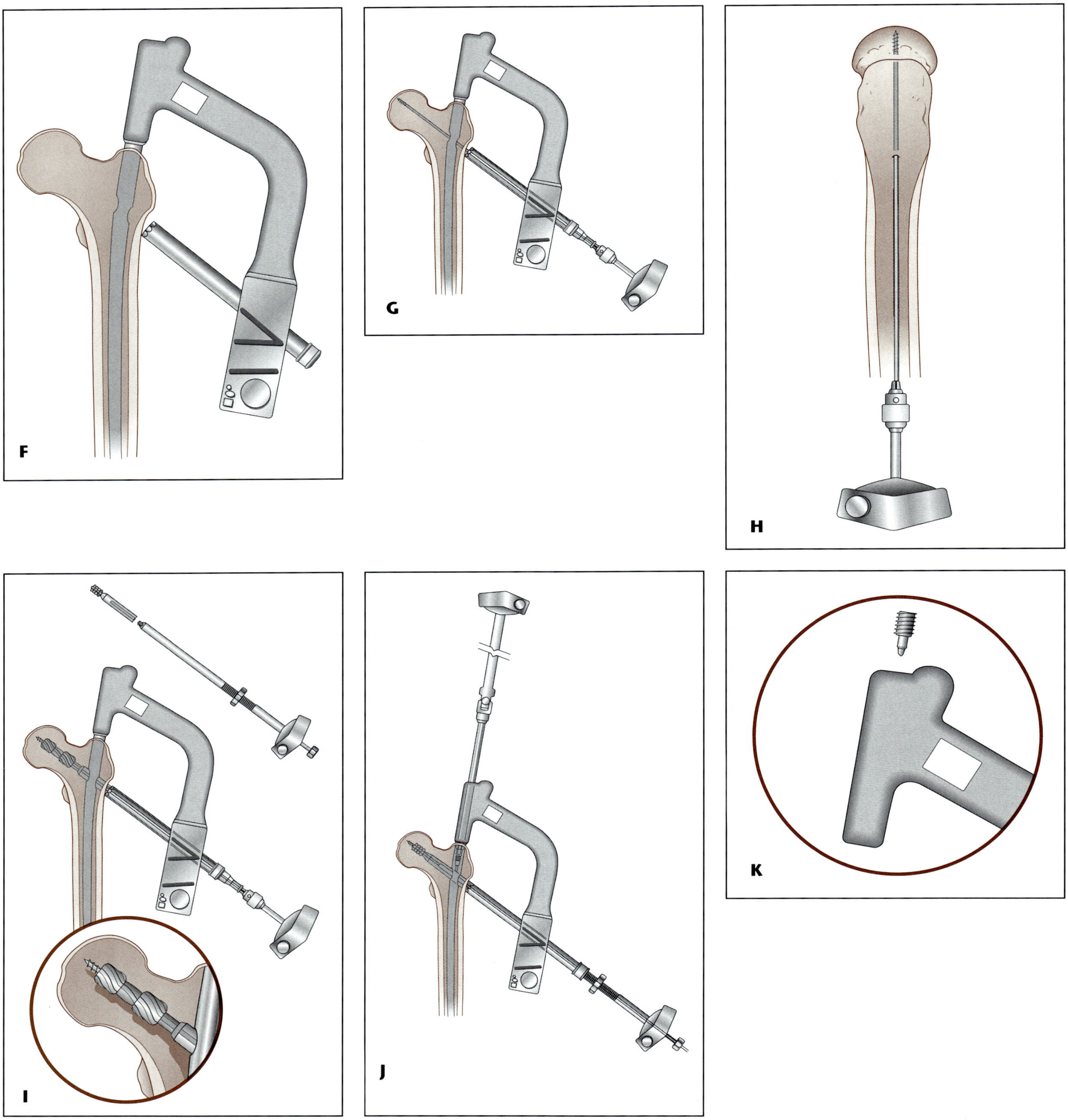

FIGURE 11-13. (*Continued*) **F**, The soft-tissue sleeve has teeth, which can be impacted into the lateral cortex to secure depth for eventual lag screw measurement. **G**, Using imaging intensification, the guide wire can be then advanced through the guide sleeve and the soft tissue protector assembly can be advanced through the femoral neck into the femoral head. **H**, The lateral projection must be checked under imaging intensification to ensure proper pin placement in the femoral head. **I**, After the guide wire has been measured for depth, the lag screw reamer can be set to that depth prior to reaming the femoral neck and head over the guide wire. The depth measured for the reamer will leave the threads of the guide wire free to maintain purchase in the femoral head. The lag screw and its insertor can then be assembled prior to lag screw insertion. **J**, The lag screw is inserted over the guide wire to the depth previously determined by the lag screw reamer. With the handle of the lag screw insertor oriented either parallel or perpendicular to the long axis of the femur, grooves in the base of the lag screw are positioned to accept a set screw to control rotation and sliding of the apparatus. **K**, The set screw is loaded through the cephalad aspect of the targeting device.

(*Continued*)

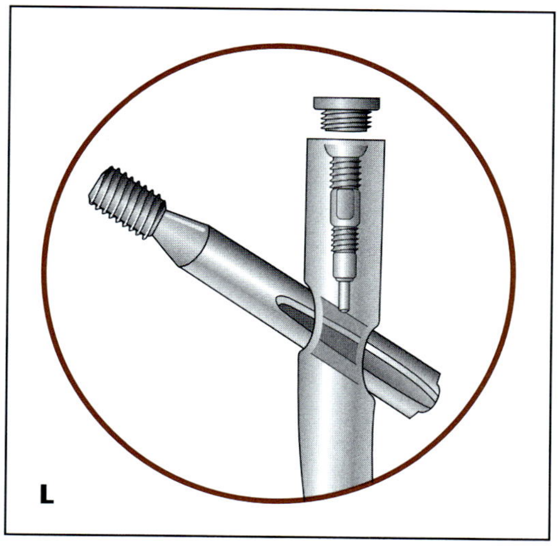

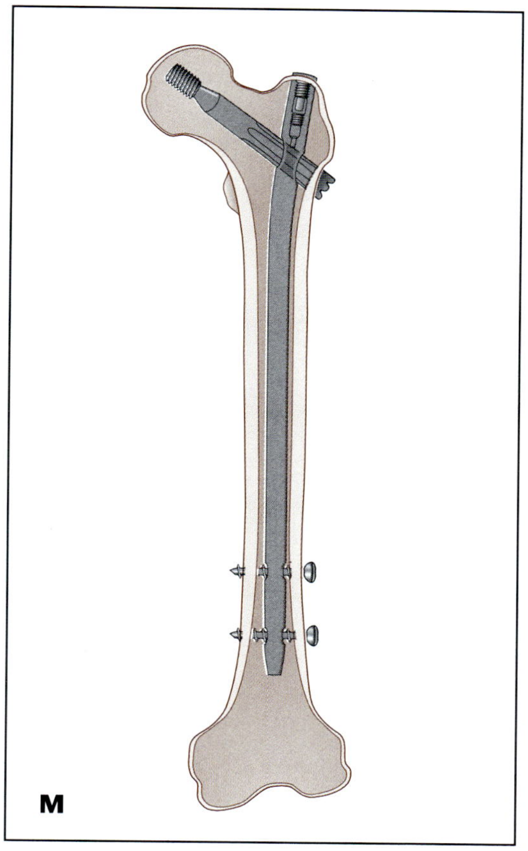

FIGURE 11-13. (*Continued*) L, When tightened, the set screw can prevent both rotation and collapse. The set screw can be loosened approximately one quarter turn to allow for collapse but still resist rotation. M, The final position of the implant following removal of the targeting device and insertion of the distal locking screws by the freehand method.

REFERENCES AND RECOMMENDED READING

Recently published papers of particular interest have been highlighted as:
- • Of interest
- •• Of outstanding interest

1. Boyd HB, Griffin LL: Classification and treatment of trochanteric fractures. *Arch Surg* 1949, 58:853.
2. DeLee J, Clanton TO, Rockwood CA: Closed treatment of subtrochanteric fractures of the femur in a modified cast-brace. *J Bone Joint Surg* 1981, 63:773–779.
3. Lechner JD, Rao JP, Stashak G, Adibe SO: Subtrochanteric fractures: a retrospective analysis. *Clin Orthop* 1990, 259:140–145.
4. Fielding JW, Magliato HI: Subtrochanteric fractures. *Surg Gynecol Obstet* 1966, 122:555–560.
5. Fielding JW: Subtrochanteric fractures. *Clin Orthop* 1973, 92:86–99.
6. Kinast C, Bolhofner BR, Mast JW, Ganz R: Subtrochanteric fractures of the femur. *Clin Orthop* 1989, 238:124–130.
7. Zickel RE:Subtrochanteric femoral fractures. *Orthop Clin North Am* 1980, 11:555–568.
8. Russel TA, Taylor JC: Subtrochanteric fractures of the femur. In *Skeletal Trauma: Fractures, Dislocations, and Ligamentous Injuries*. Edited by Browner BD, Jupiter JB, Levine AM, *et al*. Philadelphia: WB Saunders; 1992:1883–1925.
9. Bergman GD, Winquist RA, Mayo KA, Hansen ST: Subtrochanteric fracture of the femur. *J Bone Joint Surg* 1987, 69:1032–1040.
10. Haentjens P, Casteleyn PP, De Boeck H, *et al.*: Treatment of unstable intertrochanteric and subtrochanteric fractures in elderly patients. *J Bone Joint Surg* 1989, 71:1214–1225.
11. Velasco RU, Comfort TM: Analysis of treatment problems in subtrochanteric fractures of the femur. *J Trauma* 1978, 18:513–523.
12 Koch JC: The laws of bone architecture. *Am J Anat* 1917, 21:177.
13 Frankel VH, Burstein AH: *Orthopedic Biomechanics*. Philadelphia: Lea & Febiger; 1970.
14. Rybicki EF, Simonen FA, Weis EB: On the mathematical analysis of stress in the human femur. *J Biomech* 1972, 5:203–215.
15. Tordis TG: Stress analysis of the femur. *J Biomech* 1969, 2:163.
16. Tencer AF, Johnson KD, Johnston WC, Gill K: A biomechanical comparison of various methods of stabilization of subtrochanteric fractures of the femur. *J Orthop Res* 1984, 2:297–305.
17. Seinsheimer F: Subtrochanteric fractures of the femur. *J Bone Joint Surg* 1978, 60A:300–306.
18. DeLee J: Fractures and dislocations of the hip. In *Rockwood and Green's Fractures in Adults.* Edited by Rockwood, CA, Green DP, Bucholz RW, *et al.* Philadelphia: Lippincott-Raven; 1996:1741–1755.
19. Bajaj HN, Rao PS, Kumar B, Chacko V: Subtrochanteric fractures of the femur: an analysis of the results of operative and nonoperative management. *Injury* 1988, 19:169–171.
20. Dhal A, Singh SS: Biological fixation of subtrochanteric fractures by external fixation. *Injury* 1996, 27:723–731.
21. Hanson GW, Tullos HS: Subtrochanteric fractures of the femur treated with nail plate devices: a retrospective study. *Clin Orthop* 1978, 131:191–194.
22. Whatley JR, Garland DE, Whitecloud T, Wickstrom J: Subtrochanteric fractures of the femur: treatment with ASIF blade plate fixation. *South Med J* 1978, 71:1372–1375.
23. Asher MA, Tipper JW, Rockwood CA, Zilber S: Compression fixation of subtrochanteric fractures of the femur. *Clin Orthop* 1976, 117:202–208.
24. Hogh J: Sliding screw in the treatment of trochanteric and subtrochanteric fractures. *Injury* 1982, 14:141–145.
25. Mullaji AB, Thomas TL: Low-energy subtrochanteric fractures in elderly patients: results of fixation with the sliding screw plate. *J Trauma* 1993, 34:56–61.
26. Schatzker J, Waddell JP: Subtrochanteric fractures of the femur. *Orthop Clin North Am* 1980, 11:539–544.
27. Waddell JP: Subtrochanteric fractures of the femur: a review of 130 patients. *J Trauma* 1979, 19:582–592.
28. Whitelaw GP, Segal D, Sanzone CF, *et al.*: Unstable intertrochanteric/subtrochanteric fractures of the femur. *Clin Orthop* 1990, 252:238–245.

29. Kuderna H, Bohler N, Collon DJ: Treatment of intertochanteric and subtrochanteric fractures of the hip by the Ender method. *J Bone Joint Surg* 1976, 58A:604–611.
30. Levy RN, Siegel M, Sedlin ED, Sieffert RS: Complication of Ender pin fixation in basicervical, intertrochanteric, and subtrochanteric fractures of the hip. *J Bone Joint Surg* 1983, 65A:66–69.
31. Pankovich AM, Tarabishy IE: Ender nailing of intertochanteric and subtrochanteric fractures of the femur. *J Bone Joint Surg* 1980, 62A:635–645.
32. Aronoff PM, Davis PM, Wickstron JK: Intramedullary nail fixation as treatment of subtrochanteric fractures of the femur. *J Trauma* 1971, 11:637–650.
33. Kempf I, Grosse A, Beck G: Locked intramedullary nailing: its application to comminuted fractures of the femur. *J Bone Joint Surg* 1985, 67A:709–720.
34. Kang S, McAndrew MP, Johnson KD: The reconstruction locked nail for complex fractures of the proximal femur. *J Orthop Trauma* 1995, 9:453–463.
35. Pugh KJ, Morgan RA, Gorczyca JT, Pienkowski D: A mechanical comparison of subtrochanteric femur fracture fixation. *J Orthop Trauma* 1998, 12:324–329.
36. Kraemer WJ, Hearn TC, Powell JN, Mahomed N: Fixation of segmental subtrochanteric fractures: a biomechanical study. *Clin Orthop* 1996, 332:71–79.
37. French BG, Tornetta P: Use of an interlocked cephalomedullary nail for subtrochanteric fracture stabilization. *Clin Orthop* 1998, 348:95–100.
38. Thomas WG, Villar RN: Subtrochanteric fractures: Zickel nail or nail plate? *J Bone Joint Surg* 1986, 68B:255–259.
39. Winter WG, Combo CR, Lewis NV, *et al.*: Subtrochanteric fracture fixation. *Orthop Trans* 1979, 3:256.
40. Yelton C, Low W: Iatrogenic subtrochanteric fracture: a complication of Zickel nails. *J Bone Joint Surg* 1986, 68A:1237–1240.
41. Ovadia DN, Chess JL: Intraoperative and postoperative subtrochanteric fracture of the femur associated with removal of the Zickel nail. *J Bone Joint Surg* 1988, 70A:239–243.
42. Rosenblum SF, Zuckerman JD, Kummer FJ, Tam BS: A biomechanical evaluation of the Gamma nail. *J Bone Joint Surg* 1992, 74B:352–357.
43. Halder SC: The Gamma nail for peritrochanteric fractures. *J Bone Joint Surg* 1992, 74B:340–344.
44. Chevalley F, Gamba D: Gamma nailing of pertrochanteric and subtrochanteric fractures: clinical results of a series of 63 consecutive cases. *J Orthop Trauma* 1997, 11:412–415.
45. Goldhagen PR, O'Connor DR, Schwarze D, Schwartz E: A prospective comparative study of the compression hip screw and the Gamma nail. *J Orthop Trauma* 1997, 8:367–372.
46. Leung KS, So WS, Shen WY, Hui PW: Gamma nails and dynamic hip screws for peritrochanteric fractures. *J Bone Joint Surg* 1992, 74B:345–351.
47. Winter WG, Clawson DK: Complication of treatment of fractures and dislocations. In *Complications in Orthopaedic Surgery* vol 1. Edited by Epp CH. Philadelphia: JB Lippincott; 1978:439–441.

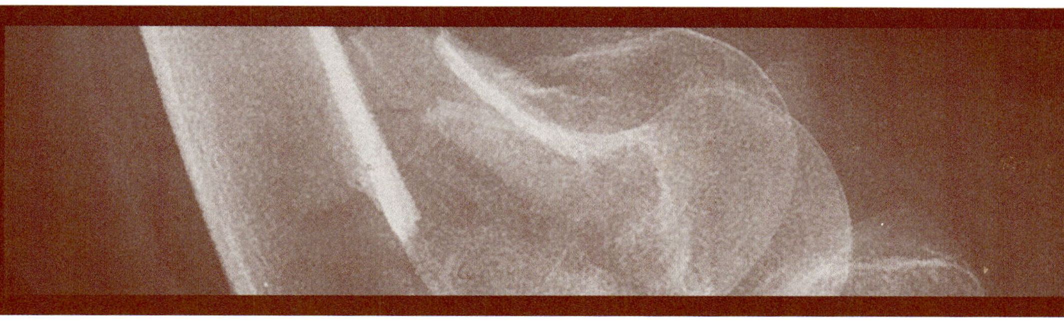

12

Fractures of the Femoral Shaft

Todd O. McKinley

Femoral shaft fractures continue to be treated successfully with intramedullary nailing. As techniques have evolved, reamed, statically locked intramedullary nailing has become the treatment of choice for most diaphyseal femur fractures. Union rates of closed fractures stabilized with closed intramedullary nailing approach 100% [1,2]. Few other fractures have been treated as successfully. As techniques have improved, indications for intramedullary fixation have expanded to metaphyseal and articular injuries. The dual focus of this chapter is to reinforce current evaluation and surgical techniques and to discuss ongoing controversies in the treatment of diaphyseal femur fractures.

PREOPERATIVE EVALUATION AND TREATMENT

The amount of energy required to fracture an adult femur is significant and must be respected. This mandates a team approach between the orthopedist, general surgeon, and anesthesiologist. Cranial, abdominal, and thoracic injuries must be promptly recognized and treated. Bleeding from femur fractures is considerable, but isolated femur fractures rarely lead to hypovolemic shock. Other potential sources of bleeding must be investigated in the hypotensive patient thought to have an isolated femur fracture. Laboratory evaluation must include determining hematocrit levels; appropriate quantities of blood must be available. Depending on associated injuries, further laboratory investigation may be necessary.

Careful inspection of the entire lower extremity is mandatory. Document a clear, concise neurologic and vascular examination. A compromise in vascularity requires further investigation with angiography. Any break in the skin is considered an open fracture until proven otherwise. Compartment syndromes are much less common in the thigh than in the leg, but they do occur. Any suspicion warrants pressure measurement of the thigh compartments. Several commercial pressure transducers are available; however, I believe using an arterial line transducer is more reliable. Open fractures and compartment syndromes should be taken to the operating room immediately. A high index of suspicion should be maintained for associated articular injuries in the proximal and distal femur. Ligamentous disruptions of the knee are common associated injuries but are difficult to evaluate until the femur has been stabilized. Pelvic ring and acetabular fractures also occur with femur fractures and such concomitant injuries affect initial and subsequent management.

A complete radiographic profile is mandatory. Anteroposterior (AP) and lateral projections of the entire femur must be obtained. Additional radiographs may be necessary in segmental or highly comminuted fractures. In addition, orthogonal views of the ipsilateral hip and knee joints must be used to evaluate for associated fractures. An internal rotation radiograph or high-quality fluoroscopic image of the femoral neck must be visualized to evaluate for a concomitant femoral neck fracture. An AP view of the pelvis is mandatory. Any suspicion, based on the pelvis radiograph, for a pelvic ring injury or acetabular fracture mandates further radiographic workup. Specialized imaging with computed tomography (CT) or magnetic resonance imaging (MRI) is not necessary for femoral diaphyseal fractures.

The mainstay of preoperative fracture treatment is maintaining length and alignment of the femur. This is especially true when a significant delay occurs before surgery. Maintenance of femur length and alignment is best accomplished with skeletal traction. Options include traction through the distal femur, proximal or distal tibia, or the calcaneus. A tensioned 0.0625-in Kirschner traction wire, inserted in the proximal tibia, works well if little delay is expected prior to surgery. The wire is inserted just below the tibial tubercle in the middle third of the sagittal diameter of the tibia. Use a larger, threaded Steinmann pin when traction is needed for several days before surgery. Distal femoral traction is used in patients with proximal tibial fractures and is inserted distal and anterior in the femur to avoid the path of an intramedullary rod. Traction through the distal tibia or calcaneus forces the knee into extension, thus adding tension to the sciatic nerve, and it should be used only when necessary.

OPERATIVE TREATMENT

The mainstay of treatment of diaphyseal fractures is antegrade, locked intramedullary nailing. Although some physicians advocate open plating for diaphyseal femur fractures, this chapter focuses on intramedullary techniques. Union rates have approached 100% in closed fractures stabilized with intramedullary nails [1,2]. Surgical techniques have become more refined, but the orthopedic principles of fracture fixation remain unchanged. An appropriate reduction must be maintained with stable internal fixation to allow early return to function. Reduction must restore length, rotation, and correct angulation.

Patients should be placed on a fracture table in either a supine or a lateral position. Lateral positioning provides more reliable access to the entry point in the piriformis fossa. This placement is advantageous in large patients and patients with proximal fractures (Figure 12-1). Properly positioned and directed entry into the proximal femur avoids varus reduction, especially in proximal fractures (Figure 12-2). I also consider distal freehand cross-locking to be easier in the lateral position. Supine nailing offers advantages in positioning patients on the fracture table and in patients with bilateral fractures. The injured leg must be adducted to afford access to the proximal femur (Figure 12-3). Access to the proximal femur can be exceedingly difficult in large patients.

McFerran and Johnson [3] have advocated femoral nailing with patients positioned free on a radiolucent table. They cite several advantages, including shorter setup and operating times. Free nailing is best performed in the acute setting. They also acknowledge that this technique should be abandoned if surgery is not performed within 72 hours and if the fracture is shortened. Patients are placed in a semilateral position with the affected buttock bumped by at least 30°. Reduction is usually performed manually but other options include skeletal traction or a femoral distractor. Their findings have been supported by two prospective studies by Wolinsky *et al.* [4] and Sirkin *et al.* [5]. The ease of setup must be

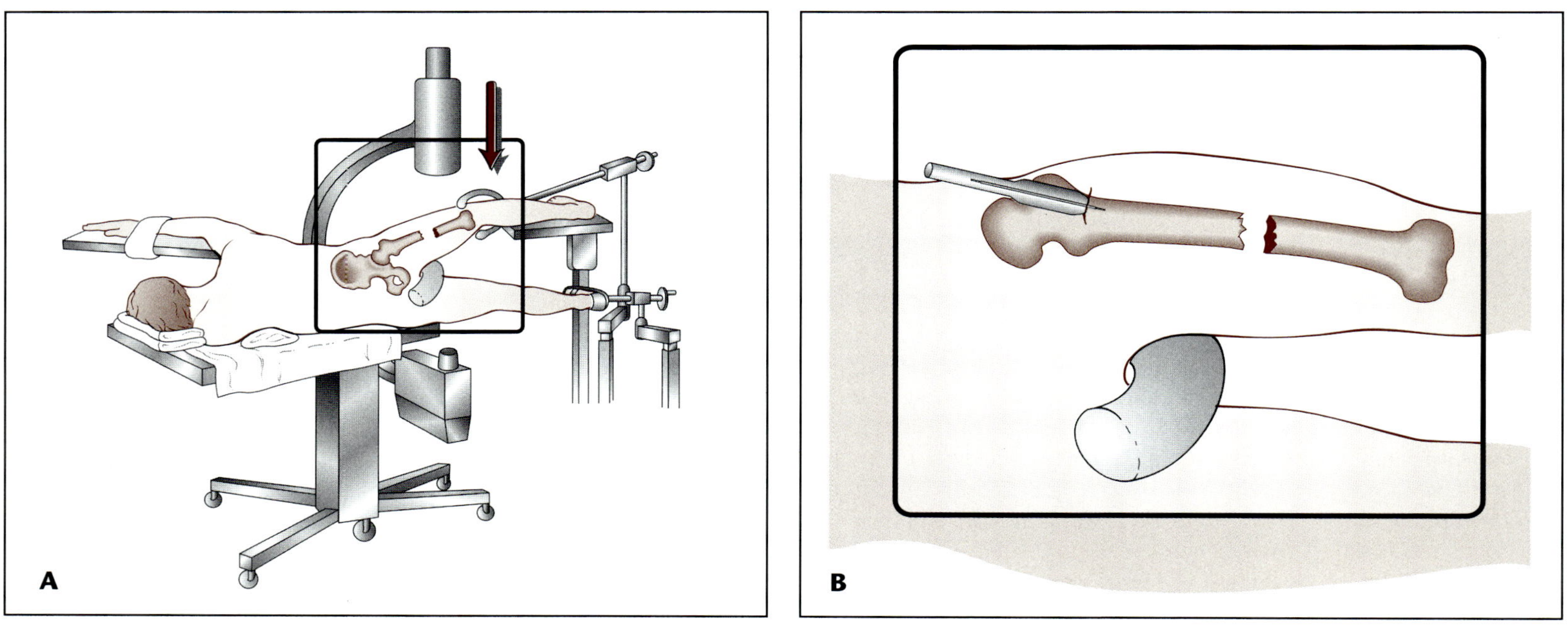

FIGURE 12-1. Lateral positioning. **A**, Patient in lateral position with good access for fluoroscopy. **B**, Enlarged view of operative area. It is easier to drill a hole in the top of the femur while the patient is positioned on his side rather than on his back.

weighed against the amount of available help. The surgeon operating with a single operative assistant must be familiar with these techniques before operating without a fracture table, because a fracture table provides an "extra set of hands" when additional help is not available.

Reduction maneuvers must be determined before surgery begins. Failure to determine a reduction strategy before surgery will prolong the operation. The fluoroscopic unit must be positioned such that clear AP and lateral views of the proximal femur, fracture site, and distal femur are easily obtained without interfering with the fracture table, opposite leg, or reduction instruments. Cortical keys seen on fluoroscopy establish correct length and rotation. Angulation can usually be determined using fluoroscopy, but if any significant doubt remains about the quality of reduction, a radiograph should be obtained.

Understanding muscular deforming forces is necessary for reduction. Shortening is overcome by longitudinal traction, but excessive traction accentuates muscular forces that increase angular deformity. The distal shaft will be pulled into extension by the gastrocnemius and into valgus angulation by the iliotibial band with increased traction (Figures 12-4 and 12-5). Gravity pulls fractures into recurvatum in supine patients and into valgus in patients who are positioned laterally. I use simple crutches positioned under fluoroscopic guidance to correct angular deformity. Fractures in the isthmal region are stable to angulation after the nail crosses the fracture site. Fractures approaching the metaphysis are not stable to angular deformity after the nail spans the fracture. Reduction in these distal fractures must be maintained during reaming, nail insertion, and cross-locking to avoid malreduction (Figure 12-6). Excellent fluoroscopic visualization of

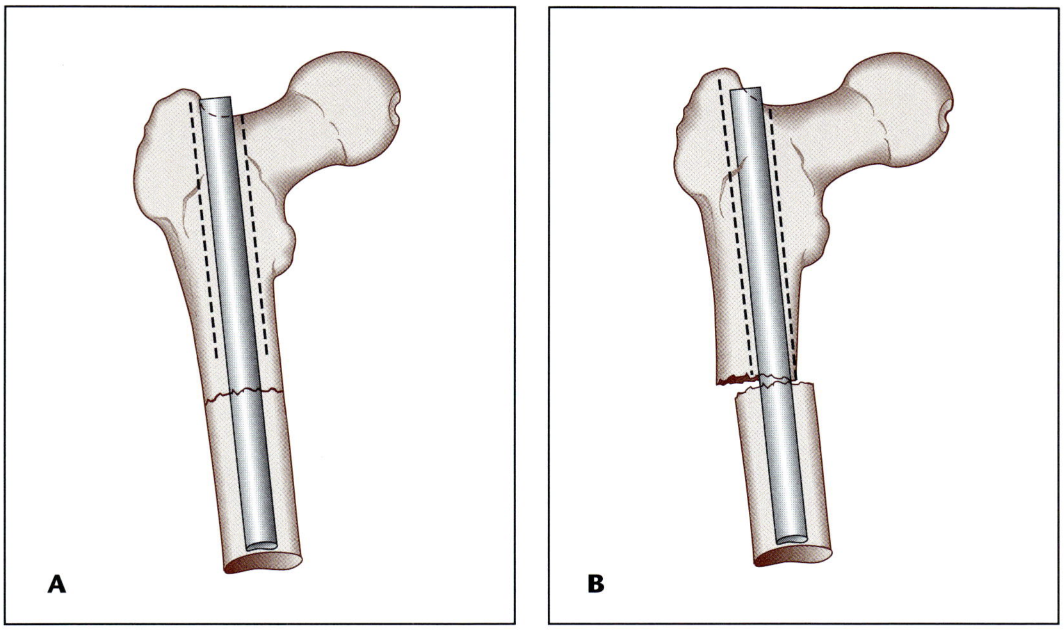

FIGURE 12-2. Entry hole into the proximal femur. **A**, Properly directed entry hole avoids varus reduction. This procedure is facilitated by the use of an end-cutting reamer over a guidewire and also by positioning the patient in the lateral position. **B**, Entry hole directed medially forces a varus reduction.

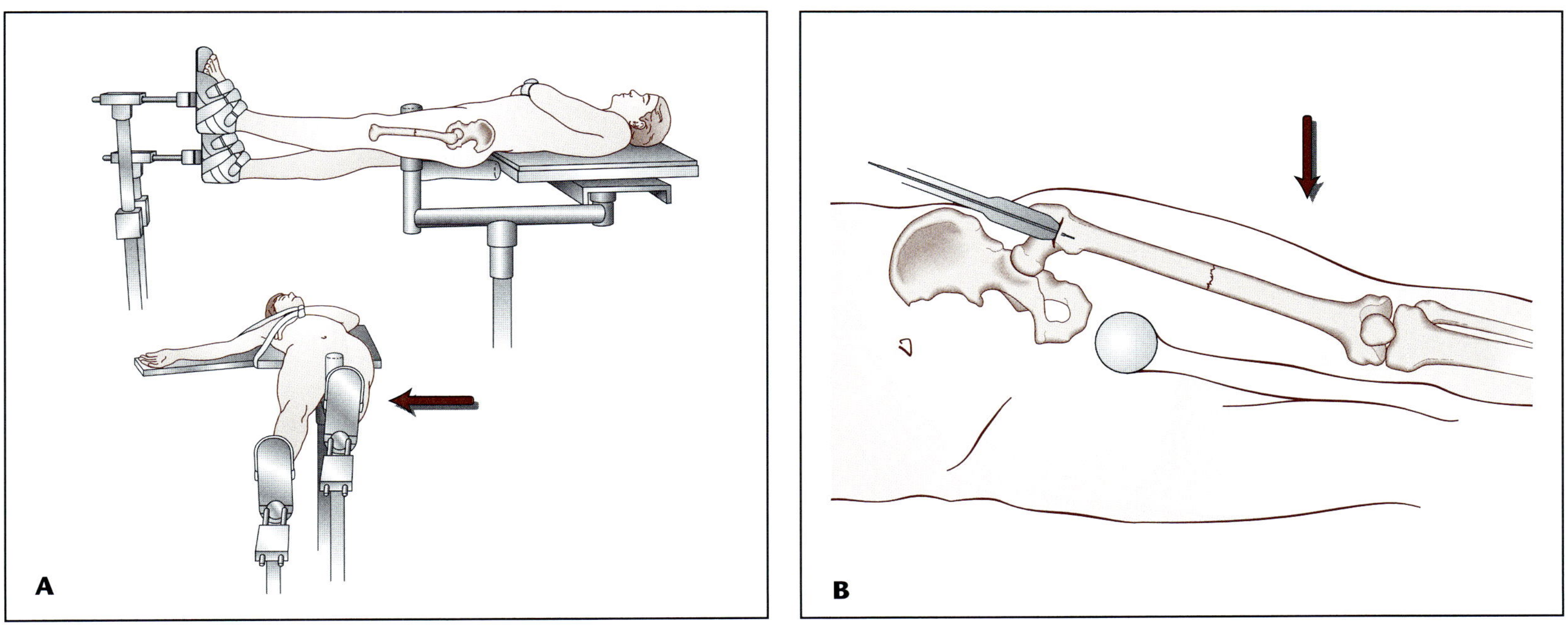

FIGURE 12-3. Supine positioning. **A** and **B**, Adduction of injured leg facilitates access to the proximal femur.

alignment in the frontal and sagittal planes or a standard radiograph must be used to confirm reduction before insertion of distal cross-locks. All patients must be examined after surgery to assess length and rotation before they are discharged from the operating room.

SEGMENTAL FRACTURES

Segmental femur fractures usually result from higher-energy injuries and affected patients have a higher incidence of associated abdominal and thoracic injuries. The soft tissue injury to the femur is greater, which increases the incidence of compartment syndrome and prolongs healing time. Evaluation for associated skeletal injuries of the ipsilateral knee and hip cannot be overemphasized.

Establishing correct length and rotation can be technically challenging. Cortical reduction keys are less obvious or often absent on fluoroscopy. Correct length can be determined by radiographic study of the uninjured femur. Scanograms establish correct length by identifying the distance between reproducible anatomic landmarks on the uninjured femur. Some systems provide a radiopaque ruler that can be superimposed on the uninjured femur to establish length and nail position. This is best done with a full-length radiograph and less reliably with fluoroscopy. Any imperfection in either centering the fluoroscopic beam or establishing the correct fluoroscopic angle on the femur and ruler distorts the image, thus rendering the test useless. Rotation should be checked clinically, comparing the injured extremity with the opposite leg. Rotation is

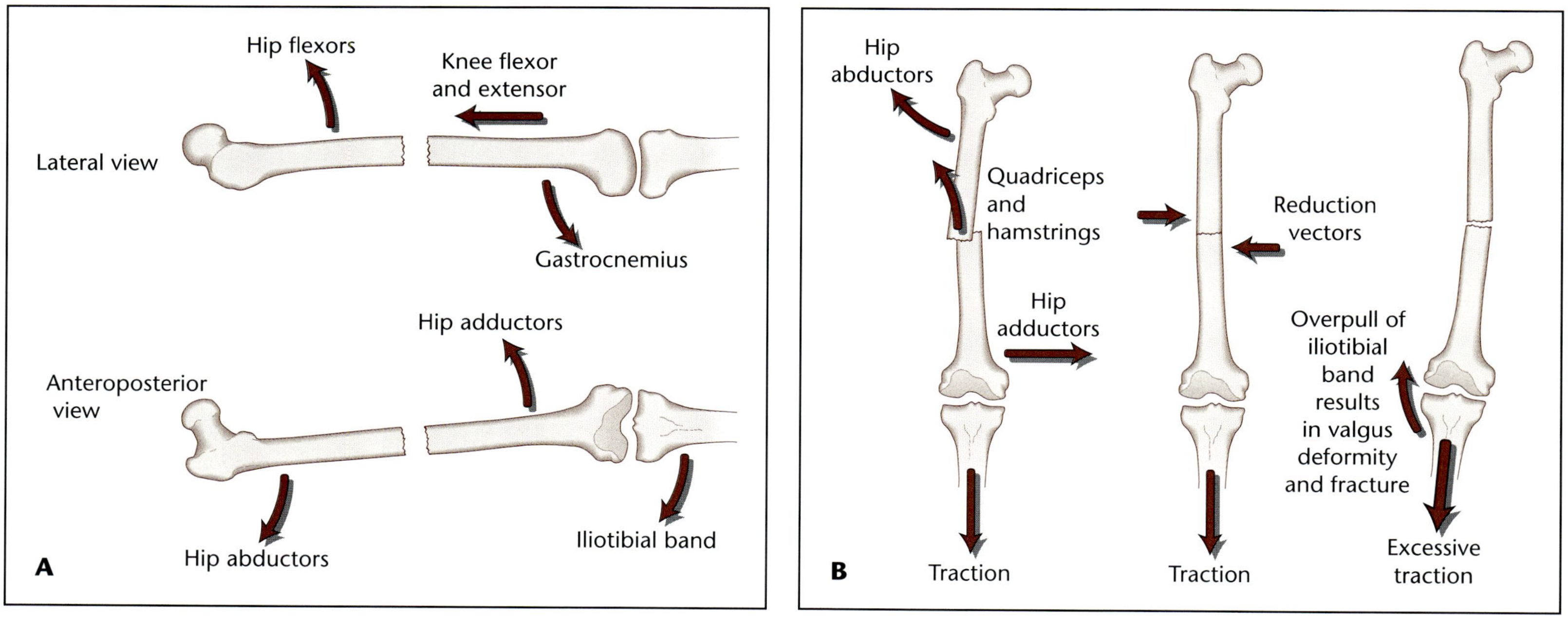

FIGURE 12-4. A, Deforming muscular forces. B, Anteroposterior view of deforming forces and reduction strategies.

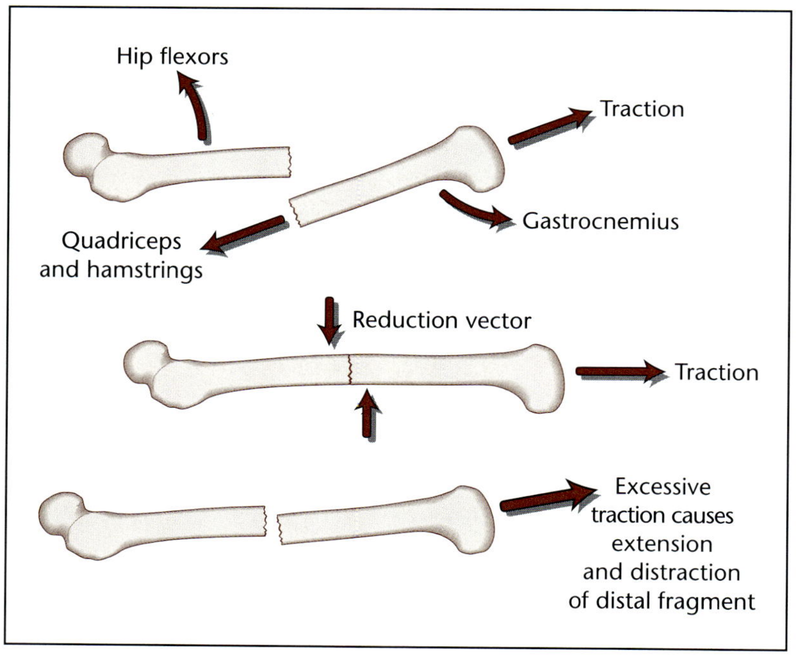

FIGURE 12-5. Lateral view of deforming muscular forces and reduction strategies. Excessive traction causes extension and distraction of distal fragment. Reduction vector should be placed as close to fracture as possible.

also checked by comparing the transcondylar axis of the distal femur with the anteversion of the femoral neck on fluoroscopy. Normally, the condylar axis of the distal femur is internally rotated approximately 10° to 15° with respect to the femoral neck (Figure 12-7). Patients with excess anteversion or retroversion of the uninjured femur must be identified and rotation of the injured femur must be adjusted accordingly.

Several technical issues deserve to be emphasized. Segmental fractures are unstable, which makes static cross-locking mandatory. An intramedullary nail does not maintain reduction in fractures with comminution that spans the isthmus. Such fractures must be held in a reduced position during reaming, nail insertion, and cross-locking. Failure to follow these steps predictably leads to malreduction.

OPEN FRACTURES

Open fractures are high-energy injuries. Even Type I injuries must be respected, because a significant amount of energy is needed for a fractured bone to fully penetrate the thick surrounding muscle sleeve in the thigh. Principles of open fracture management apply to the femur. Wounds should be cleaned of any gross debris in the emergency department and sterile povidone-iodine dressings should be applied. Therapy with appropriate antibiotics should be started immediately. First generation cephalosporins are effective against most organisms but therapy against gram-negative and anaerobic bacteria is necessary in grossly contaminated wounds or in wounds associated with severe crushing.

Patients should be taken for surgical débridement as soon as possible. Most grade I fractures can be débrided and closed during the initial surgery. Most grade II and all grade III injuries are best treated with repeated débridements that achieve a wound free of devitalized tissue before closure. Exposure of the fractured ends of the bone is mandatory during débridement. Cortical fragments free of soft tissue attachments should be removed from the wound. I believe fractures should be nailed at the initial débridement to optimize subsequent nursing care and to improve patient comfort.

Studies have consistently shown a 3% to 5% infection rate associated with open femur fractures [6,7]. Infection rates are similar for injuries treated with immediate intramedullary nailing compared with those treated with delayed nailing [7]. No evidence suggests that unreamed nails lessen infection rates in open fractures; therefore, I believe patients should be stabilized with a reamed, stable nail. External fixation plays a role in management of fractures that are severely contaminated.

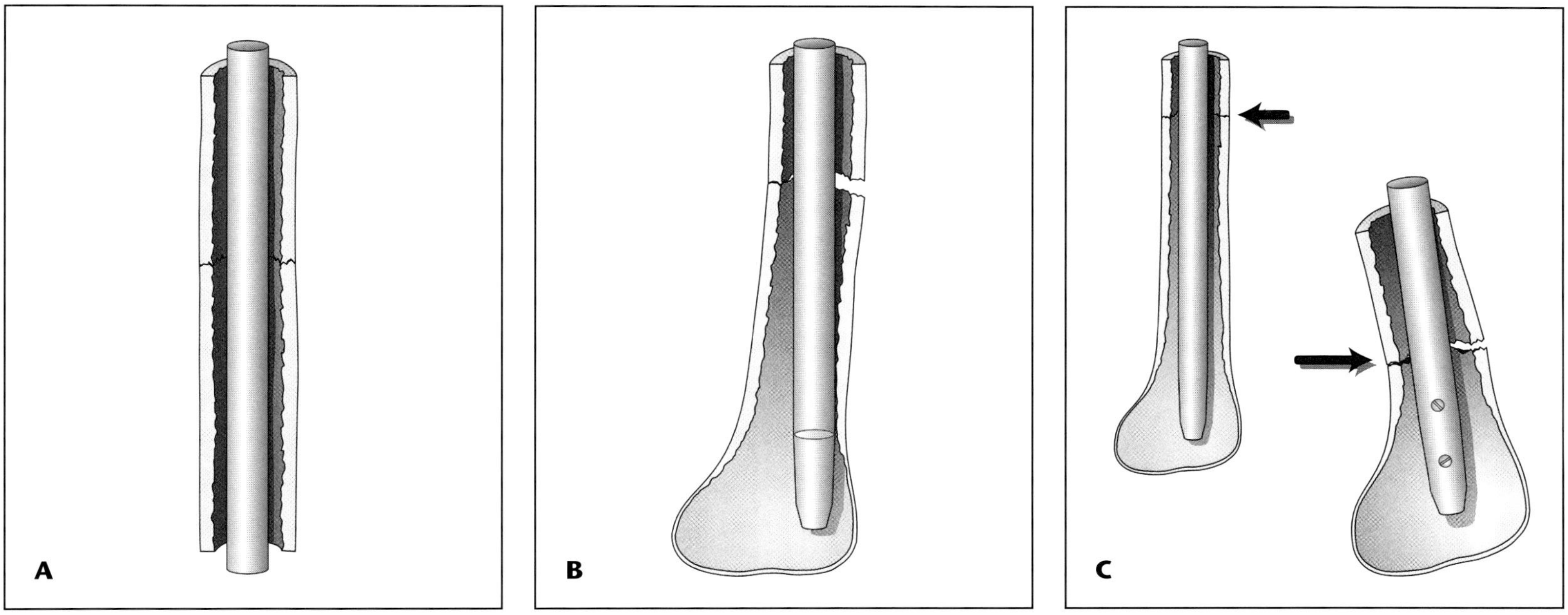

FIGURE 12-6. A, Fractures in the isthmal region are stable to angulation prior to cross-locking. B, As the canal widens in the metaphysis, the distal fragment can deform around the nail. The reduction must be maintained externally until the nail is cross-locked. C, Stable isthmal fracture (*left*, fracture indicated by *arrow*) and unstable distal fracture (*right*) with rotation around the nail (*arrow*).

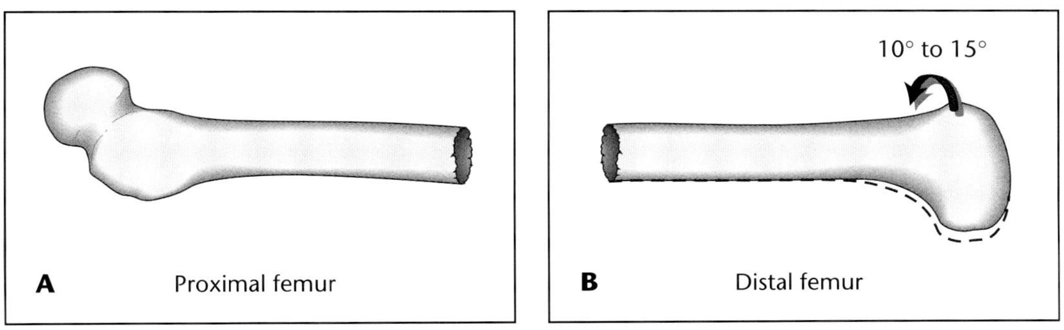

FIGURE 12-7. Fluoroscopically aided rotation reduction. A, Proximal femur. B, Distal femur. Rotation of distal fragment is adjusted until true lateral of distal femur is internally rotated 10° to 15° to the femoral neck.

RETROGRADE INTRAMEDULLARY NAILING

Retrograde techniques were originally developed to stabilize supracondylar femur fractures and periprosthetic fractures in patients with total knee prostheses. These techniques are becoming increasingly popular for treatment of diaphyseal femur fractures. Moed and Watson [8] achieved an 85% union rate using unreamed retrograde nails in diaphyseal fractures. Moed *et al.* [9] modified their original technique, using dynamization as necessary, insertion to full length of the femur, and increased fill of the femoral canal. Prospectively, their union rate improved to 94%. Herscovici and Whiteman [10] reported a similar union rate in 45 diaphyseal fractures.

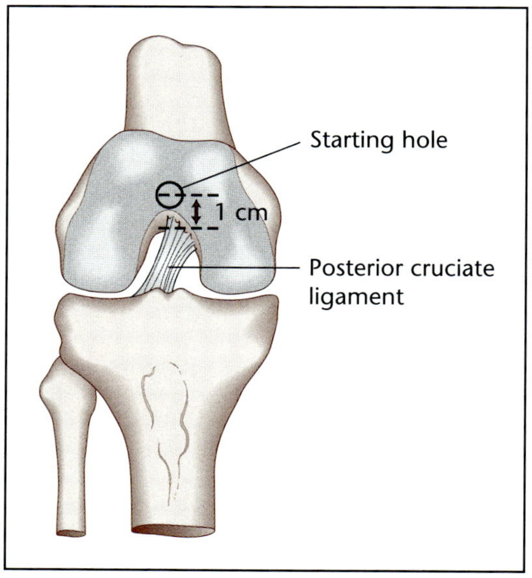

FIGURE 12-8. Starting hole for insertion of the retrograde nail, viewed from the distal end of the femur with knee flexed.

Retrograde nailing affords excellent control of the distal fragment and allows more distal placement of distal cross-locking screws. These technical advantages are important for intramedullary fixation of supracondylar and intercondylar distal femur fractures. These technical advantages are of less significance in diaphyseal fractures. Retrograde insertion requires drilling a large hole through the distal femur within the knee joint. Knee pain has not been a significant problem in early clinical reports; however, long-term clinical outcomes, specifically in terms of knee function, remain unknown. Union rates using retrograde technique are inferior to antegrade nailing for diaphyseal fractures [1,2,8–11]. Retrograde nailing of diaphyseal fractures is indicated in patients with associated proximal femur or acetabular injuries or soft tissue issues that preclude antegrade nailing. Relative indications include patients with bilateral femur fractures, multisystem trauma, ipsilateral fracture of the tibia, bilateral femur fractures, or morbid obesity. A role exists for retrograde nailing in patients with multiple orthopedic injuries who cannot undergo a prolonged operation. The surgeon must justify that the technical advantages using the retrograde technique outweigh associated intra-articular morbidity and lower union rate. Supine positioning allows access to all other extremities for concomitant fracture work.

The patient is positioned supine on a radiolucent table. Unrestricted fluoroscopic access is mandatory. Reduction maneuvers should be confirmed fluoroscopically before surgery. A firm bump placed under the flexed knee facilitates reduction of the extended distal fragment. The distal femur is opened just anterior to the femoral insertion of the posterior cruciate ligament within the notch (Figure 12-8). It is critical to insert the nail in proper sagittal and coronal orientation in the distal fragment to avoid extension and varus deformity, especially in distal fractures (Figure 12-9). The nail generally establishes length and restores alignment if the fracture is near the isthmus. More distal diaphyseal fractures, such as those near the metaphyseal junction, remain unstable until the nail is cross-locked. Sagittal and frontal plane alignment must be confirmed fluoroscopically before distal cross-

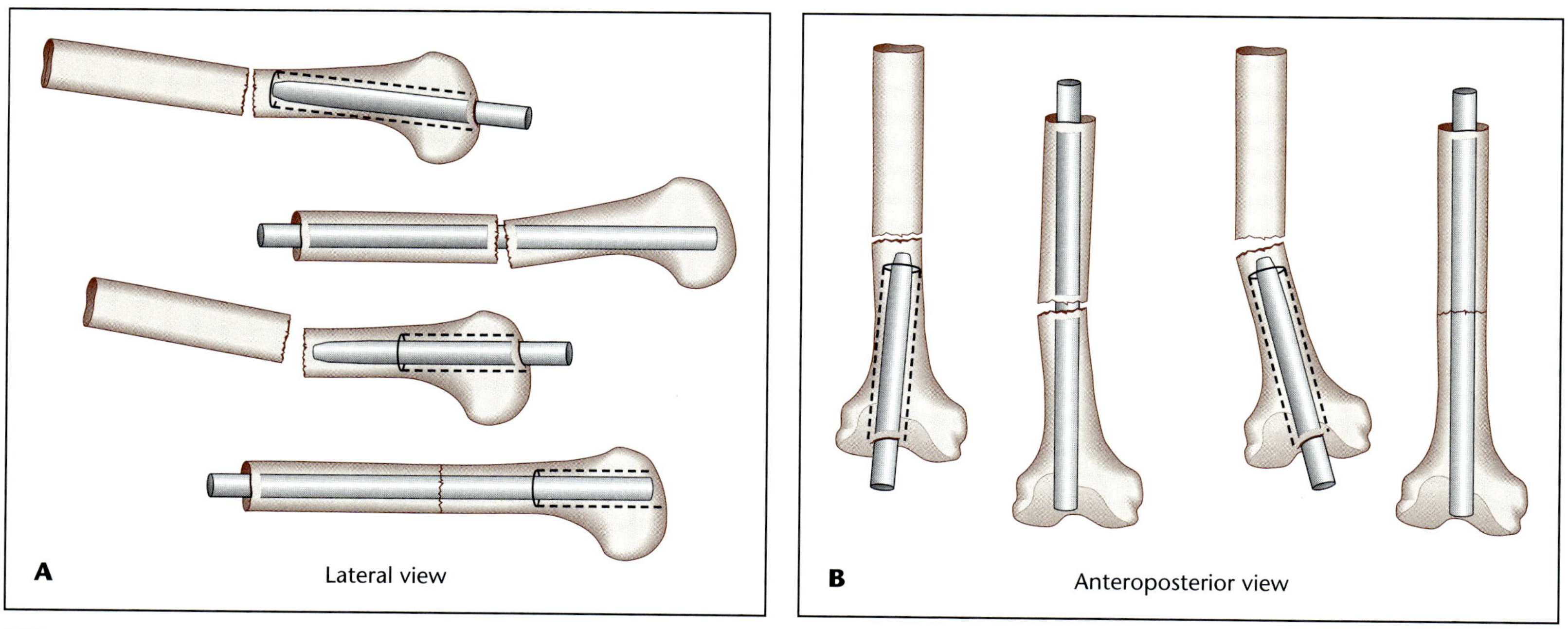

FIGURE 12-9. Aligning the opening hole in the distal fragment with the proximal fragment will lead to a malreduction. The opening in the distal fragment must be aligned anatomically with the distal fragment, not the proximal fragment, to obtain an anatomic reduction. **A**, Lateral view. **B**, Anteroposterior view.

locking to prevent malreduction. Drill guides generally aid distal cross-locking; proximal cross-locking is most commonly done with freehand technique. Proper length must be obtained before inserting proximal cross-lock screws.

CRITICALLY INJURED PATIENTS

Patients with femur fractures often have sustained concomitant cranial, abdominal, and thoracic injuries. Copeland *et al.* [12] reported that associated trauma is more severe in patients with bilateral femur fractures with a mortality rate of 26%. In a prospective, randomized study, Bone *et al.* [13] determined that patients with multiple injuries had fewer pulmonary complications when they had early stabilization (*ie*, within 24 hours of injury) of their femur fracture. Pape *et al.* [14] reported an increased incidence in adult respiratory distress syndrome (ARDS) and mortality in patients with thoracic trauma stabilized within 24 hours in a retrospective review. Bone *et al.* [15] performed a review of the more recent clinical human and animal literature and concluded that incidence of pulmonary failure and ARDS in femur fractures stabilized acutely with reamed nailing was less than 3%.

Bosse *et al.* [16], in a retrospective review, concluded that the incidence of ARDS, pneumonia, pulmonary embolism, and multiple system organ failure was not affected by insertion of a reamed nail. Furthermore, plating offered no advantages compared with reamed nailing in this review. This debate will continue, but based on the most current review and prospective evidence, I believe that patients who sustain multiple injuries, including chest trauma with femur fractures, should be stabilized as soon as possible with a reamed nail. External fixation should be reserved for use in patients with hemodynamic instability who cannot tolerate a prolonged procedure or blood loss. A high incidence of pin tract problems, loss of motion, and malreduction make external fixation undesirable, and its use must be justified by the patient's condition.

REAMED VERSUS UNREAMED NAILING

The issue of canal reaming continues to be debated, especially in patients with concomitant pulmonary injuries. It has been hypothesized that the bolus of intramedullary fat introduced into the systemic circulation can compromise oxygenation and promote lung parenchymal injury [14]. In a retrospective review of 446 patients, pulmonary morbidity was independent of reaming during femoral stabilization [16]. One advantage of using an unreamed nail is shorter operative time. However, this benefit must be weighed against several significant disadvantages associated with using unreamed technique: the incidence of implant failure is higher; the nonunion rate is higher; and the time to union is prolonged. In a recent prospective study, Clatworthy *et al.* [17] reported that unreamed patients took 11 weeks longer to unite compared with fractures in patients with reamed technique. They truncated their study early secondary to a unacceptably high incidence of implant failure in the unreamed group. Tornetta and Tiburzi [18] reported a higher incidence of delayed unions in patients treated with unreamed nailing in a prospective study. Hammacher *et al.* [19] reported a 5% nonunion rate and 3% delayed union rate using unreamed nailing. Based on recent reports, I believe the only relative indication for using an unreamed nail is in a critically injured patient to minimize operative time. In such a setting, the surgeon should ensure that the nail can be inserted at the same time that an external fixator can be applied.

CURRENT RECOMMENDATIONS

The standard of care for diaphyseal femur fractures remains a reamed statically locked antegrade intramedullary nail. Retrograde insertion has a lower union rate and long-term studies evaluating knee function are not available. This technique should be used sparingly and only with good indications in diaphyseal fractures, such as ipsilateral proximal soft tissue injuries of the femur or pelvis and acetabulum that preclude operative incisions. Retrograde insertion also has a role in the multiply injured patient to minimize operative time and in patients with bilateral femur fractures. Relative indications include floating knees, morbidly obese patients, and patients with ipsilateral fractures of the proximal femur or pelvis and acetabulum. No indication exists for use of an unreamed nail, except possibly in an open fracture that has stripped most of the femur of all soft tissue attachments. Multiply injured patients with index–injury severity scores of 18 or higher should be stabilized as soon as possible and definitely within the first 24 hours of injury. Other closed fractures should be stabilized as soon as resources become available. I have introduced some personal bias on technical issues, but "there are many roads to Rome." Surgical technique depends on the training and experience of the surgeon. However, the goal remains the same: efficient, aggressive care to stabilize the femur in anatomic alignment, restoring the patient to function as quickly as possible.

REFERENCES AND RECOMMENDED READING

Recently published papers of particular interest have been highlighted as:
- • Of interest
- •• Of outstanding interest

1. Brumback RJ, Uwagie-Ero S, Lakatos RP, *et al.*: Intramedullary nailing of femoral shaft fractures, part II: fracture-healing with static interlocking fixation. *J Bone Joint Surg* 1988, 70:1453–1462.
2. Winquist RA, Hansen ST, Clawson DK: Closed intramedullary nailing of femoral fractures: a report of five hundred and twenty cases. *J Bone Joint Surg* 1984, 66:529–539.
3. McFerran MA, Johnson KD: Intramedullary nailing of acute femoral shaft fractures without a fracture table: technique of using a femoral distractor. *J Orthop Trauma* 1992, 6:271–278.
4. Wolinsky PR, McCarty EC, Shyr Y, Johnson KD: Length of operative procedures: reamed femoral intramedullary nailing performed with and without a fracture table. *J Orthop Trauma* 1998, 12:485–495.
5. Sirkin MS, Behrens F, McCracken K, *et al.*: Femoral nailing without a fracture table. *Clin Orthop* 1996, 332:119–125.
6. Brumback RJ, Ellison PS, Poka A, *et al.*: Intramedullary nailing of open fractures of the femoral shaft. *J Bone Joint Surg* 1989, 71:1324–1331.
7. Lhowe DW, Hansen ST: Immediate nailing of open fractures of the femoral shaft. *J Bone Joint Surg* 1988, 70:812–820.
8. Moed BR, Watson JT: Retrograde intramedullary nailing, without reaming, of fractures of the femoral shaft in multiply injured patients. *J Bone Joint Surg* 1995, 77:1520–1527.
9. Moed BR, Watson JT, Cramer KE, *et al.*: Unreamed retrograde intramedullary nailing of fractures of the femoral shaft. *J Orthop Trauma* 1998, 12:334–342.

10. Herscovici D Jr, Whiteman KW: Retrograde nailing of the femur using an intercondylar approach. *Clin Orthop* 1996, 332:98–104.
11. Ostrum RF, DiCicco J, Lakatos R, Poka A: Retrograde intramedullary nailing of femoral diaphyseal fractures. *J Orthop Trauma* 1998, 12:464–468.
12. Copeland CE, Mitchell KA, Brumback RJ, *et al.*: Mortality in patients with bilateral femoral fractures. *J Orthop Trauma* 1998, 12:315–319.
13. Bone LB, Johnson KD, Weigelt J, Scheinberg R: Early versus delayed stabilization of femoral fractures: a prospective randomized study. *J Bone Joint Surg* 1989, 71:336–340.
14. Pape HC, Auf'm'Kolk M, Paffrath T, *et al.*: Primary intramedullary femur fixation in multiple trauma patients with associated lung contusion: a cause of posttraumatic ARDS? *J Trauma* 1993, 34:540–547.
15. Bone LB, Anders MJ, Rohrbacher BJ: Treatment of femoral fractures in the multiply injured patient with thoracic injury. *Clin Orthop* 1998, 347:57–61.
16. Bosse MJ, MacKenzie EJ, Reimer BL, *et al.*: Adult respiratory distress syndrome, pneumonia, and mortality following thoracic injury and a femoral fracture treated either with intramedullary nailing with reaming or with a plate: a comparative study. *J Bone Joint Surg* 1997, 79:799–809.
17. Clatworthy MG, Clark DI, Gray DH, Hardy AE: Reamed versus unreamed femoral nails: a randomized, prospective trial. *J Bone Joint Surg* 1998, 80:485–489.
18. Tornetta P III, Tiburzi D: The treatment of femoral shaft fractures using intramedullary interlocked nails with and without intramedullary reaming: a preliminary report. *J Orthop Trauma* 1997, 11:89–92.
19. Hammacher ER, van Meeteren MC, van der Werken C: Improved results in treatment of femoral shaft fractures with the unreamed femoral nail? A multicenter experience. *J Trauma* 1998, 45:517–521.

SECTION V

Fracture-Dislocations and Fractures of the Lower Limbs

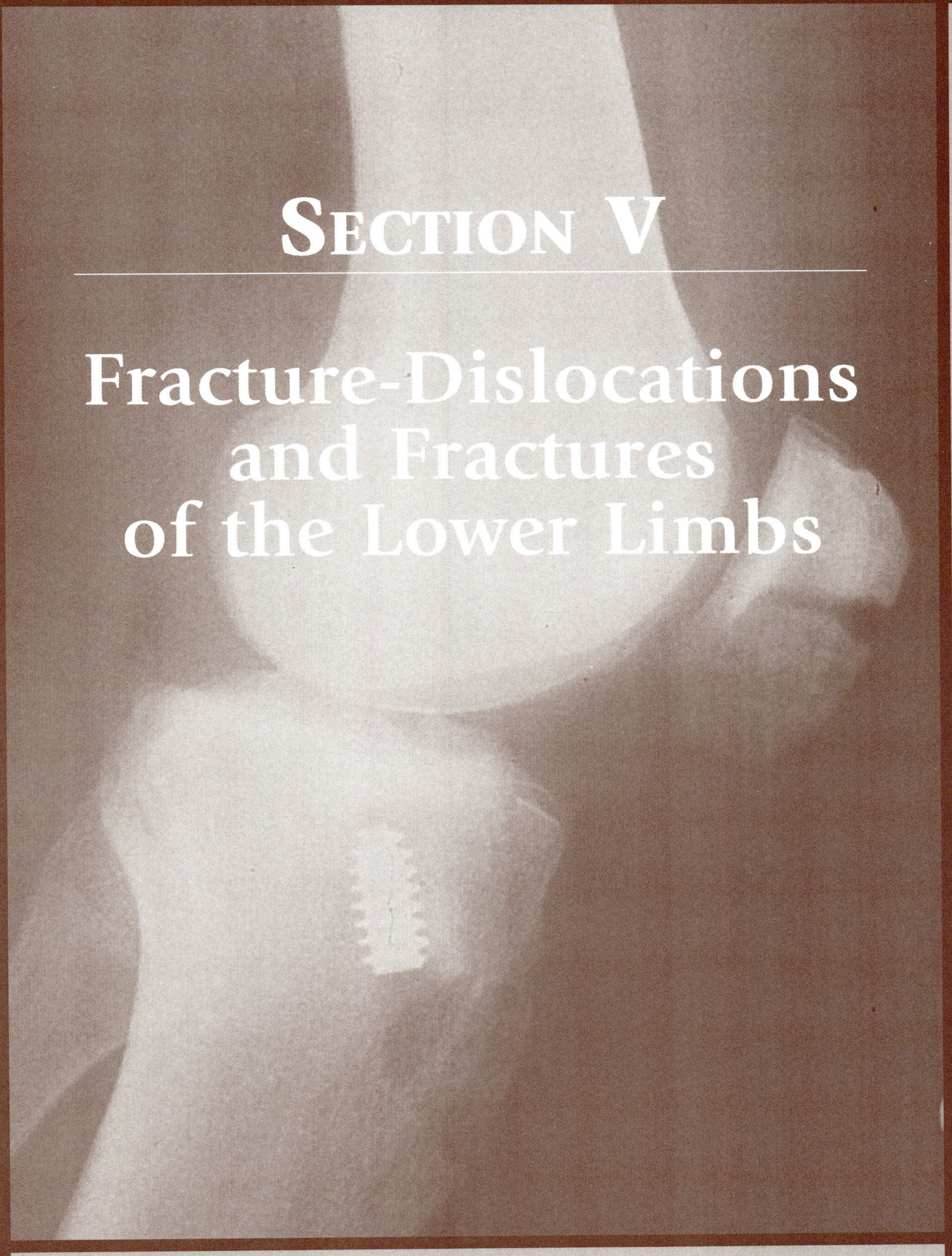

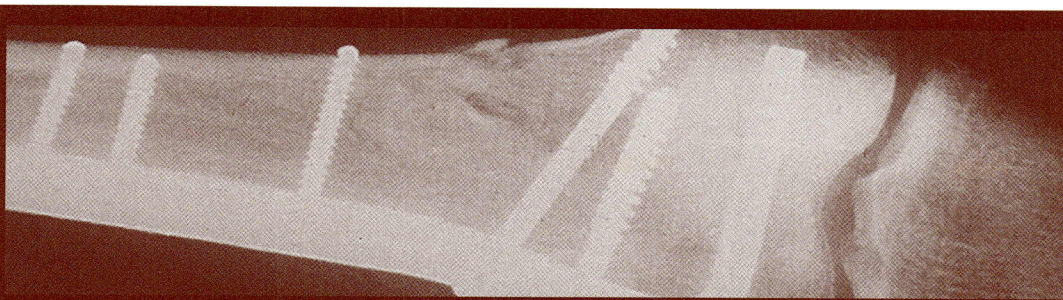

13

Supracondylar Fractures of the Femur

Christopher G. Finkemeier

Supracondylar fractures of the femur account for approximately 4% [1] of all femur fractures and approximately 31% [2] of all femur fractures after hip fractures have been excluded. These fractures tend to occur in two fairly distinct population groups: the young patient involved in moderate or high-energy trauma, such as a motor vehicle collision, and the elderly patient, typically female, involved in low-energy trauma, such as a fall onto the knee. Incidence of fractures of the distal femur increases exponentially with age and is associated with osteopenia. Two thirds of fractures caused by moderate trauma are "preceded by prior age-related fractures" (*eg*, hip, proximal humerus, distal forearm, pelvis, vertebra) or by radiographic evidence of osteopenia [2]. Supracondylar femur fractures are a challenge to treat because they frequently are comminuted, intra-articular, and associated with osteopenic bone (thin cortices and wide medullary canal).

CLASSIFICATION

Although several fracture classifications have been devised [3], the AO classification [4] (Figure 13-1) is the most commonly used system in North America and Europe. This classification separates supracondylar femur fractures into extra-articular (Type A) and intra-articular (Type B and C) fractures. Type B fractures involve a single condyle (unicondylar), whereas Type C fractures have an intracondylar fracture component that separates the condyles. Each fracture type is then categorized further into groups (*eg*, 1, 2, 3) based on increasing fracture complexity and comminution. The Type B3 pattern, or Hoffa fracture, is important to recognize because the coronal plane fracture line frequently precludes the use of a blade plate, condylar screw, or locking intramedullary nail. In such cases, the surgeon should choose a supracondylar buttress-like plate.

HISTORY AND EVOLUTION OF TREATMENT PHILOSOPHY

Prior to 1970, supracondylar fractures of the femur were treated primarily with some form of traction or splinting that required patients to stay up to 6 to 8 weeks in the hospital. The results were less than satisfactory due to malunion of the distal fragment and knee stiffness. Despite these drawbacks, open treatment with various forms of internal fixation had worse results [5,6], most likely due to unstable fixation methods, soft tissue stripping, and knee stiffness. Open reduction and internal fixation were recommended only for open fractures or fractures with an associated vascular injury that required repair.

After 1970, reports began to emerge of improved results using the principles and implants of the AO/ASIF group [7–10]. The foundational principles of anatomic reduction, stable internal fixation, limited soft tissue damage, and early range of motion became and remain the gold standard for the treatment of these fractures. Despite improved techniques and excellent results in many cases, comminuted intra-articular fractures associated with severe soft tissue injury or osteopenic bone portend a worse prognosis and present formidable challenges for surgeons limited to using plate and screw techniques.

During the late 1980s and 1990s, more surgeons noted the importance of proper soft tissue handling and began using newer techniques that emphasize anatomic reduction of the articular fractures but indirect reduction of fractures involving the metaphysis [11,12]. As surgeons' skills and experience have improved with indirect reduction techniques, new implants have been developed that allow placement of plates through minimal incisions, a technique called *minimally invasive plate osteosynthesis* (MIPO) [13,14•].

What makes management of supracondylar fractures of the femur so challenging is that not all of them can or should be treated with a single approach or implant. Surgeons treating these injuries should be capable of using several different techniques easily and of implanting systems to maximize the patient's outcome.

RELEVANT SURGICAL ANATOMY

The anatomy of the distal femur, its muscle attachments, its relationship to the anatomic and weight-bearing axes of the lower extremity, and its patellofemoral articulation have relevant implications for properly treating supracondylar fractures of the femur.

The supracondylar portion of the femur is defined as the region within 9 cm of the articular surface. When viewed from the lateral side, the femoral condyles project posteriorly to the femoral shaft (Figure 13-2). This relationship is important because a blade plate or condylar screw must be placed in the anterior half of the condyles for the plate to be aligned properly on the femoral shaft. If this does not occur, the distal fragment must be translated with or without flexation or extension to position the plate on the femoral shaft. When viewed in cross-section, the distal femur appears to be a trapezoid (Figure 13-3). The anterior articular sur-

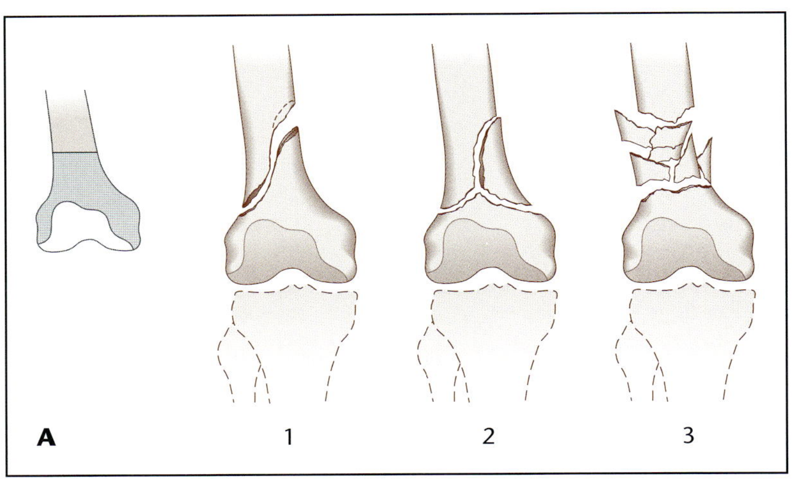

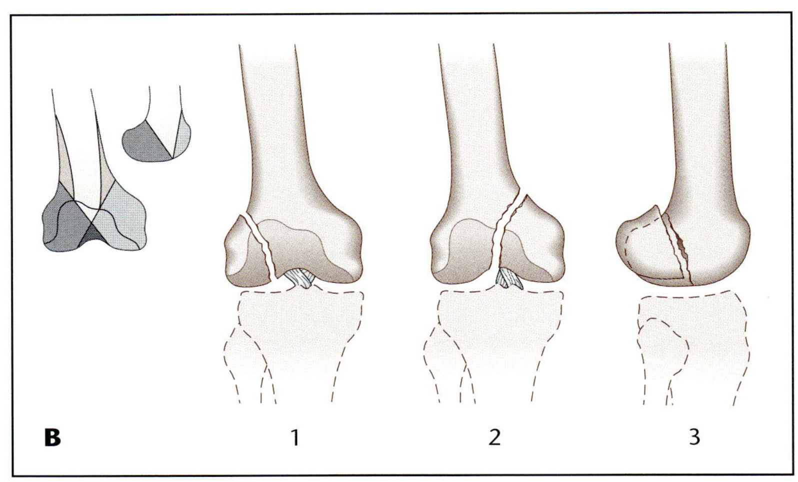

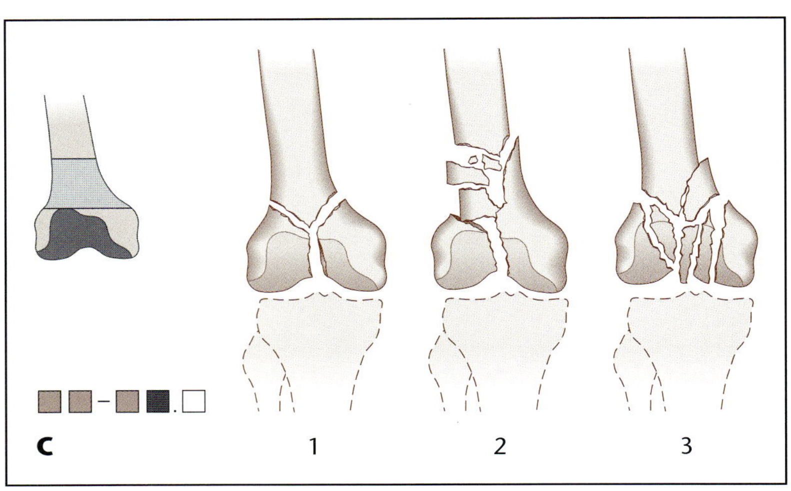

FIGURE 13-1. AO/ASIF classification of supracondylar femur fractures. (*Adapted from* Müller *et al.* [4].)

face slopes downward along a line extending from lateral to medial, whereas the posterior articular surfaces lie along a straight line. In addition, the posterior aspect of the distal femur is wider than the anterior aspect because of the inclination of the medial and lateral cortices toward one another. The medial slope is 25° and the lateral slope is 10°. Therefore, when placing screws or a blade plate from the lateral side, they must be properly inclined so as not to penetrate the intercondylar groove (Figure 13-3). In addition, anteroposterior radiographic images project the widest extent of the posterior condyles but not the distance between medial and lateral cortices more anteriorly. Therefore, to avoid overpenetration of the medial cortex and irritation of the medial collateral ligament by a blade plate or screws, they must come to lie 8 to 10 mm short of the projected image of the medial wall.

Muscular attachments and their deforming forces are important in the displacement patterns of supracondylar fractures, which must be neutralized to restore proper alignment. The quadriceps and hamstrings shorten the fracture and the gastrocnemius causes the characteristic posterior angulation of the distal fragments (Figure 13-4). Restoration of length and proper condylar rotation is important for restoring knee function.

The anatomic axis of the femur subtends an average angle of 9° to the vertical axis. Therefore, the articular surface of the distal aspect of the femur, which is parallel to the floor, subtends an angle of 81° with the femoral shaft (Figure 13-5). This anatomic relationship must be kept in mind when reducing supracondylar femur fractures, especially those that have metaphyseal comminution, to avoid fixing the distal femur in varus. If difficulty in obtaining correct alignment of the distal femur is anticipated, an anteroposterior radiograph of the opposite femur reveals normal, anatomic femoral valgus.

Finally, as the popularity of retrograde intramedullary nailing of the supracondylar and femoral shaft increases, many surgeons are rightfully concerned about patellofemoral mechanics and their long-term implications on the knee joint following retrograde nailing. As seen in Figure 13-6, the patella contacts the femoral articular surface in a linear fashion throughout knee flexion, but has increasingly more contact on the medial and lateral condyles rather than the central portion of the femoral articular surface as knee flexion increases [15]. The patella, therefore, has little to no contact with the insertion site commonly used for retrograde nailing. A recent biomechanical study revealed that mean and maximum patellofemoral contact pressures at 90° and 120° are the same between rodded and nonrodded distal femurs as long as the nail is flush or countersunk to the articular surface [16].

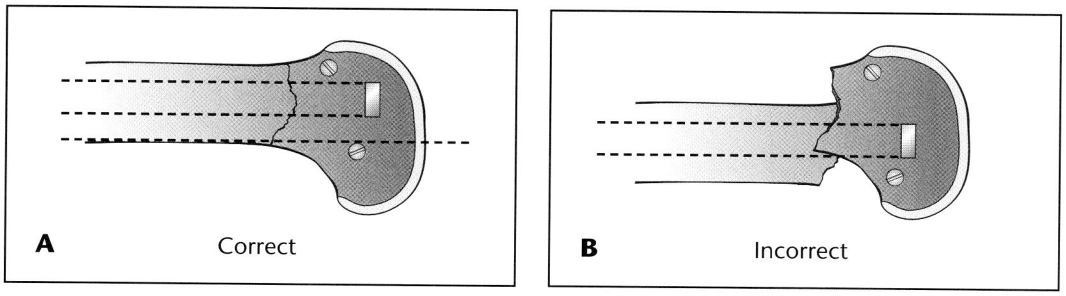

FIGURE 13-2. A, Lateral profile of supracondylar region of distal femur illustrating the posterior projection of the femoral condyles and the proper placement of a blade plate in the anterior half of the condyles. B, Incorrect placement of the blade plate too posteriorly results in anterior translation of the distal fragment.

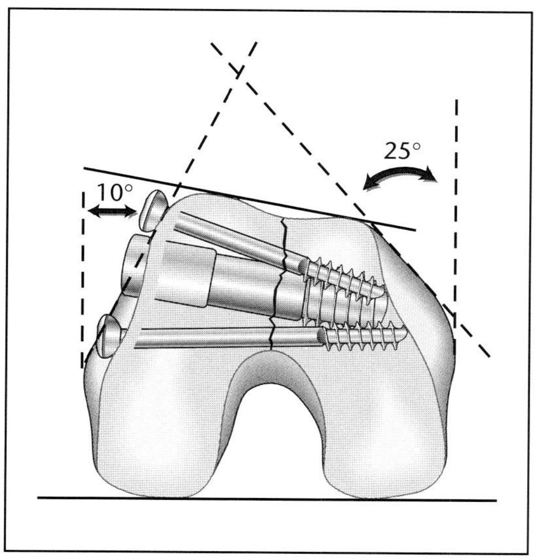

FIGURE 13-3. End-on view of distal femur reveals trapezoidal shape and proper positioning of dynamic condylar screw and two lag screws. Taking into account the lateral to medial slope of the anterior articular surface prevents cut-out into the intercondylar notch. The screws should not protrude medially beyond the cortical margin of the condyle.

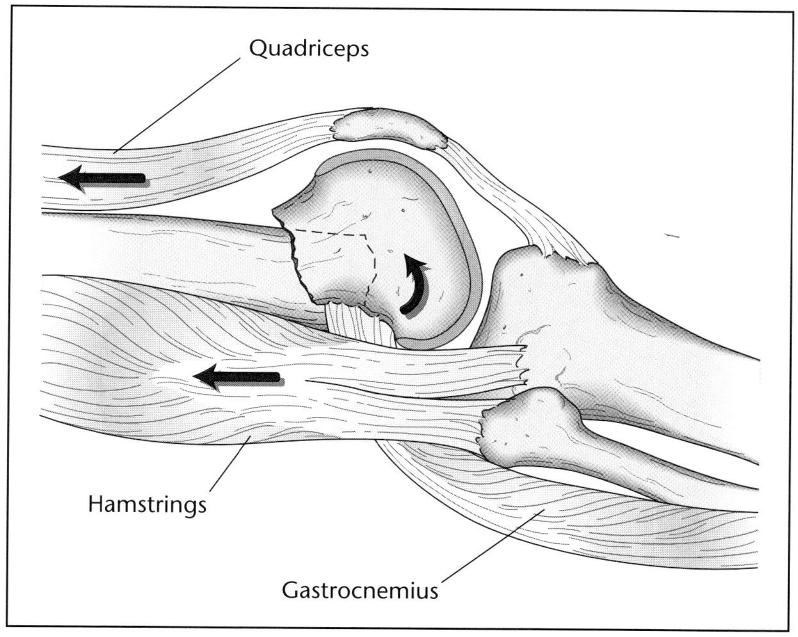

FIGURE 13-4. Lateral view of a supracondylar femur fracture showing the displacement forces of the quadriceps and hamstrings (shortening) and the gastrocnemius (extension rotation) on the distal fragment. These displacement forces need to be neutralized to restore the proper alignment and anatomy of the distal femur.

TREATMENT METHODS

NONOPERATIVE TREATMENT

With the advent of modern surgical techniques and implants, indications for nonoperative treatment of supracondylar fractures have become limited to a few unique situations (Table 13-1). If a patient has a displaced supracondylar femur fracture and is not a candidate for surgery, then I recommend two-pin traction for 2 to 4 weeks to restore length and alignment (Figure 13-7), followed by a cast brace molded with the leg in extension, external rotation, and slight valgus [3,6,17]. Nondisplaced fractures can be treated with immediate application of a cast, splint, or knee immobilizer depending on soft tissue swelling and patient compliance. Patients treated nonoperatively should not attempt to bear weight on the injured leg until clinical (*ie*, minimal pain and swelling) and radiographic (*ie*, callus) signs of healing are present. The patient may then begin protected weight bearing and progress to full weight bearing over the next several weeks as tolerated.

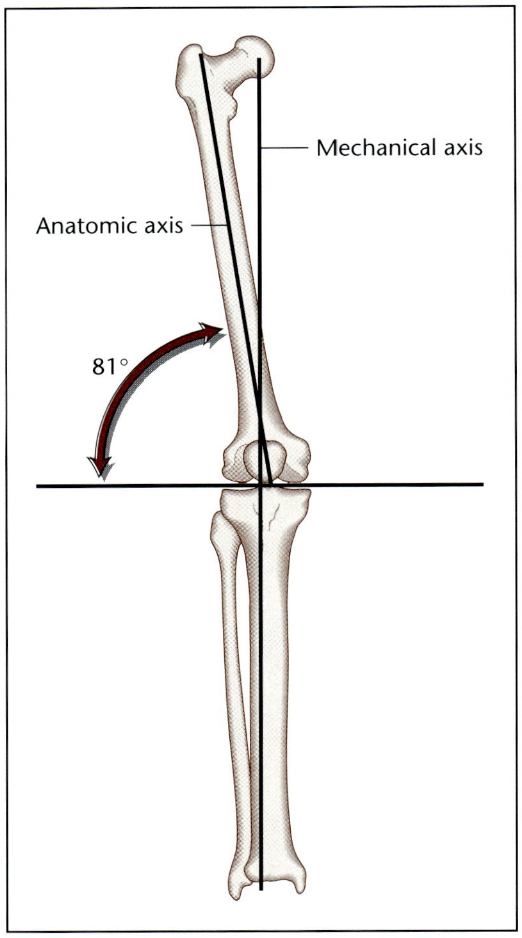

FIGURE 13-5. Anatomic and mechanical axes of the lower extremity. The anatomic axis of the femur subtends an angle of 81° with the plane of the femoral condyles. This relationship is important to restore when fixing supracondylar femur fractures to maintain the proper mechanical axis.

TABLE 13-1. INDICATIONS FOR NONOPERATIVE TREATMENT OF SUPRACONDYLAR FEMUR FRACTURES

Nondisplaced fractures
Impacted extra-articular or intra-articular fractures (less than 2 mm stepoff) in patients with osteopenic bone
Nonambulatory patients (*eg*, spinal cord disorders or severe debilitations)
Underlying medical illness that would put the patient at imminent risk of death if surgery was performed
Inexperience and unfamiliarity with the surgical techniques required

OPERATIVE TREATMENT

Indications

Properly performed operative treatment of displaced supracondylar femur fractures has many advantages compared with nonoperative treatment. Patients are more likely to have an excellent result because of anatomic restoration of articular fractures and limb

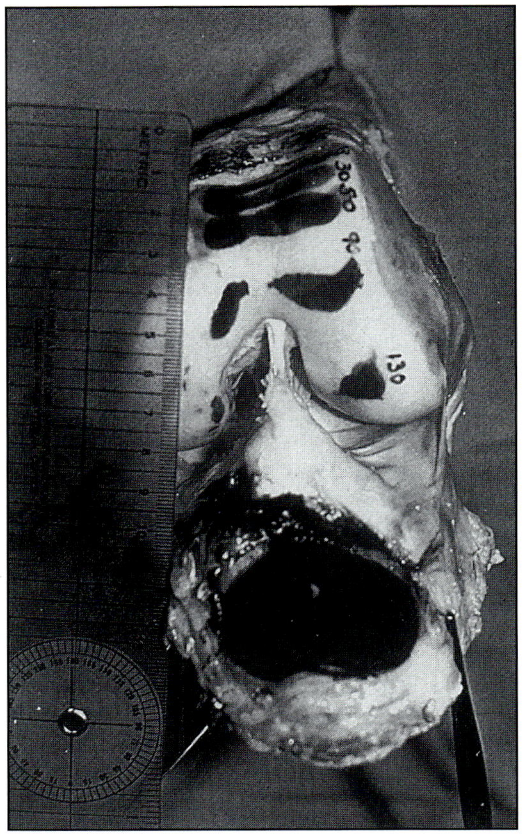

FIGURE 13-6. Photograph of experimental distal femur showing patellofemoral contact areas at different degrees of knee flexion. At 90° knee flexion, the patella has little to no contact at the entry site for a retrograde femoral nail. (*From* Carpenter *et al.* [15]; with permission.)

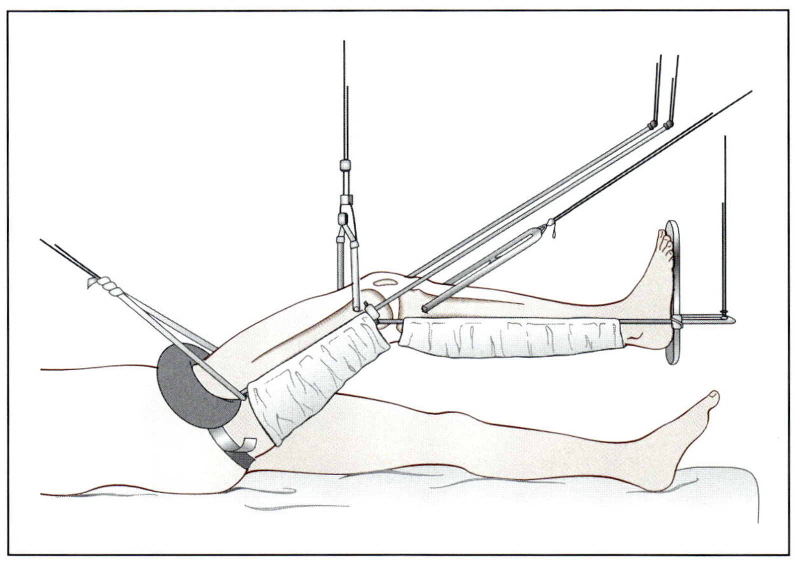

FIGURE 13-7. Example of two-pin traction. The pin in the distal femoral fragment attached to 5 or 10 lb is important to counter the extension force of the gastrocnemius.

alignment, early range of motion of the affected extremity, and improved mobility. Absolute and relative indications for surgical treatment are listed in Table 13-2.

Lateral Approach

For extra-articular fractures or simple intra-articular patterns, a traditional lateral surgical approach (Figure 13-8 and 13-9) is adequate to expose the articular surface for anatomic reduction and the lateral side of the distal femur for application of a plate.

TABLE 13-2. INDICATIONS FOR OPERATIVE TREATMENT OF SUPRACONDYLAR FEMUR FRACTURES

Displaced intra-articular fractures
Extra-articular fractures
Malaligned, displaced fractures
Comminuted (unstable) fractures
Open fractures
Fractures associated with vascular injury
Multiple trauma
Ipsilateral extremity fractures (floating knee)
Pathologic fractures
Obesity (unstable fracture in a cast)
Fracture above a total knee
Relative indications include nondisplaced intra-articular fractures

The patient is placed in a supine position on a radiolucent table and both lower extremities are prepared and draped to allow easy reference to the normal extremity for proper length and alignment. The ipsilateral anterior iliac crest should also be prepared and draped in case an autogenous bone graft is needed. A straight lateral incision is made along the distal thigh extending across the knee joint and ending just lateral to the tibial tubercle. The iliotibial band is incised and the vastus lateralis is elevated above the lateral intermuscular septum. Homan or Bennett retractors can be placed around the femoral shaft for exposure of the bone. Be careful not to unnecessarily strip soft tissue attachments anteriorly, posteriorly, and especially medially. The patella can be subluxated medially to expose the articular surface of the distal femur.

Anterior Approach

For any fracture pattern, but especially those with extensive comminution of the articular surface and medial metaphyseal region, the anterior approach (Figure 13-10) is recommended rather than a patellar tubercle osteotomy. The patient is positioned and draped as mentioned and a straight anterior incision is made from the tibial tubercle proximally as needed. The fracture is exposed through the intermuscular interval between rectus femoris and vastus lateralis. The vastus intermedius and the genu articularis comprise the deep muscular layer and are divided. The incision is extended into a lateral parapatellar arthrotomy. The patella can then be subluxated medially with complete exposure of the entire articular surface of the distal femur and all but the most medial portion of the metaphysis.

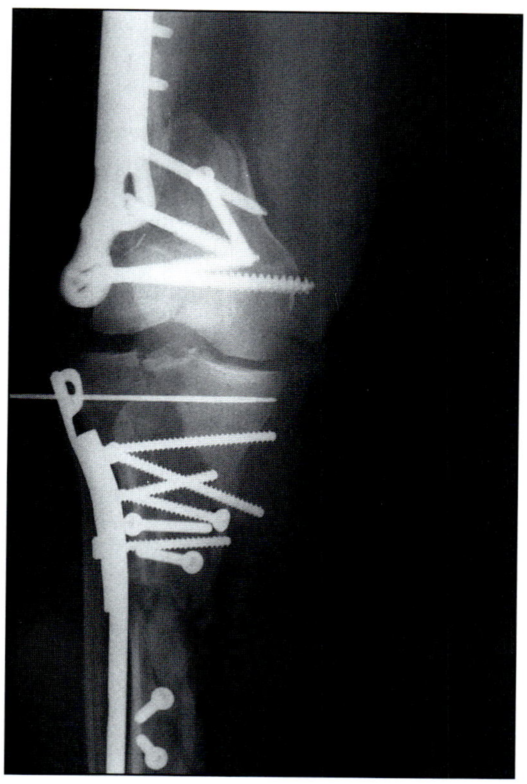

FIGURE 13-8. Intraoperative radiograph of a comminuted ipsilateral distal femoral and proximal tibia fracture treated with buttress plating. The radiograph shows temporary fixation for the tibial plateau fracture while the proper alignment is checked on the radiograph. (*Courtesy of* H. David Moehring, MD.)

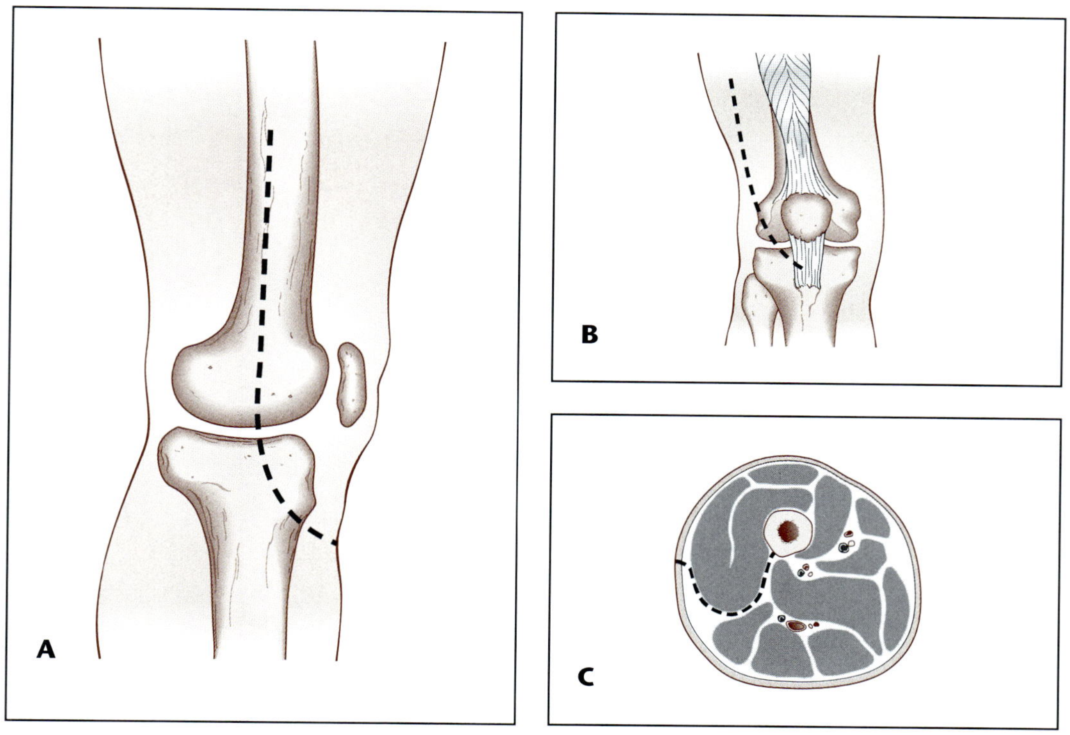

FIGURE 13-9. Lateral approach to the distal femur. **A**, Anterior view; **B**, lateral view; **C**, axial view.

Limited Anterior Approach

For placement of a retrograde intramedullary nail, a 3- to 5-cm incision is centered over the patellar tendon. The tendon can be split or retracted laterally to allow access to the intercondylar notch for placement of the nail (Figure 13-11). The exposure can be extended proximally and converted into a limited "total knee" incision to expose intra-articular fractures. The entry point for the nail is the distal intersection of Blumensaat's line and the distal extent of subchondral bone in the intercondylar notch. This location is directly in line with the femoral medullary canal and corresponds to a point just anterior to the insertion of the posterior cruciate ligament.

Fixed-angle Devices (Blade Plate and Condylar Screw and Side Plate)

The standard for most supracondylar femur fractures is a fixed-angle device: blade plate or condylar screw and side plate (Figure 13-12). A blade plate is a singular implant consisting of a blade (which is inserted into the distal fragment) and an attached plate of variable length placed at a 95° angle to the blade. Use of this implant is technically demanding because it requires proper positioning in three planes (*ie*, sagittal, coronal, axial) to avoid iatrogenic malalignment of the distal fragment. The condylar screw and side plate consist of a compression screw (which is inserted into the distal fragment) and a separate side plate of variable length attached to a barrel placed at a 95° angle to the plate. The lag screw is placed first and aligned properly in the coronal and axial planes. The side plate is placed over the lag screw through the barrel. Depending on the particular implant, the screw must be turned slightly (in a locking system) or the plate rotated to align the plate to the femoral shaft. This degree of freedom in the sagittal plane makes the condylar screw and side plate easier to use. In addition, the large compression screw provides interfragmentary compression across an intercondylar fracture line. The technique manual

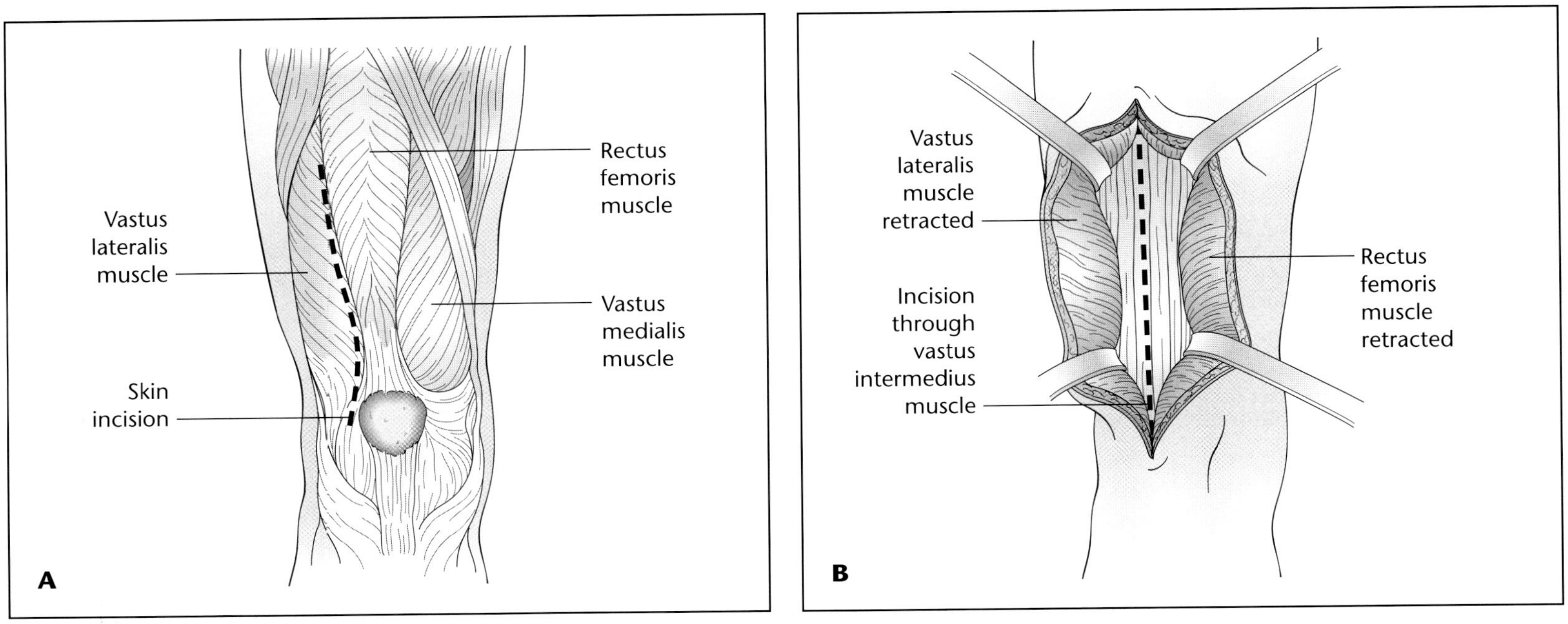

FIGURE 13-10. Anterior approach to the distal femur. **A**, After a straight anterior skin incision, the fascia is incised and the interval between vastus lateralis and rectus femoris is developed. **B**, The underlying vastus intermedius is incised down to the femur and elevated anteriorly and laterally to expose the fracture and distal articular surface.

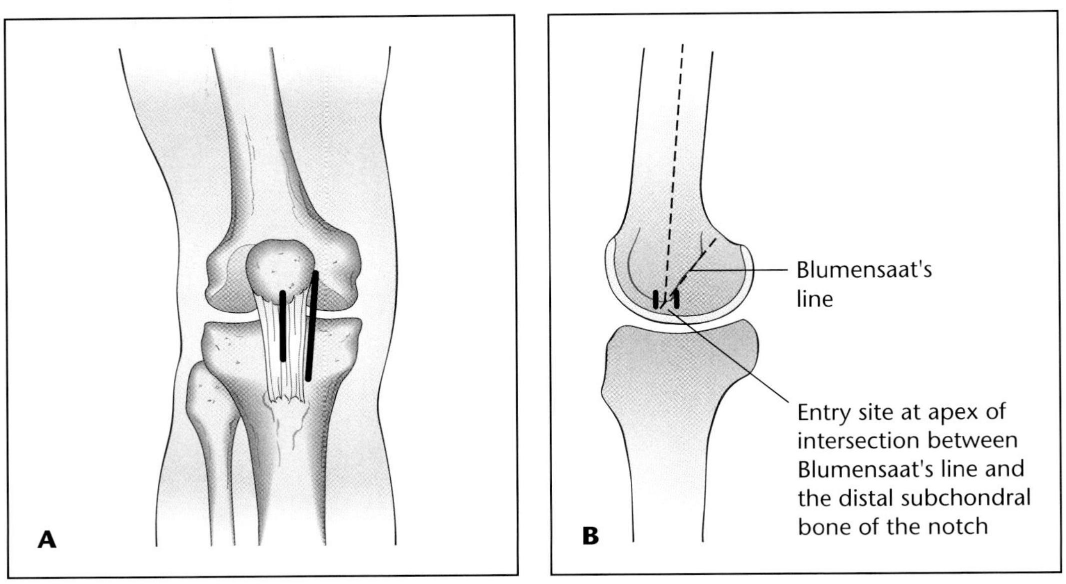

FIGURE 13-11. Limited anterior approach to the distal femur. **A**, Through a small midline skin incision, either the patella tendon can be split in its midline or the knee capsule medial to the tendon can be incised to gain access to the intramedullary nail starting point. **B**, Lateral view of distal femur showing nail entry point at the distal intersection of Blumensaat's line and the distal extent of subchondral bone in the intercondylar notch.

for the chosen implant provides additional details regarding proper insertion. Newer plate designs have an anatomically correct anterior bow to the plate to improve their fit to the femoral shaft. This modification is helpful when long plates are required. The disadvantage of the condylar screw compared with the blade plate is that bone stock must be removed through the reaming process to insert the condylar screw, whereas insertion of a blade plate does not remove any bone. This potential disadvantage of a condylar screw is most problematic if the hardware must be revised.

Regardless of the type of implant, the insertion site and placement of the blade or compression screw must be placed in the proper position within the distal femur for optimal results. The technique for placement of these devices is the same and demands accurate understanding of the anatomy of the distal femur (previously described). The implants must be inserted parallel to the articular surface of the distal femur on an anteroposterior radiograph (coronal plane). A Kirschner (K)-wire can be placed along the distal condylar surfaces for proper orientation (Figure 13-13). A second K-wire should be placed parallel to the inclination of anterior articular surface of the distal femur. Using these wires as reference, a third wire or guide pin is placed parallel to both of these wires within the distal femur. The proper location for the blade or compression screw is a point 1.5 to 2.0 cm proximal to the articular surface of the distal femur centered in the anterior two thirds of the femoral condyle. This insertion site will be directly in line with the femoral shaft.

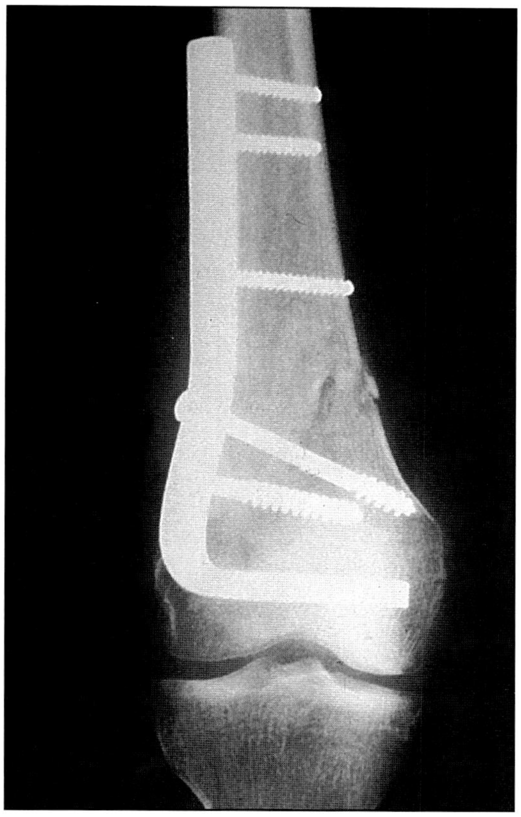

FIGURE 13-12. Example of a blade plate for treatment of an extra-articular supracondylar fracture of the femur. Because blade plates are uniconstruction implants, they must be properly oriented in three planes to ensure anatomic alignment.

Reduction and fixation of intra-articular fracture lines must be completed before a fixed-angle device can be placed. After interfragmentary hematoma and loose, unreconstructable, comminuted articular and bony pieces have been removed, the condyles can be reduced and temporarily held with K-wires. Bone grafting behind depressed articular pieces should be done next. Interfragmentary compression with 6.5- or 4.5-mm lag screws (solid or cannulated) should be placed next for definitive fixation. The surgeon must be aware of the starting point for the blade or condylar screw when inserting these screws so as to avoid interfering with its insertion. Typically, one 6.5-mm screw is placed anteriorly and another posteriorly to the expected fixed-angle device. After the distal fragment has been reconstructed, the fixed-angle device should be inserted using the technique described above. When using a blade plate, the surgeon must remember to align the chisel handle and guide with the femoral shaft. Once the blade or condylar screw has been seated in the distal fragment, the distal fragment should be brought out to length, properly aligned to the femoral shaft. An AO femoral distractor or a tensioner-distractor can be very useful in regaining proper length. The plate can then be temporarily held with a bone-holding clamp while the surgeon checks final alignment and positioning of the distal fragment in relation to the femoral shaft. Commonly, the distal fragment will still be extended by the pull of the two heads of the gastrocnemius. If this is the case, placement of two K-wires from anterior to posterior in the distal fragment can be used as joysticks to rotate the distal piece into proper position. Flexing the knee slightly to relax the gastrocnemius may be helpful as well. When the alignment is satisfactory, the screws can be placed into the proximal fragment for final fixation. Placement of an additional screw or screws into the distal piece is recommended to provide added rotational control, especially in low fractures fixed with a condylar screw and side plate (Figure 13-14).

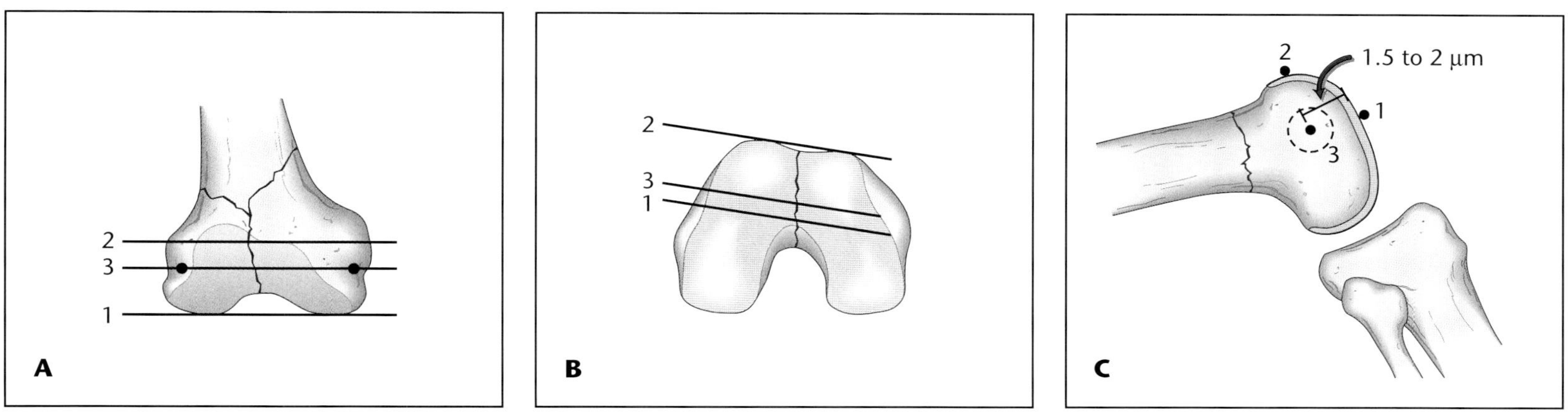

FIGURE 13-13. Proper placement of a fixed angle device requires proper orientation in three planes. Kirschner (K)-wires can be used to help orient the surgeon to the proper position of the implant. **A**, Anteroposterior view; **B**, axial view; **C**, lateral view. K-wire "C" is positioned for a dynamic condylar screw and therefore in the center of the entry site. If a blade plate were used, the K-wire would be positioned slightly distal to this location so that the blade would be positioned properly.

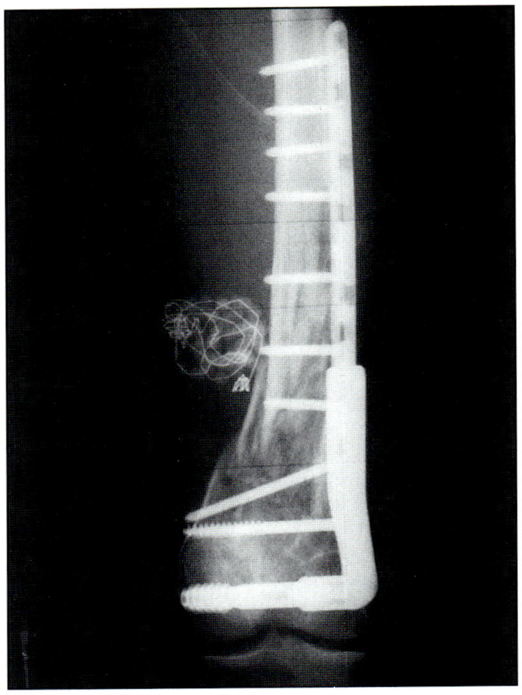

FIGURE 13-14. Anteroposterior view showing placement of a condylar screw and side plate and a string of antibiotic beads. Note the two interfragmentary lag screws placed into the distal fragment to provide additional rotational control.

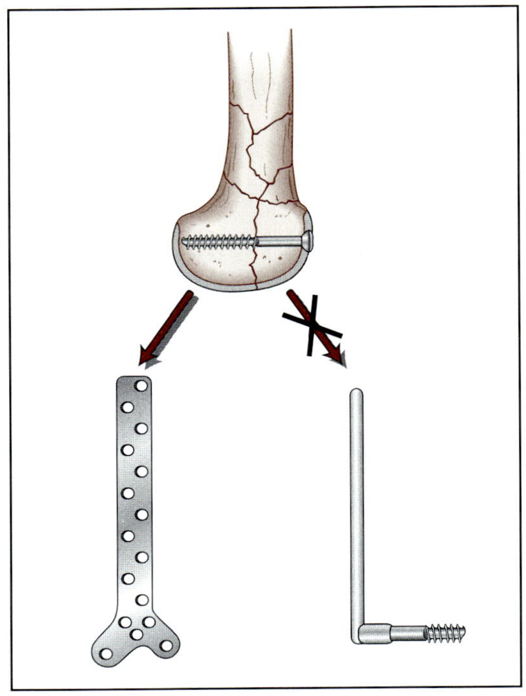

FIGURE 13-15. In supracondylar femur fractures with a coronal fracture line, a fixed-angle device or interlocking nail often cannot be used because the fracture line involves the entry point or the hardware may block the placement of the implant. In these cases, a condylar buttress plate is the implant of choice.

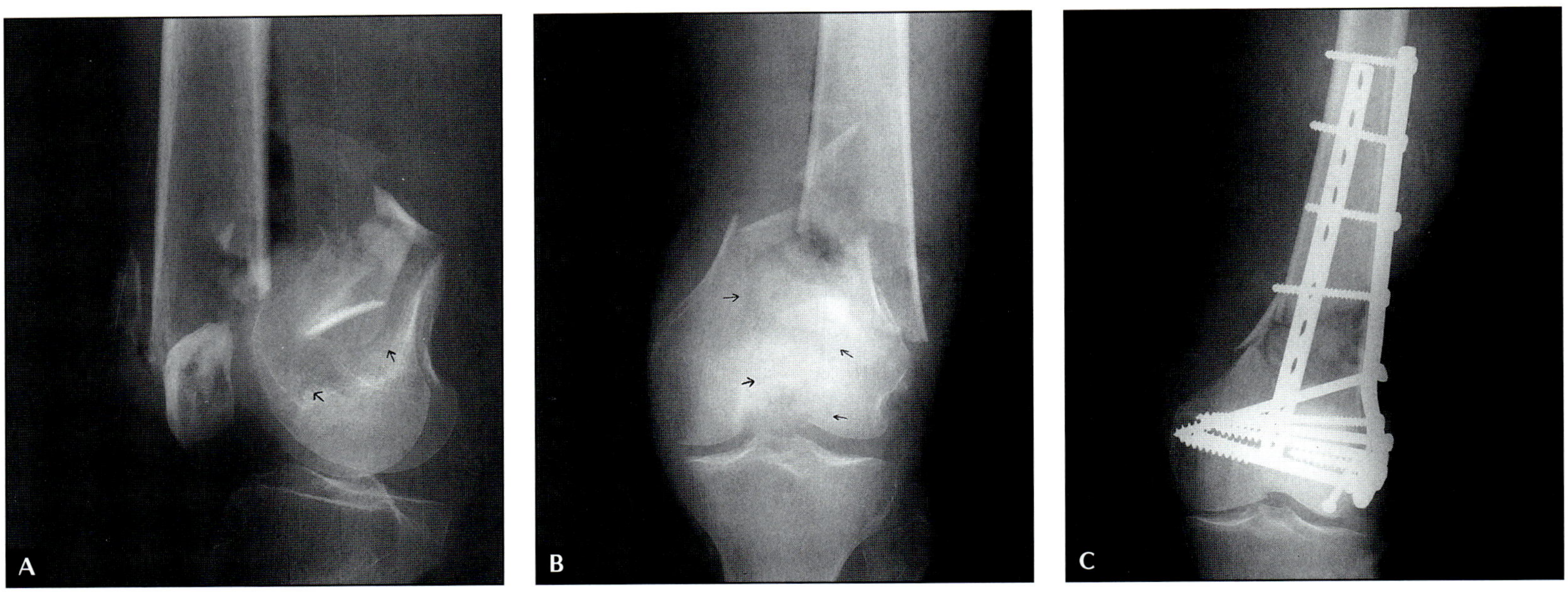

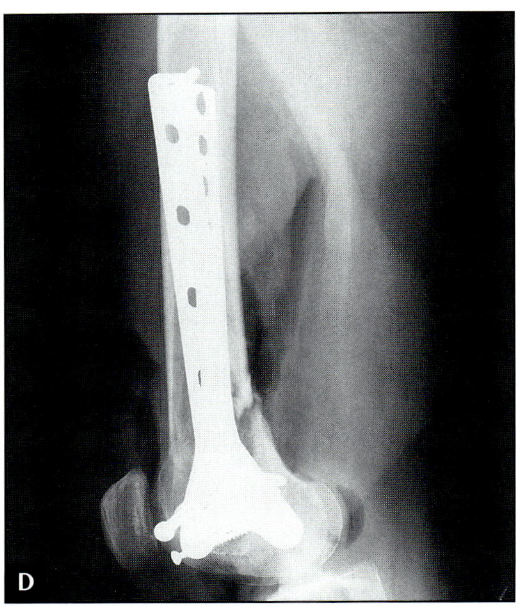

FIGURE 13-16. **A**, Preoperative anteroposterior (AP) radiograph showing supracondylar femur fracture with at least two intra-articular sagittal fracture lines. **B**, Preoperative lateral radiograph showing a subtle coronal fracture line. **C**, Postoperative AP radiograph and **D**, postoperative lateral radiograph showing lateral condylar buttress plate and an intramedullary plate substituting for the comminuted medial cortex.

In highly comminuted fractures in which no medial metaphyseal support is present, supplemental autogenous bone grafting is recommended. In addition, a small medial plate should be added if the primary fixation is tenuous because of poor bone stock or comminution. If an anterior approach was used, no significant additional exposure or stripping is needed to place a second plate anteromedially. If a lateral incision was used, then a separate medial incision should be made with elevation of the vastus medialis off the medial intermuscular septum. In severely osteoporotic bone, polymethylmethacrylate or intramedullary allograft freeze-dried cortical struts can be used to improve screw purchase.

Fixed-angle devices are my treatment of choice for most supracondylar femur fractures. There are, however, some situations in which a condylar buttress plate or a retrograde intramedullary nail are indicated.

Condylar Buttress Plating

Certain fracture patterns, such as the B3, C2, and C3 types, may have fracture lines that traverse the condyles in the coronal plane. Surgeons treating these fractures must be vigilant when looking for such fracture lines because in most instances a fixed-angle device or locking intramedullary nail cannot be used because the proper insertion site is through the plane of the fracture. In addition, the anteroposterior lag screws used to fix these fractures may block passage of the blade or condylar screw in the distal fragment. In these instances, the surgeon should choose a condylar buttress plate (Figure 13-15), which has multiple nonlocking screw holes in the distal aspect of the plate and is typically designed to fit the lateral side of right or left distal femurs. Multiple screw fixation can be obtained in the distal fragment; however, because the screws are traditionally nonlocking, they can toggle at the screw-plate interface and result in an unstable construct, especially if medial cortical comminution is evident.

The choice of surgical approach is based on intra-articular comminution as previously mentioned. The surgical tactic of anatomic reduction and provisional fixation of the distal fragment followed by distal attachment of the plate proceeds as described. After the plate has been attached to the distal fragment and the proper alignment of the condyles has been restored, the plate is secured to the femoral shaft. A femoral distractor can be used to restore length if necessary. When the plate has been secured, the fracture fixation should be tested for stability by putting the knee through a range of motion or by manipulating the condyles. If any micromotion is detected, a medial or anteromedial plate should be placed with as little additional disruption of the soft tissues as possible [18]. Another useful technique for buttressing or substituting for the medial cortex in comminuted or pathologic fractures is intramedullary plating (Figure 13-16) [11]. If medial comminution occurs and the soft tissues have been disrupted either traumatically or iatrogenically, an autogenous bone graft should be added as well.

Condylar buttress-like plates are currently being designed with threaded plate holes that allow screws to fasten tightly to the plate and prevent toggle. Koval *et al.* [19] demonstrated improved stability of a "locked buttress plate" compared with both a standard buttress plate and a blade plate in axial loading. Currently, buttress-like plates are available with better anatomic fit to the distal femur and femoral shaft (*ie*, anterior bow is precontoured into the plate).

Intramedullary Nailing

Before the late 1980s, intramedullary nailing of supracondylar femur fractures with interlocking nails was performed antegrade and usually limited to cases of femoral shaft fractures with an ipsilateral supracondylar fracture [20]. Despite acceptable results with this technique, good control of the distal fragment was at times difficult and led to malalignment. In some cases, the tip of the nail needed to be cut to obtain more distal insertion and interlocking.

In 1986, Green [21] developed an intramedullary nail for the treatment of supracondylar fractures of the femur that was to be inserted retrograde through the intercondylar notch. The advantages of this technique included improved fixation of the distal fragment, centralization of the distal fragment on the femoral shaft, better control against drifting into varus, and indirect reduction of the metaphyseal component of the fracture. Biologic osteosynthesis provided by indirect reduction decreased the need for bone grafting in many cases [22••]. Biomechanically, short retrograde nails, such as the Green–Seligson–Henry (GSH) nail, have similar bending stiffness in flexion and varus compression compared with fixed-angle devices, but are not as stiff in torsion and lateral bending [22••,23].

Indications for retrograde nailing are listed in Table 13-3. Although retrograde nailing can be used in almost any fracture (with the exception of fractures with coronal plane fracture lines), it should not be used routinely until long-term scientific data on knee function become available. I use "long" retrograde intramedullary rods for the vast majority of supracondylar fractures treated with this technique. Most manufacturers now have a retrograde nail for femur fractures, which works very nicely for supracondylar femur fractures and helps keep hospital inventory down. The ideal indication for a retrograde nail is a supracondylar fracture with proximal shaft extension or with severe metaphyseal comminution, whether it is intra-articular or not. In these situations, the advantages of biologic fixation afforded by intramedullary nailing, in addition to smaller incisions and less soft tissue dissection, outweigh the unknown risks of going through the knee. Other excellent indications for a retrograde nail are in a supracondylar fracture in an elderly patient with osteopenic bone (Figure 13-17) or in a patient with an ipsilateral total knee arthroplasty [24–28].

Many authors have reported good results using this technique [22••,29–31] in either extra- or intra-articular fractures and in young as well as elderly patients. In elderly patients with osteopenic bone, poor hold of the distal interlocking screws may be a problem. In these situations, the surgeon should use a washer or a small plate with the interlocking screws (Figure 13-18) and should not allow the patient to begin bearing weight until unequivocal signs of healing are present on follow-up radiographs. In some cases, primary femoral shortening [32] to allow impaction of the fractured surfaces and increase stability before placement of internal fixation may be helpful in situations of osteopenic bone with comminution.

TABLE 13-3. INDICATIONS FOR A RETROGRADE INTRAMEDULLARY NAIL

Supracondylar femur fracture with proximal shaft extension or separate femoral shaft fracture
Floating knee
Severe metaphyseal comminution
Osteopenic or other pathologic bone
Ipsilateral total knee arthroplasty
Relative indications for a retrograde intramedullary nail include any supracondylar femur fracture not associated with a coronal plane fracture line that would compromise interlocking

It is important to remember the anatomic relationships of the supracondylar region and the femoral shaft when reaming. If the distal fragment is reamed exactly perpendicularly to the joint line and not at 5° to 7° valgus to the femoral shaft, then the distal fragment will be fixed in varus.

External Fixation

External fixation has limited applications for the treatment of supracondylar fractures of the femur [33]. In nearly every case in which an external fixator may be indicated (*eg*, fractures requiring vascular repair and severe open fractures), a retrograde intramedullary nail will work just as well and is my treatment of choice between the two options.

External fixators may be useful as temporary fixation ("traveling traction") to stabilize a fracture initially in a patient who is too unstable to undergo definitive fixation. In many cases, the external fixator needs to span the knee joint The external fixator should be converted to either a plate or retrograde intramedullary nail within 2 weeks to decrease the risk of pin-tract infection or colonization infection.

New Trends

Although retrograde intramedullary nails provide biologic fixation, the long-term adverse effects of an intra-articular starting point remain unknown. One possible technique that may provide the benefits of minimal soft-tissue disruption but avoid placing a rod through the knee is percutaneous plating or MIPO [13,14•]. With this technique, indirect fracture reduction is followed by placement of a low-profile plate through a minimal incision at the distal lateral aspect of the knee. The plate is then slid extraperiosteally under the vastus lateralis and secured with percutaneously placed screws. MIPO is currently being used mainly in Europe, but implants for this technique will become increasingly available in the United States within the next few years.

Another trend in treatment of severely comminuted supracondylar femur fractures that are considered nonreconstructable due to severe articular comminution, osteopenia, or both is to forego fruitless attempt at open reduction with internal fixation (ORIF) and proceed directly to primary distal femoral replacement. This is truly a salvage procedure and only recommended in cases in which attempted ORIF will not result in a stable fracture and nonunion with or without debilitating stiffness seems inevitable. A primary distal femoral replacement allows immediate mobilization, weight bearing, and range of motion in the knee in patients who otherwise would be confined to bed or a wheelchair for months.

Postoperative Care

The goal of surgical treatment for these fractures is to provide anatomic reduction and stable fixation to allow early range of

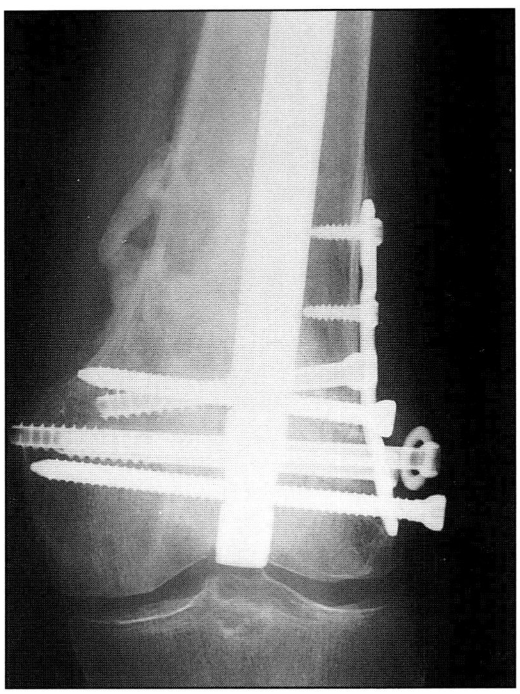

FIGURE 13-17. Postoperative anteroposterior radiograph 3 months after a closed supracondylar femur fracture showing complete union of the fracture. Due to multiple small fracture lines in the lateral methaphyseal region, a small plate was added on the lateral side to serve as an "artificial" cortex to allow more secure fixation of the cross-locking screws. Washers were also used to give better purchase of the lag screws. The patient has 0° to 115° knee range of motion and is fully weight bearing.

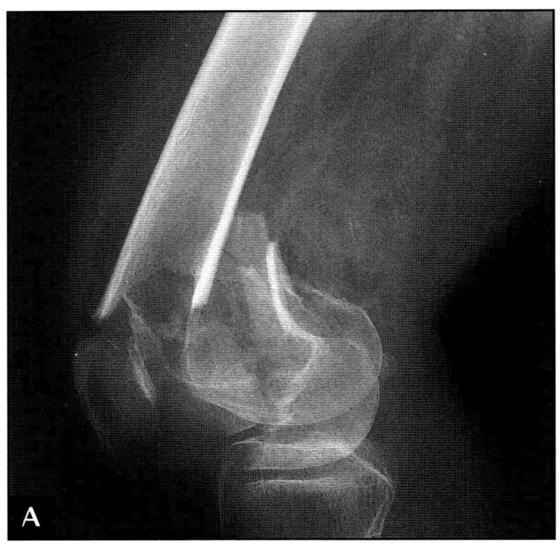

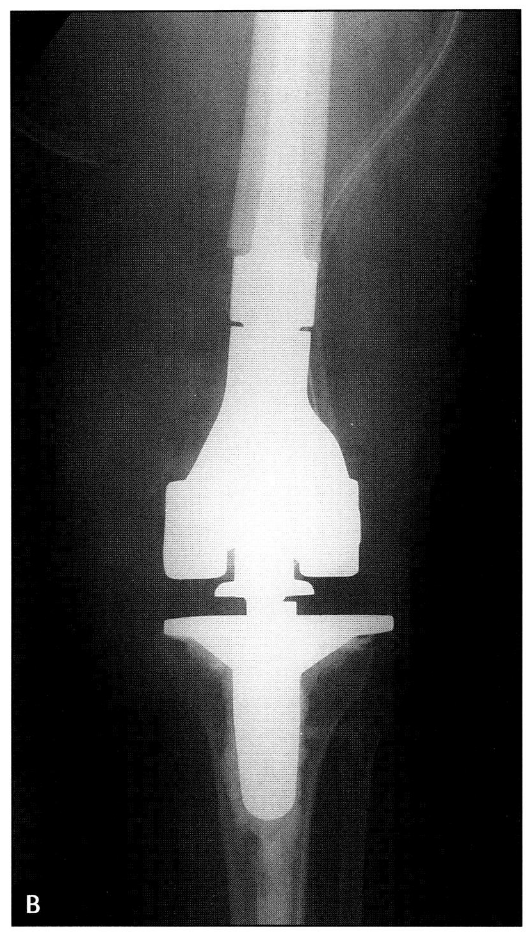

FIGURE 13-18. **A**, Lateral preoperative radiograph of a severely comminuted supracondylar femur fracture in an elderly patient with osteopenia. **B**, Postoperative radiograph showing a distal femoral replacement. (*Courtesy of* H. David Moehring, MD.)

motion and, in some cases, early weight bearing. Therefore, if the fixation is stable, I recommend starting a continuous passive motion (CPM) program within 24 hours of the operation. Although not scientifically proven to make a significant difference in the long term, CPM-treated patients regain their motion faster and are not as apprehensive about moving their knee during physical therapy. I recommend a few sessions of physical therapy to teach the patient and his or her caregivers techniques for passive- and active-assisted range of motion exercise as well as quadriceps-strengthening exercises.

Besides CPM, I recommend bilateral plantar foot pumps for prophylaxis of deep venous thrombosis (DVT) as well as to decrease limb swelling. Debilitated patients who will not be able to move independently should have some type of medical DVT prophylaxis for at least the first 2 weeks after surgery.

For stable extra-articular fractures, I allow cooperative patients to bear weight on a touch-down basis until signs that the fracture is healing are present on follow-up radiographs. This usually takes 4 to 6 weeks. At that time, I allow the patients to bear more weight progressively as tolerated. For intra-articular fractures or highly comminuted fractures in young patients, I also allow touch-down weight bearing, but if the fixation is at all tenuous such as in a patient with osteopenic bone, I will keep the patient from bearing weight until fracture consolidation and, in most cases, I will add a hinged knee brace or cast brace to protect against varus or valgus stresses.

Complications

Because supracondylar fractures of the femur are difficult to treat, complications are not infrequent. Infection, malunion, nonunion, incomplete articular reduction, loss of fixation, knee stiffness, and posttraumatic arthritis are commonly associated with these injuries. In addition, elderly patients have mortality rates approaching 22% [34] within the first year of their fracture.

Although many complications may not be avoidable, adhering to proper decision making, meticulous surgical technique, and diligent postoperative management as discussed in this chapter may prevent many of complications associated with these difficult fractures.

REFERENCES AND RECOMMENDED READING

Recently published papers of particular interest have been highlighted as:
- • Of interest
- •• Of outstanding interest

1. Kolmert L, Wulff K: Epidemiology and treatment of distal femoral fractures in adults. *Acta Orthop Scand* 1982, 53:957–962.
2. Arneson TJ, Melton LJI, Lewallen DG, *et al.*: Epidemiology of diaphyseal and distal femoral fractures in Rochester, Minnesota, 1965–1984. *Clin Orthop Rel Res* 1988, 234:188–194.
3. Wiss DA: Supracondylar and intercondylar fractures of the femur. In *Rockwood and Green's Fractures in Adults*. Edited by Rockwood CA, Green DP, Bucholz RW. Philadelphia: Lippincott-Raven; 1996:1972–1999.
4. Müller ME, Allgöwer M, Schneider R, *et al.*: *Manual of Internal Fixation*. New York: Springer-Verlag; 1979.
5. Neer CSI, Grantham SA, Shelton ML: Supracondylar fracture of the adult femur: a study of one hundred and ten cases. *J Bone Joint Surg* 1967, 49:591–613.
6. Stewart MJ, Sisk D, Wallace SL: Fractures of the distal third of the femur: a comparison of methods of treatment. *J Bone Joint Surg* 1966, 48:784–807.
7. Wenzl H, Casey PA, Hebert P, *et al.*: Die operative Behandlung der distalen Femurfraktur. *AO Bulletin* 1970, VOL:PAGES.
8. Schatzker J, Lambert DC: Supracondylar fractures of the femur. *Clin Orthop Rel Res* 1979, 138:77–83.
9. Schatzker J, Horne G, Waddell J: The Toronto experience with the supracondylar fracture of the femur, 1966–1972. *Injury* 1975, 6:113–128.
10. Giles JB, DeLee JC, Heckman JD, *et al.*: Supracondylar–intercondylar fractures of the femur treated with a supracondylar plate and lag screw. *J Bone Joint Surg* 1982, 64:864–870.
11. Mast J, Jakob R, Ganz R: *Planning and Reduction Technique in Fracture Surgery* edn 1. Berlin: Springer-Verlag; 1989.
12. Ostrum RF, Geel C: Indirect reduction and internal fixation of supracondylar femur fractures without bone graft. *J Orthop Trauma* 1995, 9:278–283.
13. Krettek C, Miclau T, Schandelmaier P, *et al.*: *Minimally Invasive Plate Osteosynthesis (MIPO) for Distal Femoral Fractures Using a Parapatellar Approach or a Percutaneous Approach and Retrograde Plate Placement*. Vancouver: Orthopaedic Trauma Association; 1998.
14.• Weller S, Hontzsch D, Frigg R: Epiperiostal, percutaneous plate osteosynthesis: a new minimally invasive technique with reference to "biological osteosynthesis." *Unfallchirurg* 1998, 101:115–121.

This is a description of the "percutaneous" plating technique and its theoretical benefits.

15. Carpenter JE, Kasman R, Matthews LS: Fractures of the patella. *Instructional Course Lectures* vol 43. Edited by Heckman JD. Rosemont, IL: The American Academy of Orthopedic Surgeons; 1994: 1550–1552.
16. Morgan E, Ostrum RF, DiCicco J, *et al.*: *Patello-Femoral Contact Forces with a Retrograde Femoral Intramedullary Nail*. Vancouver: Orthopaedic Trauma Association; 1998.
17. Mooney V, Nickel VL, Harvey JP, *et al.*: Cast-brace treatment for fractures of the distal part of the femur. *J Bone Joint Surg* 1970, 52:1563–1578.
18. Sanders R, Swiontkowski M, Rosen H, *et al.*: Double-plating of comminuted, unstable fractures of the distal part of the femur. *J Bone Joint Surg* 1991, 73:341–346.
19. Koval KJ, Hoehl JJ, Kummer FJ, *et al.*: Distal femoral fixation: a biomechanical comparison of the standard condylar buttress plate, a locked buttress plate, and the 95-degree blade plate. *J Orthop Trauma* 1997, 11:521–524.
20. Butler MS, Brumback RJ, Ellison TS, *et al.*: Interlocking intramedullary nailing for ipsilateral fractures of the femoral shaft and distal part of the femur. *J Bone Joint Surg* 1991, 73:1492–1502.
21. Green SA: Distal intramedullary fixation of supracondylar fractures of the femur. *Tech Orthop* 1988, 3:71–76.
22.•• Gellman RE, Paiement GD, Green HD, *et al.*: Treatment of supracondylar femoral fractures with a retrograde intramedullary nail. *Clin Orthop Rel Res* 1996, 332:90–97.

This is a small series of patients with open and closed supracondylar femur fractures treated with a retrograde intramedullary nail. The advantages of this technique are well outlined. The authors reported comparable functional outcomes to fixed angle devices, but with less soft tissue dissection.

23. Firoozbakhsh K, Behzadi K, DeCoster TA, *et al.*: Mechanics of retrograde nail versus plate fixation for supracondylar femur fractures. *J Orthop Trauma* 1995, 9:152–157.
24. David SM, Harrow ME, Peindl RD, *et al.*: Comparative biomechanical analysis of supracondylar femur fracture fixation: locked intramedullary nail versus 95-degree angled plate. *J Orthop Trauma* 1997, 11:344–350.

25. Rolston LR, Christ DJ, Halpern A, *et al.*: Treatment of supracondylar fractures of the femur proximal to a total knee arthroplasty: a report of four cases. *J Bone Joint Surg* 1995, 77:924–931.
26. Murrell GA, Nunley JA: Interlocked supracondylar intramedullary nails for supracondylar fractures after total knee arthroplasty: a new treatment method. *J Arthroplasty* 1995, 10:37–42.
27. Henry SL: Management of supracondylar fractures proximal to total knee arthroplasty with the GSH supracondylar nail. *Contemp Orthop* 1995, 31:231–238.
28. Smith WJ, Martin SL, Mabrey JD: Use of a supracondylar nail for treatment of a supracondylar fracture of the femur following total knee arthroplasty. *J Arthroplasty* 1996, 11:210–213.
29. Helfet DL, Lorich DG: Retrograde intramedullary nailing of supracondylar femoral fractures. *Clin Orthop Rel Res* 1998, 350:80–84.
30. Janzing HM, Vaes F, Van Damme G, *et al.*: Treatment of distal femoral fractures in the elderly: results with the retrograde intramedullary supracondylar nail. *Unfallchirurgie* 1998, 24:55–59.
31. Danziger MB, Caucci D, Zecher SB, *et al.*: Treatment of intercondylar and supracondylar distal femur fractures using the GSH supracondylar nail. *Am J Orthop* 1995, VOL:684–690.
32. Blatter G, Konig H, Janssen M, *et al.*: Primary femoral shortening osteosynthesis in the management of comminuted supracondylar femoral fractures. *Arch Orthop Traum Surg* 1994, 113:134–137.
33. Marsh JL, Jansen H, Yoong HK, *et al.*: Supracondylar fractures of the femur treated by external fixation. *J Orthop Trauma* 1997, 11:405–410.
34. Karpman RR, Del Mar NB: Supracondylar femoral fractures in the frail elderly. *Clin Orthop Rel Res* 1995, 316:21–24.

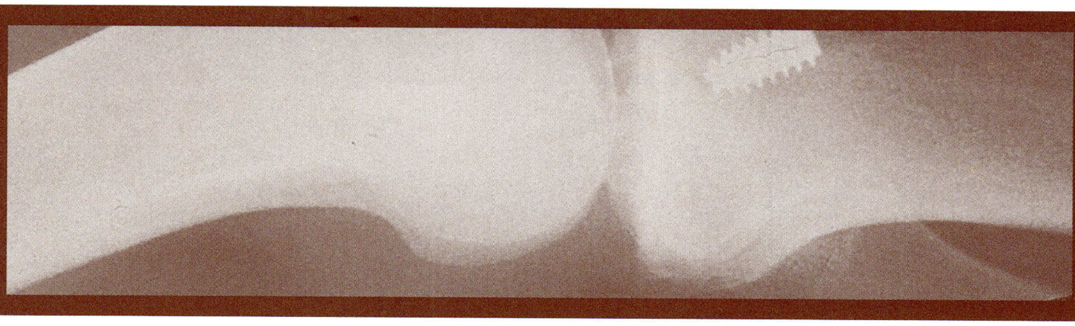

14

Patella Fractures

William I. Sterett
John M. Wright

CLASSIFICATION AND MECHANISM

There are three principal patella fracture patterns: 1) transverse, 2) vertical (longitudinal), and 3) stellate (comminuted). Polar fractures are specific forms of transverse fractures. Virtually all patella fractures (except inferior pole avulsions) are intra-articular fractures. Patella fracture patterns are a function of injury mechanism. Tensile forces characteristically produce transverse fractures. Stellate and longitudinal fractures typically stem from direct trauma.

Patella stress fractures are a relatively rare (or perhaps underdiagnosed) source of anterior knee pain [1,2]. The patella's cyclic loading pattern renders it susceptible to stress fracture. This sesamoid bone (the largest in the body) is subject to a complex combination of tension and bending forces. Tension forces are focused at the anterior patellar cortex; thus, this is the characteristic point of initiation of patella stress fractures. Because of the loading patterns responsible for this injury, most patella stress fractures have a transverse pattern.

Although some patellar stress fractures present with acute displacement, most are incomplete at the time of presentation and never propagate to completion [3]. In the absence of displacement, a high index of suspicion is necessary to avoid misdiagnosis.

CLINICAL AND RADIOGRAPHIC EVALUATION

Prepatellar skin is frequently lacerated when patella fractures are produced by direct trauma to the anterior knee. In these circumstances, the skin should be meticulously evaluated to rule out the presence of an open fracture. When doubt persists regarding potential communication between the fracture and broken skin, we recommend saline insufflation of the joint. In the presence of residual uncertainty, the fracture should be treated as open.

Because of the patella's subcutaneous position, a gap is characteristically readily palpable in cases of displaced fractures. However, minimally displaced (or nondisplaced) patella fractures present in a more subtle manner. Anterior knee tenderness is extremely nonspecific after direct trauma. Furthermore, because of continuity of the retinaculum, the presence of a displaced transverse patella fracture does not preclude the ability to perform a straight leg raise.

Accurate diagnosis of minimally displaced (and nondisplaced) fractures requires appropriate radiographs. In particular, nondisplaced longitudinal fractures are commonly overlooked unless a proper Merchant view is obtained. Scintigraphy is a useful modality when an occult stress fracture is suspected [4,5]. Magnetic resonance imaging (MRI) is valuable for detecting associated lesions, such as osteochondral fractures, ligament damage, chondral flaps, and sleeve fractures [5–7].

Although patella fractures are typically isolated injuries, a thorough knee examination should always be performed. A recent study reported that 5% of patella fractures are associated with significant knee ligament disruptions [8]. A high index of suspicion should be maintained about associated ligamentous injury, particularly in the presence of features allied with high-energy trauma (such as extensive comminution or open fractures).

NONOPERATIVE TREATMENT

Minimally Displaced Fractures

Nonoperative treatment is indicated for most nondisplaced and minimally displaced patella fractures. We define "minimal displacement" as 2 mm or less of articular incongruity and 3 mm or less of interfragmentary displacement. Our preferred method of managing these injuries consists of 6 weeks of weight bearing as tolerated in a hinged knee brace locked in full extension. After 3 weeks, we begin unlocking the brace for gentle passive range of motion exercises with flexion limited to 90°. No active knee motion is permitted until 6 weeks. The brace is discarded at 6 weeks, provided that radiographic confirmation of fracture union is available. Among compliant individuals, we have not encountered delayed fracture displacement in our experience with this form of management. Noncompliant patients are treated in a cylinder cast for 6 weeks.

Displaced Fractures

Although operative treatment is warranted for most displaced fractures, we advocate nonoperative management under select circumstances. Our indications for nonoperative management of displaced patella fractures include nonambulatory (or minimally ambulatory) baseline functional status, inability (or unwillingness) to comply with our postoperative protocol, and medical frailty.

Pritchett [9] has recently reported on the outcomes following "benign neglect" of widely displaced patella fractures in a group of similarly selected patients. He did not use immobilization in this cohort. At 2-year follow-up, none of his 12 surviving patients had severe pain. Only 3 of these patients subsequently developed severe activity limitation attributable to their patella fracture. Fracture union occurred in none of these cases, and the mean resultant extension lag was 28°. These patients all experienced a marked loss of extensor mechanism strength. Extension bracing can be prescribed to compensate for functionally limiting extensor mechanism weakness. Although this form of treatment curtails costs and avoids potential surgical complications, superior functional results are achieved with surgical intervention.

OPERATIVE TREATMENT

The primary goals of patellar fracture management are restoration and maintenance of extensor mechanism continuity and restitution of patellofemoral articular congruity. Operative stabilization offers the additional benefit of permitting early joint mobilization.

General indications for open reduction and internal fixation of patella fractures are more than 2 mm of articular incongruity or more than 3 mm of interfragmentary displacement. However, in physiologically young, active individuals, we prefer to restore anatomic articular congruity. Furthermore, in this population, we favor immediate establishment of fracture stability so that an aggressive rehabilitation program can be initiated.

TRANSVERSE FRACTURES

Several forms of internal fixation continue to have wide acceptance, including interfragmentary screws, tension-band wiring, modified AO tension-band wiring over parallel Kirschner (K)-wires, and cannulated screws plus tension-band wiring (Figure 14-1) [10]. Simple cerclage wiring has fallen into relative disfavor; however, no single method of internal fixation has garnered universal appeal. Our current preferred form of internal fixation consists of figure-eight tension-band wiring through paired parallel 4.5-mm cannulated compression screws.

Weber *et al.* [11] previously documented that transosseous (Magnusson) wires achieve superior fixation strength compared with cerclage wiring. They also reported that modified AO tension-band wiring around transosseous K-wires achieves superior fixation strength compared with transosseous wiring alone (Figure 14-2) [12].

Recent biomechanical research has suggested that tension-band wiring through parallel cannulated compression screws provides optimal stability. Specifically, in Carpenter *et al.*'s [10] cadaveric transverse patella fracture model, tension-band wiring through parallel cannulated compression screws failed at higher loads (mean = 732 N) in comparison with modified AO tension-band wiring (mean = 395 N) and compression screws alone (mean = 554 N).

An additional drawback of modified AO tension-band wiring is that it is associated with a high incidence of irritation to local soft tissues [13–16]. In this technique, the ends of the K-wires are intentionally left proud at the superior and inferior poles of the patella to serve as anchoring posts for the tension-band wire. Protrusion of the ends of the transosseous K-wires (or subsequent K-wire migration) is a common source of persistent postoperative discomfort (Figure 14-3). Reoperation for hardware removal is frequently required [15,17]. The relatively low profile of the cannulated screw plus figure-eight tension-band construct decreases incidence of irritation of peripatellar soft tissues and thus reduces the need for hardware removal.

Berg [13] has recently reported satisfactory clinical results in a series of 10 displaced transverse patella fractures treated with tension-band wiring through parallel cannulated compression screws. This construct permitted immediate passive range of motion with no associated loss of reduction (even among elderly patients with significant osteopenia). The average time to clinical union in this series was 8 weeks. The 70% good or excellent outcomes (rated by the Hospital for Special Surgery [HSS] knee score) compare favorably with previously published series of operatively managed patella fractures [18,19].

Authors' Preferred Technique for Transverse Fractures

Open Reduction and Internal Fixation

For displaced transverse fractures, the patella is exposed through a longitudinal midline incision. The joint is copiously irrigated, and the articular surfaces of the patellofemoral joint are carefully inspected. Anatomic reduction is achieved, and provisional reduction is maintained by a large tenaculum clamp with its tips at the midline of the superior and inferior poles of the patella. The articular surface is directly palpated to confirm that anatomic articular congruity has been achieved. If the size of the retinacular defect is not large enough to permit digital access to the patellar articular surface, a 2-cm longitudinal lateral parapatellar arthrotomy is created.

Two cannulated 4.5-mm partially threaded cancellous screws are inserted over parallel longitudinal guide wires (one wire on either side of the tenaculum clamp tips). A figure-eight tension-band construct is created by threading 1.25-mm wire through the two screw shafts. To facilitate tension-band wire passage into the cannulae, the guide wires are left within the screw shafts until the surgeon is prepared to insert the tension-band wire. To maximize interfragmentary compression and minimize irritation to adjacent soft tissues, the heads of the screws must be countersunk. The two limbs of the tension band are tightened anteriorly. In a further effort to minimize potential soft tissue irritation, we prefer to position the twisted portions of the wire limbs at the superior or inferior margins of the patella (rather than directly over the anterior surface of the patella). The free (twisted) ends of the wire are bent posteriorly to ensure that they will not protrude.

It is crucial to exclude intervening soft tissue from the tension-band construct. Interposed soft tissue can interfere with wire ten-

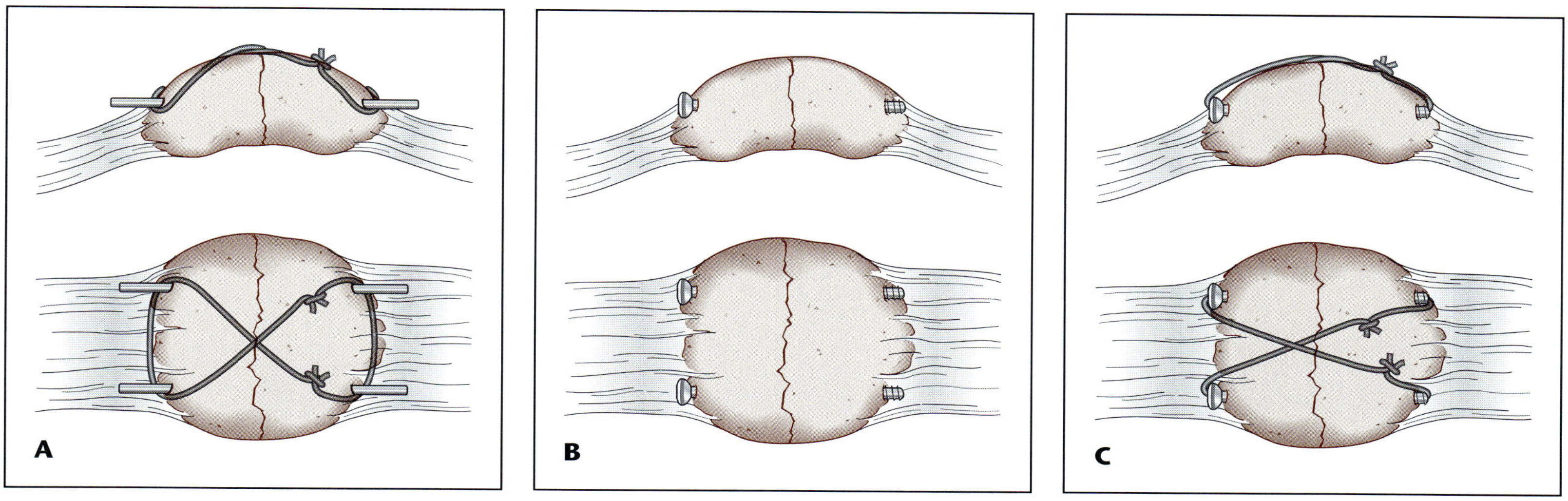

Figure 14-1. Popular methods for fixation of transverse patella fractures. **A**, Modified AO tension-band technique. **B**, Interfragmentary compression screws. **C**, Cannulated interfragmentary compression screws plus tension-band wire. (*Adapted from* Carpenter *et al.* [10].)

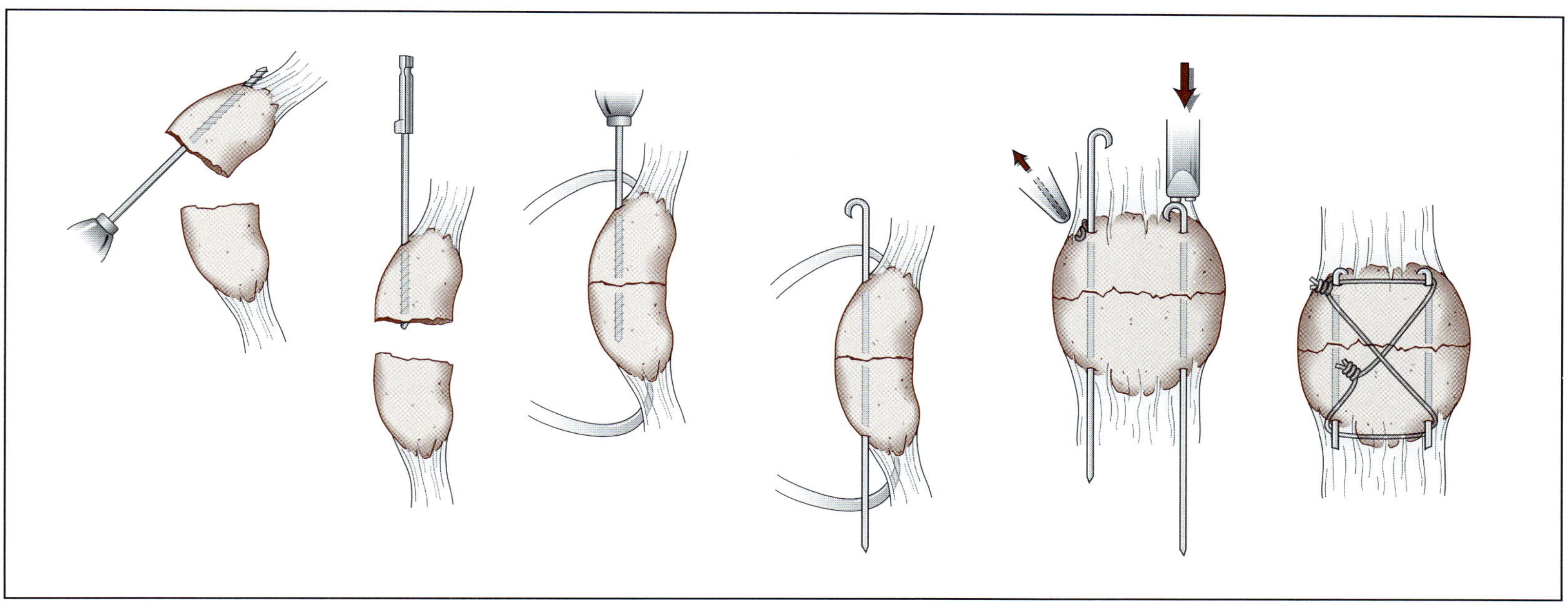

Figure 14-2. Modified AO tension band technique. (*Adapted from* Müller *et al.* [12].)

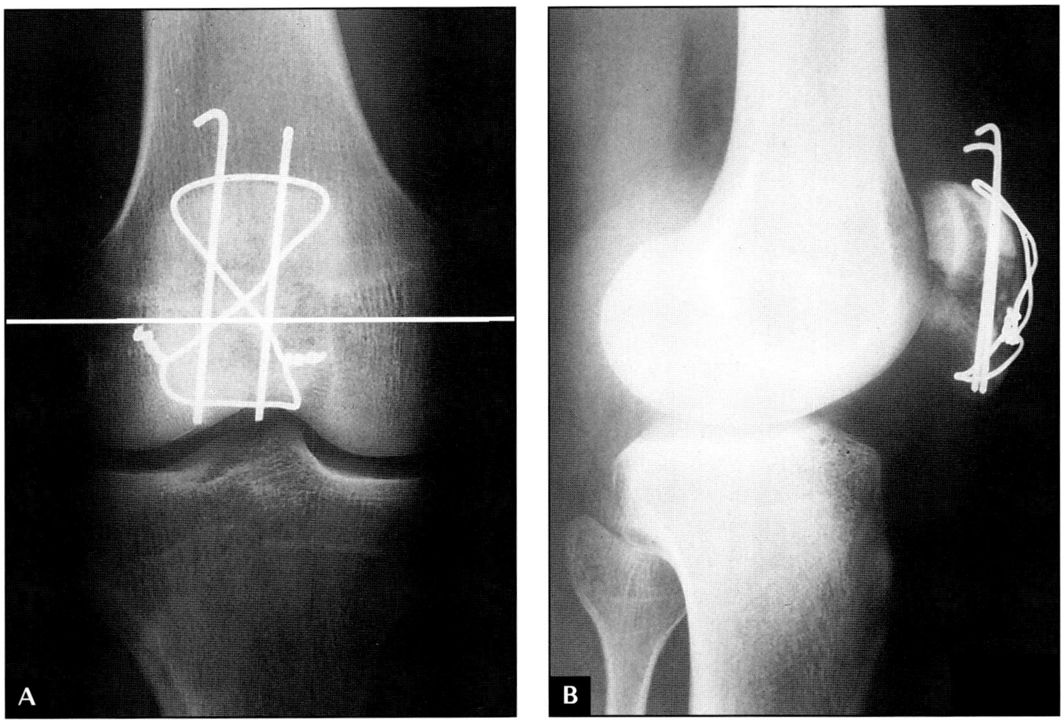

FIGURE 14-3. Hardware prominence following internal fixation of a transverse patella fracture with the modified AO tension-band technique. **A**, Anteroposterior radiograph. **B**, Lateral radiograph.

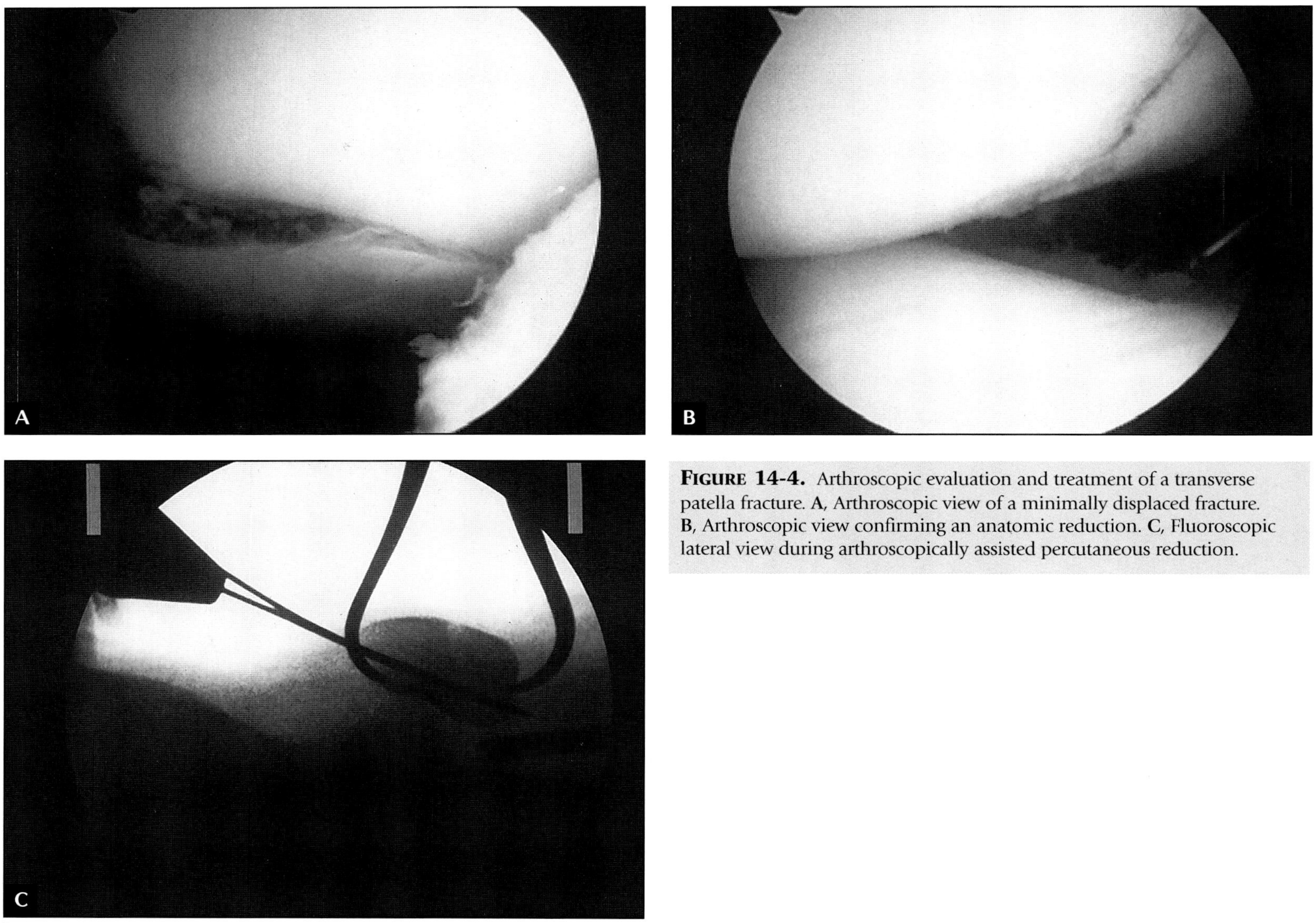

FIGURE 14-4. Arthroscopic evaluation and treatment of a transverse patella fracture. **A**, Arthroscopic view of a minimally displaced fracture. **B**, Arthroscopic view confirming an anatomic reduction. **C**, Fluoroscopic lateral view during arthroscopically assisted percutaneous reduction.

sioning. Furthermore, with cyclic loading, interposed soft tissue can atrophy and, hence, precipitate loosening of the construct [11,15].

Before wound closure, the knee is put through a full range of motion to confirm adequate rigidity of the construct. Motion limitations are determined at this point to guide postoperative rehabilitation. We prefer to repair associated retinacular tears with #0 resorbable suture. Retinacular repair has been shown to augment the stability of transverse patellar fracture fixation [11].

Arthroscopically Assisted Fixation

Nondisplaced and minimally displaced transverse fractures are amenable to a less invasive, arthroscopically assisted approach. The lack of significant retinacular injury in these cases renders arthroscopy feasible. Specifically, in the absence of retinacular disruption, fluid extravasation is less of a concern. Arthroscopy permits evacuation of the intra-articular hematoma, detection of occult osteochondral lesions, removal of intra-articular loose bodies, and evaluation of articular congruity (Figure 14-4). Furthermore, arthroscopy accomplishes these goals without surgical disruption of retinacular continuity.

A large tenaculum clamp is applied percutaneously across the fracture to achieve and maintain anatomic reduction. Arthroscopic visualization is used to confirm this reduction. Loose fragments of comminuted articular surface can be arthroscopically débrided. Dual parallel longitudinal cannulated compression screws can be inserted either percutaneously (if no tension band is desired) or through a limited anterior longitudinal incision (if a tension band is to be added). We believe that two 4.5-mm compression screws alone are sufficient to stabilize nondisplaced (and minimally displaced) fractures because the intact retinaculum offers supplemental stability. Hence, these fractures are amenable to the arthroscopically assisted percutaneous approach. In the presence of significant osteopenia, we prefer to augment the compression screws with a figure-eight tension band. Hence, we do not employ a minimally invasive approach in the osteopenic population.

Postoperative Rehabilitation

Following open reduction and internal fixation of transverse fractures, patients are allowed to bear weight as tolerated in a hinged knee brace locked in full extension. The brace is unlocked on a daily basis for passive range of motion within the limits established in the operating room. Quadriceps isometric exercises are initiated after 2 weeks and active range-of-motion exercises are commenced after 6 weeks (provided that no radiographic evidence of fracture union is found).

When no tension band is used, then passive range-of-motion is limited to 0° to 30° of flexion for the first 2 weeks; 0° to 60° of flexion for weeks 3 and 4; 0° to 90° degrees of flexion for weeks 5 and 6; and unrestricted passive motion thereafter. Active strengthening is commenced after full motion has been achieved.

Biodegradable Fixation

Although biodegradable implants have yet to gain significant popularity for patellar fixation, they offer the theoretical advantage of avoiding the potential need for a secondary operation to remove painful hardware. Literature supporting this mode of fixation is scant, but two recent investigations have reported satisfactory clinical results [20,21]. In a 2-year follow-up of 38 transverse fractures, Chen *et al.* [20] found no clinical or radiographic differences between biodegradable and metallic tension-band fixation. Likewise, Juutilainen *et al.* [21] found no difference in a prospective, randomized comparison between biodegradable and metallic tension-band wiring. Although these early results are encouraging, we have no personal experience with biodegradable forms of patellar fixation. Furthermore, we have found that the cannulated screw plus tension-band wire form of fixation is associated with a markedly lower incidence of peripatellar soft tissue irritation than the modified AO tension-band technique. Thus, the putative benefit of resorbable implants (*eg*, decreased irritation of adjacent soft tissues) is not as alluring.

Fixation with Nonabsorbable Suture

Another acceptable approach to reduce the high incidence of painful hardware associated with modified AO tension-band wiring is to substitute a #5 nonabsorbable, braided polyester suture for the stainless steel wire. Successful use of #5 nonabsorbable suture for patellar fracture fixation has recently been documented [22].

Cable Fixation

Scilaris *et al.* [23] recently performed a biomechanical analysis of the modified AO tension-band technique in a cadaver model. They demonstrated that braided cable provides superior stability in cyclic loading than monofilament wire. These findings suggest that surgeons who prefer to use the modified AO tension-band technique for transverse fracture fixation should consider using braided cable. A disadvantage of braided cable is its relatively high cost. Unfortunately, this study did not compare the fatigue properties of braided cable or monofilament wire with the #5 nonabsorbable suture method.

POLAR FRACTURES

Authors' Preferred Technique

Conceptually, polar fractures represent a subdivision of transverse fractures. Pragmatically, however, this variety of transverse fracture requires a distinct operative approach. Polar fragments are typically too small to accept dual parallel screws. For this reason, our preferred approach to standard transverse patella fractures is not applicable to polar lesions.

Most polar fractures are essentially osseous avulsion fractures. Inferior pole avulsion fractures (patellar ligament avulsions) are more common than superior pole avulsion fractures (quadriceps tendon avulsions), but our treatment algorithm is similar for lesions of both poles.

If the polar fragment is of sufficient size to accept a single screw, we prefer to apply the hybrid construct advocated by the AO group (Figure 14-5) [12]. Specifically, we augment a single, non-cannulated, 4.0-mm partially threaded compression screw with a traditional anterior tension-band wire. The screw prevents the polar fragment from rotating into the trochlea.

If the polar fragment is comminuted or too small to accept a screw, then we opt to resect the fragment and reattach the respective soft tissue element (patellar ligament for inferior polar fractures or quadriceps tendon for superior polar fractures) to the patellar remnant. The patellar ligament (or quadriceps tendon) is grasped with a pair of adjacent double-armed #5 nonresorbable modified Bunnell stitches. Both limbs of each of the Bunnell stitches are passed simultaneously to avoid inadvertent needle damage to a previously passed crossing stitch. The #5 stitches are subsequently delivered through three parallel longitudinal patellar drill holes (with the assistance of straight needles) and tied at the opposite patellar pole (Figure 14-6). After partial resection of the distal pole, it is critical to reattach the patella tendon to the *anterior* aspect of the residual patella [24].

Although some authorities advocate augmentation of inferior pole avulsion repairs with a figure-eight tension-band wire between the residual patella and the tibial tubercle (Figure 14-7), we have not experienced difficulties with our preferred technique. Furthermore, the supplemental wire frequently becomes a source of residual irritation and precipitates a secondary procedure for hardware

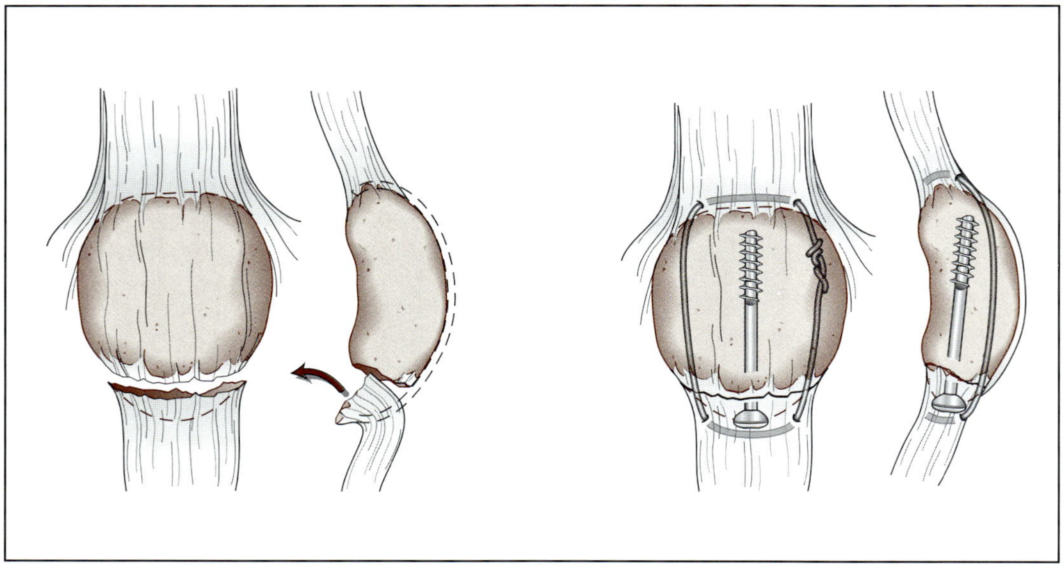

FIGURE 14-5. AO technique for internal fixation of inferior pole avulsion fractures. (*Adapted from* Müller *et al.* [12].)

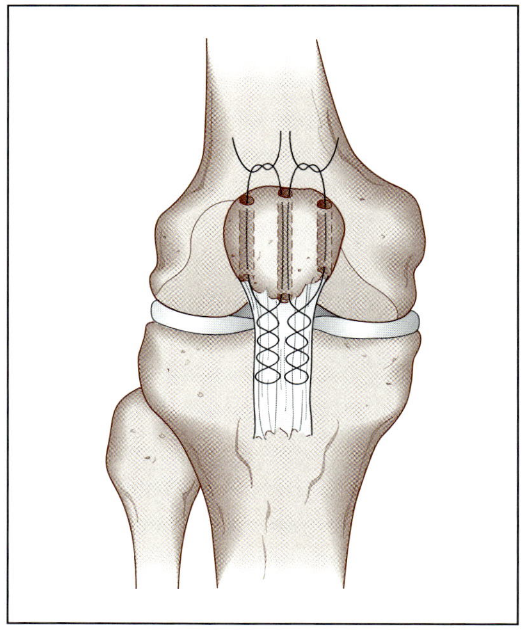

FIGURE 14-6. Technique for repair of patellar ligament avulsion from inferior pole of patella. Dual #5 nonabsorbable modified sutures are passed through three parallel drill holes and secured at the superior pole of the patella.

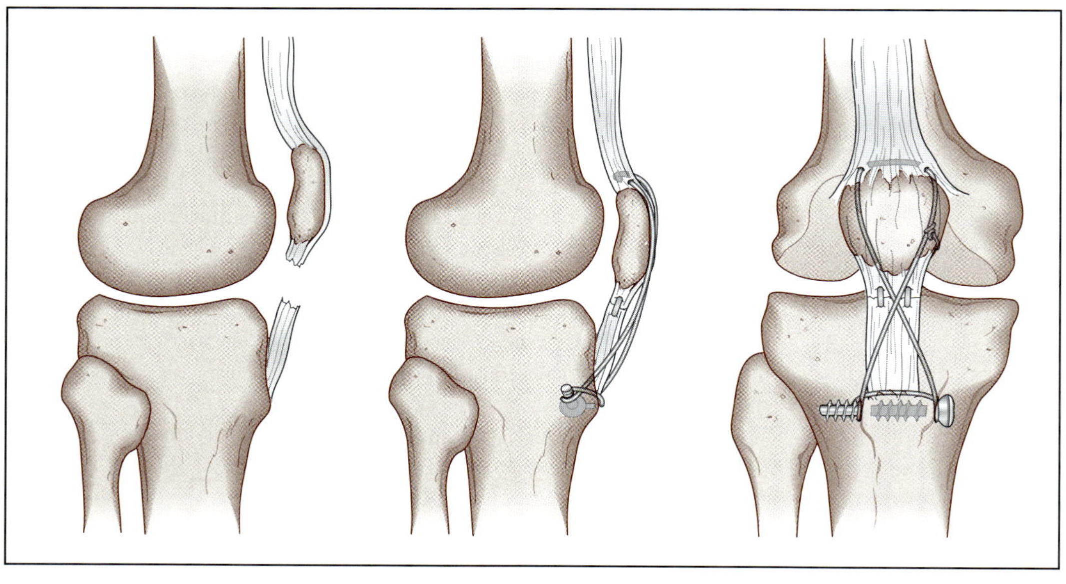

FIGURE 14-7. Augmentation of repair of patellar tendon avulsion with tension band wire.

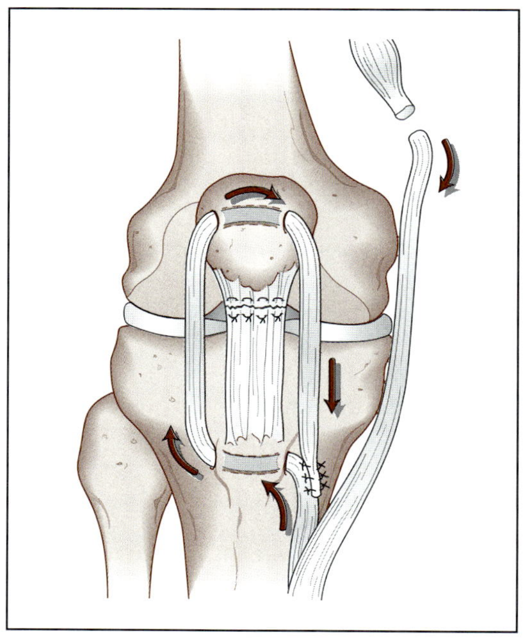

FIGURE 14-8. Augmentation of patella tendon repair with semitendinosus tendon (the Kelikian technique). (*Adapted from* Kelikian *et al.* [26].)

removal. If the strength of the repair is considered unsatisfactory, then preferable means of augmentation include figure-eight tension-band with #5 nonabsorbable suture or semitendinosus tendon autografts (Figure 14-8) [25,26].

Postoperative Rehabilitation

Our rehabilitation protocol following repair of polar avulsions is essentially identical to that of our transverse fracture protocol. One caveat is that the limitations in passive motion are more stringent because the fixation strength of the polar fracture construct is not as tenacious as that of the tension-band wire through cannulated compression screws that we apply to standard transverse fractures. In addition, when comminuted polar fragments are excised, the resting length of the extensor mechanism is shortened. To avoid excessive tension across the repaired lesion, the limit of permissible flexion is determined on the operating room table. Full weight bearing is permitted immediately postoperatively in a hinged knee brace locked in full extension. Typically, passive range of motion (*ie,* brace unlocked) is confined to 0° to 30° of flexion for the first 2 weeks, 0° to 60° of flexion for weeks 3 and 4; and 0° to 90° of flexion for weeks 5 and 6. Following week 6, unrestricted progressive passive flexion is initiated.

LONGITUDINAL FRACTURES

Authors' Preferred Technique

Our preferred mode of fixation for longitudinal (vertical) fractures consists of dual transverse 4.0-mm compression screws. Because the bending and distraction forces across longitudinal patellar fractures are considerably lower than the forces across transverse patellar fractures, we typically do not incorporate a tension band into this construct. Thus, we use noncannulated screws.

Provisional reduction is held with a transversely oriented tenaculum clamp. Because longitudinal fractures tend to be minimally displaced with no associated retinacular disruption, they are often amenable to a minimally invasive approach with percutaneous screw insertion, arthroscopic lavage of the joint space, and arthroscopic confirmation of an anatomic reduction.

Postoperative Rehabilitation

Our rehabilitation protocol following open reduction and internal fixation of longitudinal fractures is essentially identical to our transverse fracture protocol except that full passive motion is permitted immediately.

STELLATE FRACTURES

Relatively simple stellate fracture patterns are often amenable to fixation with a combination of interfragmentary compression screws and tension-band wiring. However, the presence of extensive comminution often precludes anatomic osteosynthesis. In these instances, partial patellectomy is often appropriate [16,27]. Preservation of a significant fragment of the patella offers the theoretical allure of retaining the patella's role in increasing the quadriceps' moment arm. Although partial patellectomy is capable of producing satisfactory clinical outcomes, excessive patellar resection (*ie,* more than 40%) critically alters patellofemoral contact areas and has been associated with subsequent onset of patellofemoral degenerative joint disease [28].

In a cadaveric biomechanical model, Marder *et al.* [24] recently demonstrated that excision of 60% of the native patella drastically reduces patellofemoral contact area (Figure 14-8). Resection of smaller portions (20% or 40%) of the native patella also shifted the region of patellofemoral contact proximally, decreased patellofemoral contact areas, and increased patellofemoral contact pressures. However, the authors demonstrated that attachment of the patellar tendon to the anterior aspect of the residual patella was able to minimize these mechanical alterations (Figure 14-9). Attachment of the patellar tendon to the anterior aspect of the residual patella was not able to compensate sufficiently when a 60% patellectomy was performed.

Authors' Preferred Technique

Our initial approach to stellate fractures is to attempt to achieve a stable anatomic reduction using interfragmentary compression screws (with or without supplemental tension-band wiring). When this is not feasible, our strategy is based on the study by Marder *et al.* [24]. Specifically, we resect the comminuted portion and reattach the patellar tendon to the anterior aspect of the residual patella. If excessive comminution precludes preservation of 60% or more of the native patella, then we perform a complete patellectomy.

Berg [29] has proposed a novel extensile exposure to assist with the difficult task of reestablishing articular congruity in instances of substantial patellar comminution. His approach is predicated on the improved articular visualization provided by a tibial tubercle osteotomy (Figure 14-10). He has documented successful clinical outcomes following this technique with no adverse effects related to the osteotomy. We have no experience with this approach. However, in light of Berg's outcomes, this technique is worthy of consideration. The importance of preserving patellar bone stock should not be underestimated, particularly in a patient

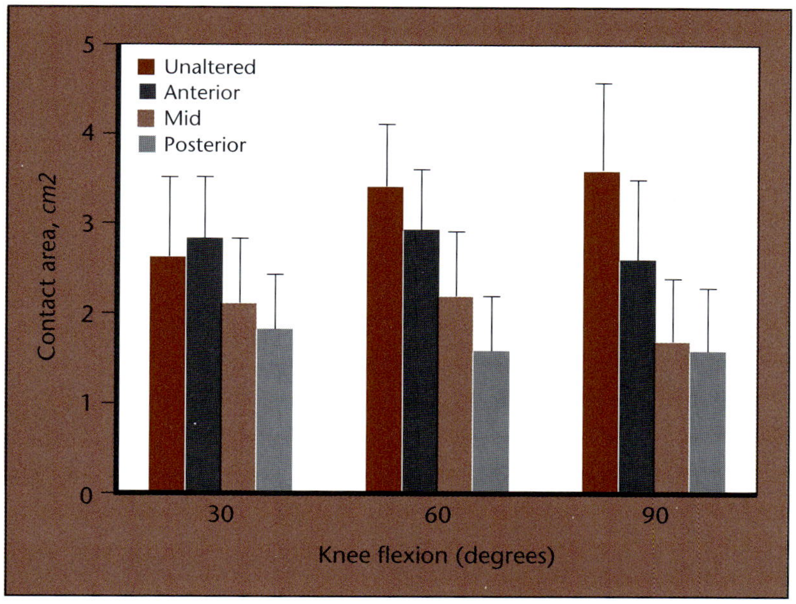

Figure 14-9. Graphic representation of patellofemoral contact areas (cm^2) for the unaltered specimens and anterior reattachment of the patellar tendon after 20% patellectomy, middle reattachment of the patellar tendon after 20% patellectomy, and posterior reattachment of the patellar tendon after 20% patellectomy. (*Adapted from* Marder *et al.* [24].)

in whom patellar resurfacing (as part of a total knee arthroplasty) is contemplated as a potential future salvage procedure.

OPEN FRACTURES

Because virtually all patella fractures are intra-articular, essentially all open patella fractures communicate with the joint space. Thus, in addition to irrigation and débridement of the fracture itself, the joint space should be irrigated and débrided in all cases. Irrigation and débridement of the joint space can be performed arthroscopically if open reduction and internal fixation of the patella is not desired [30].

Catalano *et al.* [14] have reported good to excellent functional results (rated by the HSS knee score) following irrigation and débridement with immediate open reduction and internal fixation in 17 of 22 patients (77%) at 3-year follow-up. No primary patellectomies were performed in this series (including cases with severe comminution).

Torchia and Lewallen [16] also reported 77% good to excellent results in their series of 57 open patella fractures. Unlike the series by Catalano *et al.* [14], bone stock was not universally preserved. Patellectomy (partial or total) was performed in 50% of these cases. Overall incidence of infection in this series was 10.7%. However, deep infections were confined to the more severe soft-tissue injuries. In fact, no deep infections occurred in the Type I and Type II injuries that were treated with immediate open reduction and internal fixation and primary wound closure.

OSTEOCHONDRAL FRACTURES

Large osteochondral fragments associated with comminuted fractures should be anatomically reduced and stabilized whenever possible. To accomplish this, we prefer to use either Herbert screws or absorbable pins. Successful stabilization of osteochondral fragments with biodegradable (poly-*L*-lactide) pins has been reported by Matsusue *et al.* [31]. When the osseous component of an osteochondral fragment is too small to provide successful stabilization, we excise the fragment and apply microfracture to the resultant articular defect [32].

PATELLA FRACTURE FOLLOWING ANTERIOR CRUCIATE LIGAMENT GRAFT HARVEST

Use of a bone–tendon–bone (BTB) central third patellar tendon autograft continues to be a popular, widely accepted means of performing anterior cruciate ligament (ACL) reconstruction. However, recent orthopedic literature is replete with reports of patella fracture following harvesting this type of graft (Figure 14-11) [33–41]. It is generally accepted that the defect at the patellar bone plug donor site creates a stress riser. Notably, although bone grafting of the donor site is a common practice, no proof that this decreases the incidence of subsequent patellar fracture has been documented in the orthopedic literature.

Patella fracture in the setting of BTB autograft harvest may occur intraoperatively or in a delayed fashion. The resultant fracture pattern may be transverse, longitudinal, or stellate. Rigid fixation is particularly important when treating patellar fractures associated with BTB ACL autograft harvest [34]. Under these circumstances, the stability of fracture fixation must be sufficient to allow confident restoration of knee motion so that ACL rehabilitation is not compromised. Our approach to fracture fixation in this setting is identical to the methods that have been specified above for the individual fracture patterns. An inferior quadrant fracture pattern is often encountered in this setting. This fracture pattern is readily amenable to fixation with interfragmentary compression screws (Figure 14-12).

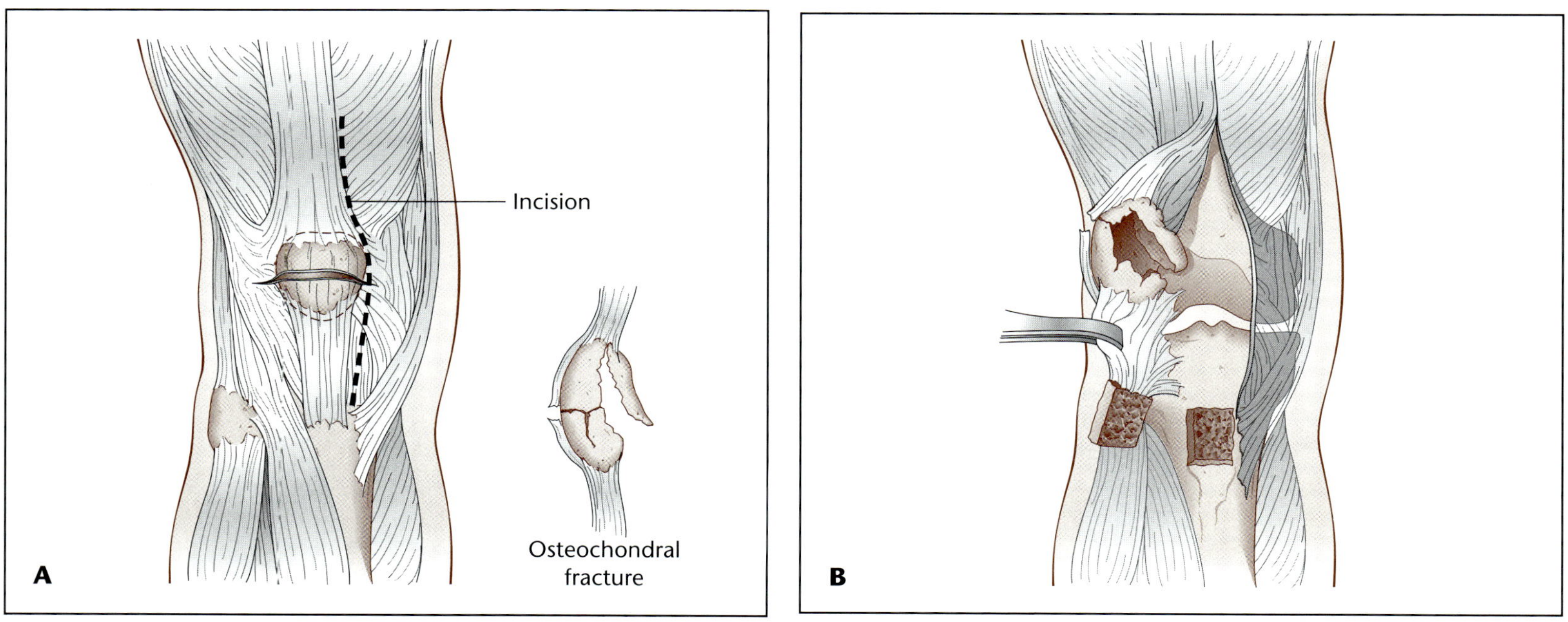

FIGURE 14-10. A and B, Tibial tubercle osteotomy technique for extensile exposure of the articular surface of the patella. (*Adapted from* Berg [29].)

PERIPROSTHETIC FRACTURES

Patella fractures are the most common form of periprosthetic fracture in the setting of total knee arthroplasty. Certain patellar implant design characteristics are associated with increased risk of periprosthetic fracture [42–45]. These include single large central pegs, inset components, and press-fit implants. Additional risk factors include revision surgery, osteolysis, excessive resection of the native patella, patellar avascularity, and thermal necrosis [44]. A triple-peg design not only enhances fixation but is also believed to decrease focal stresses within the patella [46]. Of course, the incidence of patellar fracture is considerably lower when the patella is not resurfaced. The contribution of lateral retinacular release to the risk of periprosthetic patellar stress fracture is controversial. Although Scuderi *et al.* [47] detected a higher incidence of patellar avascularity following lateral release, Ritter and Campbell [48] reported that incidence of periprosthetic patellar fracture was actually lower when a lateral release was performed (suggesting that mechanical factors were a more significant diathesis for patellar fracture than avascularity).

Although periprosthetic patellar fractures are often produced by frank trauma, patellar stress fractures are more common. Many of these lesions are asymptomatic and thus require no intervention [44].

Several factors must be considered when determining treatment of periprosthetic patellar fractures, including the integrity of the extensor mechanism, whether the fracture involves the implant interface, the implant stability, and the presence of component malalignment.

In general, nonoperative treatment is appropriate when no component loosening is present and when extensor mechanism function is intact (*ie,* no extensor lag). Periprosthetic stress fractures characteristically do not disrupt extensor mechanism function because the retinacular tissues remain in continuity. In these instances, we advocate an 8-week period of immobilization in a cylinder cast with no weight-bearing restrictions. When component malalignment (such as lateral patellar subluxation) is believed to have been a contributory factor to patellar stress fracture, then we advocate surgical realignment (*ie,* lateral retinacular release) [49].

Open reduction and internal fixation should be considered when the previously specified criteria are not met. Although some authorities advocate a period of cylinder casting to permit fracture consolidation before addressing the loose component surgically, this approach is not feasible for significantly displaced fractures associated with an extensor lag. In these instances, we prefer an immediate surgical approach to restore both extensor mechanism integrity and component stability.

Due to the decreased thickness of a resurfaced patella, periprosthetic patella fractures are typically not amenable to fixation with compression screws. Thus, the most appropriate mode of fixation for these cases is tension-band wiring (preferably with transosseous K-wires). Following fracture fixation, a new patellar implant is cemented in place. Care must be taken to exclude cement from the fracture interface. If micromotion persists at the fracture interface following fracture fixation, then patella resurfacing is delayed until after fracture union has occurred.

For cases of minimally displaced fractures associated with suspected loose implants, Insall [46] recommends arthroscopic assessment followed by arthroscopically-assisted button removal through a mini-arthrotomy. Delayed revision resurfacing of the patella can be performed subsequent to fracture union if symptoms warrant [44,50].

PATELLECTOMY

Because the patella serves a critical role by increasing the magnitude of the quadriceps' lever arm, it should not be casually sacri-

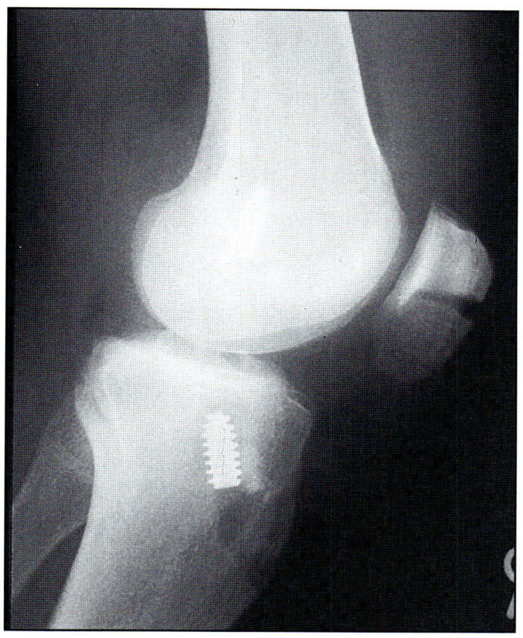

FIGURE 14-11. Transverse patella fracture following central third patellar tendon autograft harvest.

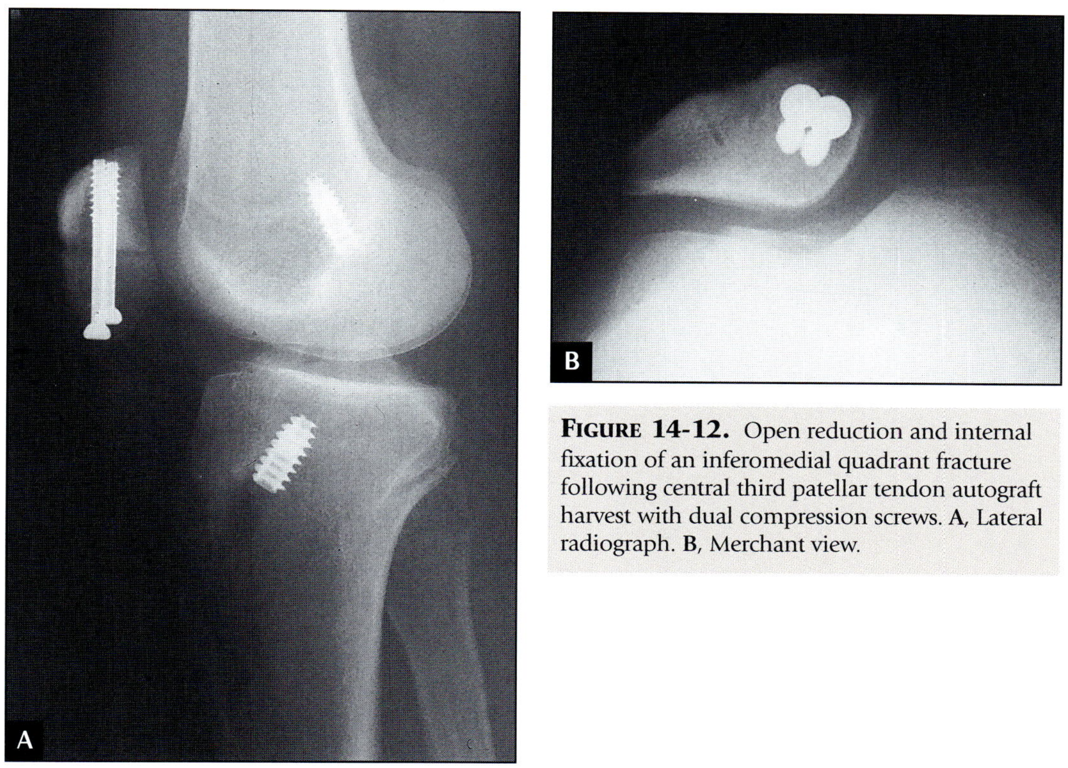

FIGURE 14-12. Open reduction and internal fixation of an inferomedial quadrant fracture following central third patellar tendon autograft harvest with dual compression screws. **A**, Lateral radiograph. **B**, Merchant view.

ficed. However, when no other reasonable option exists, patellectomy remains an effective salvage procedure [51]. We subscribe to Ficat and Hungerford's [52] statement that "a good patellectomy is better than a bad patella."

Our current indications for patellectomy include extensive comminution (requiring excision of more than 60% of the patella), recalcitrant patellar nonunion, advanced posttraumatic arthritis in physiologically young, active individuals, and anterior knee pain after periprosthetic fracture associated with insufficient residual patellar surface area to accept a revision patellar component.

Despite acceptable short-term results following isolated patellofemoral resurfacing, satisfactory long-term results are not available [53]. We do not consider isolated patellofemoral resurfacing to be an appropriate procedure for physiologically young, active patients with advanced degeneration of the patellofemoral joint.

When patellectomy is deemed appropriate, concomitant advancement of the vastus medialis obliquus should be performed. In a recent prospective, randomized trial, Gunal *et al.* [54] found that the results of simple patellectomy were significantly inferior than patellectomy with concomitant advancement of the vastus medialis obliquus. Specifically, concomitant vastus medialis obliquus advancement provided significant compensation for the functional impairment and loss of quadriceps strength associated with patellectomy alone.

Authors' Preferred Technique

For cases of advanced patellar degeneration, we prefer the Miyakawa patellectomy technique because it preserves the length of the extensor mechanism, thus minimizing resultant loss of knee flexion; permits correction of extensor mechanism malalignment; maximizes residual extension strength through advancement of the vastus medialis and lateralis; and reinforces the patellar defect (Figure 14-13) [55].

The Miyakawa technique must be modified when patellectomy is required in cases of acute patella fracture because these cases are typically associated with disruptions of the dorsal patellar aponeurosis and the patellar retinaculum. Thus, restoring proper length of the extensor mechanism is more challenging, and postoperative rehabilitation must be more conservative. After excising all patellar fragments, the defect is bridged by turndown of a superficial flap of quadriceps tendon. Distal advancements of the vastus lateralis and medialis are performed, and the retinacular tears are reapproximated. Rehabilitation following patellectomy consists of immediate ambulation (full weight bearing) in a hinged knee brace locked at full extension. Passive range of motion is confined to 0° to 30° of flexion for the first 2 weeks, 0° to 60° of flexion for weeks 3 and 4, and 0° to 90° of flexion for weeks 5 and 6.

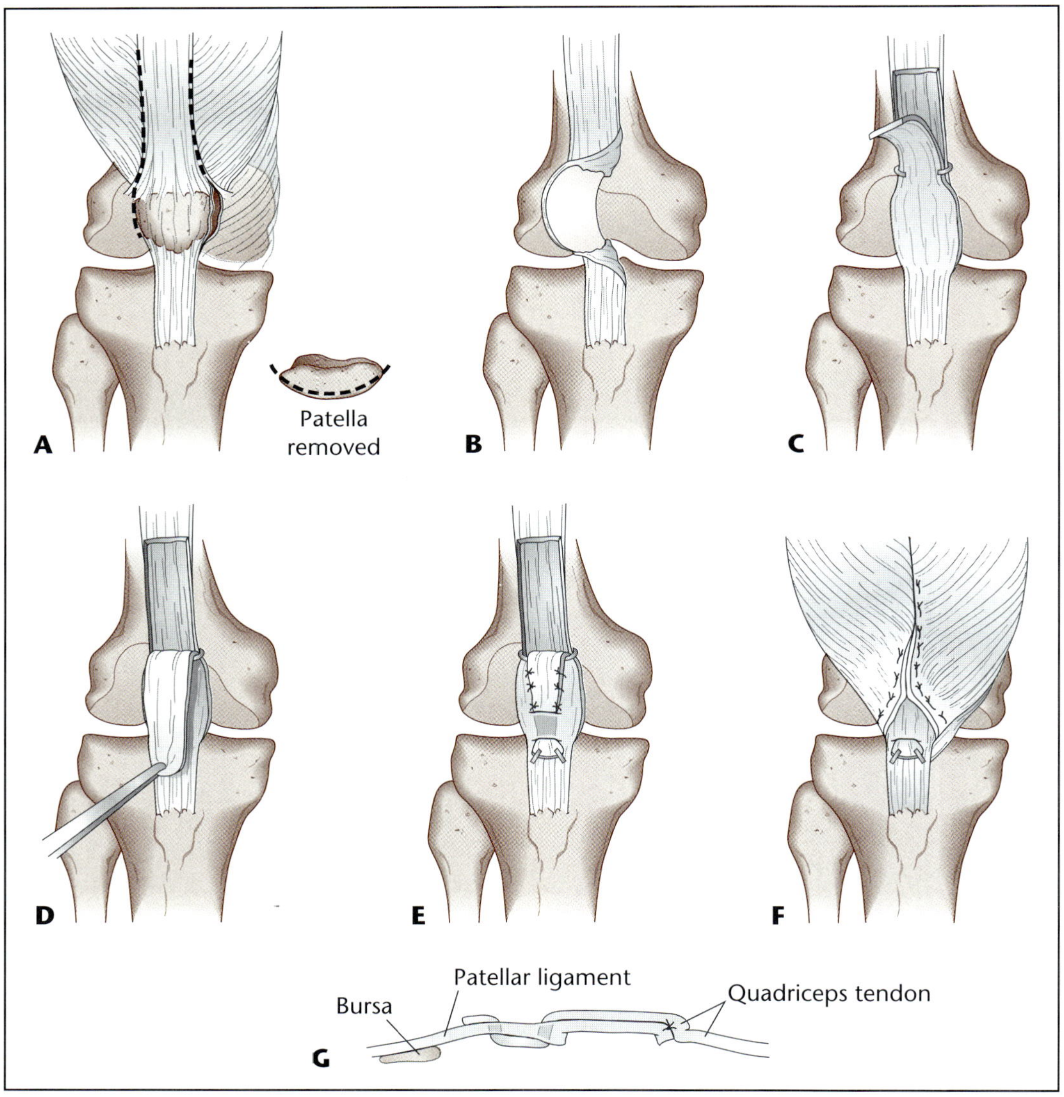

Figure 14-13. A–G, Miyakawa patellectomy technique. (*Adapted from* Baker and Hughston [55].)

Following week 6, unrestricted progressive passive flexion and quadriceps isometric exercises are initiated.

PATELLAR NONUNION

Patellar nonunion is relatively uncommon and often asymptomatic. A recent retrospective review of the results of treatment of symptomatic patellar nonunion documented functionally "successful" outcomes following both operative and nonoperative treatment of this condition [56]. The treatment preceding the establishment of nonunion was inconsistent (12 nonoperative, 8 operative). The nonunion was treated nonoperatively in seven of these patients and operatively in the remaining 13 patients. All seven patients in the nonoperative group had persistent radiographic nonunion, whereas only one of the 13 patients had persistent radiographic nonunion following open reduction and internal fixation.

REFERENCES AND RECOMMENDED READING

Recently published papers of particular interest have been highlighted as:

- • Of interest
- •• Of outstanding interest

1. Mason RW, Moore TE, Walker CW, Kathol MH: Patellar fatigue fractures. *Skeletal Radiol* 1996, 25:329–332.
2. Mata SG, Grande MM, Ovejero AH: Transverse stress fracture of the patella: a case report. *Clin J Sport Med* 1996, 6:259–261.
3. Brogle PJ, Eswar S, Denton JR: Propagation of a patella stress fracture in a basketball player. *Am J Orthop* 1997, 26:782–784.
4. Koval KJ, Kim YH: Patella fractures: evaluation and treatment. *Am J Knee Surg* 1997, 10:101–108.
5. Peterfy CG, Howard DS: Imaging of the patellofemoral joint: current status and future directions. *Am J Knee Surg* 1997, 10:110–120.
6. Shands PA, McQueen DA: Demonstration of avulsion fracture of the inferior pole of the patella by magnetic resonance imaging: a case report. *J Bone Joint Surg* 1995, 77A:1721–1723.
7. Smith AD, Tao SS: Knee injuries in young athletes. *Clin Sports Med* 1995, 14:629–650.
8. Kosanovi M, Komadina R, Batista M: Patella fractures associated with injuries of the knee ligament. *Arch Orthop Trauma Surg* 1998, 117:108–109.
9. Pritchett JW: Nonoperative treatment of widely displaced patella fractures. *Am J Knee Surg* 1997, 10:145–147.
10. Carpenter JE, Kasman RA, Patel N, Goldstein SA: Biomechanical evaluation of current patella fracture fixation techniques. *J Orthop Trauma* 1997, 11:351–356.
11. Weber MJ, Janecki CJ, McCloud P, *et al.*: Efficacy of various forms of fixation of transverse fractures of the patella. *J Bone Joint Surg* 1980, 62A:215–220.
12. Muller ME, Allgower M, Schneider R, Willenegger H: *Manual of Internal Fixation* edn 3. New York: Springer-Verlag; 1992.
13. Berg EE: Open reduction internal fixation of displaced transverse patella fractures with figure-eight wiring through parallel cannulated compression screws. *J Orthop Trauma* 1997, 11:573–576.
14. Catalano JB, Iannacone WM, Marczyk S, *et al.*: Open fractures of the patella: long-term functional outcome. *J Trauma* 1995, 39:439–444.
15. Smith ST, Cramer KE, Karges DE, *et al.*: Early complications in the operative treatment of patella fractures. *J Orthop Trauma* 1997, 11:183–187.
16. Torchia ME, Lewallen DG: Open fractures of the patella. *J Orthop Trauma* 1996, 10:403–409.
17. Us AK, Kinic H: Self-locking tension band technique in transverse patellar fractures. *Int Orthop* 1996, 20:357–358.
18. Hung LK, Chan KM, Chow YN, Leung PC: Fractured patella: operative treatment using the tension band principle. *Injury* 1985, 16:343–347.
19. Levack, B, Flannagan, JB, Hobbs, S: Results of surgical treatment of patella fractures. *J Bone Joint Surg* 1985, 67B:416–419.
20. Chen A, Hou C, Bao J, Guo S: Comparison of biodegradable and metallic tension-band fixation for patella fractures: 38 patients followed for 2 years. *Acta Orthop Acand* 1998, 69:39–42.
21. Juutilainen T, Patiala H, Rokkanen P, Tormala P: Biodegradable wire fixation in olecranon and patella fractures combined with biodegradable screws or plugs and compared with metallic fixation. *Arch Orthop Trauma Surg* 1995, 114:319–323.
22. Chatakondu SC, Abhaykumar S, Elliot DS: The use of non-absorbable suture in the fixation of patellar fractures: a preliminary report. *Injury* 1998, 29:23–27.
23. Scilaris TA, Grantham JL, Prayson MJ, *et al.*: Biomechanical comparison of fixation methods in transverse patella fractures. *J Orthop Trauma* 1998, 12:356–359.
24. Marder RA, Swanson TV, Sharkey NA, Duwelius PJ: Effects of partial patellectomy and reattachment of the patellar tendon on patellofemoral contact areas and pressures. *J Bone Joint Surg* 1993, 75A:35–45.
25. Haas SB, Callaway H: Disruptions of the extensor mechanism. *Orthop Clin N America* 1992, 23:687–695.
26. Kelikian H, Riashi E, Gleason J: Restoration of quadriceps function in neglected tear of the patellar tendon. *Surg Gynecol Obstet* 1957, 104:200.
27. Saltzman CL, Goulet JA, McClellan RT, *et al.*: Results of treatment of displaced patellar fractures by partial patellectomy. *J Bone Joint Surg* 1990, 72A:1279–1285.
28. Bostman O, Kiviluoto O, Nirhamo J: Comminuted displaced fractures of the patella. *Injury* 1981, 13:196–202.
29. Berg EE: Extensile exposure of comminuted patella fractures using a tibial tubercle osteotomy: results of a new technique. *J Orthop Trauma* 1998, 12:351–355.
30. Perry DJ, Sanders DP, Nyirenda CD, Lezine-Hanna JT: Gunshot wounds to the knee. *Orthop Clin North Am* 1995, 26:155–163.
31. Matsusue Y, Nakamura T, Suzuki S, Iwasaki R: Biodegradable pin fixation of osteochondral fragments of the knee. *Clin Orthop* 1996, 322:166–173.
32. Steadman JR, Rodkey WG, Singleton SB, Briggs KK: Microfracture technique for full-thickness chondral defects: technique and clinical results. *Op Tech Orthop* 1997, 7:300–304.
33. Benson ER, Barnett PR: A delayed transverse avulsion fracture of the superior pole of the patella after anterior cruciate ligament reconstruction. *Arthroscopy* 1998, 14:85–88.
34. Berg EE: Management of patella fractures associated with central third bone-patella tendon-bone autograft ACL reconstruction. *Arthroscopy* 1996, 12:756–759.
35. Bonatus TJ, Alexander AH: Patella fracture and avulsion of the patellar ligament complicating ACL reconstruction. *Orthop Rev* 1991, 20:770–774.
36. Brownstein B, Bronner S: Patella fractures associated with accelerated ACL rehabilitation in patients with autogenous patella tendon reconstructions. *J Orthop Sports Phys Ther* 1997, 26:168–172.
37. Christen B, Jakob R: Fractures associated with patellar ligament grafts in cruciate ligament surgery. *J Bone Joint Surg* 1992, 74B:617–619.
38. Graf B, Uhr F: Complications of intra-articular anterior cruciate ligament reconstruction. *Clin Sports Med* 1988, 7:835–848.
39. McCarroll JR: Fracture of the patella during a golf swing following reconstruction of the anterior cruciate ligament. *Am J Sports Med* 1983, 11:26–27.

40. Ouweleen KM, McElror JJ: A unique complication following arthroscopic anterior cruciate ligament reconstruction. *Arthroscopy* 1995, 11:225–8.
41. Simonian PT, Mann FA, Mandt PR: Indirect forces and patella fracture after anterior cruciate ligament reconstruction with the patellar ligament: case report. *Am J Knee Surg* 1995, 8:60–64.
42. Healy WL, Wasilewski SA, Takei R, *et al.*: Patellofemoral complications following total knee arthroplasty: correlation with implant design and patient risk factors. *J Arthroplasty* 1995, 10:197–201.
43. Rorabeck CH, Angliss RD, Lewis PL: Fractures of the femur, tibia, and patella after total knee arthroplasty: decision making and principles of management. *Instr Course Lect* 1998, 47:449–58.
44. Vince KG, McPherson EJ: The patella in total knee arthroplasty. *Orthop Clin North Am* 1992, 23:675–686.
45. Younger AS, Dunwoody I, Duncan CP: Periprosthetic fractures of the hip and knee: the scope of the problem. *Instr Course Lect* 1998, 47:251–256.
46. Insall JN: Knee arthroplasty: limits and other problems: extensor mechanism complications. *Orthopedics* 1996, 19:809–811.
47. Scuderi G, Scharf SC, Meltzer LP, *et al.*: The relationship of lateral releases to patella viability in total knee arthroplasty. *J Arthroplasty* 1987, 2:209–214.
48. Ritter MA, Campbell ED: Postoperative patellar complications with or without lateral release during total knee arthroplasty. *Clin Orthop Rel Res* 1987, 219:163–168.
49. Singerman R, Heiple KG, Davy DT, Goldberg VM: Effect of tibial component position on patellar strain after total knee arthroplasty. *J Arthroplasty* 1995, 10:651–656.
50. Engh GA, Ammeen DJ: Periprosthetic fractures adjacent to total knee implants: treatment and clinical results. *Instr Course Lect* 1998, 47:437–448.
51. Kelly MA, Brittis DA: Patellectomy. *Orthop Clin North Am* 1992, 23:657–663.
52. Ficat P, Hungerford D: *Disorders of the Patellofemoral Joint.* Baltimore: Williams & Wilkins; 1977.
53. Kolettis GT, Stern SH: Patellar resurfacing for patellofemoral arthritis. *Orthop Clin North Am* 1992, 23:665–673.
54. Gunal T, Taymaz A, Kose N, *et al.*: Patellectomy with vastus medialis obliquus advancement for comminuted patellar fractures: a prospective randomized trial. *J Bone Joint Surg* 1997, 79B:13–16.
55. Baker CL, Hughston JC: Miyakawa patellectomy. *J Bone Joint Surg* 1988, 70A:1489–1495.
56. Klassen JF, Trousdale RT: Treatment of delayed and nonunion of the patella. *J Orthop Trauma* 1997, 11:188–194.

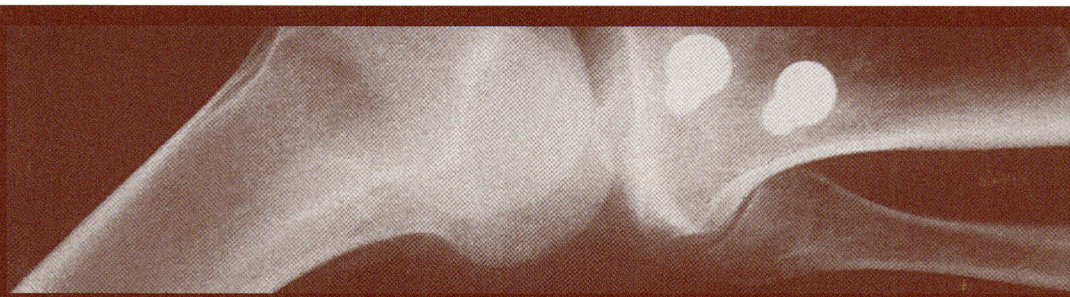

15

Fractures of the Tibial Plateau

Edward A. Perez
Paul J. Duwelius

Tibial plateau fractures comprise 1% of all fractures and 8% of fractures in the elderly. These have long been a controversial and difficult intra-articular fracture for the orthopedic surgeon to treat. The objective in treatment of tibial plateau fractures is to obtain a stable, pain-free knee joint with a functional range of motion. Several authors advocate open reduction and internal fixation [1–5]. Other authors have reported good results with limited internal fixation in combination with functional bracing or various traction techniques [6–13]. Regardless of the treatment method, the fracture must be stable enough in a reasonable amount of time to allow for early range of motion to prevent arthrofibrosis and unacceptable stiffness of the knee.

ANATOMY

A fracture of the tibial plateau is an intra-articular fracture of a major weight-bearing joint. It occurs as a result of a combination of lateral bending and an axial load. This mechanism of loading and fracture results in depression of the articular surface and shearing off of portions of the metaphysis.

The tibial plateau is composed of a 10° posteriorly sloped medial and lateral flare of the proximal tibia that results in the medial and lateral condyles. The anatomic differences between the weight-bearing surfaces of the lateral and medial tibial plateaus should be considered when treating these fractures. In cadaver experiments, Walker and Erkman [14] demonstrated that almost the entire load borne on the lateral compartment is carried by the lateral meniscus (Figure 15-1) [15]. In contrast, load distribution on the medial side is shared equally by the medial meniscus and exposed articular cartilage. The weight-bearing function of the lateral meniscus may explain why functional results after lateral plateau fractures are usually good to excellent despite not achieving a perfect roentgenographic appearance. This may also explain the relatively high frequency of less-satisfactory functional results in bicondylar and medial plateau fractures. A complete understanding of the soft tissues prone to injury in addition to the bony disruption is essential for evaluation and optimal care of tibial plateau fractures.

ASSOCIATED INJURIES

Several authors have reported on the number of associated injuries seen with tibial plateau fractures. Bennett and Browner [16] reported a 56% incidence of associated soft tissue injuries in a series of 30 tibial plateau fractures [17,18]. The medial collateral ligaments were injured in 20%, the lateral collateral ligaments in 3%, the menisci in 20%, the peroneal nerve in 3%, and the anterior cruciate ligaments in 10% [16].

Delamarter *et al.* [17] reported on ligament injuries associated with tibial plateau fractures. In that study, 39 patients with tibial plateau fractures and concomitant ligament injury were evaluated at least 1 year after injury. An additional 22 isolated medial collateral, 8 lateral collateral, 1 isolated anterior cruciate, and 8 combined ligament injuries were found. All types of tibial plateau fractures were associated with ligamentous injury, although split-compression and local-compression types were most common. This study confirms the view that instability is a major cause of unaccepted results in tibial plateau fractures. Operative repair of medial and lateral collateral ligaments, with appropriate treatment of the bony plateau fracture, may reduce late instability and may improve overall morbidity in these concomitant injuries. Cruciate ligament injury associated with a tibial plateau fracture carries a poor prognosis in this series [17].

CLASSIFICATION

Several tibial plateau fracture classifications exist and no single fracture classification system is all encompassing. The AO, Rasmussen [12], and Hohl [19] classification systems are similar and describe most plateau fractures quite well. The Schatzker classification describes in more detail the plateau fracture that extends distally into the metaphyseal region of the tibia [4]. This classification (Figure 15-2) has been the mainstay of radiographic categorization [4]. Six types exist, each representing a group of fractures that are similar in mechanism of injury, fracture pattern, and prognosis. Although we now espouse several treatment modalities that differ from original recommendations, the classification still stands as a valuable tool in the evaluation of tibial plateau fractures.

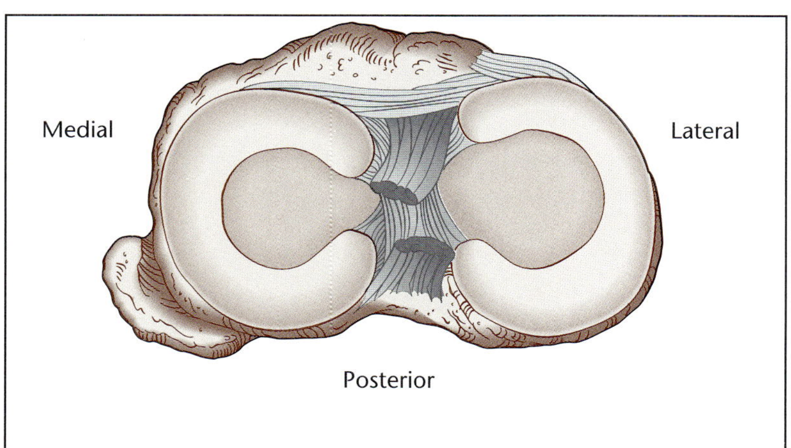

FIGURE 15-1. Tibial plateau seen from above showing exposed surface areas. (*Adapted from* Duwelius and Templeman [15].)

TYPE I FRACTURES

Type I fractures are a split or wedge fracture of the lateral plateau resulting from an axial load coupled with a valgus (medially directed) stress at the knee. These present predominantly in younger patients with good bone stock. The strong cancellous bone resists the articular depression seen in older patients, leaving the less-supported lateral condyle vulnerable to fracture. Displacement can signify meniscal tears, entrapment of the meniscus in the fracture, or disruption of the tibial or fibular collateral ligaments.

TYPE II FRACTURE

Type II fractures are similar to Type I fractures with the additional finding of articular depression. These split-depression injuries are more common in the elderly because osteoporotic cancellous bone cannot support the axial load transmitted through the lateral femoral condyle. These fractures are subject to the same soft tissue injury as described in the Type I classification.

TYPE III FRACTURE

Type III injuries are pure depression fractures of the articular surface of the lateral tibial plateau, again seen mainly in an older population because of the less dense cancellous bone present in such patients. Soft tissue disruption similar to that of Types I and II lesions is possible.

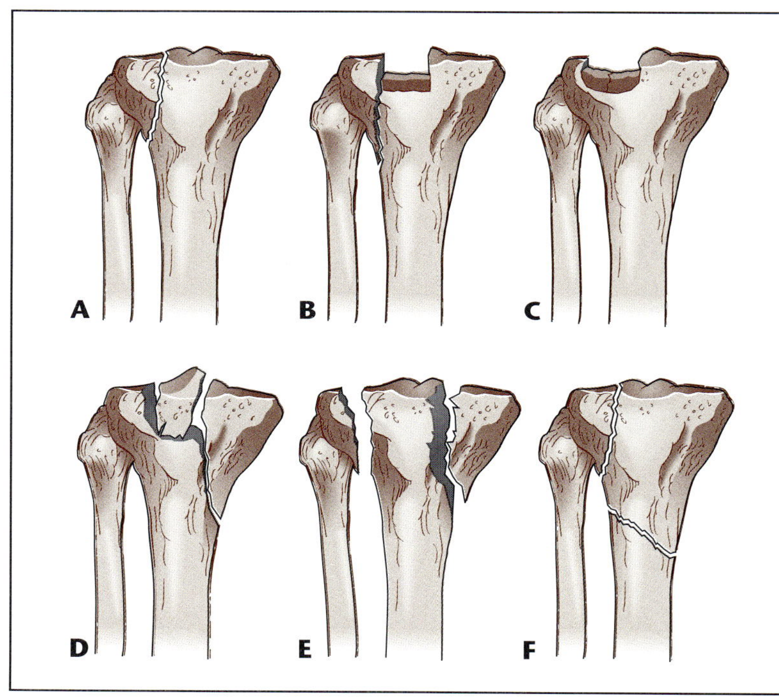

FIGURE 15-2. Schatzker classification of tibial plateau fractures [4]. A, Type I—lateral plateau split fracture. B, Type II—lateral plateau split-depression fracture. C, Type III—lateral plateau central depression fracture. D, Type IV—medial plateau fracture. E, Type V—bicondylar split fracture. F, Type VI—associated plateau and proximal shaft fracture. (*Adapted from* Koval and Helfet [20].)

Type IV Fractures

Type IV injuries are medial plateau split or split-depression fractures that result from compression with the varus forces. These are not to be confused with a traction avulsion of the medial plateau from a valgus force transmitted through the tibial collateral ligament, commonly known as "the ultimate fracture by valgus." Type IV medial plateau fractures are often associated with avulsion of the tibial intercondylar eminence, signifying disruption of the anterior and possibly the posterior cruciate ligaments. Continued varus force can disrupt the fibular collateral ligament. The concern with this type of fracture pattern, however, is the increased possibility of stretch injury to the popliteal neurovascular bundle. Neuropraxia or more severe injury of the common peroneal nerve occurs, as well as intimal tears or disruption of the popliteal artery.

Type V Fractures

Type V is a bicondylar split fracture, consistent with a pure axial load on the extended knee. The diaphysis and metaphysis remain in continuity, whereas the medial and lateral plateaus split off. Because the tibial condyles are sloped posteriorly, the compressive force can develop a shearing force that directs the femoral condyles posteriorly. This results in disruption of the soft tissues.

Type VI Fractures

Type VI injuries are high-energy, complex fractures involving both medial and lateral plateaus as well as separation of the metaphysis from the diaphysis. Disruption of any and all of the soft tissue constraints is possible, along with varying amounts of articular condylar comminution. The involvement of the metaphyseal–diaphyseal fracture often precludes the effective use of traction or ligamentotaxis as reduction techniques because the diaphysis is drawn away from the metaphysis with the application of force.

CLINICAL EVALUATION

After evaluation and stabilization of the patient from life-threatening and concurrent injuries, initial examination of tibial plateau fractures must consist of circumferential inspection of the skin around the knee. Open fractures occur about 5% of the time, and this finding will change management significantly. An open fracture is an absolute indication for emergency-basis débridement and irrigation [21]. Benirschke *et al.* [22] have shown good results with aggressive débridement and early internal fixation of open tibial plateau fractures.

All tibial plateau fractures are clinically evaluated with an examination of the knee in extension and are determined to be either stable or unstable. Unstable fractures have more than 1 cm of opening to varus or valgus stress testing [12]. The knee must also be stressed from 0° to 90° to evaluate for occult instability. If pain precludes an adequate examination, the patient then requires an examination under anesthesia to document stability in extension. Unstable fractures with a more than 1-cm opening in extension are deemed unstable. Examination under general anesthesia also allows an attempt at reduction using only ligamentotaxis.

Examination of the neurovascular status is mandatory. If discrepancies occur in comparison with the contralateral extremity or if a knee fracture-dislocation is suspected, arteriography should be performed. Compartment syndromes are possible with these types of fractures. Radiographic evaluation starts with standard dedicated knee lateral and 10° to 15° caudal tilt anteroposterior (AP) (Moore view) radiographs. The Moore view takes into account the posterior slope of the plateau for better visualization. Oblique 45° views help to delineate the plateaus further; internal rotation shows the lateral plateau and the external rotation view, thus demonstrating the medial plateau. Fractures that are unstable should have conventional tomography or computed tomography (CT) scan with sagittal and coronal reconstruction. These radiologic studies allow the surgeon to formulate a three-dimensional preoperative planning scheme that will facilitate accurate placement of screws, plates, or external fixation devices into good bone.

If the patient will not receive emergency surgery or if abrasions and skin lesions such as fracture blisters preclude surgery, then the knee can be aspirated and a local anesthetic injected. The leg should then be splinted and evaluated.

TREATMENT

Tibial plateau fracture treatment is primarily based on the examination of the knee in extension. The goal of treatment is to restore the fractured knee anatomically and functionally to a condition that is as near normal as possible. With a stable examination result, cast bracing is all that is therapeutically necessary. For fractures that are more complex, a molded, hinged cast brace is applied after longitudinal traction. For simpler fractures, a Bledsoe-type cast brace is used.

Rasmussen [12] revealed that unstable knees with tibial plateau fractures treated surgically and stable knees treated nonsurgically did well. Lansinger *et al.* [23] supported Rasmussen's classic work with 20-year follow-up using these principles based on the examination of the knee in extension. These authors believe no incisions should be made until an examination of the knee using ligamentotaxis and fluoroscopic evaluation has been completed. This gives the surgeon the critical preoperative planning information.

Several previous studies have advocated open reduction and internal fixation with plates and screws. Although good radiographic results sometimes are achieved, several report high rates (25% to 30%) of fair to poor results [2–4]. Others advocate more limited types of internal fixation, possibly in association with ring or external fixation [9,10,12,23,24]. Despite the treatment used, the surgeon must have established criteria for the surgical indications. We think examination of the knee in extension is the best indicator for surgical intervention. Regardless of which type of treatment is chosen, the knee must be allowed immediate and protected free range of motion postoperatively in a hinged brace.

ARTHROSCOPY

The arthroscope for diagnosis and visualized repair is a useful tool in the arsenal of techniques used to repair tibial plateau fractures [11,25]. Using the commercially available anterior cruciate ligament placement guides, a Steinmann pin can be accurately placed directly under the central area of articular depression, and a directly visualized reduction through a cortical window can ensue. Cannulated core cutters and bone tamps greatly facilitate this reduction technique [11]. Bone graft may be needed for large defects, but the cortical window driven up under the defect with a less than 10-mm depression is usually sufficient. The graft and condylar fragment can be supported with percutaneous cannulated screws. A washer used as an antiglide or buttressing "one-hole plate" works well in patients with good bone stock and a noncomminuted condylar fragment if placed at the distal apex of the fragment.

The arthroscope can be a worthwhile adjunct in the treatment of low-energy tibial plateau fractures. With skill, its use can help limit incisions and bone stripping. Arthroscopy has been shown to be safe, with no increase in wound problems. Use of the scope for meniscal repair or limited débridement is another modality [25]. Arthroscopy lends itself especially well to the unstable Schatzker Types I, II, and III. Because of disruption of restraining soft tissues, the resultant articular step-off is often more than acceptable. Open repair of the affected collateral ligaments should be accomplished through a limited incision. With poor bone stock or comminution, formal open plating with a buttress plate is recommended.

OUR PREFERRED SURGICAL TECHNIQUE

Indirect reduction techniques play an important role in the management of tibial plateau fractures. When successful, this results in a minimal amount of additional trauma to the soft tissues while achieving the goal of an anatomic articular reduction. The key to operative reduction is ligamentotaxis, using longitudinal traction or a femoral distractor (Figure 15-3). In addition, specially designed bone reduction clamps are of great assistance in reducing the articular block, thus facilitating an indirect reduction. If reduction is satisfactory, percutaneous screw fixation is then used. Multiple screws serve as one-hole plates and the washer acts as a buttress. Schatzker Types IV, V, and VI tibial plateau fracture patterns with extensive metaphyseal comminution require a buttress plate or external fixator. The current trend for these high-energy injuries with compromised soft tissues has been to minimize any additional trauma to the soft tissue envelope. The practice of limited internal fixation to reduce the articular surface in conjunction with a circular or hybrid external fixator has been increasing in popularity. The goal is to decrease wound complications and deep infection while maintaining stable fixation that allows range of motion [26].

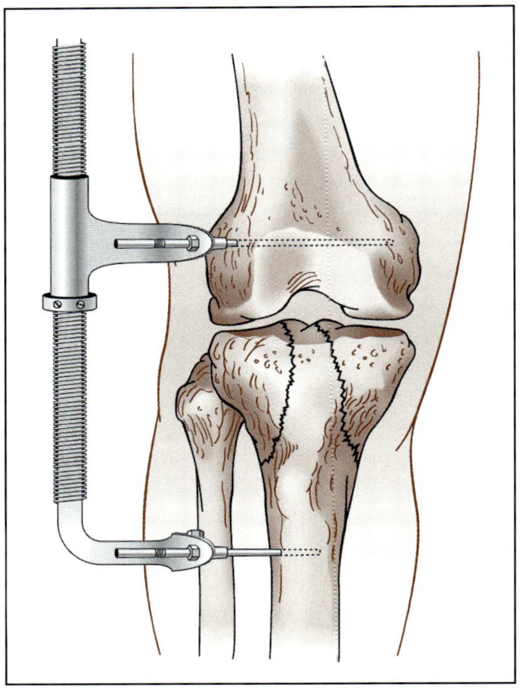

FIGURE 15-3. The femoral distractor is used to achieve reduction using ligamentotaxis. (*Adapted from* Duwelius and Templeman [15].)

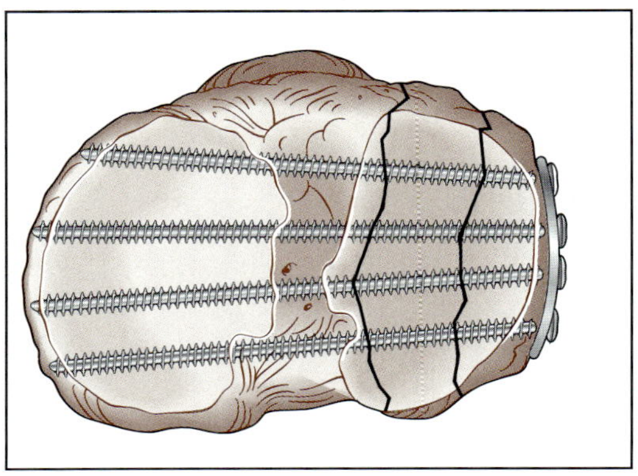

FIGURE 15-4. Orientation of 3.5-mm screws and small fragment "T" plate as seen from above in a split-depression fracture. (*Adapted from* Benirschke and Swiontkowski [27].)

Most plateau fractures can be reduced well by ligamentotaxis alone. Fixation with percutaneous screws placed under fluoroscopy maintained the reduction. Preferably, screws are placed parallel, although a more distal screw with a washer to catch the apex of the fracture may serve as a buttress support.

When ligamentotaxis is unsuccessful in reducing the fracture (*ie*, trapped meniscus or split central depression bone fragments precluding reduction), then a limited arthrotomy using a parapatellar medial or lateral incision is made for the respective medial or lateral plateau fractures, and stabilization with a buttress plate or cannulated screws and iliac crest bone graft is accomplished. There is a trend toward the use of lower-profile plates with four 3.5-mm screws versus the larger plates with 6.5-mm screws [27]. The smaller plates and screws promote less irritation and the four screws provide more subchondral support (Figure 15-4). Herriott and Hubbard [28] found no difference in mechanical stability when comparing the 3.5-mm cortical screws and small fragment "T" plates with more traditional constructs in cadaveric split-depression fractures. We believe that 3.5-mm cortical screws and low-profile plates offer the best construct for supporting the subchondral bone in split-depression or bicondylar fracture patterns.

TYPE I OR SPLIT FRACTURES

Most often, these are wedge-type fractures of the lateral tibial plateau in young adults whose good bone quality resists depression. Undisplaced types can be placed in a cast brace immediately with full range of knee motion. If displaced, most of these fractures are ideal candidates for percutaneous screw fixation using ligamentotaxis, fluoroscopy, and possibly arthroscopy. Displaced fractures occasionally have a trapped meniscus that precludes reduction. Arthroscopy or limited open reduction can allow reduction of the fracture (Figure 15-5).

TYPE II OR SPLIT-CENTRAL DEPRESSION FRACTURES

These fractures, in addition to the wedge split, have varying amounts of central depression of the lateral plateau (Figure 15-6). The mechanism of injury is similar to the first type. Generally, the quality of the bone is not as good; therefore, the weakened bone fails in a compressive load. These fractures commonly occur in older patients with some degree of osteoporosis. If the knee during examination is stable in extension, then no treatment is necessary. The lateral meniscus covers most of the joint surface and the fracture will do well if the joint is moved. Unstable fractures result in joint incongruity and need to be addressed by an attempt at closed reduction using ligamentotaxis followed by percutaneous fixation. Usually, a limited anterior incision is required, with care being taken not to undermine any soft tissue or strip any periosteum. The incision should be centered over the split fragment so that maximum visualization of the depressed fragment as well as joint surface can be used. The central depressed portion needs to be elevated with a bone tamp and supported by bone graft or a bone graft substitute [29]. The fracture can be stabilized with percutaneous screws to avoid further dissection or with a buttress plate and screws if the depressed area is significant or if the lateral wedge is thin so as not to allow for screw fixation with washes alone. The 3.5-mm low-profile buttress plate construct is ideal in this situation.

TYPE III OR CENTRAL DEPRESSION FRACTURES

Depression of the central portion of the lateral plateau occurs without an associated wedge fracture. Generally, those with such fractures are older patients with significant osteoporosis. The knee examination in extension determines which of these fractures need surgery. The treatment protocol is the same as for split or split-central depression fractures. Arthroscopy can be particularly useful in these fractures.

TYPE IV OR MEDIAL PLATEAU FRACTURES

Type IV fractures are particularly prone to problems (Figure 15-7). They are generally found in younger patients with a higher degree of injury. They are almost always unstable. Fractures of the medial plateau that are nondisplaced, especially with an intact fibula, are prone to fall into varus, necessitating that the fracture be stabilized regardless of results found in examination of the knee [30]. Depending on the fracture pattern, percutaneous screws or plates are indicated to reconstruct the joint surface and prevent subsequent varus deformity. The poor prognosis associated with these injuries is caused by the amount of joint surface exposed on the medial plateau compared with the lateral plateau [28]. In addition, soft tissue injury may cause knee instability as well as peroneal nerve or popliteal artery injury.

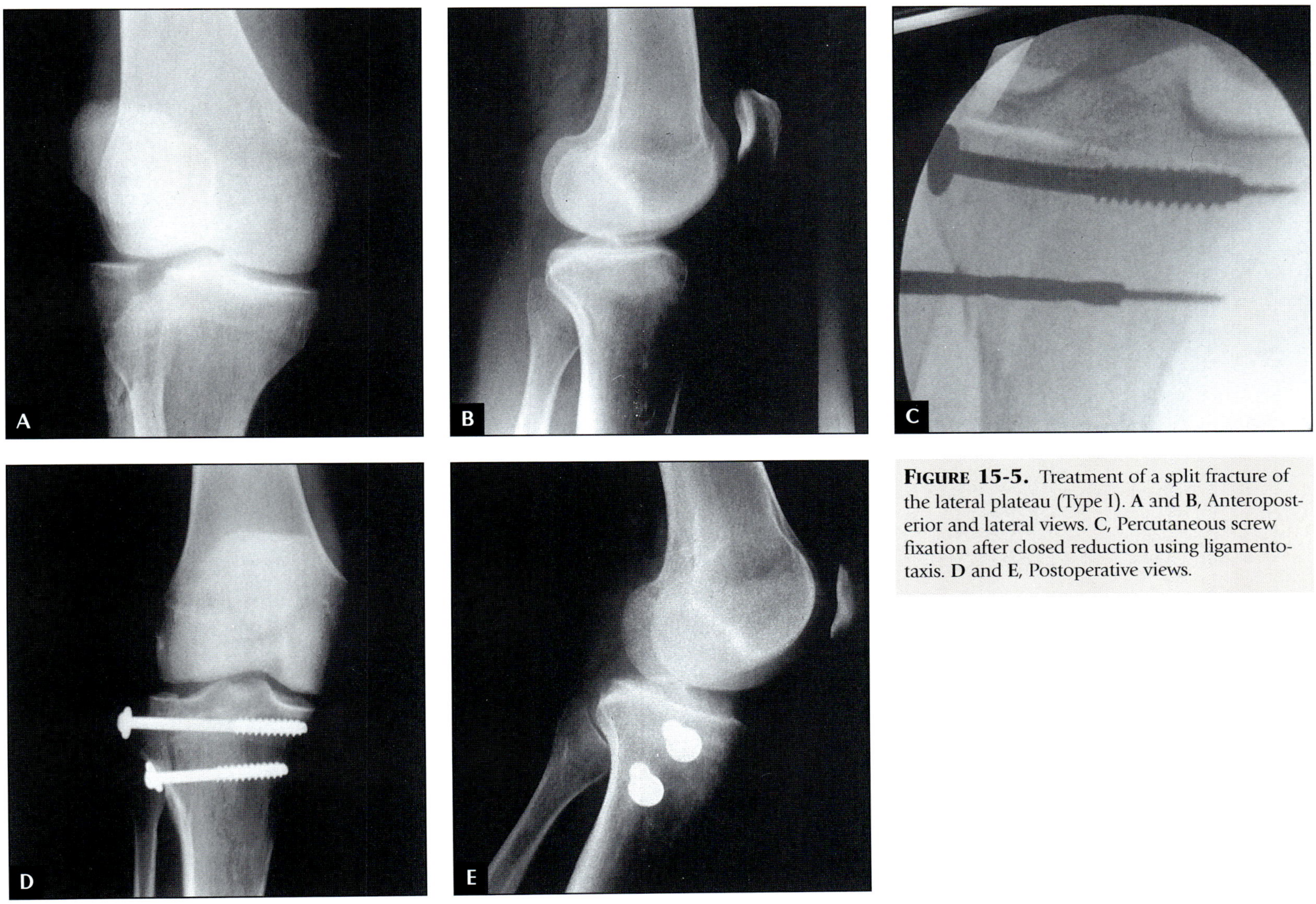

FIGURE 15-5. Treatment of a split fracture of the lateral plateau (Type I). **A** and **B**, Anteroposterior and lateral views. **C**, Percutaneous screw fixation after closed reduction using ligamentotaxis. **D** and **E**, Postoperative views.

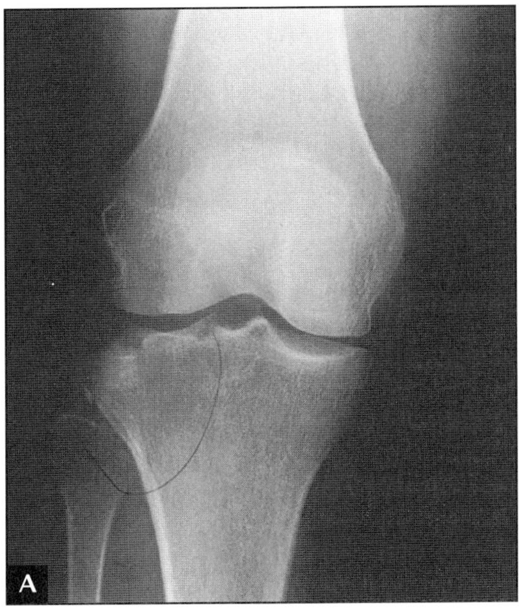

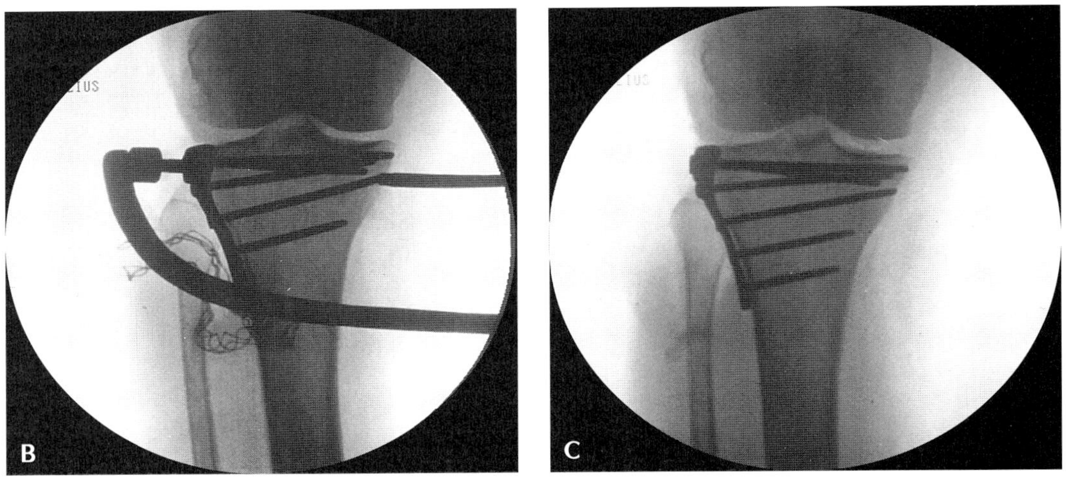

FIGURE 15-6. Treatment of a split-central depression fracture of the lateral plateau. A, Anteroposterior view. B, After indirect reduction and elevation of the articular surface, fixation is achieved with a low-profile plating system. C, Postoperative anteroposterior view.

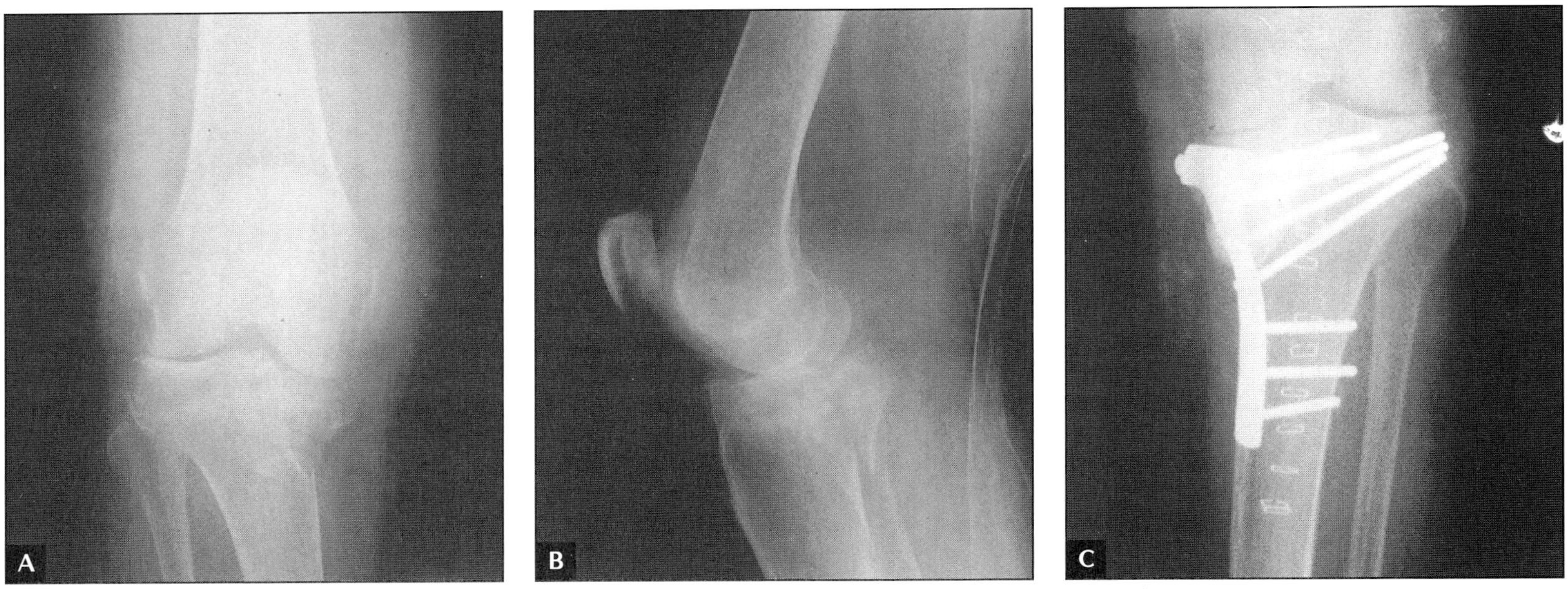

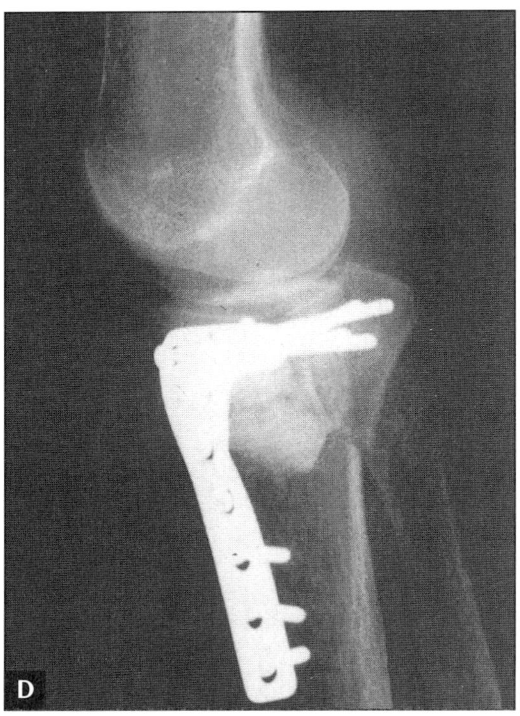

FIGURE 15-7. Treatment of a medial plateau fracture (Type IV) in a woman aged 63 years with severe rheumatoid arthritis. A and B, Anteroposterior and lateral views with significant medial and posterior displacement. C and D, Postoperative views after indirect reduction with a femoral distractor and internal fixation with a low-profile plating system.

TYPE V OR BICONDYLAR FRACTURES

Bicondylar fractures have many different types of fracture patterns. Generally, these fractures are unstable in extension because of the medial condyle involvement. If traction can align these fractures, many can be treated by cast bracing. For unstable fracture patterns, we advocate plating the condyle with the most severe articular involvement with an anterior incision (Figure 15-8). Most commonly, this is the lateral plateau and can be addressed using a Tscherne extensile incision [5]. The other condyle can be treated with percutaneous screw fixation or small plates using a limited medial incision. Limited fixation of the less injured condyle avoids the soft tissue dissection and subsequent vascular problems associated with double plating. Alternatively, limited internal fixation of the condyles with screws and hybrid external fixation to stabilize the articular block to the shaft is effective with severe comminution or high-energy soft tissue injury. Many Type V and VI plateau injuries are associated with significant cartilage injury.

TYPE VI FRACTURES

The hallmark of the Type VI fracture (Figure 15-9) is a fracture line that separates the metaphysis from the diaphysis (Figure 15-10). These fractures usually are extremely high-energy mechanisms of injury with resultant complex fracture patterns. The resultant separation of the condyles from the metaphyseal–diaphyseal junction makes nearly all of them unstable during examination; therefore, this severe injury almost always requires surgical intervention.

The best surgical approach involves an incision over the fractured condyle with the most involved fracture pattern. If the condyles can be assembled with limited internal fixation to restore condylar widening and joint depression, this is optimal. The shaft component can be restored to the condyles through a circular or hybrid external fixator. If plates are chosen, then external fixation is out of the question because of the high incidence of infection. If a plate is chosen to reestablish the condyles to the shaft, then percutaneous fixation of the less injured plateau is optimal. Double plating should be used only in instances in which a small, separate counter incision is made with limited internal fixation to avoid soft tissue and bone necrosis from the excessive surgical dissection required in placement of double plates. These significant injuries require anatomic reduction, bone grafting, and early mobilization of the knee for best results.

RESULTS

Much difficulty exists in comparing literature reports of results. The reasons for this are multiple. Different classification systems and functional result scales are routinely employed, making direct comparison impossible. Bearing this in mind, several important series are listed here. As a rule, the lesser or nondisplaced lower energy injuries of Schatzker Types I, II, and III have a better prognosis than

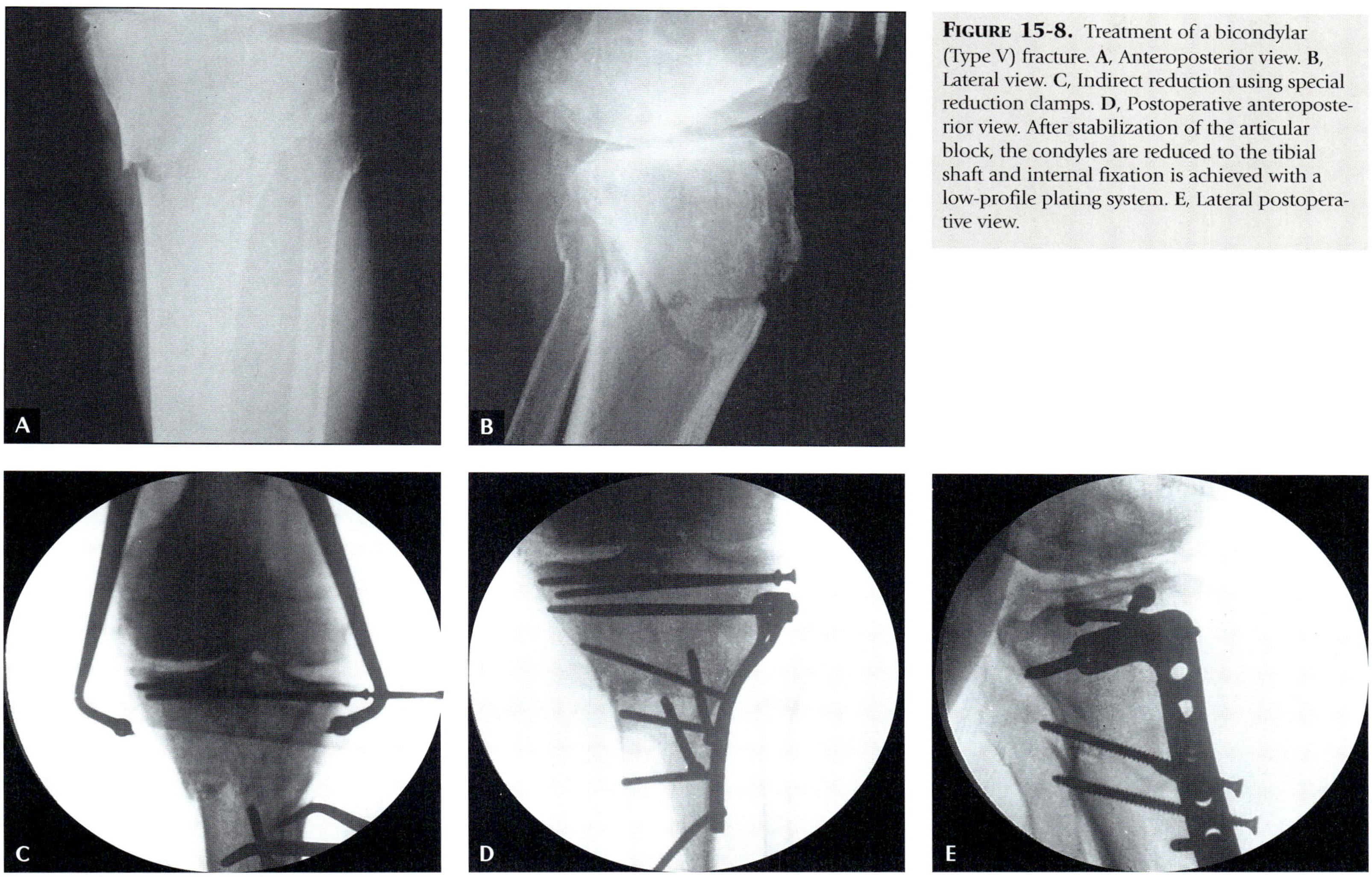

FIGURE 15-8. Treatment of a bicondylar (Type V) fracture. **A**, Anteroposterior view. **B**, Lateral view. **C**, Indirect reduction using special reduction clamps. **D**, Postoperative anteroposterior view. After stabilization of the articular block, the condyles are reduced to the tibial shaft and internal fixation is achieved with a low-profile plating system. **E**, Lateral postoperative view.

the more complicated fractures. Lansinger *et al.* [23] observed 102 patients during follow-up using Rasmussen's [12] operative indications (with 20-year minimal follow-up) with 90% good-to-excellent results. Duwelius and Connolly [9], Duwelius *et al.* [10••], and Koval *et al.* [23] report similar 2-year follow-up using limited internal fixation combined with appropriate external support. Schatzker *et al.* [4] report nearly 90% acceptable results based on aggressive stabilization with buttress plates. Koval *et al.* [24] reported 90% good or excellent results on 21 patients with percutaneous fixation. Delmarter *et al.* [17] confirm that instability is a major cause of unacceptable results in tibial plateau fractures.

COMPLICATIONS

Complications are myriad and best handled with prevention and strict adherence to gentle tissue handling and limited incisions. Maintenance of viable skin coverage and prophylactic antibiotics for closed wounds and appropriate débridement, irrigation, antibiotic therapy, and flap coverage if needed within 1 week are all required to reduce infection. Early range of motion, regardless of treatment selected, must be instituted as soon as possible after surgery to limit the development of stiffness due to ankylosis. To prevent deep venous thrombosis, we prefer the use of sequential compression devices; if a deep venous thrombosis occurs, treatment with warfarin anticoagulation or placement of a Greenfield filter are matched to the patient's needs.

Tibial plateau fractures have a low incidence of nonunion; if it occurs, however, infection must be carefully excluded as a cause. For malunion, failure of fixation is less of a concern than missed diagnosis of unstable fractures that are then undertreated. Stability must be evaluated from 0° to 90° with every injury.

Pauwels [31] has demonstrated that exceeding a certain force on articular surfaces causes degeneration of the cartilage, or posttraumatic osteoarthritis. Patients must be forewarned of this distinct possibility. Early range of motion is essential to preserve as much articular function as possible.

The formation of painful bursas is a frequent result of prominent hardware. Care must be taken to limit hardware as much as possible, provide adequate soft tissue coverage, and be meticulous with screw measurement. For complaints of hardware pain, other sources of pain such as occult infection, nonunion, malunion, neuroma, and arthritic pain must be ruled out before hardware removal. Avoidance of prominent screws is important to avoid unnecessary future surgical removal of implants.

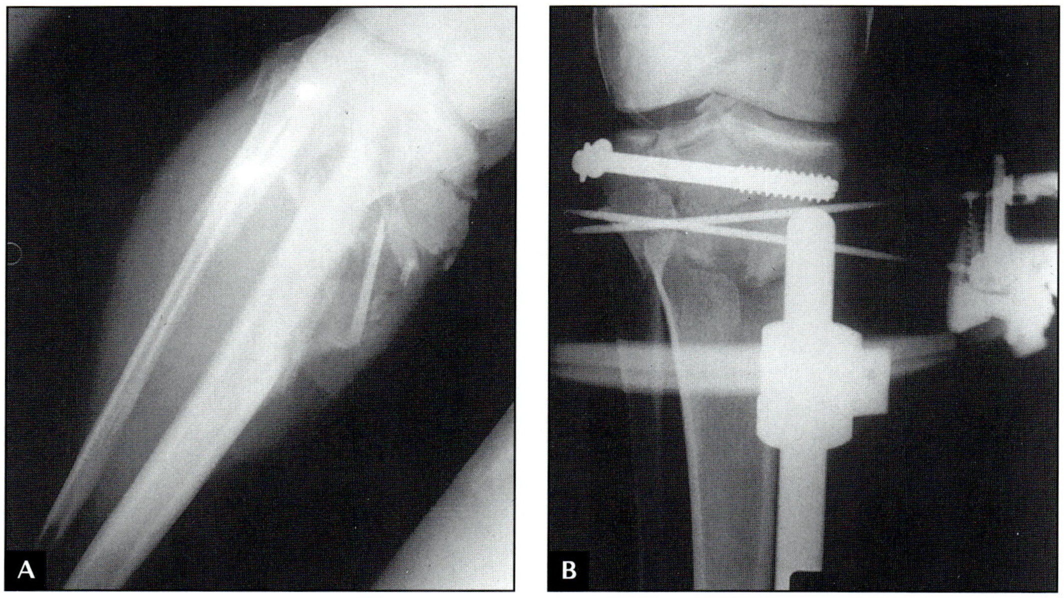

FIGURE 15-9. Treatment of a Type VI fracture secondary to a high-energy injury with a poor soft tissue envelope. **A**, Anteroposterior view. **B**, Postoperative anteroposterior view after limited internal fixation and fine-wire external fixation.

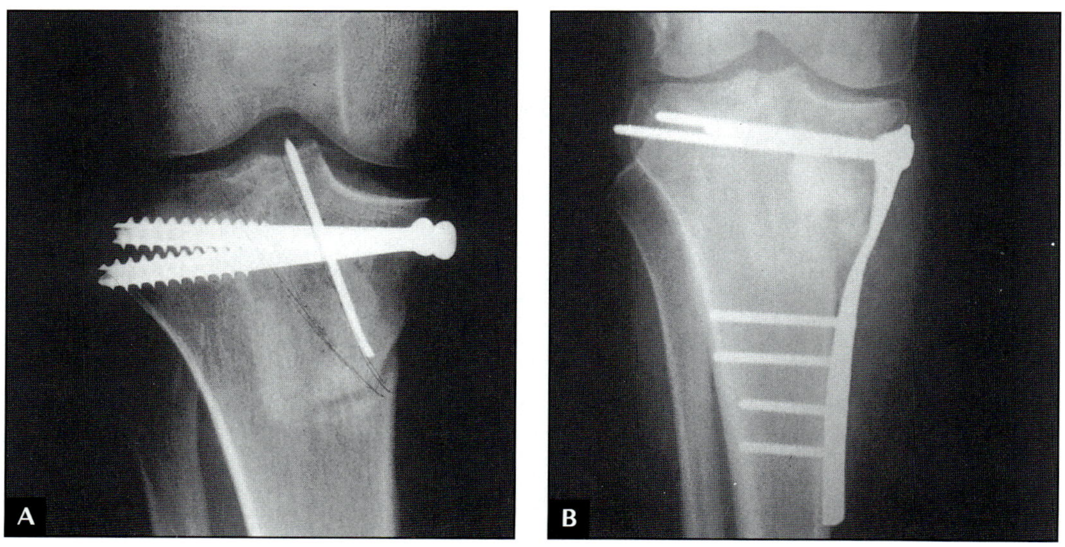

FIGURE 15-10. **A**, Treatment of varus malunion in a man aged 29 years with a medial condyle fracture treated with limited internal fixation. The patient had pain and a marked varus thrust. **B**, Postoperative anteroposterior view after an intra-articular osteotomy, placement of a bone graft substitute, and rigid fixation using a low-profile plating system.

CONCLUSIONS

The goal of treatment of fractures of the tibial plateau is a stable, pain-free joint with a functional range of motion. Immediate range of motion is obligatory regardless of operative or nonoperative treatment. The personality of the fracture and associated injuries must be considered before rendering treatment. In the low-energy injuries, operative trends have leaned toward indirect reduction techniques, limited internal fixation, and the use of lower profile plates with 3.5-mm cortical screws. In high-energy injuries, the state of the soft tissues dictates treatment choice. With good soft tissues, buttress plating of the more involved side with contralateral limited internal fixation or small counterincision with small plates has been successful. In situations in which the soft tissues are in poor condition, limited internal fixation with ring or hybrid external fixators is recommended. Tibial plateau fractures remain a challenge to the orthopedic surgeon; however, by adhering to basic principles, good outcomes can be expected.

REFERENCES AND RECOMMENDED READING

Recently published papers of particular interest have been highlighted as:
- • Of interest
- •• Of outstanding interest

1. Agnew SG, Benirschke SK, Mayo KA, *et al.*: Open reduction internal fixation of complex proximal tibial fractures. *J Orthop Trauma* 1991, 5:236.
2. Blokker CP, Rorabeck CH, Bourne RB: Tibial plateau fractures: an analysis of the results of treatment in 60 patients. *Clin Orthop* 1984, 182:193–199.
3. Rombold C: Depressed fractures of the tibial plateau: treatment with rigid internal fixation and early mobilization. A preliminary report. *J Bone Joint Surg Am* 1960, 42:783–797.
4. Schatzker J, McBroom R: The tibial plateau fracture: the Toronto experience 1968–1975. *Clin Orthop* 1979, 138:94–104.
5. Tscherne H, Lobenhoffer P: Tibial plateau fractures: management and expected results. *Clin Orthop* 1993, 292:87–100.
6. Apley AG: Fractures of the lateral tibial condyle treated by skeletal traction and early mobilization: a review of sixty cases with specific reference to the long-term results. *J Bone Joint Surg Br* 1956, 38:699–708.
7. Brown GA, Sprague BL: Cast brace treatment of plateau and bicondylar fractures of the proximal tibia. *Clin Orthop* 1976, 119:184–193.
8. Drennan DB, Locher FG, Maylahn DJ: Fractures of the tibial plateau: treatment by closed reduction and spica cast. *J Bone Joint Surg Am* 1979, 61:989–995.
9. Duwelius PJ, Connolly JF: Closed reduction of tibial plateau fractures: a comparison of functional and roentgenographic end result. *Clin Orthop* 1988, 230:116–126.
10. Duwelius PJ, Rangitsch MR, Colville MR, *et al.*: Treatment of tibial plateau fractures by limited internal fixation. *Clin Orthop* 1997, 339:47–57.
11. Holzach P, Matter P, Minter J: Arthroscopically assisted treatment of lateral tibial plateau fractures in skiers: use of a cannulated reduction system. *J Orthop Trauma* 1994, 8:273–281.
12. Rasmussen PS: Tibial condylar fractures: impairment of knee joint stability as an indication for surgical treatment. *J Bone Joint Surg Am* 1973, 55:1331–1350.
13. Scotland T, Wardlaw D: The use of cast-bracing as treatment for fractures of the tibial plateau. *J Bone Joint Surg Br* 1981, 63B:575–578.
14. Walker PS, Erkman MJ: The role of menisci in force transmission across the knee. *Clin Orthop* 1975, 109:184–192.
15. Duwelius PJ, Templeman DC: The knee: tibial plateau fracture reduction techniques utilizing cannulated screw fixation. In *Cannulated Screw Fixation.* Edited by Asius SE, Kyle RF. New York: Springer Verlag; 1996:171.
16. Bennett WF, Browner B: Tibial plateau fractures: a study of associated soft tissue injuries. *J Orthop Trauma* 1994, 8:183–188.
17. Delmarter RB, Hohl M, Hopp E Jr: Ligament injuries associated with tibial plateau fractures. *Clin Orthop* 1990, 250:226–233.
18. Vangsness CT Jr, Ghaderi B, Hohl M, *et al.*: Arthroscopy of meniscal injuries with tibial plateau fractures. *J Bone Joint Surg* 1994, 76:488–490.
19. Hohl M, Luck V: Fractures of the tibial condyle. *J Bone Joint Surg* 1956,38A:1001–1018.
20. Koval JK, Helfet DI: Tibial plateau fractures: evaluation and treatment. *J Am Acad Orthop Surg* 1995, 3:86–93.
21. Gustilo RB: Current concepts in management of open fractures. *Instruct Course Lect* 1987, 36:357–369.
22. Benirschke SK, Agnew SG, Mayo KA, *et al.*: Immediate internal fixation of open, complex tibial plateau fractures: treatment by a standard protocol. *J Orthop Trauma* 1992, 6:78–86.
23. Lansinger O, Bergman B, Korner L, *et al.*: Tibial condylar fractures: a twenty-year follow-up. *J Bone Joint Surg Am* 1985, 68:13–19.
24. Koval KJ, Sanders R, Borrelli J, *et al.*: Indirect reduction and percutaneous screw fixation of displaced tibial plateau fractures. *J Orthop Trauma* 1992, 6:340–346.
25. Fowble CD, Zimmer JW, Schepsis AA: The role of arthroscopy in the assessment and treatment of tibial plateau fractures. *Arthroscopy* 1993, 9:584–590.
26. Weiner LS, Kelly M, Yang E, *et al.*: The use of combination internal fixation and hybrid external fixation in severe proximal tibia fractures. *J Orthop Trauma* 1995, 9:244–250.
27. Benirschke SK, Swiontkowski MF: Proximal tibia fractures. In *Orthopaedic Trauma Protocols.* Edited by Hansen ST, Swiontkowski MF. New York: Raven Press; 1993:313–325.
28. Herriott GE, Hubbard DF: Low-profile fixation of tibial plateau fractures. Paper presented at Orthopaedic Trauma Association Annual Meeting, Vancouver, BC; 1998.
29. Bucholz RW, Carlton A, Holmes R: Interporous hydroxyapatite as a bone graft substitute in tibial plateau fractures. *Clin Orthop* 1989, 240:53–62.
30. Sarmiento A, Kinman PB, Latta LL: Fractures of the proximal tibia and tibial condyles: a clinical and laboratory comparative study. *Clin Orthop* 1979, 145:136–145.
31. Pauwels F: Neve Richtlinien Fuer Die Operative Behndlung der Coxarthrose. *Ver Dtsch Orthop Ges* 1932, 48:332–336.

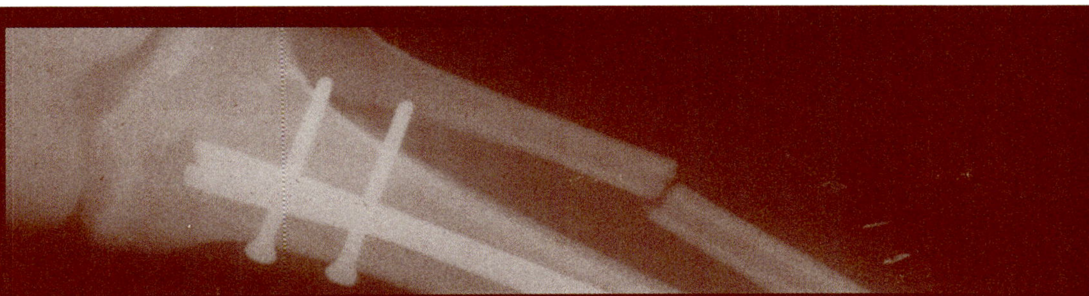

16

Fractures of the Tibial Shaft

Thomas A. Russell

Fractures of the tibia and fibula comprise a spectrum of injuries united by a common loss of unrestricted load bearing of the extremity. This spectrum ranges from fatigue-type injuries (stress fractures), which are primarily osseous failures, to extreme energy-absorbing injuries that result in the loss of soft tissue envelope continuity, neurologic dysfunction, vascular insufficiency, and loss of bone. With sufficient damage to the different tissue groups, viability of the limb may be lost, resulting in amputation of the leg.

Fractures of the tibia and fibula are the most common long-bone fractures in adults. The risk of sustaining this injury in the United States is 1 to 2 per 125,000 population with approximately 25% of the fractures presenting as open injuries [1]. All forms of treatment have a place in individual cases, but the functional outcomes from these fractures vary widely. Fractures of the tibia and fibula continue to represent a source of debate regarding optimal treatment, not only in medical literature and scientific forums but also increasingly in the politics of the "healthcare insurance complex," in which physicians must contend with attempts by insurance companies to dictate patient treatment.

PERTINENT ANATOMY

A thorough knowledge of both the topographic and structural anatomy of the leg is essential for successful nonoperative and operative treatment of injuries to the leg. Each of the four leg compartments (anterior, lateral, superficial, and deep posterior) comprises specific neurologic, vascular, and musculotendinous units that may contribute to significant functional loss through the complications of compartment syndrome, neural damage, and tissue disruption. These complications may preclude reconstructive options after tibial injury and produce significant functional loss even though the fracture may unite satisfactorily.

The medullary canal of the tibia is more triangular than circular in cross-section. The lack of curvature of the tibial medullary canal compared with the femur makes a longitudinal interference fit difficult using an intramedullary nail. Some medullary canals are small, which may preclude use of conventional intramedullary nailing. In patients with small canals, excessive reaming may lead to thermal injury and secondary infection; intramedullary implants less than 8 mm in diameter frequently do not have sufficient fatigue life for treatment of the tibial fracture.

At the proximal and distal metaphyseal–diaphyseal transitions, the cortex thins and the medullary canal expands. Clinically, this often presents difficulties when intramedullary or external fixation is required for proximal and distal one-quarter fractures. In this region, external fixation half-pins engage less cortex and thus have less stress resistance. Intramedullary nails that do not fill the canal offer little or no resistance to deforming forces without interlocking screw supplementation. Biplanar interlocking nail and external fixation systems offer little resistance to deforming forces in the metaphyseal–diaphyseal junction regions. The move toward multiplanar external fixation for increased stability has recently been applied to intramedullary nails with placement of interlocking screws in different planes to enable these devices to better control forces in the metaphyseal regions.

Complications related to the anatomy of the tibia specific to external fixation relate to pin-site osteomyelitis, fracture through pin sites after removal of external fixation (usually diaphyseal pins), and neurovascular complication from damage during pin insertion. Cross-sectional anatomy of the leg is important in the application of conventional external fixators and recently introduced circular fixators using transfixion wires to avoid neurologic and vascular injury. Green [2] defined "safe-zones" for the insertion of transfixing pins; a cross-sectional atlas should be consulted when planning to use these devices.

The intramedullary vascular supply is the most important in normal bone; however, after an injury that disrupts the intramedullary vascular pattern, periosteal blood vessels increase their contribution and become prominent in the formation of new bone [3]. The nutrient artery of the tibia arises from the posterior tibial artery and enters the posterolateral cortex of the bone at the origin of the soleus muscle just below the oblique line of the tibia posteriorly. This artery divides into three ascending branches and a single main descending branch, which gives off smaller branches to the endosteal surface. The periosteum has an abundant blood supply from branches of the anterior tibial artery as it courses down the interosseous membrane. Periosteal vascular network development after fracture increases from its normal 25% contribution to nearly 100% contribution to bone viability at the fracture site.

The five major venous structures of the leg are the greater and lesser saphenous veins, the posterior and anterior tibial veins, and the peroneal vein. These structures are important in revascularization techniques and are a source of possible thromboembolic disease after lower-extremity trauma.

FRACTURE CLASSIFICATIONS

Classifications for tibial fractures that can be replicated from physician to physician are currently elusive. Most classification systems include some type of bony injury grade, soft tissue injury grade, and a locational description for the fracture. Johner and Wruhs [4] reported results of tibial plating using a classification

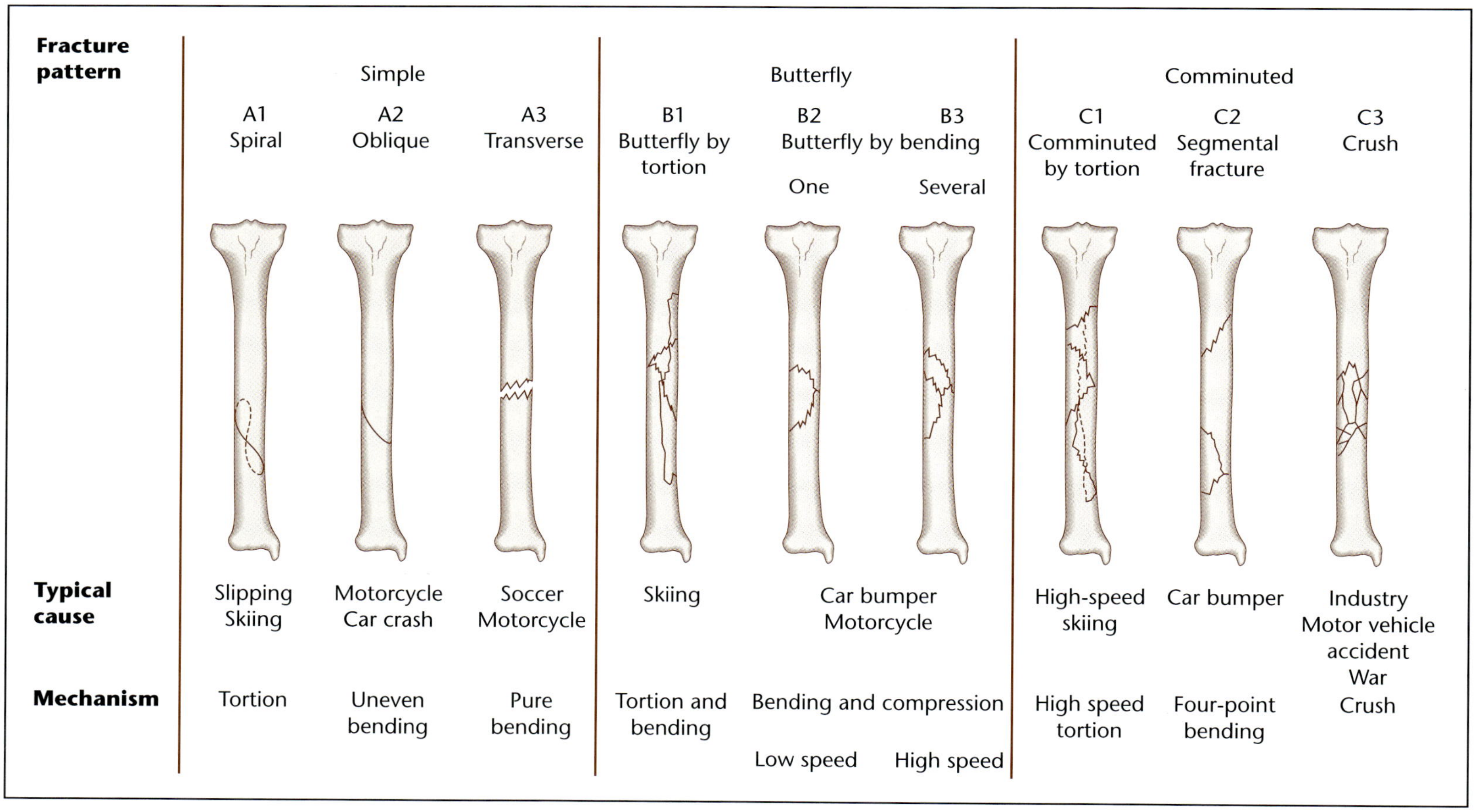

FIGURE 16-1. Johner and Wruhs classification. (*Adapted from* Johner and Wruhs [4].)

that evaluated the mechanical forces resulting in various fracture patterns (Figure 16-1). Torsional injuries are more common with low-energy trauma in which the foot becomes fixed and the body rotates about this fixed point, as seen in skiing injuries. Radiographically, these injuries appear spiral with varying degrees of comminution depending on the energy applied and absorbed by the tibia at the time of failure. Three- and four-point bending forces produce short oblique and transverse fractures. As the points of bending are spread apart and the energy applied is increased, comminution increases and even segmental fractures may develop. Direct-force applications are crushing in nature with high concentrations of energy to a smaller area with resulting increased damage to the bone and soft tissues.

Johner and Wruhs' [4] alphanumeric classification and correlation with these mechanistic fracture descriptions was expanded and modified by Müller *et al.* [5]. The Orthopedic Trauma Association [6] has published a classification of fractures that draws heavily from Müller *et al.*'s work in an attempt to standardize the literature for the future (Figure 16-2). However, until these systems are validated in clinical settings with regard to reproducibility and interobserver agreement, the validity and comparability of the literature remain open to speculation.

Gustilo and Anderson's 1976 [7] classification of Types I, II, and III injuries in conjunction with Gustilo's 1984 modification [8] that subgrouped Type III injuries into IIIA, IIIB, and IIIC patterns is still the most widely used system in North America and has been shown to correlate with the rates of infection, nonunion, and amputation (Table 16-1). The ability to reproduce the interobserver agreement with the Gustilo classification has been demonstrated to approximate 60% even after initial débridement and irrigation.

INITIAL INJURY ASSESSMENT

Bony stability and soft tissue injury are the main determinants for the type of treatment selected for the individual tibial fracture. Because the tibia is subcutaneous for most its length, deformity is usually readily apparent. Stability of the fracture is one of the first assessments required during any physical examination. An obvious deformity or shortening confirms the diagnosis of mechanical instability of the tibial diaphysis. However, minimally displaced or nondisplaced fractures may be tested by application of careful varus or valgus stress of the extremity during examination and ini-

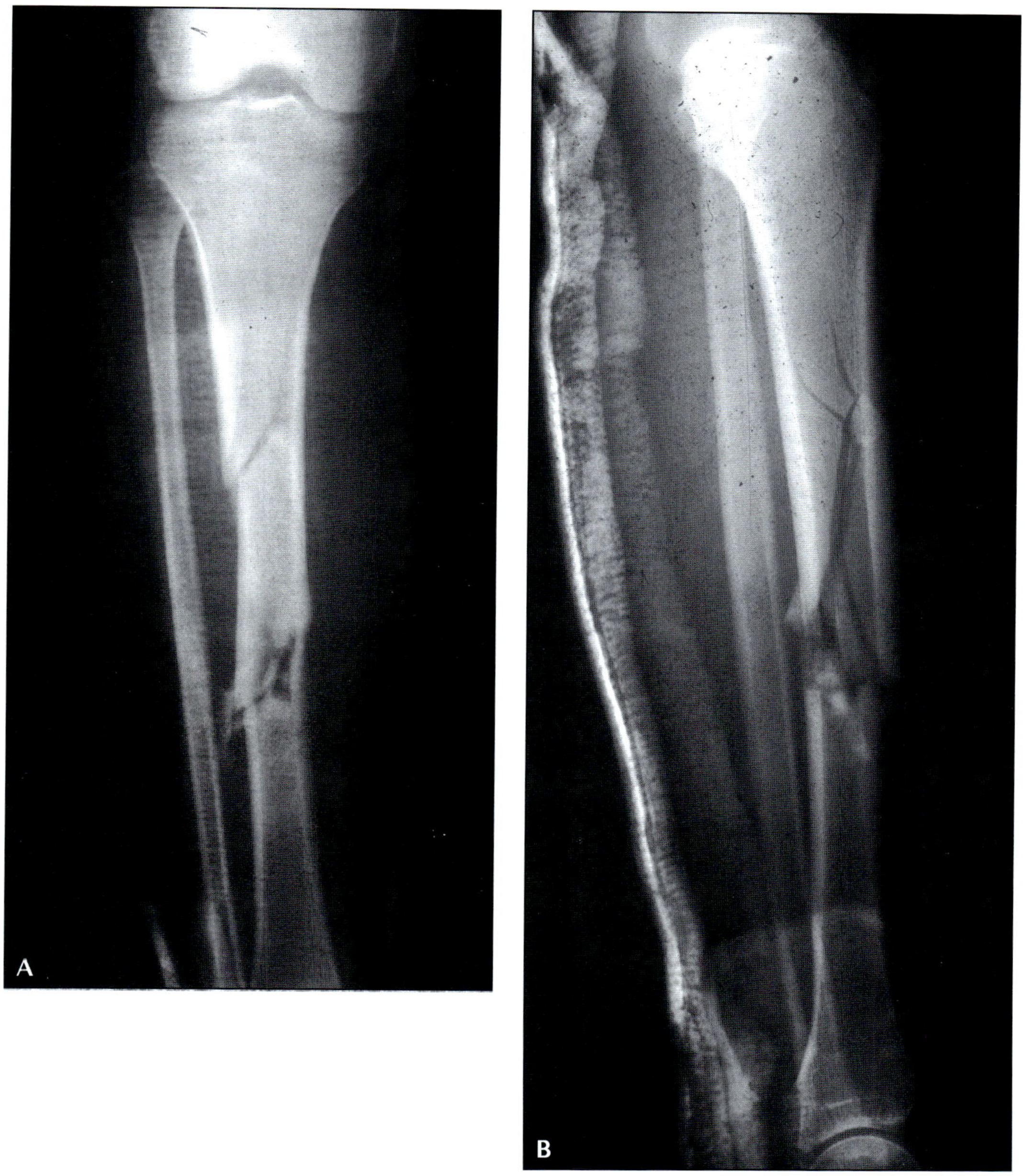

FIGURE 16-2. Segmental Orthopedic Trauma Association-C type closed fracture tibia from motor vehicular trauma. **A**, Anteroposterior radiograph. **B**, Lateral radiograph.

tial splinting, which are then followed by standard anteroposterior and lateral radiographic evaluation from the knee to the ankle.

The soft tissue envelope of the tibia must be inspected throughout its circumference for ecchymosis, open wounds, and tissue turgidity. Associated fractures of the fibula may provide insight into the degree of initial displacement during the injury, show the potential for instability of the tibial fracture, and aid in reduction evaluation, especially with regard to length correction. Documentation and continued observation of neural motor and sensory function in the four compartments and vascularity of the limb are critical.

TREATMENT OPTIONS FOR CLOSED DIAPHYSEAL FRACTURES

A shift has occurred in the appreciation of outcome results for tibial injuries by the surgeon with increased regard for the patient's perception of the result of treatment with a resultant decreased tolerance for malunion and functional loss. Most texts and articles still reference acceptable but arbitrary guidelines of less than 1 cm of shortening, alignment within 5° to 10° varus and valgus with anterior posterior 5° to 10° tolerance, and less than 20° of external rotation and 10° of internal rotation. Often with these strict criteria, results of nonoperative treatment become less desirable (Table 16-2).

Nonoperative management of tibia fractures with long leg casts and braces have been in existence for hundreds of years. Closed treatment offers the advantages of lack of surgical risks, decreased risk of infection in closed fractures, decrease in some treatment associated costs, and widespread availability. Disadvantages of closed treatment are prolonged treatment, work and recreation restrictions, greater residual deformity, and contractures.

Oni *et al.* [9] in 1988 and Sarmiento *et al.* [10] in 1989 reviewed nonrandomized selected studies with initial cast immobilization with a weight-bearing program. Sarmiento *et al.* concluded that bracing was contraindicated in fractures with excessive initial shortening or showed increasing angular deformity while in the cast. They also expressed the belief that patients with significant neurologic or vascular damage, segmental bone loss, or those requiring soft tissue flaps were not candidates for bracing. Other complications of casting and bracing, including skin irritation and maceration, occasionally require discontinuation of bracing. Most series report a range of 25% to 40% incidence of joint stiffness in the ankle and subtalar joint after prolonged casting and immobilization. Although nonoperative modalities can work in a certain percentage of patients, the surgeon must inform the patient of the possible conversion to operative modalities if stabilization cannot

TABLE 16-1. GUSTILO CLASSIFICATION OF OPEN FRACTURES

Type	Description
I	Skin opening of 1 cm or less, quite clean. Most likely from inside to outside. Minimal muscle contusion. Simple transverse or short oblique fractures.
II	Laceration longer than 1 cm, with more extensive soft tissue damage, flaps, or tissue avulsion. Minimal-to-moderate crushing component. Simple transverse or short oblique fractures with minimal comminution.
III	Extensive soft tissue damage including muscles, skin, and neurovascular structures. Often a high-velocity injury with a severe crushing component.
IIIA	Extensive soft tissue laceration, adequate bone coverage. Segmental fractures and gunshot injuries.
IIIB	Extensive soft tissue injury with periosteal stripping and bone exposure. Usually associated with massive contamination.
IIIC	Vascular injury requiring repair.

Data from Gustilo and Anderson [7] and Gustilo *et al.* [8].

TABLE 16-2. RESULTS OF NONOPERATIVE TREATMENT

Treatment	Oni *et al.* [9]	Sarmiento *et al.* [10]
Time to union	19% delayed	21.5 wk
Nonunion	4%	2.5%
Malunion	34%	50%
Failed change	Unknown	6%
Treatment	Unknown	17% LTFU
Loss length significant	5.3%	60% average 7.1 mm
Loss of motion ankle	43%	Unknown

LTFU—lost to follow-up.

be maintained with casts or bracing. Frequent clinical visits and radiographs are required with this type of surveillance.

Open reduction with plates and screws is rarely used in North America except for unstable metaphyseal fractures or polytrauma patients with ipsilateral lower extremity injuries in which other techniques are not possible. Interest continues in this area with emphasis on indirect reduction techniques and even percutaneous plate application even though these efforts are still investigational. Ruedi *et al.* [11], using anatomic reduction and stable fixation with a dynamic compression plate as described by Müller *et al.* [5], achieved 93% good functional results in a closed group with a 6% failure rate. Johner and Wruhs [4], using plate and screw fixation also as described by Müller *et al.* [5], noted an increase in complications to 9.5% with simple fracture patterns and to 48% with comminuted fractures with a respective increase in infection rates from 2.1% to 10%. Nonunion was twice as common and infection five times as common when open fractures were plated compared with closed fractures. These difficulties and the inability of many surgeons to obtain the excellent results of Ruedi *et al.* [11] have dampened enthusiasm in North America for open reduction and plate and screw fixation for tibial diaphyseal fractures.

External fixation has been applied primarily to open fractures but advocates exist for its application in closed tibial fracture treatment [12]. The anterior crest of the tibia and the medial aspect of the tibia are preferred sites for percutaneous half-pin external fixation systems for two reasons. First, because of the unobstructed area, the external fixator can be placed very close to the extremity, thus increasing its mechanical stability. Second, because no muscle tendon units are transfixed by the pins, functional movement of the foot and ankle is not impaired. With external fixation techniques, when the diaphysis is intact above and below the fracture, the diaphyseal portions of the tibia are best managed with half-pin bicortical fixation, but in the metaphyseal regions, transfixion techniques with small wires have demonstrated greater mechanical stability and longevity. This modality is of use in patients with tibial fractures in conjunction with compartment syndrome and multitrauma patients with head injuries, burns, or impaired sensation.

Dynamization of the fracture treated with external fixation has been reported with passive and active techniques. Research and clinical studies thus far have been inconclusive on the advantage of passive dynamization. Dynamization seems to aid primarily in closing gaps at fracture sites if activated within the first 6 weeks. Kenwright *et al.* [13] have shown a significant improvement in time to union with active dynamization, but it has not yet reached clinical utility in North America. Richardson *et al.* [14] reported on a series of 219 patients with closed and open injuries in which they were able to use the external fixator to measure the fracture stiffness by strain gauge measurement through the fixator. Interestingly, they found that the stiffness of 15 Newton meters per degree in the sagittal plane provided a useful definition for union of the tibial fracture. With this protocol, they were able to eliminate refractures in the study group that achieved 15 Newton meters per degree of stiffness. These two aspects of external fixation, active dynamization, and telemetry through the frame are potential benefits for clinical use in the future.

Reamed interlocking intramedullary nailing for closed tibial fractures most closely realizes the optimal solution for surgical treatment of diaphyseal tibial fractures. Use of intramedullary nails for tibial fracture stabilization effectively began with the techniques of Kuntscher and Lottes [15]. Unlocked nails were frequently unable to maintain the reduction of the fracture even when reaming was used to place larger implants for better fatigue life. Ender-type nails were used in the 1970s and 1980s with good results in stable fractures but have been surpassed by the interlocking nail. These specialized interlocking nails with custom wall and section modulation were designed to withstand stresses incurred with healing tibial fractures. The addition of interlocking screws to aid in prevention of axial and rotational deformities became widely accepted. Bone and Johnson [16] reported on 112 fractures of the tibia treated by reamed and intramedullary nailing. They obtained a 99% union rate, a 6% infection rate, and a nonunion rate of less than 3%. Only 5% of patients had shortening of 1 cm or more. These results have been replicated by a number of surgeons from different countries and institutions. Using interlocking nails with nonreamed techniques in closed fractures has met with mixed results. Because of a higher screw breakage rate, sometimes up to 40% with weight bearing programs with small diameter nails, some authors have tried unreamed interlocking nail technique combinations with delayed weight bearing or none at all [17]. Riemer *et al.* [18] used a nonreamed interlocking nail technique with non–weight bearing with prolonged time to union of 32 weeks with 42% requiring reoperations including exchange nailing, dynamization, and bone grafting to obtain union. These patients were in a delayed weight-bearing program because of the concern for implant failure with small-diameter interlocking nail designs. Most authors now recommend minimal reaming to 1 mm larger than the nail diameter and reaming only 1 mm of cortex if possible with early weight-bearing.

Difficulties have been encountered when surgeons have tried to extend tibial intramedullary nailing techniques to proximal and distal metaphyseal fractures and when trying to decide when to statically rather than dynamically interlock the nail. Intramedullary nails that do not fill the medullary canal offer little or no resistance to deforming forces without interlocking screw supplementation [19]. Even with interlocking screws, if the nail does not prevent translational deformation of the fracture, instability will result in higher implant failure rates and loss of fracture position.

Interlocking nails do not provide sufficient stability in metaphyseal fractures alone. This can result in higher malunion and nonunion rates, particularly when the proximal and distal limits are pushed to the extreme. These problems are exacerbated when the surgeon dynamizes the interlocking nail construct, resulting in increased instability of the nail bone construct and increased rate of fatigue failure and loss of reduction. Templeman *et al.* [20] have found that segmentally comminuted and long spiral fractures benefit from static locking. Another complication unique to intramedullary nailing is residual knee pain. Not all pain is related to the nail prominence and not all knee pain will be resolved with nail removal [21,22]. The solution to this complication remains elusive.

Recently, prospective data are becoming available comparing nonoperative treatment with intramedullary nailing. Hooper *et al.* [23] performed a prospective randomized study comparing traditional conservative management and a weight-bearing program with reamed interlocking intramedullary nailing of the tibia. The study groups included patients with isolated tibial fractures displaced 50% or more or angulated 10° or more, closed and grade I open fractures in skeletally mature patients with the fracture zone at least 5 cm from the knee and ankle. During the study, 24% of the cast group failed and were treated with intramedullary nailing. The nonoperative group required 200% more radiographs, 62% more office visits, 70% more time off from work, and experienced a malunion rate 10 times greater than that of the nail group. The authors concluded that nonoperative treatments were indicated only in nondisplaced fractures. They placed significant importance on the decreased time to union, rate of malunion, and the improved functional rehabilitation of the patients in the intramedullary nail treatment group.

In another comparative series by Bone *et al.* [24], the authors found a significant increase in time to union for casted patients compared with reamed interlocking intramedullary nail patients with 26 weeks required on average for casted patients and 18 weeks required for the nail group. Nonunion rates were also significant, with a 10% rate for casted patients compared with a 2% rate for nailed patients. This study also applied functional outcome measurements, which confirmed better function and patient satisfaction with intramedullary nailing. Downing *et al.* [25] have found that the differences in cost between casting and nailing disappear when the total costs of lost work time and benefits during treatment are added to the hospitalization charges; nails then become less expensive than closed treatment.

For closed, isolated tibia–fibula fractures in the diaphyseal region within 5 cm of the joint proximally and distally, the treatment with the highest recorded rate of success and functional improvement of the patients is the reamed interlocking intramedullary nail with a closed technique.

OPEN FRACTURES

Treatment of open fractures of the tibia may best be considered as an exercise in applied microbiology and host defense mechanisms. There are five key procedures for successful treatment of the open fracture. First, radical débridement and pulsed lavage irrigation are necessary to dilute the bacterial innoculum and remove necrotic tissue, which can serve as a site of bacterial adherence required for bacterial replication. Second, the fracture must be stabilized with minimal further devascularization of injured soft tissues to maximize the vascularity of the remaining zone of injury and provide stability for soft tissue repair. Third, antibiotic therapy (usually cephalosporins and, in Gustilo and Anderson [7] Type III open fractures, the addition of an aminoglycoside in bactericidal doses for 3 to 5 days) reduces the surviving population of reproducing bacterial cells that escaped débridement. The remaining bacterial population, in addition to tissue that undergoes necrosis after the first débridement, makes repeat débridements mandatory in crush and severely contaminated wounds, because all necrotic tissue will not be evident at the initial débridement. Fourth, soft-tissue coverage should be obtained within 4 to 7 days with whatever plastic procedure will yield the most stable wound environment with the least functional compromise to the patient. Reconstitution of skin coverage restores an effective barrier to secondary bacterial contamination. Fifth, functional rehabilitation and preemptive bone grafting in high-energy trauma and bone loss maximize the fatigue life of the internal or external fixation and shorten the time of recovery for the patient.

Burgess *et al.* [26] demonstrated the need for removal of all avascular tissue, including bony fragments. They reported a decrease in time to union of 64% (from 58.4 weeks to 37.6 weeks) for ordinary Type III open tibial fractures during the evolution of their protocol. They recommended sharp débridement, copious pulsed lavage, scheduled repeat débridement every 24 hours, judicious use of internal fixation, early grafting or free-flap coverage of soft-tissue defects, anterior half-pin external fixation, early prophylactic bone grafting by 3 to 4 weeks after injury, and gradual disassembly of the external frame. Retention of large avascular bony fragments has been advocated for structural considerations, but with newer techniques of antibiotic bead pouches and bone grafting and intercalary limb regeneration, as described by Ilizarov [27], bony reconstruction is usually attainable without the increased risk of sepsis by retention of avascular fragments.

Stabilization of the extremity benefits the treatment of the fracture and soft tissues. External fixation and interlocking intramedullary nails with a nonreamed technique have gained widespread acceptance over cast and plate-and-screw techniques in the open fracture. Behrens *et al.* [28] outlined the general principles of external fixation of the tibia using half-pin techniques. Loss of reduction and a higher malunion rate using initial external fixation and then transition to long leg casting have led most surgeons to ascribe to one of three fixation strategies: treat the open fracture to union with external fixation, attempt to convert the external fixation to intramedullary nailing as soon as a stable

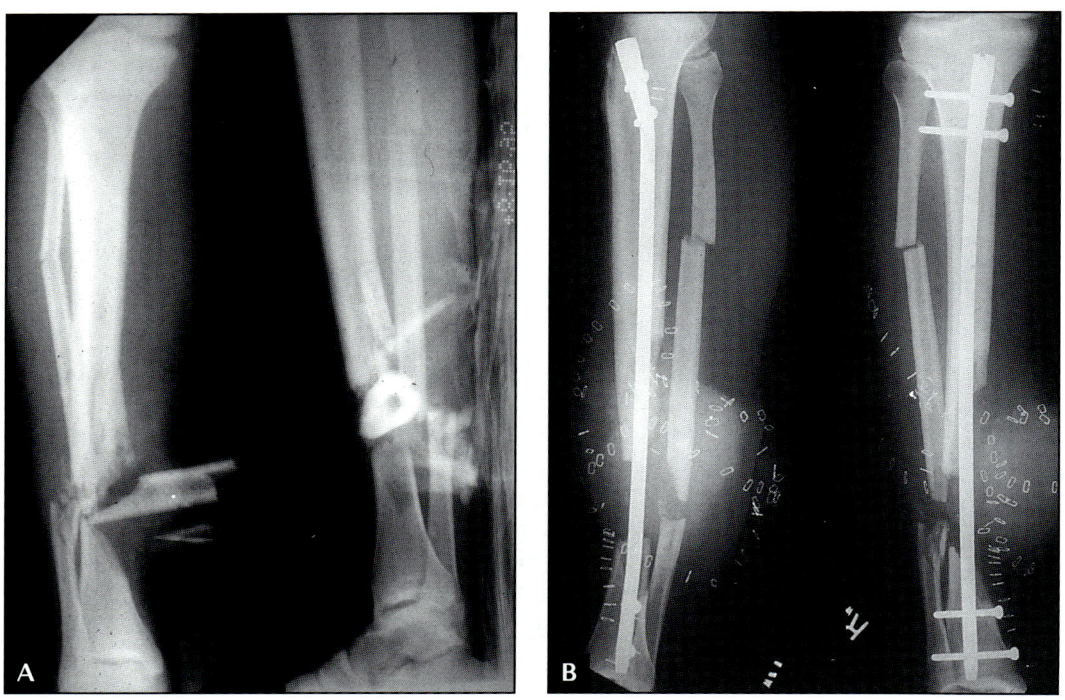

FIGURE 16-3. A and B, Type IIIB open fracture treated with nonreamed interlocking tibial nailing. Free flap has been applied for wound closure. Segmental loss will be grafted at 8 weeks post injury.

wound is obtained or treat the open fracture with acute interlocking nailing with or without reaming [21–37].

Caudle and Stern [29], reviewing 62 Type III open fractures treated with external fixation noted a correlation with Gustilo *et al.*'s [8] classification of Type III injuries with significant difference in these groups. The Type IIIA fractures had no infections and a 28% nonunion rate. The 42 Type IIIB fractures had a 35% nonunion rate, 39% infection rate, and 17% amputation rate. In the IIIB subgroup that had early flap coverage, the nonunion rate, infection rate and amputation rate decreased the infection rate to 21% and the amputation rate to 8%. In the Type IIIC fractures, 78% resulted in amputation and the remaining 22% were considered poor results.

Whittle *et al.* [31] reported the on the development and use of closed-section interlocking intramedullary nails designed with smaller diameters and modified section modulus characteristics to allow insertion with nonreamed techniques. In 50 open tibial fractures with 68% Type III (A-22, B-12), the infection rate was 0% for grade I and II fractures, 5% for Type IIIA fractures, and 25% in Type IIIB fractures. The union rate was 96% and 36% were dynamized or bone grafted. No malunions were evident at follow-up (Figure 16-3).

Henley *et al.* [38], in a prospective randomized study comparing external fixation with intramedullary nails, found the primary differences between external fixation and nonreamed interlocking intramedullary nails to be a higher malunion rate, pin-tract infection problems, and more operations required to obtain union with external fixation. In Type II, IIIA, and IIIB open fractures, union rates for the nail group were 92% compared with 88% for external fixation; 0.6 secondary procedures were required for the nail group compared with 2.5 for the external fixation group. Malunions occurred in 24% of the external fixation group with and no malunions occurred in the nail group. It is believed that the loss of reduction during the course of treatment of the tibia with the external fixator system implies loss of stability of the fracture construct due to slippage of the connections with external fixation systems. As such, all connections should be checked at frequent follow-up visits to prevent loss of reduction. Several authors have confirmed Henley *et al.*'s [38] finding that nonreamed interlocking intramedullary nailing for acute open tibial fractures is equivalent, if not superior, to conventional external fixation [39–40]. Debate now centers on which Type III fractures can be treated with reaming in addition to interlocking nailing to avoid some complications of small diameter nails without increasing the infection rate [41]. However, minimal reaming without the use of a tourniquet with sharp reamers with low pressure must be strictly enforced as part of the technique. It does appear from the work of Marsh *et al.* [30] and others that there may be a difference in the new generation of external fixators with regard to control of the fracture to avoid malunions. A Type IIIA fracture may be treated effectively with either external fixation or intramedullary nailing with fairly low complication rates if the biologic principles are maintained. The Type IIIB fracture in most series an infection rate between 5% and 50% depending on soft tissue viability, a malunion rate between 5% and 30%, and a nonunion rate between 10% and 20%. The Type IIIC injury evokes the most controversy regarding limb salvage versus amputation because the surgeon is compromised by the emotional impact of amputation on the patient and concerns about possible litigation (Figure 16-4). Conversely, unsuccessful limb salvage may truly compromise a patient's return to being a functioning member of society, resulting in loss of employment, continuing medical problems such as drug addiction, and loss of family unit integrity.

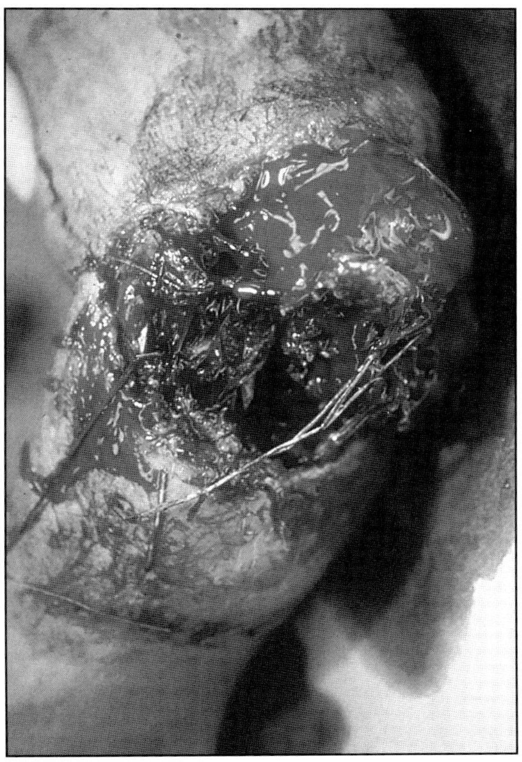

FIGURE 16-4. Severe open tibial fracture with gross contamination and 12 hours of ischemic time from four-wheeler accident. Amputation was performed as definitive treatment acutely.

Current prospective studies have documented the ability to salvage the severe open tibia fractures frequently. In a study by Georgiadis *et al.* [42] comparing functional outcome, they found that patients who underwent a long limb salvage viewed themselves as more disabled than patients with below-the-knee amputation. They also documented a higher economic cost and a longer period of disability in limb-salvage patients over that of patients with below-the-knee amputations. The *American Medical Association Guidelines for Permanent Physical Impairment* [cited in 43] assign the patient a lower permanent physical impairment for limb salvage over amputation. This may reflect less sensitivity in the rating system rather than improvement over the functional results of limb salvage over amputation.

Most authors currently recommend amputation in Type IIIC open tibial fractures. The limb salvage scoring system advocated by Helfet *et al.* [44] relates amputation versus limb salvage success based on time from injury, warm ischemia time, presence of shock, and severity of injury. McNamara *et al.* [45] modified the mangled extremity severity score (MESS) to include neural injury and to separate soft tissue and bone grading with a preliminary increased incidence of sensitivity. Although helpful in decision making, it has not been sufficiently validated by other studies to permit its endorsement by the general orthopedic community for prospective amputations.

COMPLICATIONS

NONUNION

Wiss *et al.* [46] reported excellent results with compression plating technique for nonunion of the tibia with deformity. Helfet *et al.* [47], in another study, used the femoral distractor for reduction and plate fixation with indirect reduction for displaced nonunion, which offers significant advantages over intramedullary nailing if previous external fixation has left previous sites of occult pin-site osteomyelitis that might be exacerbated with reamed nailing techniques. Reamed intramedullary nailing has also been shown to be effective with or without fibular osteotomy for deformity correction [48]. If impaired biologic response is evident by poor callus formation or atrophic bone, autologous bone grafting should be added to the mechanical construct. For the nonunion complicating a previous nailed fracture, exchange-reamed interlocking nailing in a dynamic mode (if axial stability is obtained) or static mode (if axial stability is not present) is an elegant solution to the nonunion (Figure 16-5) [49].

Infection

All external fixation series for open tibial fractures demonstrate a fairly constant rate of pin tract infection, usually 50%. These problems generally respond to local conservative measures or exchange of pin or wire fixation. Pin tract infections are a source of concern because of the use of intramedullary nailing as a salvage procedure for nonunion. This has led some surgeons to recommend plate fixation for nonunion following failed external fixation because of concern about intramedullary sepsis. This relationship relates more to previous pin tract infection and the time of external fixation application before nail treatment than any other factor. Intramedullary nailing is rarely recommended in the presence of an acute infection. If preexisting pin-tract deep sepsis exists, an exchange treatment from external fixation to nailing should probably be avoided.

The issue of infection with intramedullary nailing now seems to be more a factor of initial surgical débridement and soft tissue coverage rather than the nail technique. Infection rates of between 1% and 5% are frequently reported in closed tibial nail studies. Infection after intramedullary nailing has found to be more readily treatable than previously thought [50]. Current recommendations are to maintain the nail in place if it is providing stability and to suppress the infection until fracture healing occurs and then proceed with removal of the nail and débridement of the canal. If the implant is unstable, it should be removed with débridement; irrigation should be performed and the extremity stabilized with external fixation along with appropriate antibiotics and soft tissue treatment. In dealing with infection of the tibia after a fracture, treatment should be based on the extent of the infection and the tissue planes involved; this is best handled in centers specializing in these techniques.

Compartment Syndromes

The surgeon must have a high index of suspicion and a low threshold for intervention for compartment syndrome even in open fractures. Compartment pressure monitoring has become readily available and is especially helpful in patients who are comatose or unresponsive because of other injuries. A patient with symptoms and signs of compartment syndrome does not require compartment pressure measurements before proceeding with fasciotomy. The issue of compartment syndromes induced by intramedullary nailing has received a great deal of attention; however, studies have documented increased compartment pressure primarily at the time of reduction of the fracture with both closed and operative treatments.

Compartment syndromes, if unrecognized, frequently result in contractures of the leg and foot, but contractures may also occur from trapping of muscle-tendon units in fracture fragments or fixation systems. Functional treatment of the extremity with early mobilization of the joints of the foot and ankle help minimize this problem or alert the physician to its presence. Neurologic deficits occur with tibial fractures whether they are treated with closed or operative modalities. Frequently, these are neuropraxic injuries resulting in a peroneal nerve palsy. They can be quite troublesome to the patient, for whom they are a source of continued disability. Overdistraction of the tibia should especially be avoided (Figure 16-6).

CONCLUSIONS

With all the technologic advances in the treatment of tibial fractures, much work still remains. The literature has too few studies intended to select the optimal treatment for the individual; it must therefore be left to the judgment of the orthopedic surgeon attending the individual patient [51]. Continuing development of better functional outcome rating systems and better classification agreement between surgeons is required.

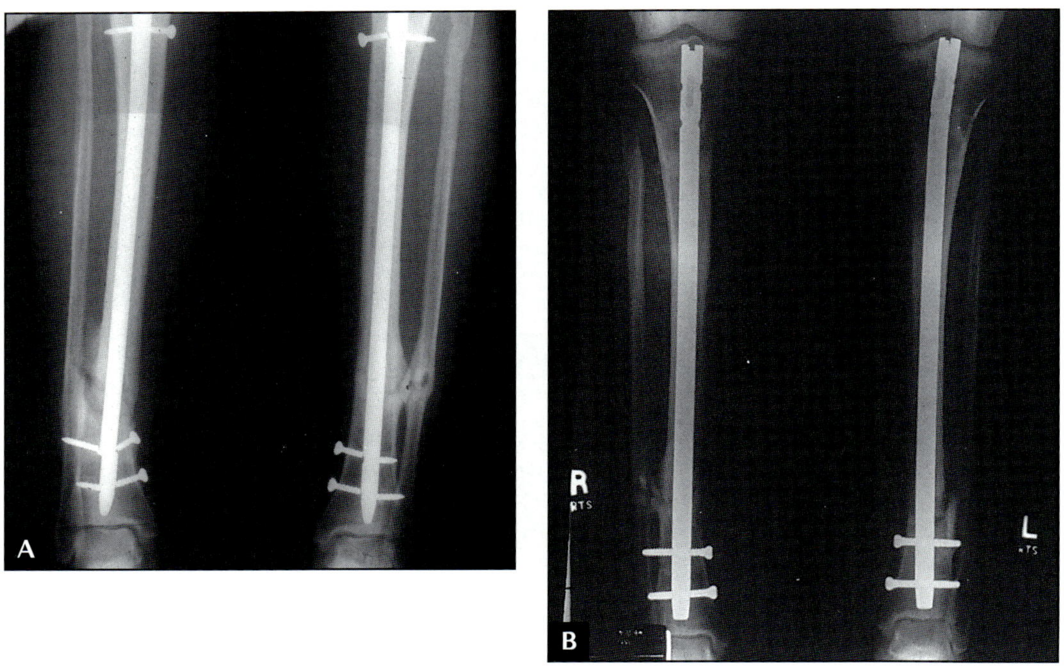

Figure 16-5. A, Nonunion of both tibial fractures with broken interlocking screws and right nail. B, Patient was treated with exchange nailing after open removal of broken nails and screws.

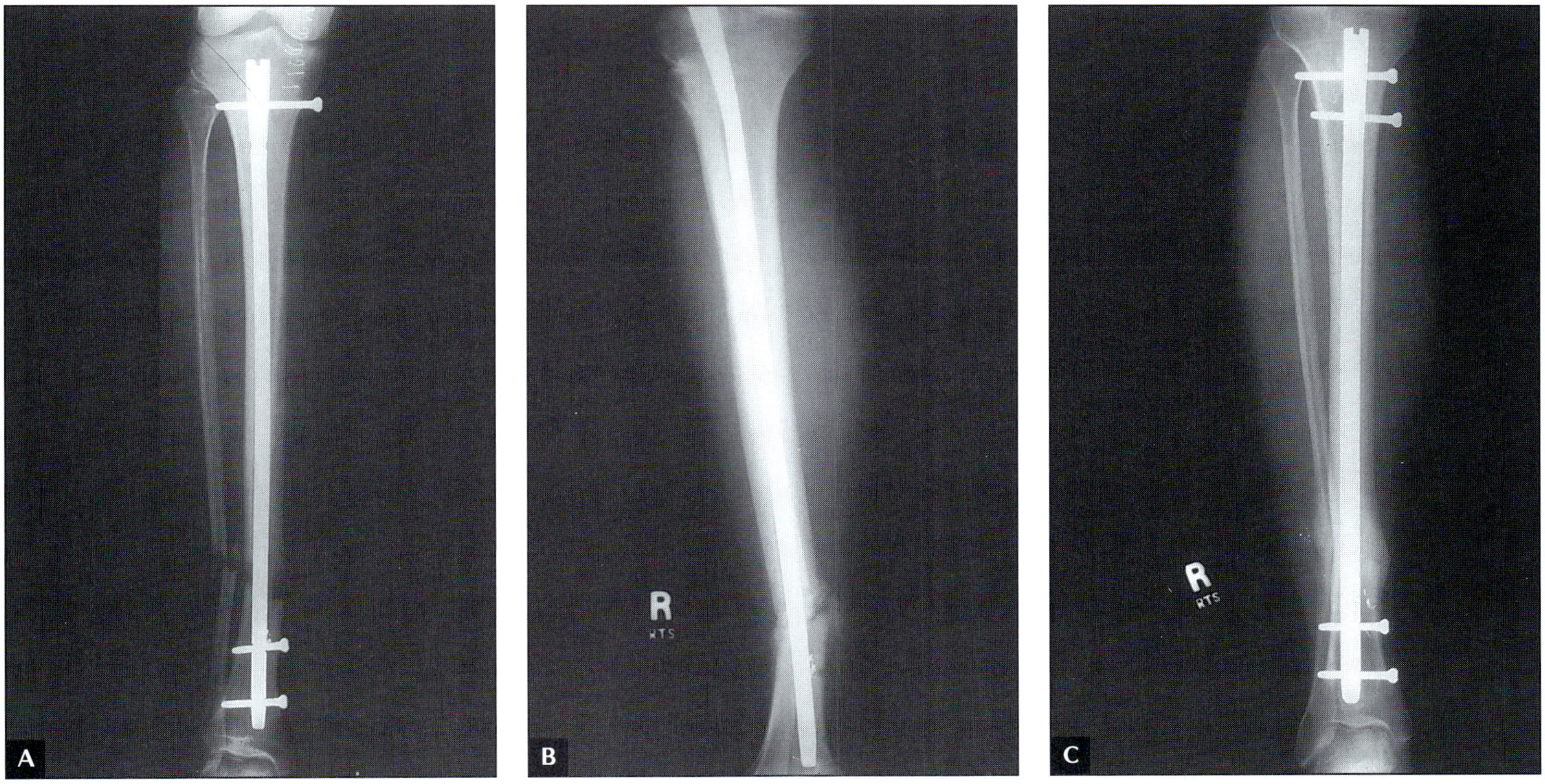

FIGURE 16-6. A, Distraction from nonreamed nailing of closed tibial fracture. Note one screw proximal with slight backing out and fibula distracted along with tibia. B, Loss of alignment with removal of screws with valgus malposition and proximal migration of nail. Gap was closed, but with loss of stability and alignment after dynamization. C, Union and correction of deformity with reamed static interlocking nail.

REFERENCES AND RECOMMENDED READING

Recently published papers of particular interest have been highlighted as:
- • Of interest
- •• Of outstanding interest

1. Court-Brown CM, McBirnie J: The epidemiology of tibial fractures. *J Bone Joint Surg* 1995, 77:417–421.
2. Green SA: *Complication of External Fixation*. Springfield, IL: Charles C. Thomas; 1981.
3. Macnab I, de Haas WG: The role of periosteal blood supply in the healing of fractures of the tibia. *Clin Orthop* 1974, 105:27–34.
4. Johner R, Wruhs O: Classification of tibial shaft fractures and correlation with results of rigid internal fixation. *Clin Orthop* 1983, 178:7–25.
5. Müller ME, Nazarian S, Koch P, *et al.*: *The Comprehensive Classification of Fractures of Long Bones*. New York: Springer-Verlag; 1990.
6. Orthopedic Trauma Association Committee for Coding and Classification: Fracture and dislocation compendium. *J Orthop Trauma* 1996, 10(suppl):1–154.
7. Gustilo RB, Anderson JT: Prevention of infection in the treatment of 1025 open fractures of log bones. *J Bone Joint Surg* 1976, 58:453–458.
8. Gustilo RB, Mendoza RM, Williams DN: Problems in the management of type III (severe) open fractures: a new classification of type III open fractures. *J Trauma* 1984, 24:742–746.
9. Oni OOA, Hui A, Gregg PJ: The healing of closed tibial shaft fractures: the natural history of union with closed treatment. *J Bone Joint Surg* 1988, 70:787–790.
10. Sarmiento A, Gersten LM, Sobol PA, *et al.*: Tibial shaft fractures treated with functional braces: experience with 780 fractures. *J Bone Joint Surg* 1989, 71:602–609.
11. Ruedi T, Webb JK, Allgower M: Experience with the dynamic compression plate (DCP) in 418 recent fractures of the tibial shaft. *Injury* 1976, 7:252–257.
12. De Bastinani G, Aldegheri R, Renzi-Brivio L: The treatment of fractures with a dynamic axial fixator. *J Bone Joint Surg* 1984, 66:538–545.
13. Kenwright J, Richardson JB, Cunningham JL, *et al.*: Axial movement and tibial fractures. *J Bone Joint Surg Br* 1991, 73:654–659.
14. Richardson JB, Cunningham JL, Goodship AE, *et al.*: Measuring stiffness can define healing of tibial fractures. *J Bone Joint Surg* 1994, 76:389–394.
15. Lottes JO: Blind nailing technique for insertion of the triflange medullary nail. *JAMA* 1954, 155:1039.
16. Bone LB, Johnson KD: Treatment of tibial fractures by reaming and intramedullary nailing. *J Bone Joint Surg* 1986, 68:877–887.
17. Gregory P, Sanders R: The treatment of closed, unstable tibial shaft fractures with unreamed interlocking nails. *Clin Orthop* 1995, 315:48.
18. Riemer BL, DiChristina DG, Cooper A, *et al.*: Nonreamed nailing of tibial diaphyseal fractures in blunt polytrauma patients. *J Orthop Trauma* 1995, 9:66–75.
19. Court-Brown CM, Christie J, McQueen MM: Closed intramedullary tibial nailing: its use in closed and type I open fractures. *J Bone Joint Surg* 1990, 72:605–611.
20. Templeman D, Larson C, Varecka T, Kyle RF: Decision making errors in the use of interlocking tibial nails. *Clin Orthop* 1997, 339:65–70.
21. Koval, KJ, Clapper MF, Brumback RJ, *et al.*: Complications of reamed intramedullary nailing of the tibia. *J Orthop Trauma* 1991, 5:184–189.
22. Court-Brown CM, Gustilo T, Shaw AD: Knee pain after intramedullary tibial nailing: its incidence, etiology, and outcome. *J Orthop Trauma* 1997, 11:103–105.
23. Hooper GJ, Keddell RG, Penny ID: Conservative management or closed nailing for tibial shaft fractures: a randomised prospective trial. *J Bone Joint Surg* 1991, 73:83–85.

24. Bone LB, Sucato D, Stegemann PM, Rohrbacher BJ: Displaced isolated fractures of the tibial shaft treated with either a cast or intramedullary nailing: an outcome analysis of matched pairs of patients. *J Bone Joint Surg* 1997, 79A:1336–1341.
25. Downing ND, Griffin DR, Davis TR: A comparison of the relative costs of cast treatment and intramedullary nailing for tibial diaphyseal fractures in the UK. *Injury* 1997, 28:373–375.
26. Burgess AR, Poka A, Brumback RJ, *et al.*: Pedestrian tibial injuries. *J Trauma* 1987, 27:596–601.
27. Ilizarov GA: The tension-stress effect on the genesis and growth of tissues. *Clin Orthop* 1989, 239:263–285.
28. Behrens F, Comfort TH, Searls K, *et al.*: Unilateral external fixation of severe open tibial fractures: preliminary report of a prospective study. *Clin Orthop* 1983, 178:111–120.
29. Caudle RJ, Stern PJ: Severe open fractures of the tibia. *J Bone Joint Surg* 1987, 69:801–807.
30. Marsh JL, Nepola JV, Wuest TK, *et al.*: Unilateral external fixation until healing with the dynamic axial fixator for severe open tibial fractures. *J Orthop Trauma* 1991, 5:341–348.
31. Whittle AP, Russell TA, Taylor JC, Lavelle DG: Treatment of open fractures of the tibial shaft with the use of interlocking nailing without reaming. *J Bone Joint Surg* 1992, 74:1162–1171.
32. Keating JF, O'Brien PJ, Blachut PA, *et al.*: Locked intramedullary nailing with and without reaming for open fractures of the tibial shaft: a prospective randomized study. *J Bone Joint Surg* 1997, 79:334–341.
33. Blachut PA, Meek RN, O'Brien PJ: External fixation and delayed intramedullary nailing of open fractures of the tibial shaft: a sequential protocol. *J Bone Joint Surg* 1990, 72:729–735.
34. McGraw JM, Lim EVA: Treatment of open tibial shaft fractures: external fixation and secondary intramedullary nailing. *J Bone Joint Surg* 1988, 70:900–911.
35. Mauer DJ, Merkow RL, Gustilo RB: Infection after intramedullary nailing of severe open tibial fractures initially treated with external fixation. *J Bone Joint Surg* 1989, 71:835–838.
36. Fischer MD, Gustilo RB, Varecka TF: The timing of flap coverage, bone-grafting, and intramedullary nailing in patients who have a fracture of the tibial shaft with extensive soft-tissue injury. *J Bone Joint Surg* 1991, 73:1316–1322.
37. Antich-Androver P, Marti-Garin D, Murias-Alvarez J, Puente-Alonso C: External fixation and secondary intramedullary nailing of open tibial fractures: a randomized prospective trial. *J Bone Joint Surg* 1997, 79:433–437.
38. Henley MB, Chapman JR, Agel J, *et al.*: Treatment of type II, IIIA, and IIIB open fractures of the tibial shaft: a prospective comparison of unreamed interlocking intramedullary nails and half-pin external fixators. *J Orthop Trauma* 1998, 12:1–7.
39. Schandelmaier P, Krettek C, Rudolf J, *et al.*: Superior results of tibial rodding versus external fixation in grade 3B fractures. *Clin Orthop* 1997, 342:164–172.
40. Tornetta P III, Bergman M, Waknik N, *et al.*: Treatment of grade-IIIb open tibial fractures: a prospective randomized comparison of external fixation and non-reamed locked nailing. *J Bone Joint Surg* 1994, 76B:13–19.
41. Whittle AP, Wester W, Russell TA: Fatigue failure in small diameter interlocking tibial nails: implications for postoperative care. *Clin Orthop* 1995, 136:119–128.
42. Georgiadis G, Behrens F, Joyce M, *et al.*: Open tibial fractures with severe soft tissue loss: limb salvage compared with below-the-knee amputation. *J Bone Joint Surg* 1993, 1:75.
43. Kemp A, van Niekerk J, van Meurs P: Impairment scores of type III open tibial fractures. *Injury* 1993, 24:161–162.
44. Helfet CK, Howey T, Sanders R, Johansen K: Limb salvage versus amputation: preliminary results of the mangled extremity severity score. *Clin Orthop* 1990, 256:80–86.
45. McNamara MG, Heckman JD, Corley FG: Severe open fractures of the lower extremity: a retrospective evaluation of the mangled extremity severity score (MESS). *J Orthop Trauma* 1994, 8:81–87.
46. Wiss DA, Johnson DL, Miao M: Compression plating for non-union after failed external fixation of open tibial fractures. *J Bone Joint Surg* 1992, 74:1279–1285.
47. Helfet DL, Jupiter JB, Gasser S: Indirect reduction and tension-band plating of tibial non-union with deformity. *J Bone Joint Surg* 1992, 74A:1286–1295.
48. Wiss DA, Stetson WB: Nonunion of the tibia treated with a reamed intramedullary nail. *J Orthop Trauma* 1994, 8:189–194.
49. Court-Brown CM, Keating JF, Christie J, McQueen MM: Exchange intramedullary nailing. *J Bone Joint Surg* 1994, 77:407–411.
50. Court-Brown CM, Keating JF, McQueen MM: Infection after intramedullary nailing of the tibia: incidence and protocol for management. *J Bone Joint Surg* 1992, 74:770–774.
51. Littenberg B, Weinstein LP, McCarren M, *et al.*: Closed fractures of the tibial shaft: a meta-analysis of three methods of treatment. *J Bone Joint Surg* 1998, 80:174–183.

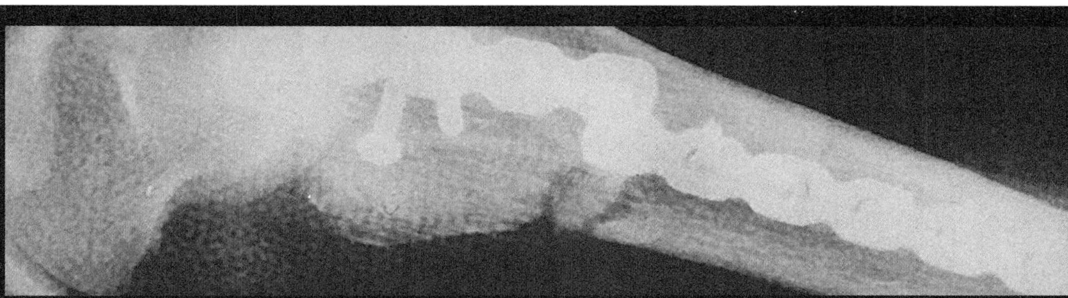

17

Pilon Fractures

Vasilios Mathews
Lon S. Weiner

Fractures of the distal tibia are among the most challenging injuries to treat in orthopedic surgery. Fracture patterns, articular involvement, and associated soft tissue injuries are confounding factors of variable involvement in each of these fractures. The common saying that each fracture has its "own personality" is one that each orthopedic surgeon should keep in mind when confronted with a pilon fracture. Even so, certain basic tenets, which are reviewed and commented on in this chapter, should be recognized by physicians treating these fractures.

Pilon fractures are produced by a force that causes impaction of the talus against the distal tibia. In general, the greater the force, the more damage that will be done. The position of the foot during this vertical force affects the fracture pattern: plantarflexion causes more posterior injuries, and dorsiflexion causes more anterior injuries. Angulation and rotatory forces at the foot during injury play a key role in the pattern of metaphyseal involvement [1].

The fundamental characteristic of these fractures is involvement of the distal tibial metaphysis, proximal to the articular surface. Degrees of articular involvement, comminution, cartilage damage, and soft tissue injuries further confound the picture.

PRINCIPLES OF TREATMENT

Despite the individual variability of pilon fractures, certain fundamental principles must be observed to address them in a systematic, logical fashion. Initial treatment consists of identification of all injuries, attention to soft tissue and neurovascular status, reduction, immobilization, and traction. Finally, the principles of definitive fixation come into play. These include anatomic restoration of the articular surface and sufficiently stable fixation for early range of motion. These principles must be weighed against the desire for soft tissue integrity and limited further stripping for adequate bony healing.

CLASSIFICATION

Several classification schemes for fractures involving the distal tibial region have been proposed. These include Ruedi and Allgower's [2] descriptive system (*ie,* I to III), centered on the presence or absence of articular displacement and comminution, and its subsequent various modifications by other authors. A more common method of classification is the AO system, which has been shown to have moderate interobserver agreement [3,4]. This construct separates fractures according to pattern of articular involvement, pattern of metaphyseal involvement, and the relationship of the articular surface to the distal tibial metaphysis. Type B3 and all Type C fractures have significant articular and metaphyseal components and thus should be considered pilon fractures [5•].

ASSOCIATED INJURIES

This aspect of diagnosis is critical to the management of pilon fractures. The forces capable of producing extensive comminution and displacement of bone have the same potential for causing severe damage to the overlying relatively sparse soft tissue of the distal tibial area. Important aspects to note include skin integrity and swelling. An open fracture or a fracture with potential for skin bullae and necrosis are potentially devastating determinants of outcome. Neurologic, vascular, and tendinous injuries are often found with careful examination (Figure 17-1). Attention should be placed on the possibility of an ensuing compartment syndrome.

IMAGING

Radiographic evaluation of pilon fractures must include anteroposterior (AP), lateral, and mortise views of the ankle. A 45° external rotation view can greatly aid in visualizing fragments and patterns in the oblique plane. Finally, a computed tomography (CT) scan with sagittal and coronal reconstructions is, in most cases, essential for preoperative planning before beginning definitive treatment. Recent studies have demonstrated that CT scans can improve clinical understanding of fracture pattern and can change the operative plan or add additional information in most cases (Figure 17-2) [6,7].

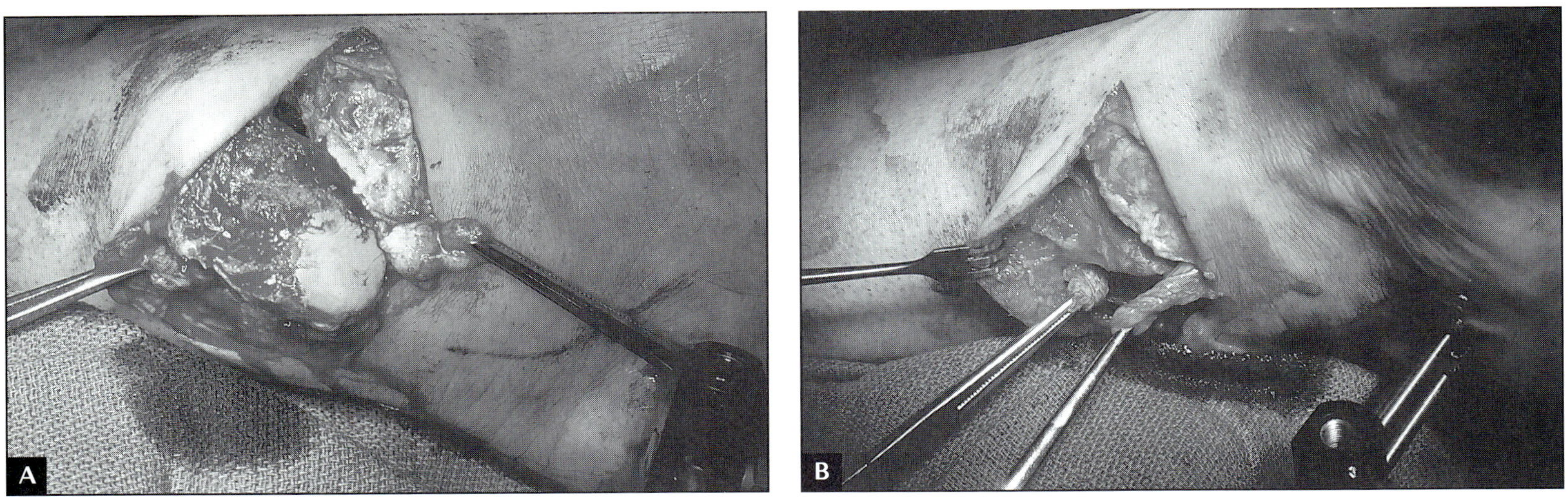

FIGURE 17-1. Open pilon fracture. Careful inspection revealed a tibialis posterior tendon rupture without damage to the neurovascular bundle. The tendon was repaired primarily at original operative débridement to avoid retraction and scarring. The patient eventually had excellent return of function.

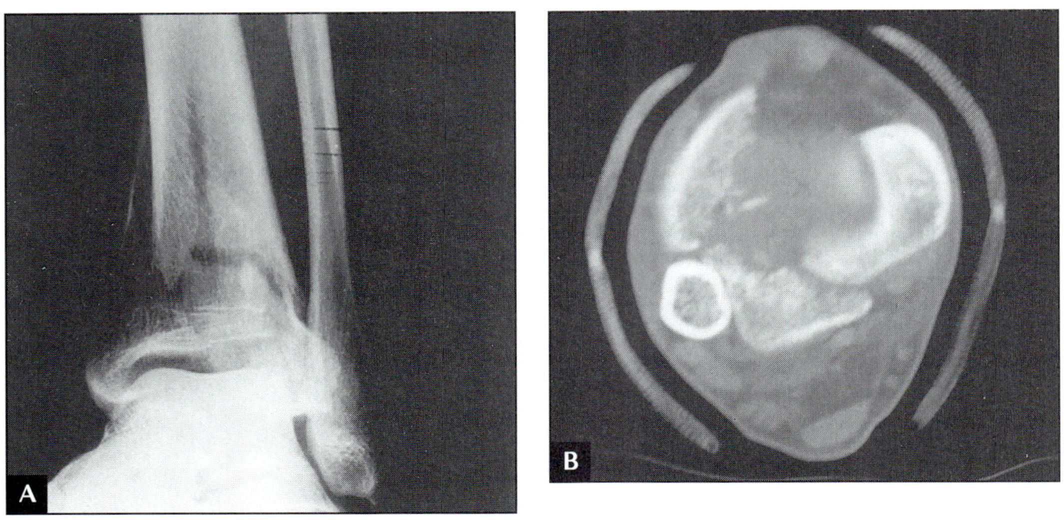

FIGURE 17-2. **A**, Pilon fracture with comminution at the articular surface. **B**, Computed tomography scan provides a more extensive illustration of the amount and nature of the comminution.

ANALYSIS CHECKLIST

An analysis checklist can be used to explore each of the various issues surrounding each pilon fracture and to fashion a plan of treatment.

SOFT TISSUES

Management of the surrounding soft tissue envelope is paramount. On presentation, immobilization and elevation are essential to prevent further compromise of the soft tissues.

Fracture hematoma and later intradermal edema cause significant swelling of the overlying soft tissues. Onset is almost immediate. Fracture blisters are common and can develop within hours to days. Ischemia of this swollen tissue can continue for almost a week and can be in the transitional zone well beyond the fracture site or open injury. Treatment of fracture blisters has been studied; aspiration, deroofing, sulvidine, open-air, and nonadherent dressing treatments were compared in a prospective study and showed no difference in infection or healing rates [8].

A decision as to when to intervene with surgery is critical and related to outcome. Excellent markers of soft tissue compromise include marked edema, contusions, abrasions, loss of skin wrinkles and palpable bony landmarks, and the presence of fracture blisters.

It is always acceptable to wait, in the absence of an open injury or compartment syndrome, because not doing so can be disastrous. No controversy has been raised about delayed open reduction with internal fixation (ORIF) in patients with severe fractures or with signs of severe soft tissue compromise. Numerous studies have reaffirmed the poor wound results obtained with immediate reconstruction in severe fractures [9]. The waiting period can be anywhere from a few days to 3 weeks. Markers of skin safety include the resolution of skin glossiness, epithelialization of blisters, and return of skin creases.

Fracture reapproximation and lengthening in the emergency department or operating room are two of the best things that the clinician can do to improve soft tissue compromise. Temporary traction is also important for disimpaction of metaphyseal comminution, which becomes more difficult as time passes (Figure 17-3).

When planning incisions, 7-cm skin bridges must be maintained to ensure that further soft tissue ischemia will not occur.

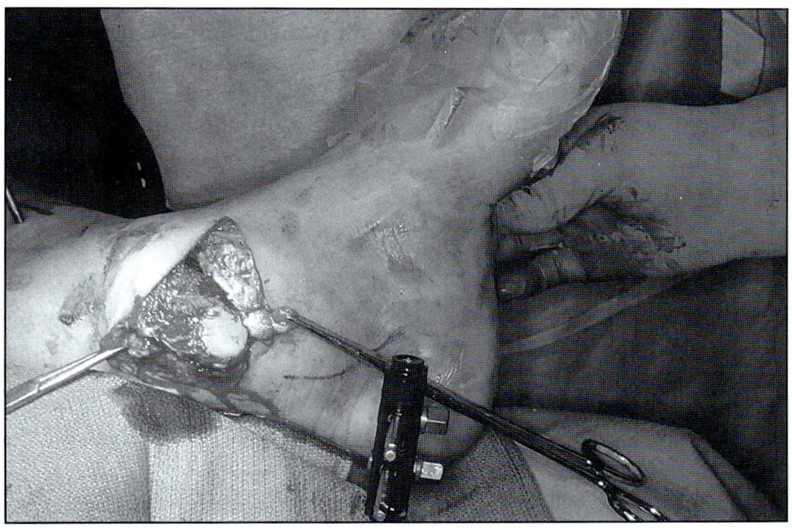

FIGURE 17-3. Use of the external fixator as primary fixation and traction device.

OPEN INJURIES

Although the general principles regarding the initial care of pilon fractures are the same, open injuries often require more thought, diligence, and care in the long run. They are, first of all, emergencies. The open fracture introduces certain important concepts, such as tetanus status, antibiotic coverage, and early— often multiple—débridements.

The importance of performing the definitive treatment in a sterile, healthy operative field is a basic principle known to all orthopedic surgeons. Some controversy exists as to the timing of final fixation in open fractures. Most recent studies advocate immediate definitive fixation in open fractures. These reviews in ankle fractures have shown good-to-excellent results of up to 87% with minimal infective complications [10,11]. However, caution must be used when extrapolating data from ankle fractures for guidance in the management of pilon fractures. A recent study of open pilon fractures treated definitively in an immediate fashion resulted in no infections [12]. These recent studies have shown that open injuries do not necessarily increase the risk of postoperative infection. The decision of primary versus delayed fixation in open fractures should depend on the degree of contamination and the severity of injury, which are qualitative rather than absolute judgments. A very recent study by Sirkin *et al.* [13•] demonstrated comparably minimal wound problems in severe open and closed fractures treated in a staged manner.

FRACTURE CHARACTERIZATION

Classification of the fracture highlights the individual anatomic characteristics that must be addressed so that crucial preoperative planning can be performed.

NONDISPLACED FRACTURES

The reflex response is to treat these fractures in a conservative manner, because very often they will heal with traction and immobilization. Frequently, however, the fracture pattern may not maintain its structural integrity with conservative treatment. In addition, it is well recognized that prolonged traction and immobilization contribute to joint stiffness, further articular damage, and atrophy [5•]. Although traction and immobilization are essential parts of treatment, their role is predominantly to temporize to obtain general stability of the patient or soft tissue recovery.

If possible, therefore, nondisplaced metaphyseal or articular fractures should be fixed to prevent the aforementioned complications.

UNRECONSTRUCTABLE FRACTURES

Among clinicians, there is often a reluctance to discuss this topic. The surgeon must recognize that primary amputation of the severely affected limb is a viable option, in the face of a result that will clearly be unacceptable, despite the most valiant efforts at limb salvage. In addition, arthrodesis, although not a good option primarily because of reported difficulties, is an acceptable procedure after soft tissue recovery and some return of bone stock [14].

PRINCIPLES OF OPERATIVE TREATMENT

Ruedi and Allgower [2] have outlined the four main issues of surgery in pilon fractures. These include restoration and maintenance of fibular length, anatomic restoration of the articular surface, attention to bone loss, and buttressing of the medial tibial column.

FIBULAR FRACTURE

Some authors believe that restoration of the tibial articular surface and metaphysis are not possible without restoration of fibular length [15]. In selected cases, this alone can be sufficient for tibial reduction. In addition to its role in reduction, fibular reconstruction is also considered critical for restoring the lateral distal tibiofibular architecture, thus preventing a valgus deformity.

Some confusion exists in the literature about the proper way to treat the fibula. In one study by multiple authors [16], no specific way of treating the fibula could be decided. Most authors advocate fibular reduction and fixation as long as the associated incision will not cause further soft tissue compromise.

The cautions with fibular fixation include taking care to leave an adequate skin bridge when making the posterolateral incision and avoiding overdistraction or varus of the tibial components of the fracture. If these occur, then fibular fixation should be abandoned in that specific case. One way to avoid a large lateral incision and possible exposure of hardware is intramedullary fibular fixation with a rod.

Articular Comminution

Reference points for the anatomic reconstruction of the tibial articular surface are the tibiofibular syndesmotic region and the talar articular surface. Often, these intact surfaces can give a hint as to the appropriate level of the joint. Provisional fixation can be achieved using minimally traumatic Kirschner wires and, after anatomic reduction has been confirmed, permanent fixation with screws can be performed [5•].

Metaphyseal Comminution and Bone Loss

In a fashion similar to that used in articular surface restoration, metaphyseal comminution can be provisionally fixed using wires and then transitioned to a more permanent fixation. Metaphyseal bone defects must be filled in with bone graft, preferably autologous, so that further stability and healing may be obtained. This is best performed as early as possible.

Articular–Metaphyseal–Diaphyseal Dissociation

Type C pilon fractures require reconstruction and buttressing of the longitudinal connection of the diaphysis to the articular surface. The two general ways to achieve this fixation are through plate fixation or external fixation. Care must be taken to avoid tibial devascularization, even at the expense of absolute stability, and to leave adequate skin bridges between incisions.

Plate fixation is the classic approach to these fractures. It remains appropriate, even as sole fixation, in the situations in which minimal soft tissue violation and predominantly metaphyseal involvement are present. Various plates can be used and fashioned to fit according to the specific fracture pattern. Most commonly, a 3.5-mm dynamic compression plate is applied for support of the medial column. Other techniques include cloverleaf or T plates or the *en-peigne* technique with fixation through the fibula and into the tibia in cases with severe soft tissue compromise medially.

External fixation allows further indirect reduction and does not further damage or inhibit access to soft tissues. Numerous options are available for external fixation. These include the choice of spanning the joint if necessary. Also occasionally used is the articulated external fixator, although questions still remain with respect to movement across the fracture site, infection, and loosening [17].

Hybrid external fixation using light-gauge wires is less traumatic to the soft tissues, requires less intact cancellous bone, and can capture smaller metaphyseal fragments. These fixators are best used in situations without significant articular comminution [5•,14,18].

A combination of external fixation with limited internal fixation is a significant recent trend in pilon fracture treatment, especially in the more severe AO Type C3 fractures. This combination allows the surgeon to take advantage of the benefits of both types of fixation. Limited internal fixation includes interfragmentary screws or a dynamic compression plate (DCP) (Figure 17-4).

Controversy still exists as to the choice of fixation. The key to understanding the treatment of these fractures is to understand some of the history, and thus the way in which new treatment concepts have evolved. Classic ORIF with plating along the anteromedial tibia was first popularized when Ruedi and Allgower [2] showed 74% good-to-excellent results. Authors in the 1980s were unable to repeat these superior results and actually demonstrated awful outcomes, ranging in the 75% fair-to-poor range [9]. The main criticism of Ruedi's study was that most of the injuries were rotational skiing injuries rather than high-energy impact injuries and thus more amenable to immediate fixation because of reduced soft tissue compromise.

One of the only direct comparative clinical trials on this subject showed that patients with limited ORIF had better wound healing and less arthrosis than patients with formal ORIF [16,19]. Thus, in the early 1990s, the trend swung toward immediate external fixation with accessory limited internal fixation. Tornetta *et al.* [20] prospectively looked at Ruedi Type III fractures treated with this method and found 70% good-to-excellent results with infrequent wound complications.

Wyrsch *et al.* [21••] has very recently published the only prospective, randomized study on this subject, showing that external fixation with limited internal fixation produced significantly fewer wound complications and reoperations, in addition to a trend toward a better clinical postoperative ankle score, when compared with formal ORIF.

As more information shows soft tissue integrity to be the rate-limiting factor, more authors are advocating patience. This trend advocates a staged approach, with immediate fibular fixation and medial tibial external fixation and ORIF only after an extended wait for soft tissue improvement [12,21••]. The study by Patterson and Cole

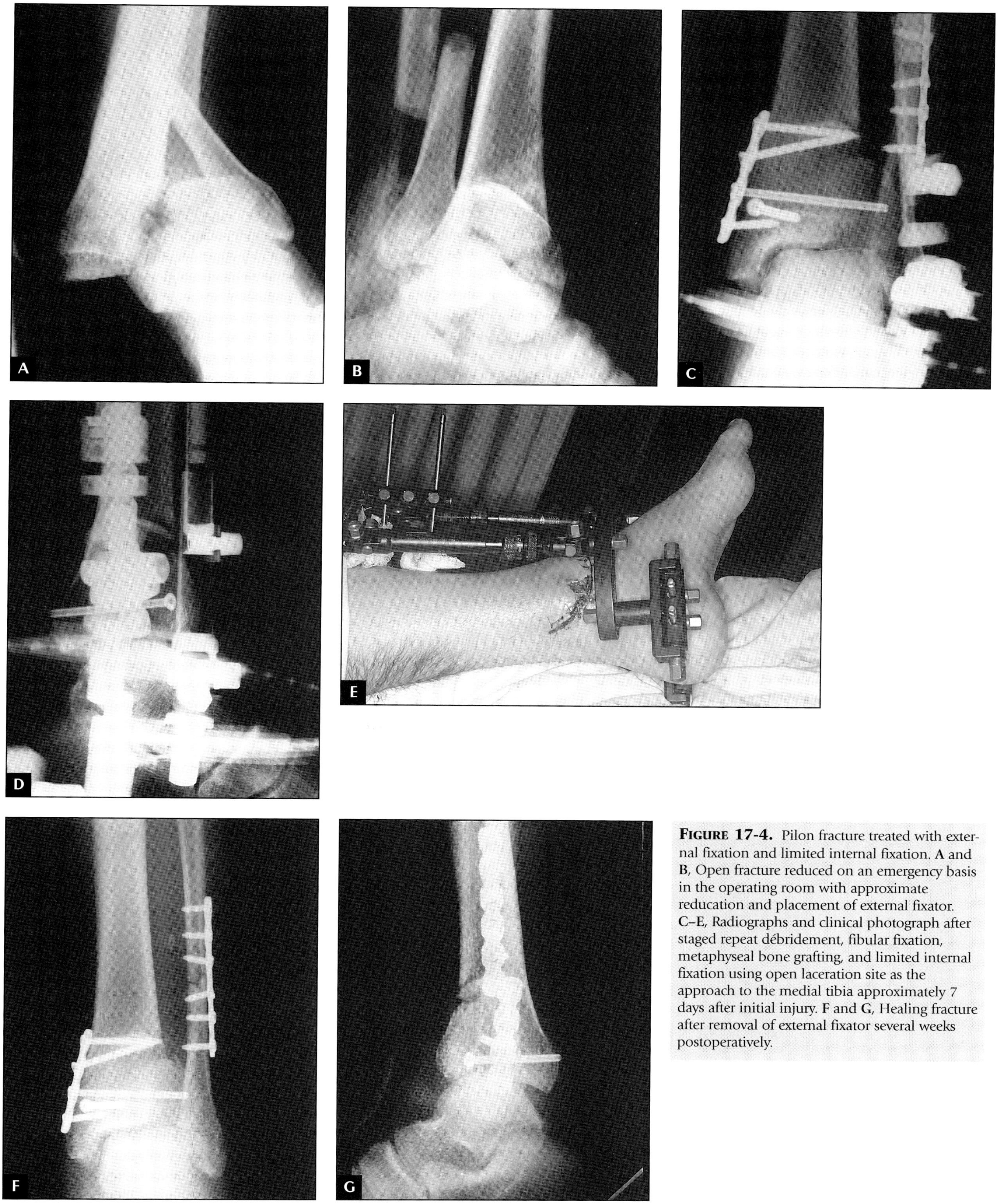

FIGURE 17-4. Pilon fracture treated with external fixation and limited internal fixation. A and B, Open fracture reduced on an emergency basis in the operating room with approximate reducation and placement of external fixator. C–E, Radiographs and clinical photograph after staged repeat débridement, fibular fixation, metaphyseal bone grafting, and limited internal fixation using open laceration site as the approach to the medial tibia approximately 7 days after initial injury. F and G, Healing fracture after removal of external fixator several weeks postoperatively.

[22•] averaged a formal ORIF at 24 days postinjury, with almost 80% good-to-excellent results and *no* wound complications. Although acknowledging the increase in difficulty at 3 weeks postinjury, these authors argue that awaiting soft tissue recovery can only be beneficial and that ORIF also has advantages over direct visualization of the articular surface (Figure 17-5).

AUTHORS' PREFERRED METHOD OF MANAGEMENT

There are basically three main categories of pilon fracture treatment: ORIF, internal fixation with a spanning external fixator, and hybrid external fixation. Choosing which treatment method to apply to which fracture pattern is the key to optimizing results. Important elements of the pilon fracture include the size and displacement of the articular fragments, metaphyseal–diaphyseal comminution and fracture extension, and the presence or absence of a fibular fracture. The choice of treatment modality also depends heavily on the status of the overlying soft tissues and preferences and experience of the surgeon.

Open Reduction and Internal Fixation

This procedure may be staged with preliminary reduction of the fibula and external fixation prior to final definitive fixation. Fractures best suited to ORIF include AO Types B3, C1, and C2. Type B3 fractures require an anterior plate for fixation to keep the talus from subluxating forward. Type C1 or C2 fractures with joint displacement also require ORIF; it works best in cases in

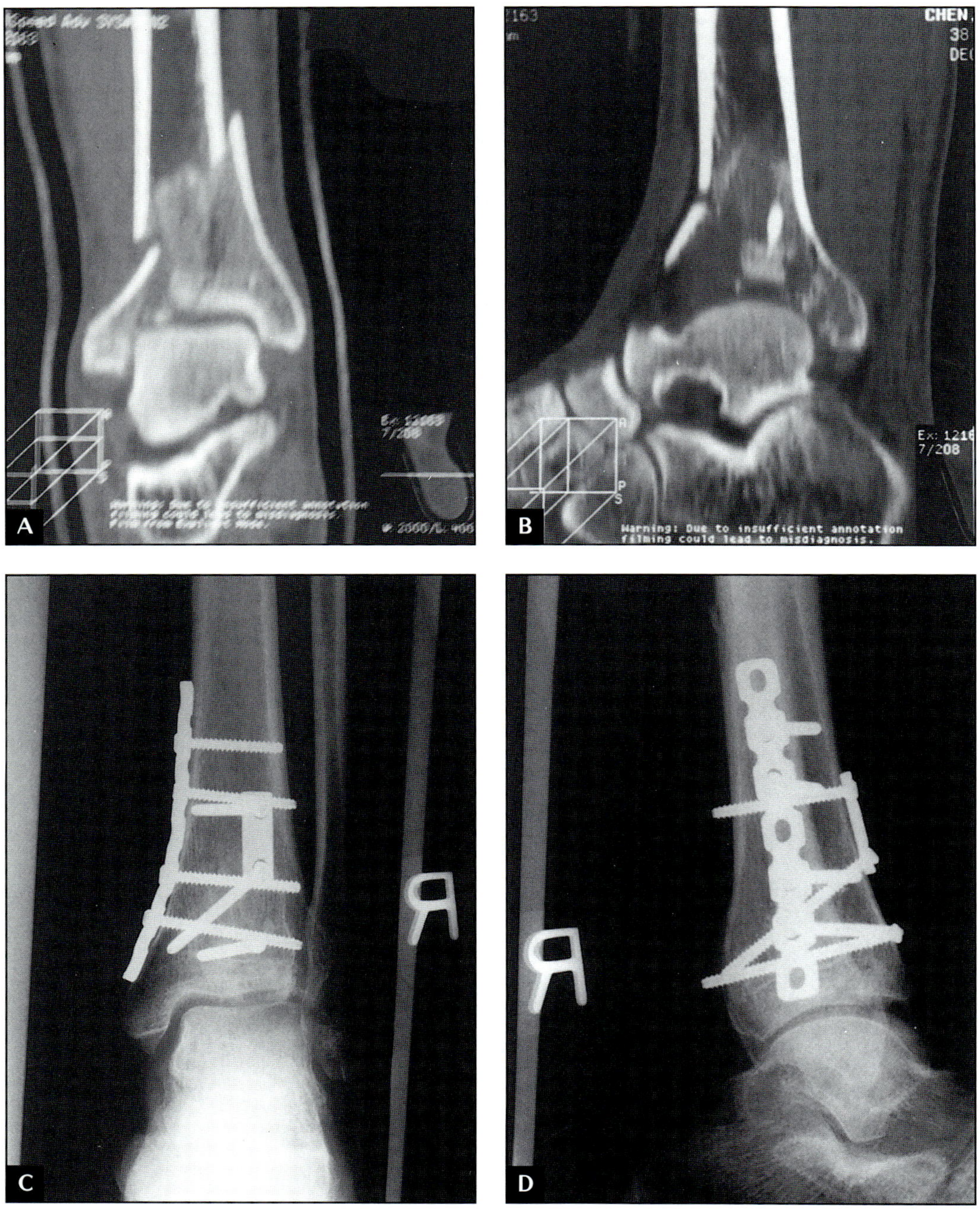

Figure 17-5. A–D, Pilon fracture treated solely with plate fixation after awaiting soft tissue recovery.

which a bony column of tibia can be reconstructed. Plates are less effective when they span an area of severe comminution (Figure 17-5).

Open Reduction and Internal Fixation with Spanning External Fixation

Spanning external fixators provide a number of advantages in pilon fracture treatment. Distraction across the joint can be used as temporary traction while awaiting soft tissue recovery. Ligamentotaxis can be applied intraoperatively to assist with fracture reduction. Finally, a spanning external fixator can be used to align and stabilize the metaphyseal-to-diaphyseal component of the pilon.

Fractures best suited to this method of treatment include those with comminution severe enough to make stable fixation with ORIF alone not feasible. The fixator augments and protects the repair. This is especially useful in the "low" Type C3 fracture in which crushing is present within 3 cm of the joint (Figure 17-4).

Hybrid External Fixation

Hybrid external fixation can be applied with three modalities: percutaneous, mini-open, or arthrotomy. Advantages of this method include anatomic reduction and stable fixation with less soft tissue dissection. Disadvantages are similar to those of external fixators—*ie,* pin-tract problems and the inconvenience of the external device.

Indications for hybrid fixation have become more specific. One of these is feasible reconstruction of the metaphysis into a stable segment. This allows for good fixation using a combination of wires and half-pins. Pilon fractures with diaphyseal extension are also treatable in this manner. Minimally displaced articular fractures can be treated percutaneously or with a limited open approach with definitive hybrid external fixation. Conversely, fractures with significant articular comminution should not be treated with a hybrid fixator. Fractures best suited to hybrid fixation include Types C1, C2, and C3 with diaphyseal extension (Figure 17-4).

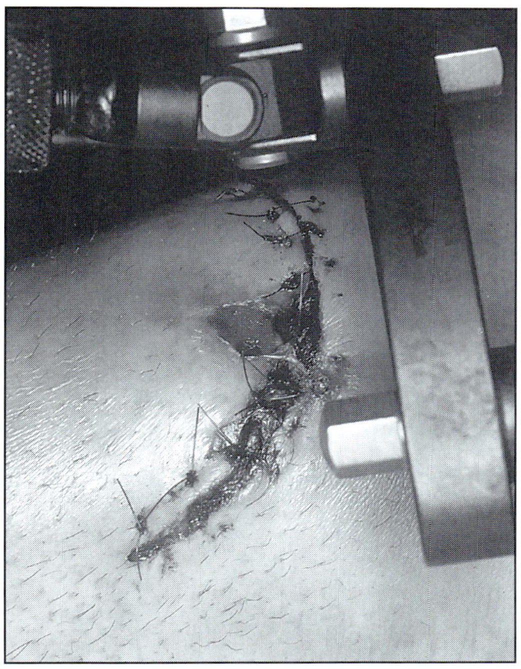

Figure 17-6. Marginal skin necrosis and one small avascular area after treatment of an open fracture with open reduction and internal fixation and a spanning external fixator. There was necrosis of this small area. With meticulous monitoring and care, the wound granulated in without incident.

CLOSURE

Wound closure is often a difficult feat to accomplish. It first requires good judgment about skin integrity. The aforementioned skin markers are guides to whether an attempt at closure is feasible. Careful attention to the viability of skin edges, a layered closure without dead space, and tensionless wound edges are all part of good surgical technique required for pilon fracture closure.

If prudence dictates that immediate primary closure cannot be accomplished, delayed primary or soft tissue coverage can be performed within a week. Usually implants can at least be covered with paratenon or subcutaneous tissue. With careful postoperative wound care, even temporary exposed metal should not get infected. Bare tendon or bone does not accept tissue transfers well and should be avoided.

Often, soft tissue transfer procedures must be performed, especially in the face of large defects from open fractures. These methods must be done in the absence of infection and when soft tissue compromise has resolved—usually within 1 week.

POSTOPERATIVE CARE

The diligence of care during the immediate postinjury period continues into the postoperative period. Once again, elevation and attention to the viability of soft tissues are essential to a good result. The usual postoperative antibiotic coverage, pin-site care, and deep venous thrombosis prophylaxis should be employed. Smoking and alcohol use by patients should be minimized. Early range-of-motion exercises of the ankle and non–weight bearing ambulation should start when the soft tissues have recovered. Dorsiflexion is very difficult to recover, and this should be stressed during rehabilitation [23]. Weight bearing should start months down the line, when radiographic tests provide evidence of progressive healing, especially at the metaphyseal–diaphyseal junction.

COMPLICATIONS

Various aspects of pilon fractures can end as complications. Wound complications include marginal-to-major skin necrosis. The amount of necrosis is related, first of all, to the severity of the injury. Placement of operative incisions can also have a tremendous effect on an already hypovascular soft tissue setting (Figure 17-6).

Infections are also commonly reported in pilon fractures. As mentioned earlier, several recent studies have not been able to demonstrate a difference in infection rates between open and closed fractures. Other factors that have been reported in association with postoperative infection include surgeon inexperience and reconstruction during soft tissue compromise. Finally, pin tracts are a common site of superficial infection, and although easily treated, can occasionally lead to deep infections of the soft tissue, bone, and joints.

Acute postoperative infections can develop into the more dreaded chronic osteomyelitis, which can become very difficult to treat. The treatment principles in osteomyelitis include extremely thorough débridement, therapy with local and systemic antibiotics, and eventual reconstruction.

Infections can cause nonunion, malunion, and delayed union. Other causes of these entities include poor fixation and overdistraction. These are also extremely specialized problems to deal with, involving revision fixation, bone grafting, and, often, multiple procedures (Figure 17-7).

Finally, some posttraumatic arthrosis is unavoidable, especially in the more severe fractures. The magnitude of these injuries itself causes damage to the articular cartilage, in the form of comminution or vascular insult. Immobilization also has a role. Many patients can recover with minimal or no symptoms. Fusion must be considered in those patients with severe, persistent symptomatology.

CONCLUSIONS

Various options are available for the treatment of pilon fractures. The choice often depends on the surgeon's preference. However, certain principles must be remembered. These include paramount consideration of soft tissues, because often their poor condition is the primary obstacle to a good result. Reconstruction of the articular surface, maintenance of reduction, and early motion can thus be achieved in various manners with acceptable results, as even the most recent literature shows.

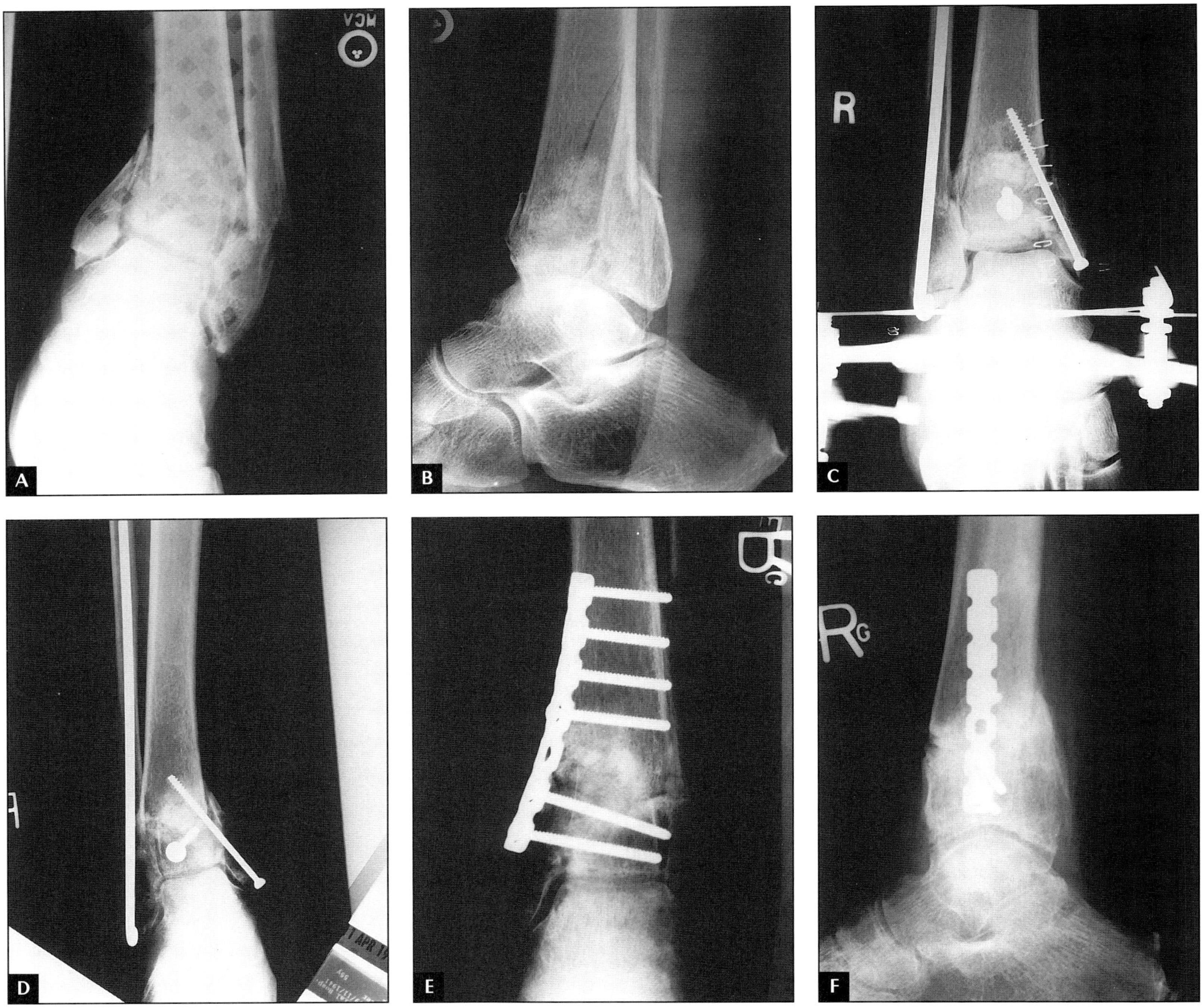

FIGURE 17-7. A–D, Nonunion of pilon fracture originally treated with external fixation and limited internal fixation. E and F, Fracture healing after débridement, bone grafting, and revision fixation with medial tibial buttressing. Rodding of metaphyseal fibular fracture caused excessive straightening of the fibula leading to tibia vara.

REFERENCES AND RECOMMENDED READING

Recently published papers of particular interest have been highlighted as:
- • Of interest
- •• Of outstanding interest

1. Gay R, Evard: Les fractures récentes du pilon tibial chez l'adulte [in French]. *Rev Chir Orthop* 1963, 49:397–512.
2. Ruedi T, Allgower M: Fractures of the lower end of the tibia into the ankle joint. *Injury* 1969, 1:92–99.
3. AO/ASIF Documentation Center: *Comprehensive Classification of Fractures.* Davos, Switzerland: AO/ASIF Documentation Center; 1996.
4. Swiontkowski MF, Sands AK, Agel J, *et al.*: Interobserver variation in the AO/OTA fracture classification system for pilon fractures: is there a problem? *J Orthop Trauma* 1997, 11:467–470.
5.• Bartlett C, D'Amato MJ, Weiner LS: Fractures of the tibial pilon. In *Skeletal Trauma: Fractures, Dislocations, Ligamentous Injuries* edn 2. Edited by Browner BD, Levine AM, Jupiter JB. *et al.* Philadelphia: WB Saunders; 1998.

This is an excellent, comprehensive review of the pilon fracture.

6. Tornetta B, Gorup J: Axial computed tomography of pilon fractures. *Clin Orthop Rel Res* 1996, 323:273–276.
7. Martin JS, Marsh JL, Bonar SK, *et al.*: Assessment of the AO/ASIF fracture classification for the distal tibia. *J Orthop Trauma* 1997, 11:477–483.
8. Giordano CP, Koval KS: Treatment of fracture blisters: a prospective study of 53 cases. *J Orthop Trauma* 1995, 9:171–176.
9. Teeny SM, Wiss DA: Open reduction and internal fixation of tibial plafond fractures: variables contributing to poor results and complications. *Clin Orthop Rel Res* 1993, 292:108–117.
10. Franklin JL, Johnson KD, Hansen ST Jr: Immediate internal fixation of open ankle fractures: report of 38 cases treated with a standard protocol. *J Bone Joint Surg* 1984, 66:1349–1356.
11. Johnson EE, Davlin LB: Open ankle fractures: the indications for immediate open reduction and internal fixation. *Clin Orthop Rel Res* 1993, 292:118–127.
12. Bone L, Stegemann P, McNamara K, Seibel R: External fixation of severely comminuted and open tibial pilon fractures. *Clin Orthop Rel Res* 1993, 292:101–107.
13.• Sirkin M, Sanders R, DiPasquale T, Herscovici D Jr: A staged treatment protocol for soft tissue management in the treatment of complex pilon fractures. *J Orthop Trauma* 1999, 13:78–84.

This is a retrospective review comparing the results between open and closed fractures and one of the only studies reviewing pilon fractures rather than ankle fractures.

14. Stiehl JB, Dollinger B: Primary ankle arthrodesis in trauma: a report of three cases. *J Orthop Trauma* 1988, 2:277–283.
15. Tile M: Fractures of the distal tibial metaphysis involving the ankle joint: the pilon fracture. In *The Rationale of Operative Fracture Care.* Edited by Schatzker J, Tile M. Berlin: Springer-Verlag; 1987:343–369.
16. Karas E, Weiner L: Displaced pilon fractures: an update. *Orthop Clin North Am* 1994, 25:651–663.
17. Kim HS, Jahng JS, Kim SS, *et al.*: Treatment of tibial pilon fractures using ring fixators and arthroscopy. *Clin Orthop Rel Res* 1997, 334:244–250.
18. Marsh JL, Bonar S, Nepola JV, *et al.*: Use of an articulated external fixator for fractures of the tibial plafond. *J Bone Joint Surg* 1995, 77:1498–1509.
19. Nast-Kolb D, Betz A, Rodel C, *et al.*: Minimal osteosynthesis of the tibial pilon fracture [in German]. *Unfallchirurgie* 1993, 96:517–523.
20. Tornetta P III, Weiner L, Bergman M, *et al.*: Pilon fractures: treatment with combined internal and external fixation. *J Orthop Trauma* 1993, 7:489–496.
21.•• Wyrsch B, McFerran MA, McAndrew M, *et al.*: Operative treatment of fractures of the tibial plafond: a randomized prospective study. *J Bone Joint Surg* 1996, 78:1646–1657.

This article is one of the only randomized and prospective studies on pilon fractures.

22.• Patterson MJ, Cole JD: Two-staged open reduction and internal fixation of severe pilon fractures. *J Orthop Trauma* 1999, 13:85–91.

This is one of the most recent studies, which reports on the recent trend of sole internal fixation as definitive treatment after a protracted waiting period for soft tissue recovery.

23. Brumback RJ, McGarvey WC: Fractures of the tibial pilon: evolving treatment concepts for the pilon fracture. *Orthop Clin North Am* 1995, 26:273–285.

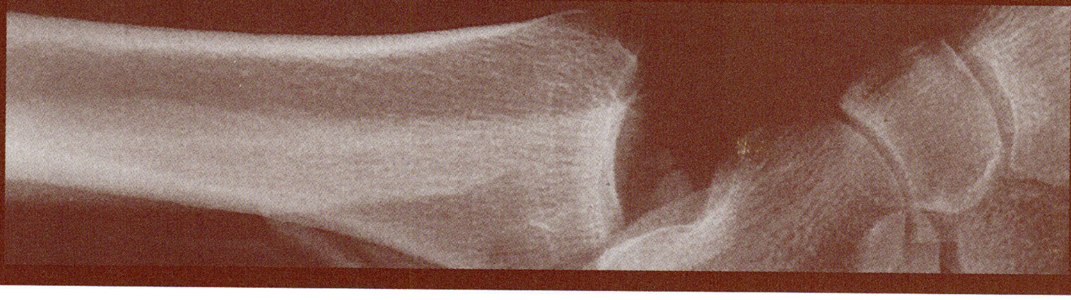

18

Ankle Fractures and Ankle Fracture-Dislocation

Bruce H. Ziran
Franklin D. Shuler

Ankle fractures are the injury most frequently treated by orthopedic surgeons. Studies indicate a steady increase in the prevalence of severe injuries [1,2]. This chapter provides the reader with information critical to determining which injury patterns respond well to conservative or nonoperative treatment compared with those injuries that respond more favorably to operative intervention.

The classification of ankle fractures based on radiographic presentation has been well described. The Lauge-Hansen [3] system is based on fracture patterns produced in cadavers using the position of the foot at the time of injury and the direction of the deforming force to define and describe the type of fracture. The importance of this system for the orthopedic surgeon is its ability to provide an understanding of the mechanism of injury so that thoughtful reduction can be performed to reduce or reverse the injury pattern identified.

The Danis-Weber (or AO) classification is based on the position of the fibular fracture in relation to the lateral malleolus. This system is not prognostic and also does not consider bony and soft-tissue injuries to the medial ankle joint, which can cause biomechanical disruption of normal ankle joint kinematics. It does, however, provide some therapeutic guidelines; most Weber A fractures can be treated conservatively, whereas most Weber C fractures require some type of operative intervention. The AO classification system elaborates on the Danis-Weber classification to incorporate medial injuries. Ultimately, the classification scheme used by the orthopedist is more directly related to training and education, and unfortunately all systems are associated with poor interobserver reliability [4–6]. Although a basic understanding of functional ankle anatomy and biomechanics is assumed, separate coverage is beyond the scope of this chapter, and the reader is directed to several excellent references [7,8].

ANKLE FRACTURE EVALUATION

A thorough history and physical and radiographic examination are required in all ankle fractures, although some information may be impossible to ascertain depending on the severity of injury in a polytraumatized patient. History should focus on mechanism of injury, previous ankle or leg problems (*eg,* ulcers, infection, pain, instability, deformity, disuse as a result of stroke), systemic illness (*eg,* peripheral vascular disease and claudication, cardiovascular or respiratory compromise, smoking, psychiatric diseases, and diabetes), and the possibility of associated injuries. The examination should fully assess the location and extent of injury, neurovascular status, skin integrity, and soft-tissue compromise.

Radiographic evaluation of fractures is covered in Chapter 1. Ankle radiographic evaluation includes anteroposterior (AP), mortise (15° internal oblique), and lateral views. Published studies indicate that the lateral and mortise views are sufficient to detect 95% of all ankle fractures [9]. Particular attention should be paid to evaluation of the entire fibula because of the possibility of a Maisonneuve-type injury. A mortise that appears stable can be surreptitiously unstable because of a high fibula fracture associated with disruption of the interosseous soft-tissue stabilizers. More specialized radiographic examination including stress views may be needed. If inconclusive, radiographs may be compared with those obtained on the unaffected side. Plain radiographs may not demonstrate articular cartilage injury of the talar dome that accompanies 49% of malleolar fractures [10]. Therefore, computed tomography (CT) and magnetic resonance imaging (MRI) studies may be needed to evaluate the injury fully.

MANAGEMENT OF SPECIFIC FRACTURES

General Considerations

The specific injuries described in this chapter range from isolated closed patterns to open fractures in polytraumatized patients. Appropriate treatment of an ankle injury depends on the presence of other injuries; the application of life-saving and limb-saving measures takes precedence over other therapy. The individual surgeon's decision to proceed with a treatment plan must depend on appropriate patient selection and timing. It was once thought that surgical treatment of such injuries be either immediate (*ie,* before maximal swelling) or delayed (*ie,* after subsidence of swelling). Several studies have examined this topic and the conclusions remain inconclusive. The injury patterns discussed in this chapter are lateral malleolar, medial malleolar, bimalleolar, and trimalleolar ankle fractures. Sections addressing injuries to the syndesmosis, management of open ankle fractures, and associated ankle fracture-dislocations are also included.

Lateral Malleolus Fractures

Evaluation

The lateral malleolus serves as the attachment site for the fibular collateral ligament complex composed of the anterior talofibular, posterior talofibular, and calcaneofibular ligaments (Figure 18-1)[11]. These ligaments are frequently damaged in ankle injuries, and functional testing of lateral ankle stability should be attempted [12]. Functional testing is derived from understanding the individual ligament contribution in restraining talar motion. The anterior talofibular ligament resists talar inversion when the ankle is plantarflexed and resists anterior talar subluxation when the foot is in a neutral position. The calcaneofibular ligament resists talar inversion when the ankle is dorsiflexed. Functional testing of lateral ankle stability should therefore be performed with the ankle in neutral flexion, plantarflexion, and dorsiflexion.

Isolated lateral malleolar fractures are classified using the Danis-Weber classification as Type B fractures, comprising up to 90% of all fractures about the ankle [13,14]. Although these fractures are common, open reduction and internal fixation (ORIF) of isolated lateral malleolar fractures remains controversial. Closed treatment of isolated lateral malleolar injuries yields more than 94% successful outcomes with long-term follow-up [15,16]. Operative treatment does not improve outcome over casting or bracing [17,18]. Biomechanical analysis of lateral malleolar injury supports nonoperative treatment, with isolated lateral fractures not producing dynamic incongruity/instability [19–21]. Additional support for nonoperative intervention is obtained from CT scans demonstrating that an isolated lateral malleolus fracture is not associated with changes in tibiofibular articulation with the apparent displacement of the fracture site on plain radiographs due to the relative external rotation of the proximal fibular shaft [20]. However, 15% of lateral malleolar fractures are accompanied by medial joint injury either as a bony fracture or deltoid ligament disruption that produce dynamic joint incongruity and should be addressed operatively [22].

Treatment

Various methods of lateral malleolar fixation can be used, depending on fracture pattern, with considerations of anatomic reduction and maintenance of fibular length of paramount importance (Figures 18-2 and 18-3)[23]. Treatment of a Weber A

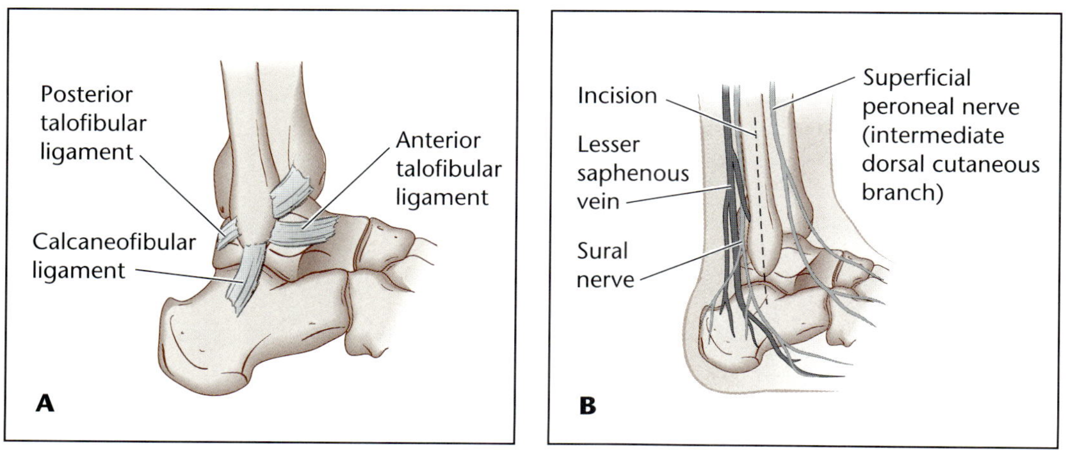

Figure 18-1. Lateral ankle anatomy. **A,** Fibular collateral ligament complex. **B,** Important surgical anatomy of the lateral approach demonstrating the short saphenous vein and sural nerve posterior and the superficial peroneal nerve anterior to the lateral incision. (*Adapted from* Rockwood *et al.* [11].)

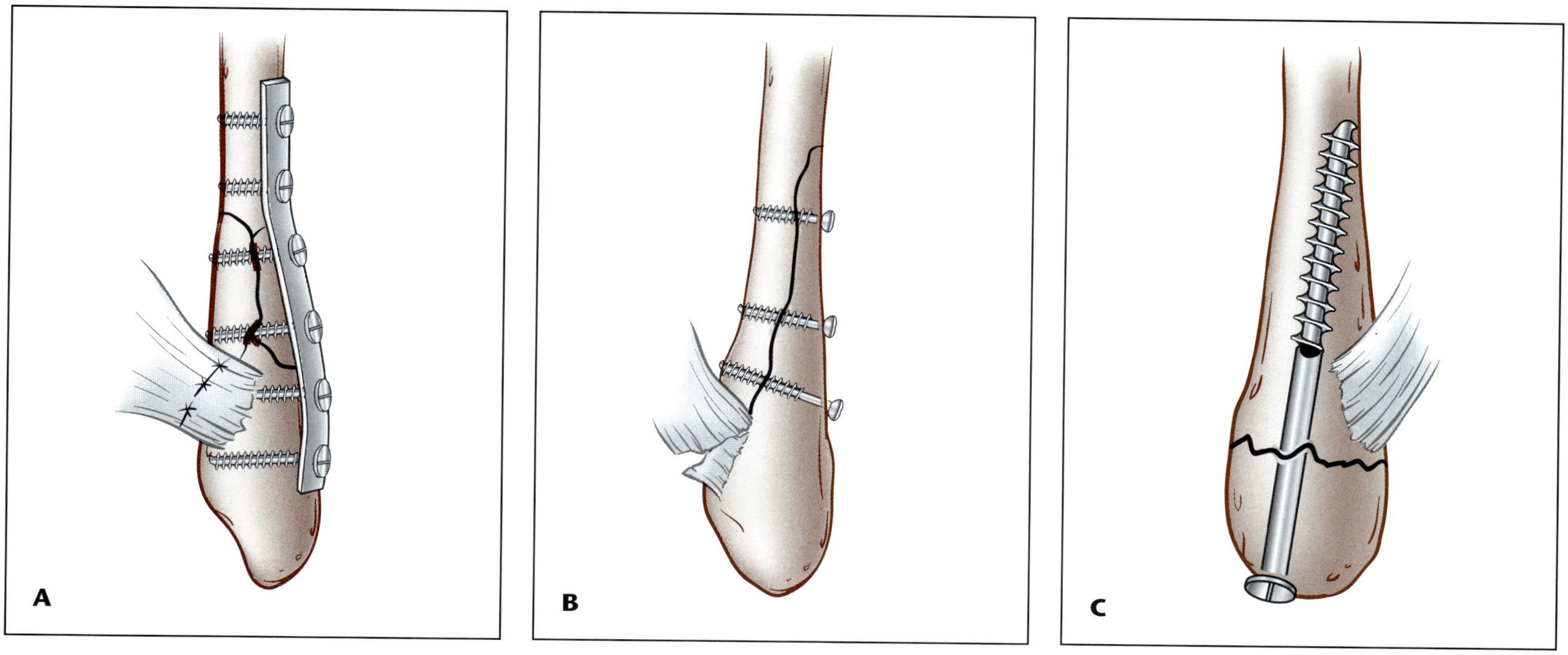

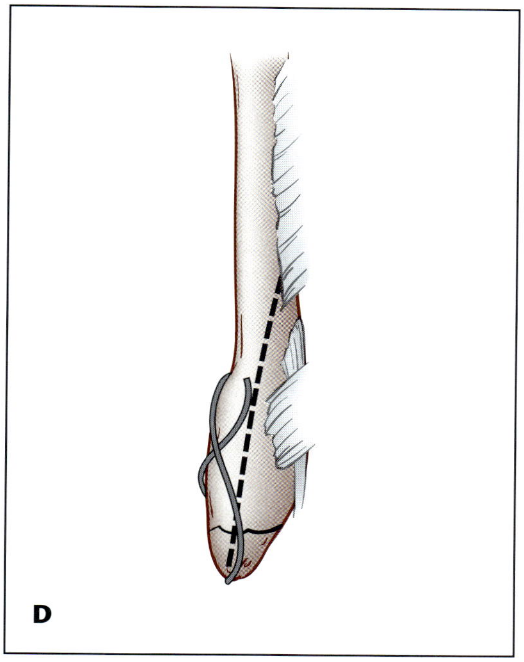

FIGURE 18-2. Techniques for fixation of lateral malleolar fractures. **A**, Standard fixation of fibular fracture with one-third semitubular 3.5-mm plate and screws. **B**, Multiple 3.5-mm lag screw fixation. **C**, Single 4.5-mm malleolar screw for low transverse fracture. **D**, Tension-band wiring. (*Adapted from* Johnson and Davlin [23].)

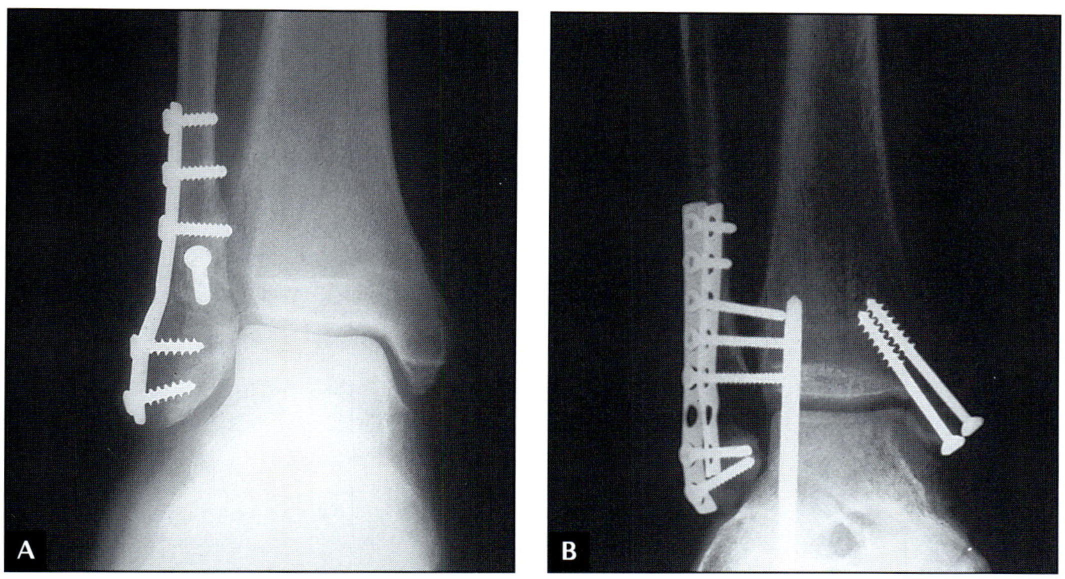

FIGURE 18-3. Surgical examples of fixation of lateral malleolar fractures. **A**, Surgical treatment of an isolated lateral malleolus fracture. An interfragmentary lag screw was used to achieve tentative fracture reduction before placement of the precontoured semitubular plate. **B**, Surgical treatment of this complex ankle fracture employs several techniques described in this chapter. Treatment of the lateral malleolar fracture associated with segmental comminution was performed by use of both extraosseous and interosseous plating with three screws engaging the lateral cortex of the tibia to improve stability of the construct. Use of a Childress pin is described in the text.

fracture as an isolated displaced injury is usually with closed treatment followed by functional rehabilitation. If marked displacement or instability is present, fixation can be done with 3.5- to 4.5-mm screws or tension-band wiring. When part of a bimalleolar fracture pattern, the lateral malleolus is usually approached first. The surgical approach to the lateral malleolus needs to consider fixation technique. If a posterolateral plate is used, the patient should be semilateral and the incision more posterior to allow placement of the plate and screws. Ziran prefers this method because the plate and screws are less prominent. Peroneal tendon irritation has not been problematic with this technique. For straight lateral plating, care should be taken not to avoid damage to the superficial branch of the peroneal nerve because its anatomy has been shown to vary considerably. Recent reports have discussed using bioabsorbable fixation in many circumstances. With newer polymers, the previous complication of aseptic abscess related to the presence of the biomaterials has been significantly decreased. Treatment of a Weber B fracture as an isolated displaced injury or part of a bimalleolar fracture pattern focuses on reduction and stabilization with lag screws perpendicular to the fracture line. Neutralization of the fracture is then performed with a one-third tubular plate contoured to accommodate the distal fibular lateral bow and fixed with 3.5-mm cortical screws. In patients with mild osteopenia, a more posteriorly oriented antiglide plate can be used [24,25]. In patients with severe osteopenia, or segmental comminution, Ziran prefers to engage the fibular screws into the lateral tibia using it as the "far" cortex of fixation, and thereby improving the stability of the construct. Alternatively, external fixation can be employed using any of the commercially available brands. Treatment of Weber C fracture patterns is covered in the following section on syndesmosis injuries.

Syndesmosis Injuries

Evaluation

The syndesmotic ligament complex is responsible for the attachment of the distal tibia to the fibula. This complex is composed of four ligaments: anterior inferior tibiofibular, posterior inferior tibiofibular, inferior transverse tibiofibular, and interosseous (Figure 18-4). Although the potential for syndesmosis instability exists in Weber C fracture patterns, dynamic instability and widening of the distal tibia/fibula articulation are not appreciated unless accompanied by medial joint injury or talar subluxation [26–28]. A critical zone of syndesmotic disruption leading to talar instability has recently been described [26,29], located 3 to 4.5 cm above the mortise when the deltoid ligament has been torn. Syndesmotic fixation is based on radiographic evidence of widening or intraoperative assessment of stability of the intact or internally fixed fibula. Radiographic evidence of diastasis is demonstrated when the tibiofibular overlap is less than 10 mm on an AP projection or less than 1 mm on the mortise projection (Figure 18-5) [30]. Other signs of disruption include evidence that the fibula is displaced posteriorly on a lateral neutral flexion view, or when the talomalleolar joint space is more than 4 mm on the mortise view. Studies have demonstrated that lateral stress radiographs are more reliable than the mortise or AP stress radiograph [31]. Intraoperatively, a clamp can be placed on the distal fibula and a distracting force can be applied. A posteriorly directed force, as well as a rotational force, should be done so that subtle but significant injuries can be identified.

Treatment

Operative stabilization of disrupted syndesmosis is accomplished by lateral placement of a transverse 3.5-, 4.0-, or 4.5-mm fully threaded screw from fibula to tibia 2 cm above the plafond and parallel to the joint space (Figure 18-6). This screw is angled 30° anteriorly from posterolateral to anteromedial because the fibula is posterior to the tibia. During screw placement, the ankle is held in 5° to 10° of dorsiflexion to engage the widest part of the talar dome to avoid any overtightening of the screw that will limit the dorsiflexion obtained postoperatively. Much debate focuses on whether to engage 3 or 4 cortices with the syndesmotic screw [32]. Biomechanical studies of fibular motion demonstrate that dorsiflexion of the ankle produces external rotation of the fibula, and three-cortex fixation allows for this motion [33–35]. However, in the presence of a Maisonneuve-type injury, operative stabilization of the syndesmosis employs four-cortex fixation

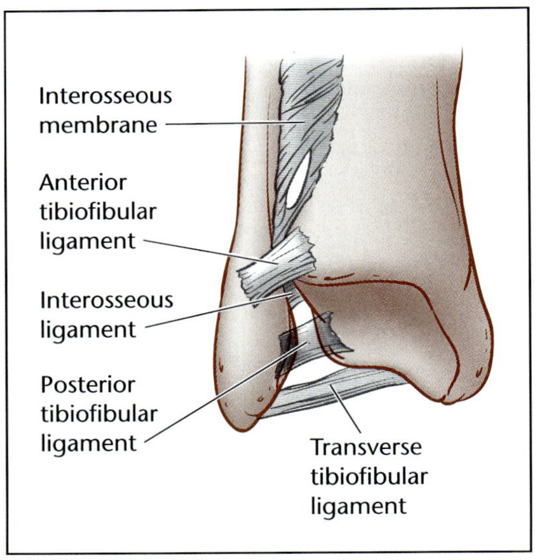

Figure 18-4. Syndesmotic ligaments of the ankle (*Adapted from* Rockwood *et al.* [11].)

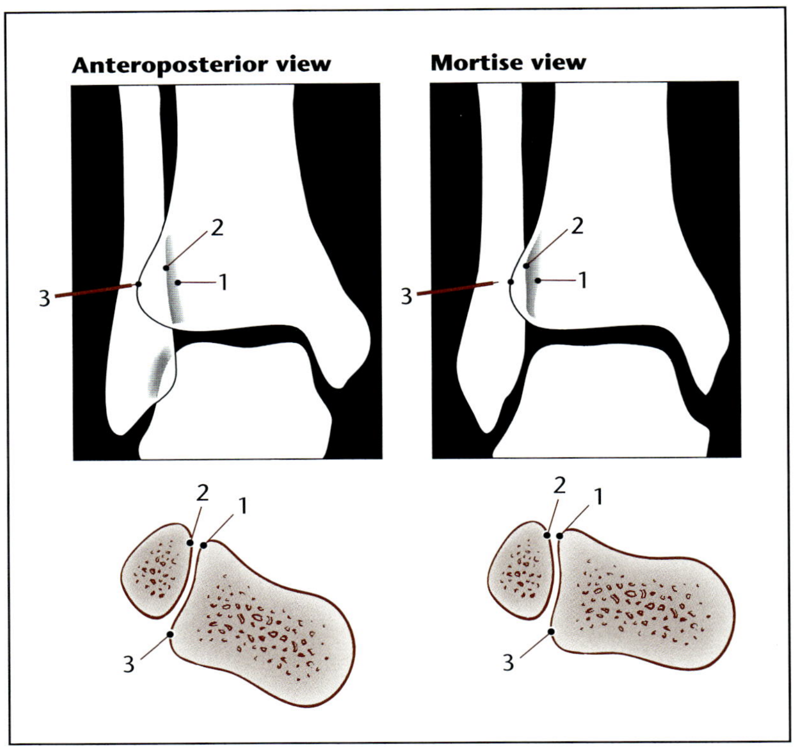

Figure 18-5. Landmarks to assess syndesmotic injury. (*Adapted from* Pettrone *et al.* [30].)

with screw removal occurring at 4 to 6 months. We also prefer to use fully threaded 4.0-mm cancellous screws because they are less likely to loosen in cancellous bone and because we believe that a 4.5-mm screw creates too large a stress riser in the event of complete metal removal. If the syndesmotic screw needs to be removed, we do not remove it sooner that 4 months postoperatively. When using these techniques, screw breakage is generally not a problem. Patients have reported a subjective improvement in gait and slightly increased dorsiflexion after screw removal or breakage. Because ligament healing does not occur before 6 to 8 weeks, postoperative immobilization is continued until week 6, when partial weight bearing is resumed. Bioabsorbable fixation is being used more frequently in treating this injury pattern and may avoid some of these concerns.

Medial Malleolus and Bimalleolar Fractures

Evaluation

The medial malleolus is smaller than the lateral malleolus and serves as the attachment site for important ankle stabilizers. The medial deltoid ligament is composed of superficial and deep com-

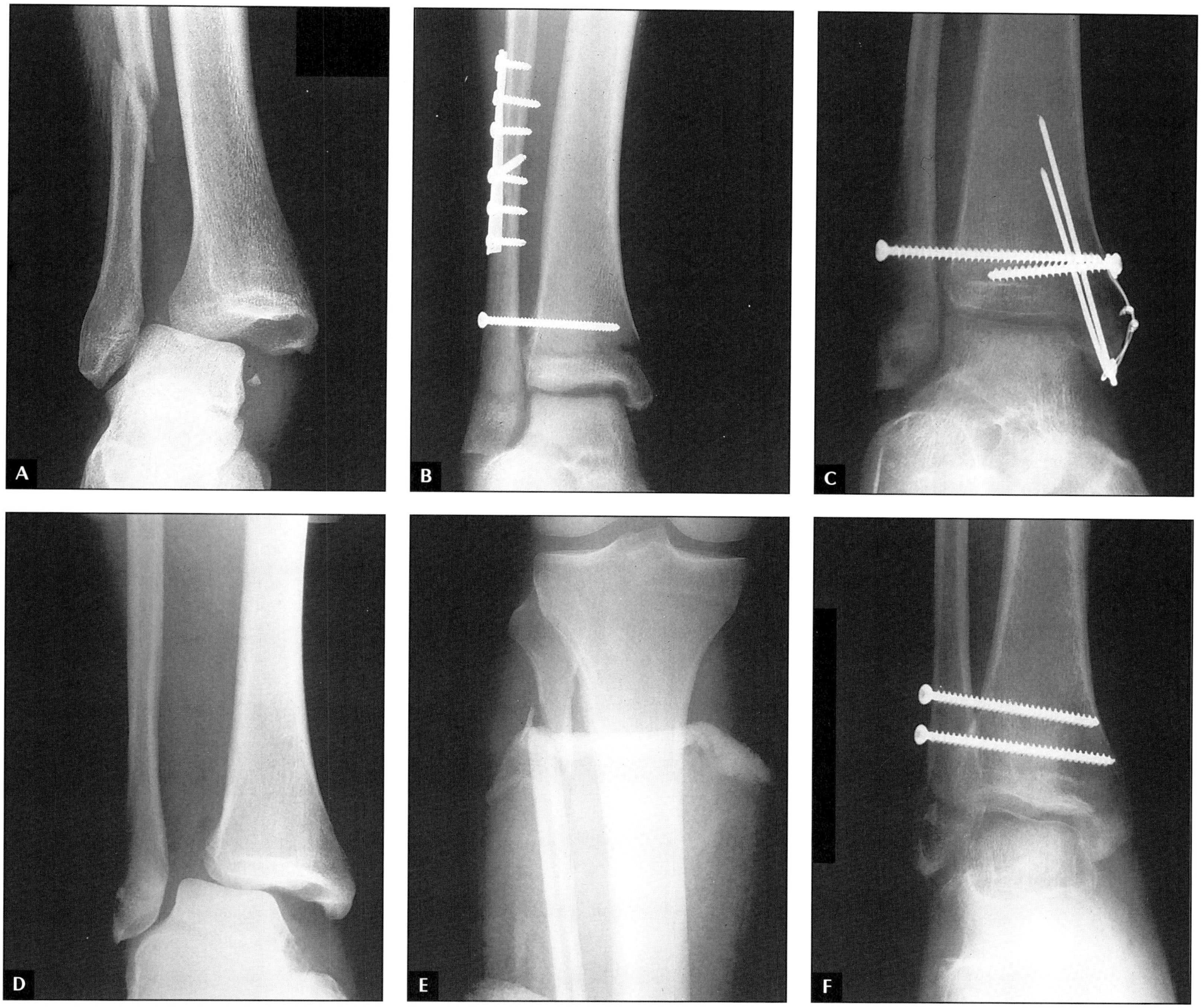

Figure 18-6. Stabilization of tibiofibular syndesmosis injury. **A**, Preoperative radiograph demonstrating lateral malleolus fracture with evidence of medial malleolus disruption associated with lateral subluxation of the talus. **B**, Postoperative radiograph demonstrating the stabilization of the lateral malleolus along with placement of a syndesmotic screw that engages 3 cortices. **C**, Postoperative radiograph demonstrating an intact mortise following fixation with a four-cortex syndesmosis screw along with tension-band wiring of the medial malleolus. **D** and **E**, Preoperative radiographs demonstrating syndesmotic injury in the Maisonneuve fracture. **F**, Postoperative radiograph reveals the use of dual four cortical fixation to enhance stability of the construct. These screws are removed at 4 to 6 months after operative stabilization.

ponents (Figure 18-7) [36]. The superficial deltoid ligament is composed of calcaneotibial, talotibial, and naviculotibial fibers, which describes its attachment from the anterior colliculus of the medial malleolus to the calcaneous, talus, and navicular bones, respectively. This superficial ligament complex provides little ankle stability. The deep deltoid ligament is the primary medial ankle stabilizer. Fibers of the deep deltoid run transversely from both colliculi to the nonarticular medial talus and restrain external rotation of the talus in the mortise. Soft tissue disruption of the medial deltoid ligament complex is assumed if more than a 4-mm space is seen between the medial malleolus and talus in a mortise or medial stress view. Diagnosis of medial ligament disruption is important in a lateral malleolus fracture because both the bony and the soft tissue injury patterns alter ankle contact area and kinematics prompting ORIF of the lateral malleolus [19,21,27]. This point highlights the fact that the key to ankle stability in the presence of medial injury is the reduction and fixation of the lateral malleolus. In the bimalleolar equivalent fracture pattern (lateral malleolus fracture with radiographic evidence of deltoid ligament disruption), operative stabilization of the lateral malleolar fracture obviates the need for deltoid ligament repair with no reports demonstrating clinical advantage of deltoid ligament repair [37,38]. If the medial joint space remains wide, then the clinician must consider interposition of small chondral fragments, ligament interposition, or rarely, entrapment of the posterior tibial tendon.

Treatment

Isolated medial malleolar fractures are treated with cast immobilization if nondisplaced and with ORIF if displaced. Displaced fractures may allow talar displacement and are approached surgically using an anteromedial exposure that allows for direct inspection of the ankle joint. Fixation can be made with lag screws, tension-band wiring, or buttress plating (Figure 18-8). Internal fixation of displaced medial malleolar fractures can also be accomplished through the use of absorbable implants with results equivalent to those of metallic implants in prospective, randomized studies [39,40].

Bimalleolar fractures, usually displaced at presentation, are unstable injuries requiring operative fixation. The key principle in treatment of these injuries is maintenance of lateral malleolar

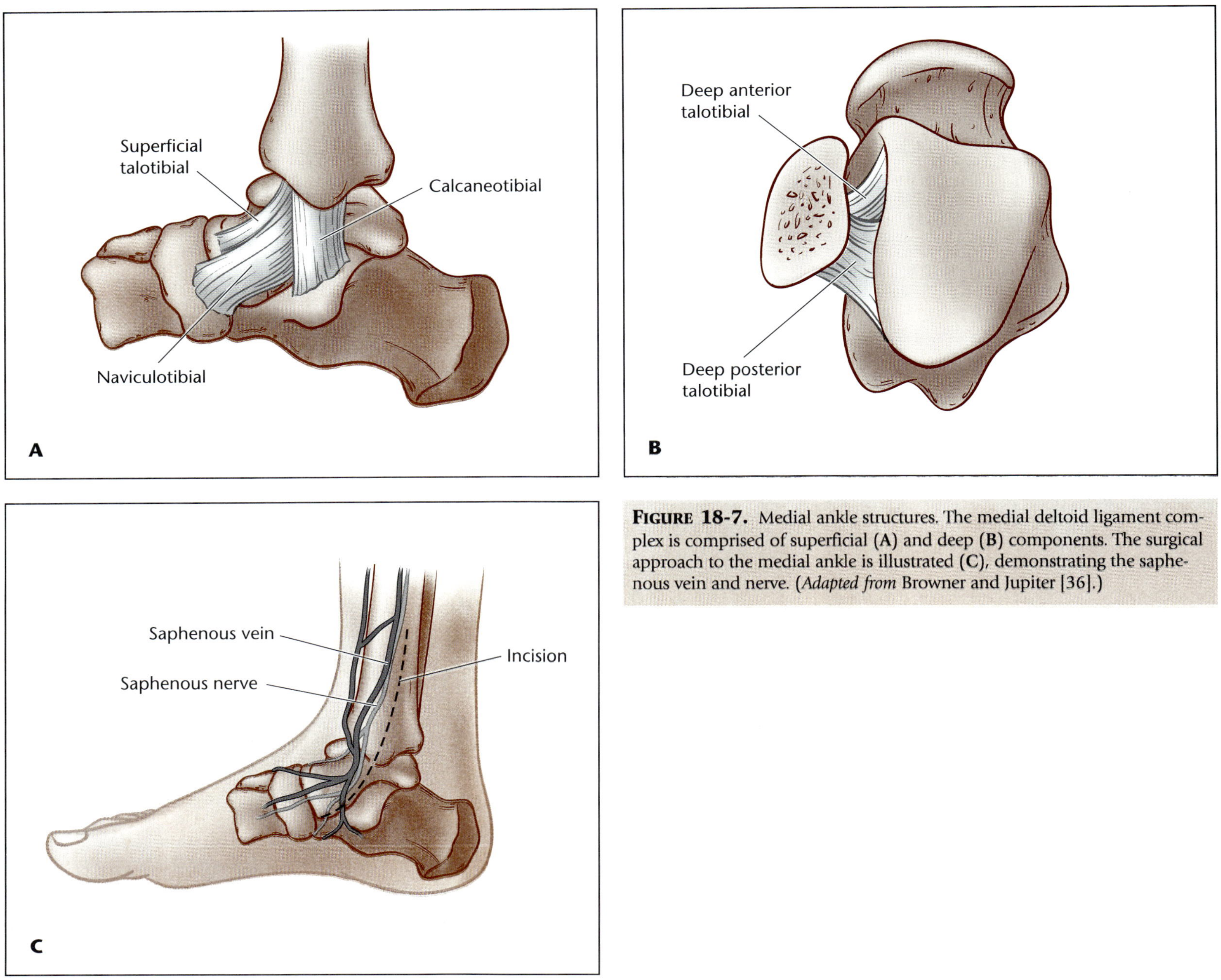

FIGURE 18-7. Medial ankle structures. The medial deltoid ligament complex is comprised of superficial (A) and deep (B) components. The surgical approach to the medial ankle is illustrated (C), demonstrating the saphenous vein and nerve. (*Adapted from* Browner and Jupiter [36].)

reduction, which is difficult with closed treatment. Another key principle in the treatment of these injuries is timing, because of the large amount of soft tissue swelling that accompanies them. It is well established that more severe ankle fractures and open fractures benefit from earlier surgical intervention [41–44]. However, studies in Weber B bimalleolar fractures challenge this premise; Konrath *et al.* [45] concluded that delayed surgery can be justified in patients with severe soft tissue injury. Examples of bimalleolar fracture treatment are shown in Figure 18-9.

Trimalleolar Fractures

Evaluation

Bimalleolar fracture of the ankle with fracture of the posterior lip of the tibial plafond is called a *trimalleolar fracture.* The posterior lip of the plafond is the attachment for inferior tibiofibular syndesmotic ligament (Figure 18-4). This ligament is responsible for the avulsion fractures associated with disruption between the tibia and the fibula. This fracture can occur in the latter stages of supination-eversion rotation and pronation-eversion rotation injuries. Biomechanical instability of the ankle has been demonstrated in cases in which the posterior fragment is more than 30% of the posterior tibial surface with some studies demonstrating that the amount of articular surface involvement seen on the lateral radiograph underestimates the actual surface area as compared with findings gathered using CT studies [46,47]. Clinically, closed reduction of fractures involving less than 25% of the posterior tibial surface produces generally good outcomes with worse results obtained when the fragment size is larger [48]. In a recent study, however, patients with trimalleolar fractures who also had a posterior malleolar fracture comprising more than 25% of the articular surface were all treated with ORIF of the medial and lateral malleolar fractures. The posterior malleolar fractures were either treated with ORIF or not treated, with results demonstrating no posterior talar subluxation in either group and no clinical difference in outcome.

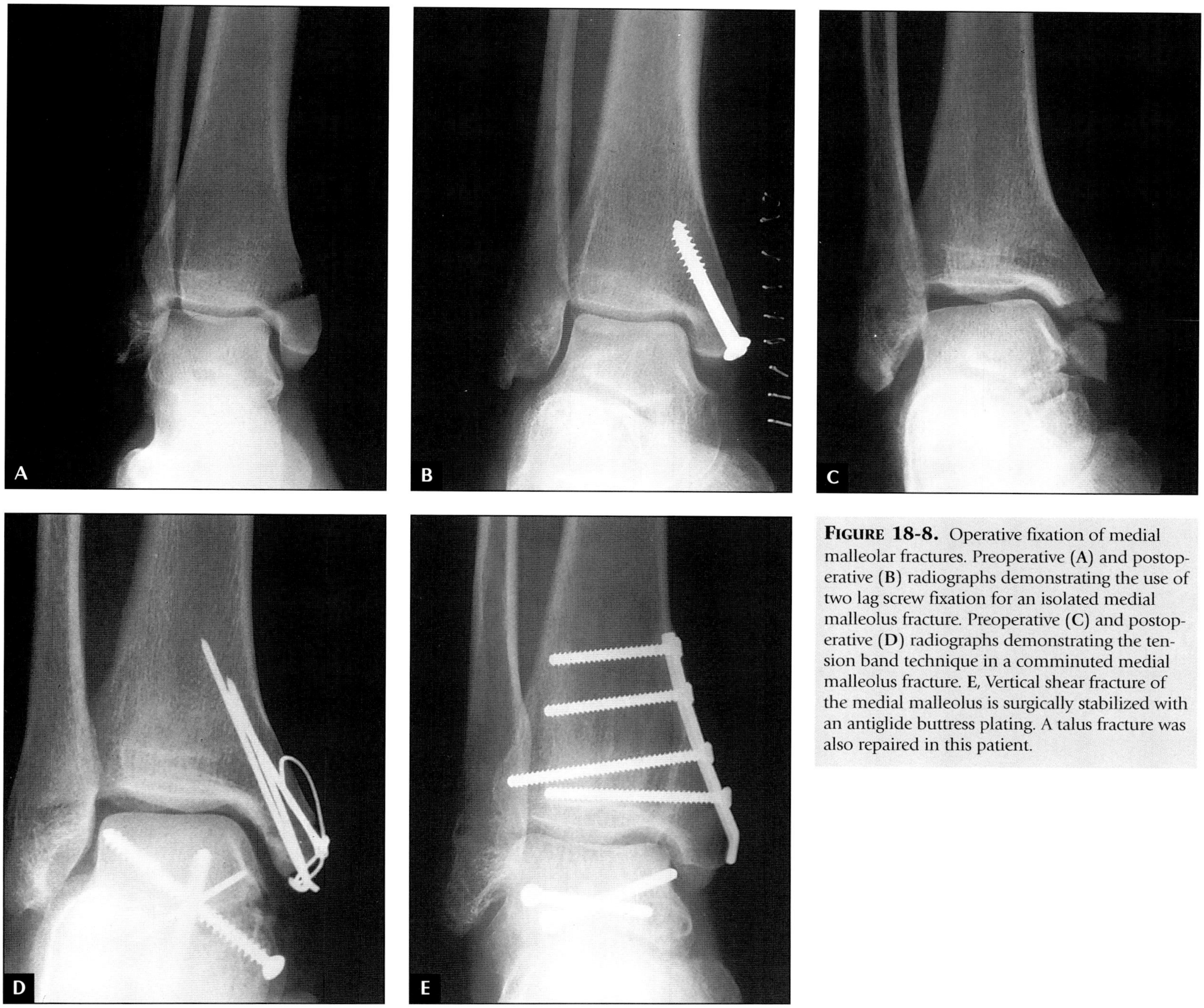

Figure 18-8. Operative fixation of medial malleolar fractures. Preoperative (**A**) and postoperative (**B**) radiographs demonstrating the use of two lag screw fixation for an isolated medial malleolus fracture. Preoperative (**C**) and postoperative (**D**) radiographs demonstrating the tension band technique in a comminuted medial malleolus fracture. **E**, Vertical shear fracture of the medial malleolus is surgically stabilized with an antiglide buttress plating. A talus fracture was also repaired in this patient.

Treatment

Ziran performs ORIF of the posterior malleolar fragment only if a greater than 2-mm residual step off after ORIF of the medial and lateral structures exists. In practice, reduction of the medial and lateral malleoli frequently satisfactorily reduces the fracture of the posterior malleolus through ligamentotaxis through the posterior tibiofibular ligament [49]. In addition, the flexor hallucis longus traverses over this area of the tibia, so that dorsiflexion of the great toe occasionally helps reduce this fragment. It is generally easier to gain access to the posterior fragment through the medial wound by extending the subperiosteal dissection carefully around the back of the tibia using a dental pick or reduction clamp. Examples of trimalleolar fixation are shown (Figure 18-10) with 3.5-mm screws used in an anterior-to-posterior direction to secure a large posterior malleolar fragment.

SPECIAL CONSIDERATIONS

Open Fractures and Soft-Tissue Management

Skeletal considerations for open fractures are similar to those of closed fractures, but when a fracture is open, it generally indicates more severe injury, and the focus shifts to the soft tissues. After initial evaluation, reduction and possible decontamination in open fractures may be needed along with tetanus prophylaxis (when needed) and appropriate antibiotic therapy with immobilization, elevation, and application of ice used to avoid additional compromise to the region while definitive treatment is planned. With any open wound, the clinician must consider the

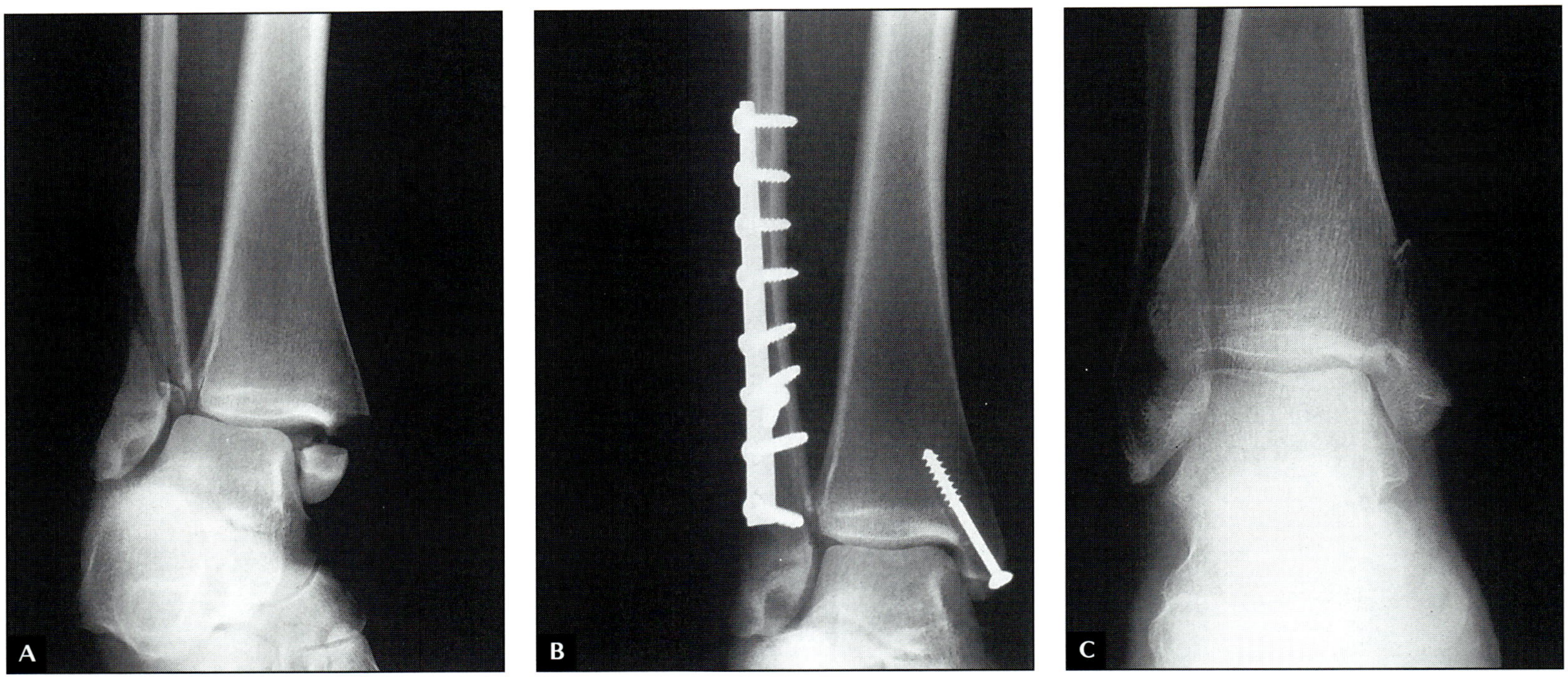

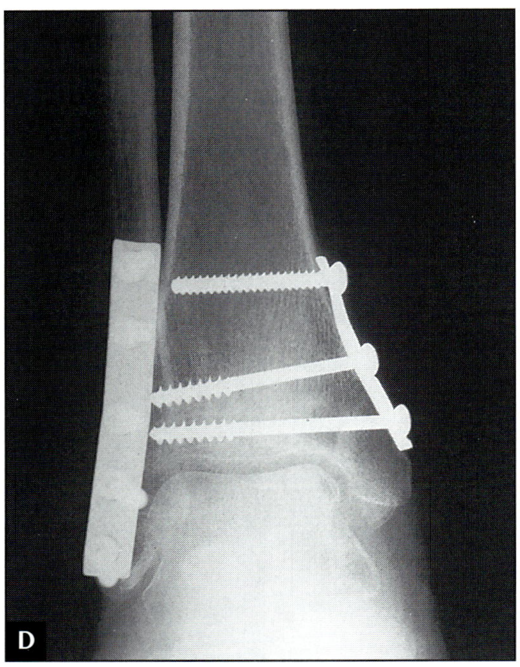

Figure 18-9. Operative fixation of bimalleolar fractures. **A**, Preoperative radiograph demonstrates a bimalleolar fracture with a medial malleolus fracture accompanied by a comminuted fracture of the lateral malleolus having a proximal extension and a small free fragment at the level of the lateral mortise. **B**, Postoperative radiograph demonstrates single screw fixation of the medial malleolus with lateral plating restoring fibular length. **C** and **D**, Bimalleolar fracture with a vertical fracture of the medial malleolus was treated with lateral malleolar plating and buttress plating of the medial malleolus.

zone of injury and must not hesitate to explore beyond the immediate traumatic wound to properly determine the nature of the soft tissue damage. Standard principles of open fracture management are followed. Frequently, a transverse wound is present just at or above the medial malleolus usually associated with lateral dislocation of the talus. The medial soft tissues are thin and tenuous, especially in the elderly, and soft tissue coverage options are limited or may be contraindicated in the debilitated elderly. If necessary, the wound can be extended to provide fracture exposure or to allow exploration of neurovascular structures, which are occasionally injured. It is not uncommon to find tendon injuries; injuries to the posterior tibialis tendon are the most common and should be addressed at the time of final closure. We have found at our institution that a vascular injury can often be overlooked when exploration is not performed. Depending on the condition of the foot, this lesion may need to be addressed expeditiously.

Adequate débridement generally requires extension of the traumatic wound. Because of the linearity of the cutaneous blood flow, Ziran extends the wound by bisecting it because the distances from the intact skin to the edges of the wound are smaller with bisection than with a Z extension. Nonetheless, complication rates of these injuries are significant and must be taken into consideration when planning treatment. In the young patient with significant injury, a microvascular soft tissue procedure may be necessary. Unfortunately, in the elderly, this may be less well tolerated

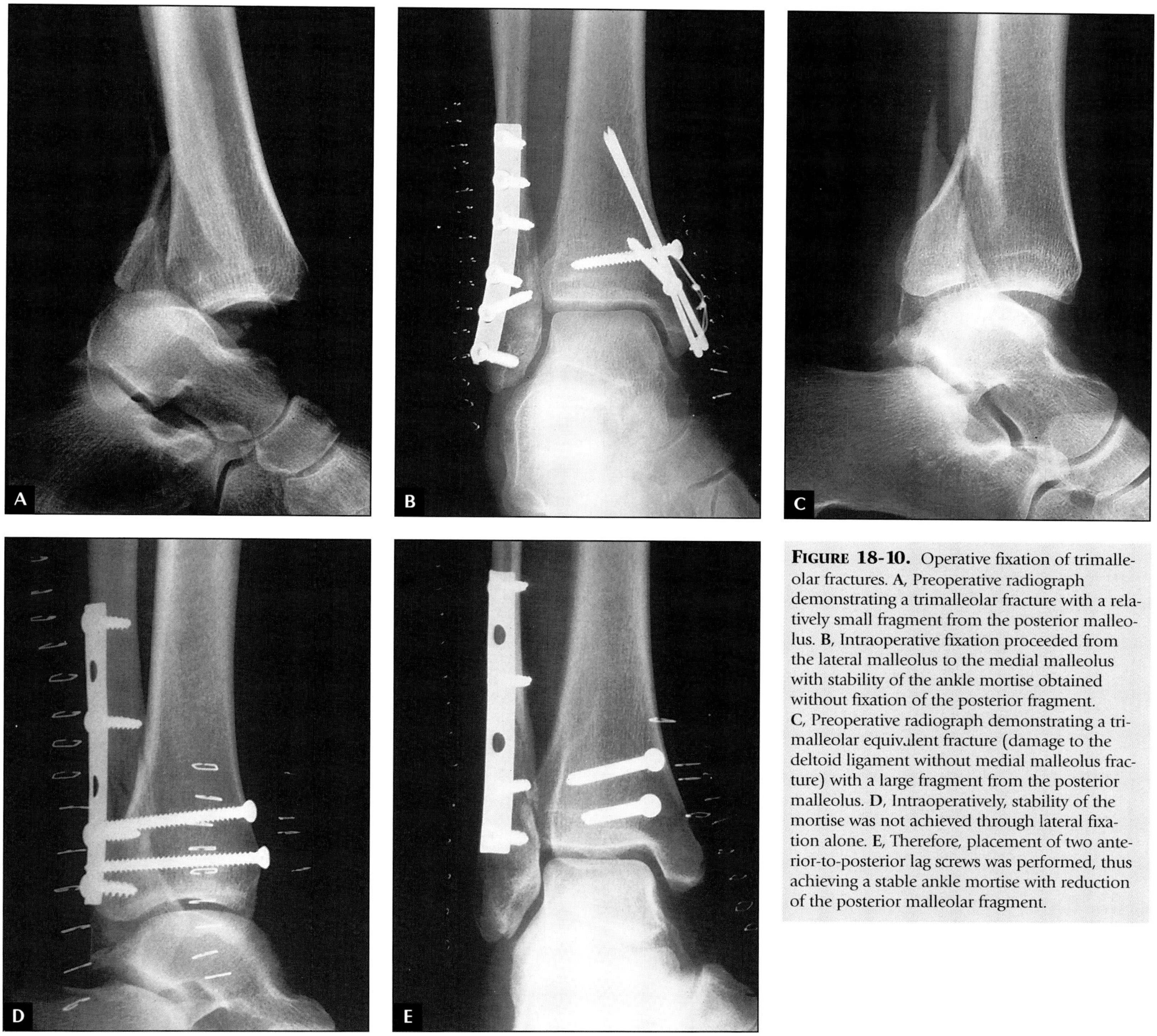

FIGURE 18-10. Operative fixation of trimalleolar fractures. A, Preoperative radiograph demonstrating a trimalleolar fracture with a relatively small fragment from the posterior malleolus. B, Intraoperative fixation proceeded from the lateral malleolus to the medial malleolus with stability of the ankle mortise obtained without fixation of the posterior fragment. C, Preoperative radiograph demonstrating a trimalleolar equivalent fracture (damage to the deltoid ligament without medial malleolus fracture) with a large fragment from the posterior malleolus. D, Intraoperatively, stability of the mortise was not achieved through lateral fixation alone. E, Therefore, placement of two anterior-to-posterior lag screws was performed, thus achieving a stable ankle mortise with reduction of the posterior malleolar fragment.

and the fate of the leg may depend on the viability of the remaining tissues. In any case, initial treatment is aimed at the soft tissue, with provisional stabilization of the ankle with an external fixator, returning later for definitive stabilization once the soft tissues have been stabilized. The use of a Childress pin [50,51]—a large smooth Steinmann pin inserted retrograde from the calcaneus into the talus and tibia (Figure 18-11)—is reserved for unstable ankles with tenuous soft tissue. It does not provide rotational stability and is used only in situations with severe injuries that preclude the use of other techniques.

Ankle Dislocations

Ankle dislocations (Figure 18-12) usually occur in association with fractures but need not [52]. Initial treatment of this injury focuses on immediate reduction with open injuries prompting

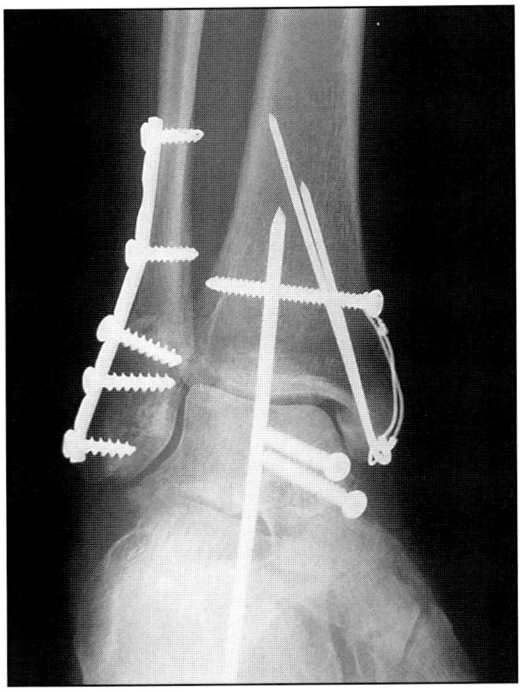

Figure 18-11. Childress' pin. In patients with unstable ankles following initial reduction, a calcaneotalotibial/Childress pin can be used to help provide additional stability. The postoperative radiograph in demonstrates the use of a Childress pin in a bimalleolar ankle fracture. The postoperative radiographs in Figure 18-2 demonstrate the use of the Childress' pin in a patient who had segmental loss of bone from the lateral malleolus resulting from open injury. Concerns over stability of the lateral malleolus were addressed intraoperatively with the use of both intra- and extramedullary plating along with screw fixation to the lateral tibial cortex. Additional stability of this construct was achieved by using a Childress' pin.

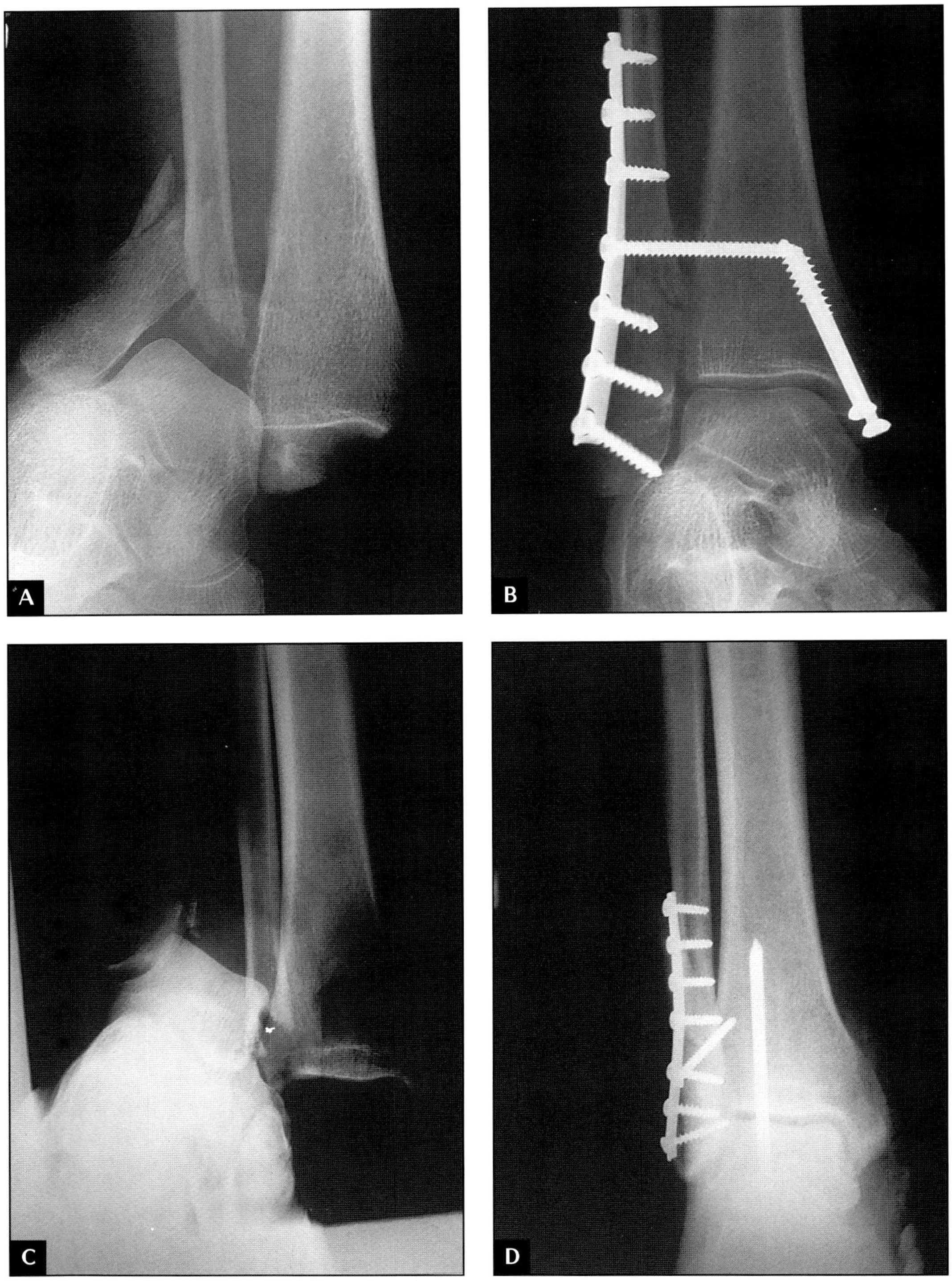

Figure 18-12. Ankle fracture-dislocation. **A**, Preoperative radiograph demonstrating an ankle fracture-dislocation with disruption of lateral and medial malleoli. **B**, Postoperative radiograph demonstrates plating of the lateral malleolus with screw fixation of the medial malleolus with congruity of the mortise achieved. **C**, Preoperative anteroposterior radiograph demonstrating a fracture-dislocation in a patient with an intact medial malleolus. Operative fixation of the lateral malleolus restored fibular length. Additional stability was provided by the use of a Childress' pin (**D**).

meticulous débridement, possible ligamentocapsular repair, and possible delayed closure [53]. Difficulty with initial closed reduction may indicate soft-tissue entrapment or Bosworth fracture-dislocation where the posteriorly dislocated and trapped fibula impedes reduction [54]. Location of the dislocation helps determine which tendon may be entrapped, thereby precluding closed reduction. Following reduction, ankle stability is assessed. If any asymmetry or loss of motion is noted, the clinician ought suspect soft tissue interposition that would then prompt surgical treatment. After reduction has been achieved, the ankle should be stabilized for a period of 6 weeks. If the reduction is stable and no fracture is present, then simple casting will be sufficient. If a fracture does exist, the stability must be assessed after skeletal stabilization. If still unstable, then either external fixation or a Childress pin (Figure 18-12) can be used for stabilization [55,56].

ACKNOWLEDGMENTS

We would like to thank Marshall L. Balk for critical review of this chapter.

REFERENCES AND RECOMMENDED READING

Recently published papers of particular interest have been highlighted as:
- • Of interest
- •• Of outstanding interest

1. Bauer M, Bengner U, Johnel O, *et al.*: Supination-eversion fractures of the ankle joint: changes in incidence over 30 years. *Foot Ankle* 1987, 8:26–28.
2. Praemer A, Furner S, Rice DP: *Musculoskeletal Conditions in the United States.* Park Ridge IL: American Academy of Orthopaedic Surgeons; 1992.
3. Lauge-Hansen N: Fractures of the ankle, II: combined experimental-surgical and experimental-roentgenologic investigations. *Arch Surg* 1950, 60:957–985.
4. Nielsen JO, Dons Jensen H, Sarensen TT: Lauge-Hansen classification of malleolar fractures: an assessment of the reproducibility in 118 cases. *Acta Orthop Scand* 1990, 61:385–387.
5. Rasmussen S, Madsen PV, Bennicke K: Observer variation in the Lauge-Hansen classification of ankle fractures: precision improved by instruction. *Acta Orthop Scand* 1993, 64:693–694.
6. Thompson NOB, Overgaard S, Olsen LH, *et al.*: Observer variations in the radiographic classification of ankle fractures. *J Bone Joint Surg Br* 1992, 73:676–678.
7. Carr BJ, Trafton PG: Malleolar fractures and soft tissue injuries of the ankle. In *Skeletal Trauma: Fractures, Dislocations, Ligamentous Injuries,* edn 2. Edited by Browner BD, Jupiter JB, Levine AM. Philadelphia: WB Saunders; 1998:2327–2404.
8. Donatto K: Fractures of the ankle. In *OKU: Foot and Ankle* vol 2. Edited by Mizel MS, Miller RA, Scioli MW. Park Ridge IL: American Academy of Orthopaedic Surgeons; 1998:185–199.
9. Vangsness CT Jr, Carter V, Hunt T, *et al.*: Radiographic diagnosis of ankle fractures: are three views necessary? *Foot Ankle Int* 1994, 15:172–174.
10. Lantz BA, McAndrew M, Scioli M, *et al.*: The effect of concomitant chondral injuries accompanying operatively reduced malleolar fractures. *J Orthop Trauma* 1991, 5:125–128.
11. Rockwood CA Jr, Green DP, Bucholz, *et al.*: *Rockwood and Green's Fractures in Adults* edn 4. Philadelphia: Lippincott-Raven Publishers; 1996:2207–2211.
12. Whitelaw GP, Sawka MW, Wetzler M, *et al.*: Unrecognized injuries of the lateral ligaments associated with lateral malleolar fractures of the ankle. *J Bone Joint Surg Am* 1989, 71:1396–1399.
13. Mueller ME, Allgower M, Schneider R,*et al.*: *Manual of Internal Fixation: Techniques Recommended by the AO Group* edn 2. New York: Springer-Verlag; 1979:282–299.
14. Weber BG: Die verletzungen des oberen spurnggelenkes. In *Aktuelle Probleme in der Chirurgie.* Berne: Verlag Hans Huber; 1966:CHAPTER PAGES.
15. Bauer M, Jonsson K, Nilsson B: Thirty-year follow-up of ankle fractures. *Acta Orthop Scand* 1985, 56:103–106.
16. Kristensen KD, Hanson T: Closed treatment of ankle fractures: stage II supination-eversion fractures followed for 20 years. *Acta Orthop Scand* 1985, 56:107–109.
17. Harper MC: An anatomic study of the short oblique fracture of the distal fibula and ankle stability. *Foot Ankle* 1983, 4:23–29.
18. Stuart PR, Brumby C., Smith SR: Comparative study of functional bracing and plaster cast treatment of stable lateral malleolar fractures. *Injury* 1989, 20:323–326.
19. Michelson JD, Helgemo SL, Ahn UM: Dynamic biomechanics of the normal and fractured ankle. *Trans Orthop Res Soc* 1994, 40:253.
20. Michelson JD, Magid D, Ney DR,*et al.*: Examination of the pathologic anatomy of ankle fractures. *J Trauma* 1992, 32:65–70.
21. Clarke HJ, Michelson JD, Cox QGK,*et al.*: Tibio-talar stability in bimalleolar ankle fractures: a dynamic in vitro contact area study. *Foot Ankle* 1991, 11:222–227.
22. Yablon IG, Heller FG, Shouse L: The key role of the lateral malleolus in displaced fractures of the ankle. *J Bone Joint Surg Am* 1977, 59:169–173.
23. Johnson EE, Davlin LB: Open ankle fractures: indications for immediate open reduction and internal fixation. *Clin Orthop* 1993, 292:118–127.
24. Schaffer JJ, Manoli A: The antiglide plate for distal fibular fixation. *J Bone Joint Surg Am* 1987, 69A:596–604.
25. Winkler B, Weber BG, Simpson LA: The dorsal antiglide plate in the treatment of Danis Weber type B fractures of the distal fibula. *Clin Orthop* 1990, 259:204–209.
26. Boden SD, Labropoulos PA, McGowin P,*et al.*: Mechanical considerations for the syndesmotic screw: a cadaver study. *J Bone Joint Surg Am* 1989, 71:1548–1555.
27. Burns WCII, Prahash K, Adelaar R,*et al.*: Tibiotalar joint dynamics: indications for the syndesmotic screw-a cadaver study. *Foot Ankle* 1993, 14:153–158.
28. Leeds HC, Ehrlich MC: Instability of the distal tibiofibular syndesmosis after bimalleolar and trimalleolar ankle fractures. *J Bone Joint Surg Am* 1984, 66:490–503.
29. Chissell HR, Jones J: The influence of a diastasis screw on the outcome of Weber C ankle fractures.*J Bone Joint Surg Br* 1995, 77:435–438.
30. Pettrone FA, Gail M, Pee D, *et al.*: Quantitative criteria for prediction of the results after displaced fracture of the ankle. *J Bone Joint Surg* 1983, 65A:667–677.
31. Xenos JS, Hopkinson WJ, Mulligen ME,*et al.*: The tibiofibular syndesmosis: evaluation of the ligamentous structures, methods of fixation, and radiographic assessment. *J Bone Joint Surg Am* 1995, 77:847–856.
32. Amendola A: Controversies in diagnosis and management of syndesmosis injuries of the ankle. *Foot Ankle* 1992, 13:44–50.
33. Procter P, Paul JP: Ankle joint biomechanics. *J Biomechanics* 1982, 15:627–634.
34. Peter RE, Harrington RM, Henley MB: Effects of implants on the motion of the distal tibio-fibular syndesmotic joint: comparison of screw versus K-wire fixation of Weber "C" injuries. *Trans Orthop Res Soc* 1992, 38:264.
35. Kaye RA: Stabilization of ankle syndesmosis injuries with a syndesmosis screw. *Foot Ankle* 1989, 9:290–293.
36. Browner BD, Jupiter JB, Levine AM: *Skeletal Trauma: Fractures, Dislocations, Ligamentous Injuries* edn 2. Philadelphia: WB Saunders; 1997.

37. Baird RA, Jackson ST: Fractures of the distal part of the fibula with associated disruption of the deltoid ligament: treatment without repair of the deltoid ligament. *J Bone Joint Surg Am* 1987, 69:1346–1352.
38. Stromsoc K, Hoqevold HE, Skjeldal S, *et al.*: The repair of a ruptured deltoid ligament is not necessary in ankle fractures. *J Orthop Trauma* 1995, 9:377–380.
39. Bucholz RW, Henry S, Henley MB: Fixation with bioabsorbable screws for the treatment of fractures of the ankle. *J Bone Joint Surg Am* 1994, 76:319–324.
40. Rokkanen P., Bostman O, Vainionpaa S, *et al.*: Biodegradable implants in fracture fixation: early results of treatment of fractures of the ankle. *Lancet* 1985, 1:1422–1424.
41. Carragie EJ, Csongradi JJ, Bleck EE: Early complications in the operative treatment of ankle fractures: influence of delay before operation. *J Bone Joint Surg Br* 1991, 73:79–82.
42. Fogel GR, Marrey BF: Delayed open reduction and fixation of ankle fractures. *Clin Orthop* 1987, 215:187–195.
43. Wiss DA, Gilbert P, Merritt PO, *et al.*: Immediate internal fixation of open ankle fractures. *J Orthop Trauma* 1988, 2:265–271.
44. Bray TJ, Endicott M, Capra SE: Treatment of open ankle fractures: immediate internal fixation versus closed immobilization and delayed fixation. *Clin Orthop* 1989, 240:47–52.
45. Konrath G, Karges D, Watson JT, *et al.*: Early versus delayed treatment of severe ankle fractures: a comparison of results. *J Orthop Trauma* 1995, 9:377–380.
46. Raasch WG, Larkin JJ, Droganich LF: Assessment of the posterior malleolus as a restraint to posterior subluxation of the ankle. *J Bone Joint Surg Am* 1992, 74:1201–1206.
47. Scheidt KB, Stiehl JB, Shrade DA, *et al.*: Posterior malleolar ankle fractures: an in vitro biomechanical analysis of stability in the loaded and unloaded states. *J Orthop Trauma* 1992, 6:96–101.
48. McDaniel WJ, Wilson FC: Trimalleolar fractures of the ankle and end result study. *Clin Orthop* 1977, 122:37–45.
49. Elliott JS, Larkin JJ, Lange EC, *et al.*: The role of the fibula in reducing ankle instability following bimalleolar fractures. *Trans Orthop Res Soc* 1994, 40:256.
50. Childress HM: Vertical transarticular-pin fixation for unstable ankle fractures. *J Bone Joint Surg Am* 1965, 47:1323–1334.
51. Childress HM: Vertical transarticular pin fixation for unstable ankle fractures. Impressions after 16 years of experience. *Clin Orthop* 1965, 120:164–171.
52. Moehring HD, Tan RT, Marder RA,*et al.*: Ankle dislocation. *J Orthop Trauma* 1994, 8:167–172.
53. Kelly PJ, Peterson FP: Compound dislocations of the ankle without fractures. *Am J Surg* 1986, 103:170–174.
54. Hoblitzell RM, Ebraheim NA, Merritt T, *et al.*: Bosworth fracture-dislocation of the ankle: a case report and review of the literature. *Clin Orthop Rel Res* 1990, 255:257–262.
55. Wroble RR, Nepola JV, Malvitz TA: Ankle dislocations without fracture. *Foot Ankle* 1988, 2:64–74.
56. Toohey JS, Worsing RA: A long-term follow-up study of tibio-talar dislocations without associated fractures. *Clin Orthop Rel Res* 1989, 239:207–210.

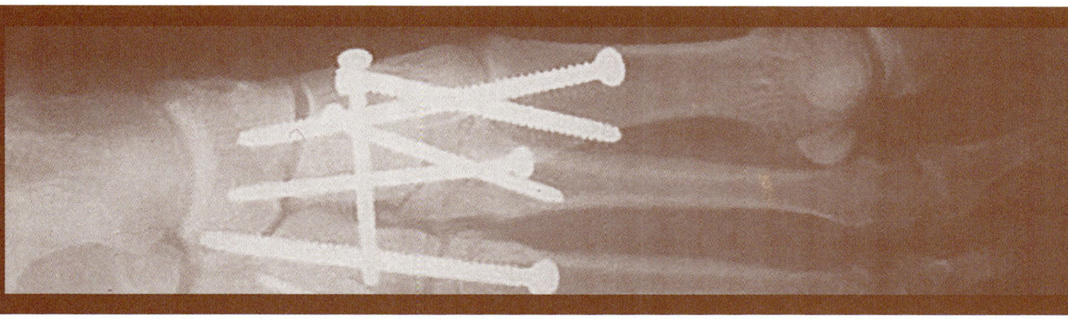

19

Foot Fractures

David S. Levine
Sigvard T. Hansen, Jr

The number of foot fractures seen in the emergency department of busy level 1 trauma centers appears to be increasing. Motor vehicle accidents (MVAs) account for a significant percentage of these injuries. Enhanced passenger safety restraint systems (*ie,* airbags, shoulder/lap belts) and improved emergency medical services have resulted in an increasing number of victims of high-energy trauma who survive their injuries [1]. With the diminishing incidence of fatal injuries to the head, chest, and abdomen, those patients with concomitant injuries to the lower extremity, including the foot, are being seen with increasing frequency. The orthopedic surgeon must, therefore, become increasingly aware and capable of treating such injuries.

Over the past two to three decades, advances in the field of orthopedic traumatology have increased understanding of the management of the polytraumatized patient. Early management of long-bone fractures has become standard in this patient population. As such, immediate emphasis is placed on management of femoral and tibial shaft fractures. "Less urgent fractures" are often diagnosed and treated as part of a secondary or tertiary survey once injuries regarded as more life threatening have been treated. Recent evidence suggests, however, that the presence of fractures involving the foot adversely affects the functional outcome of the polytraumatized patient [2]. In two groups of patients with matched Injury Severity Scores (ISS), the cohort with foot fractures had a significantly lower functional outcome when compared with those who had not experienced such fractures. Simply stated, although fractures of the foot cannot kill the polytraumatized patient, they may leave such a patient significantly disabled.

Fractures of the foot are among the more challenging fractures to treat. With an increasing incidence and the recognition that such fractures significantly influence the outcome of the traumatized patient, the orthopedic surgeon needs to be increasingly aware of their existence and capable of treating these fractures effectively.

CALCANEUS FRACTURES

Perhaps no other fracture has elicited as much controversy in terms of its management than the calcaneus fracture. Its unique shape, multiple articulations, unforgiving soft tissue environment, and traditionally unpredictable outcome are among the reasons such controversy persists.

Falls from a height and MVAs account for most fractures of the calcaneus. The energy absorbed can vary widely; such variability is responsible for the wide array of bony and soft tissue injuries encountered. Associated injuries of the musculoskeletal system, particularly the spine, are frequent and must be carefully evaluated.

Plain radiographs, including lateral, axial (Harris), and anteroposterior (AP) views, are important in establishing the primary and secondary fracture lines. Broden's radiographs have been largely replaced by preoperative computed tomography (CT) scanning; however, they are still quite valuable for assessing intraoperative articular reduction. Axial and semicoronal CT scanning have greatly contributed to the understanding of these difficult fractures. CT-based classification of Sanders is used most frequently for communication and research purposes [3]. However, classification of intra-articular fractures into joint depression and "tongue" types, as originally described by Letournel [4], has proven most helpful in our experience.

Broadly defined, management of calcaneus fractures revolves around intra-articular and extra-articular derangement. Intra-articular incongruity of the talocalcaneal (subtalar) articular facets often results in limited motion and painful weight bearing. Loss of height and length coupled with the increase in the width of the heel following calcaneal fracture makes use of standard footwear difficult if at all possible. The extra-articular fracture as well as the nondisplaced intra-articular fracture of the calcaneus may be treated nonoperatively. Early, aggressive range-of-motion exercises coupled with the avoidance of weight bearing until fracture consolidation has taken place may result in a satisfactory outcome. The displaced intra-articular calcaneus fracture should be treated operatively, unless contraindicated, to restore articular congruity and extra-articular dimensions of the heel. Occasionally, a nondisplaced or minimally displaced intra-articular fracture may have significant extra-articular derangement. Limited or percutaneous fixation is being used to restore the height, length, and width of the calcaneus in these special cases without the morbidity of an extensile exposure. The outcomes of these percutaneous procedures awaits further investigation.

After the soft tissue envelope has become amenable to surgical intervention, typically 10 days to 2 weeks following injury, the displaced intra-articular calcaneus fracture is approached through a lateral extensile exposure popularized by Benirschke and Sangeorzan [5]. Meticulous handling of the soft tissues is imperative because soft tissue slough with or without infection can be disastrous. The lateral wall of the calcaneus is reflected and the lateral portion of the posterior articular facet is temporarily removed. The anterior portion of the calcaneus is then reduced provisionally with Kirschner (K)-wires. The tuber fragment is subsequently reduced to the sustentacular fragment, thus restoring the extra-articular anatomy. Finally, posterior facet congruity is restored and the lateral wall replaced. The provisional reduction is verified intraoperatively, including taking a Broden's view to assess posterior facet congruity. Provisional fixation is then exchanged for low-profile implants, such as a 2.7-mm calcaneal reconstruction plate and screws. Closure is performed in layers over a suction drain. Plaster immobilization for 48 hours is followed by aggressive subtalar range-of-motion exercises. Non–weight bearing is maintained until fracture consolidation occurs, typically after about 12 weeks. Postoperative rehabilitation is essential, and has been noted in our experience to improve for up to 18 months following surgical intervention.

Ongoing prospective, randomized trials comparing operative and nonoperative management of displaced intra-articular calcaneus fractures can provide further insight into the management of these difficult fractures. In addition, the role of percutaneous or limited fixation of calcaneus fracture is certain to be further defined (Figure 19-1).

TALUS FRACTURES

Fractures of the talus, like the calcaneus, are a challenge for even the most experienced orthopedic traumatologist. The talus is covered by articular cartilage over most of its surfaces, which limits its blood supply. Its unusual, asymmetric shape and its relatively inaccessible position within the center of the hindfoot make assessment of the fracture reduction particularly difficult.

In addition to the standard foot radiograph series, a Canale view (taken in maximum equinus, 15° of internal rotation and 15° of cephalad tilt) is particularly helpful in evaluating the talar neck alignment. CT scanning is also helpful in assessing intra-articular involvement and fracture morphology.

Fractures of the talus are classified based on location in the head, neck, body, and process. Fractures of the talar head are uncommon. Principles of management include the restoration of the congruity of the talonavicular joint with stable, low-profile internal fixation to allow controlled early range-of-motion activity until fracture consolidation is observed.

Fractures of the talar neck are the most common. Often, the result of a fall or MVA, the energy involved may vary widely. Hawkins' classification, modified by Canale and Kelly [6], is useful for descriptive as well as prognostic purposes. The incidence of disruption of the talar body blood supply and therefore the incidence of avascular necrosis are predicted by the classification system. Nondisplaced talar neck fractures (Type I) may be treated nonoperatively. However, in our experience, most of these supposedly nondisplaced neck fractures have rotational and angular displacement that warrants surgical intervention. Type II (displacement of the subtalar joint) neck fractures are best treated with surgical stabilization to accurately verify an anatomic reduction of the fracture fragments. Type III (displacement of both the subtalar and tibiotalar articulations) talar neck fractures may present with internal or external extrusion of the talar body. They should be considered surgical emergencies and can have disastrous soft tissue consequences if displacement remains for greater than a few hours. Type IV fractures, which include a dislocation of the talonavicular joint, result in a nearly certain occurrence of avascular necrosis of the talar body.

Anteromedial and anterolateral approaches are used simultaneously at our institution. This dual exposure is required to ensure anatomic reduction of the displaced fracture and restoration of the complex subtalar articulation that is essential for its normal function. In cases without significant comminution, two crossed lag screws are used to maintain the reduction. If significant comminution of the talar neck is present, precluding compression, low-profile bridging fixation using miniblade plates and screws is particularly helpful. Postoperatively, immobilization for 48 hours is followed by controlled early range-of-motion exercises.

Non–weight bearing for 12 weeks is routine. Periodic radiographs are obtained to evaluate for radiographic signs of revascularization (Hawkins' sign).

Fractures of the talar body, like those of the talar head, are uncommon. Principles of periarticular fracture management are employed, including restoration of articular congruity and stable internal fixation followed by early motion. Medial or lateral malleolar osteotomy often provides needed exposure. Careful placement of lower-profile implants has increased the accuracy of our articular reduction. Improved outcome as a result of these advances remains theoretic, because a prospective evaluation of these uncommon fractures has not been recently reported.

Fractures of the lateral process of the talus are common. They require a high index of suspicion and may be overlooked by the unwary. Fragments that involve a significant portion of the posterior subtalar articular facet should be reduced and internally fixed. Smaller and extra-articular fracture fragments may be observed or excised if symptomatic.

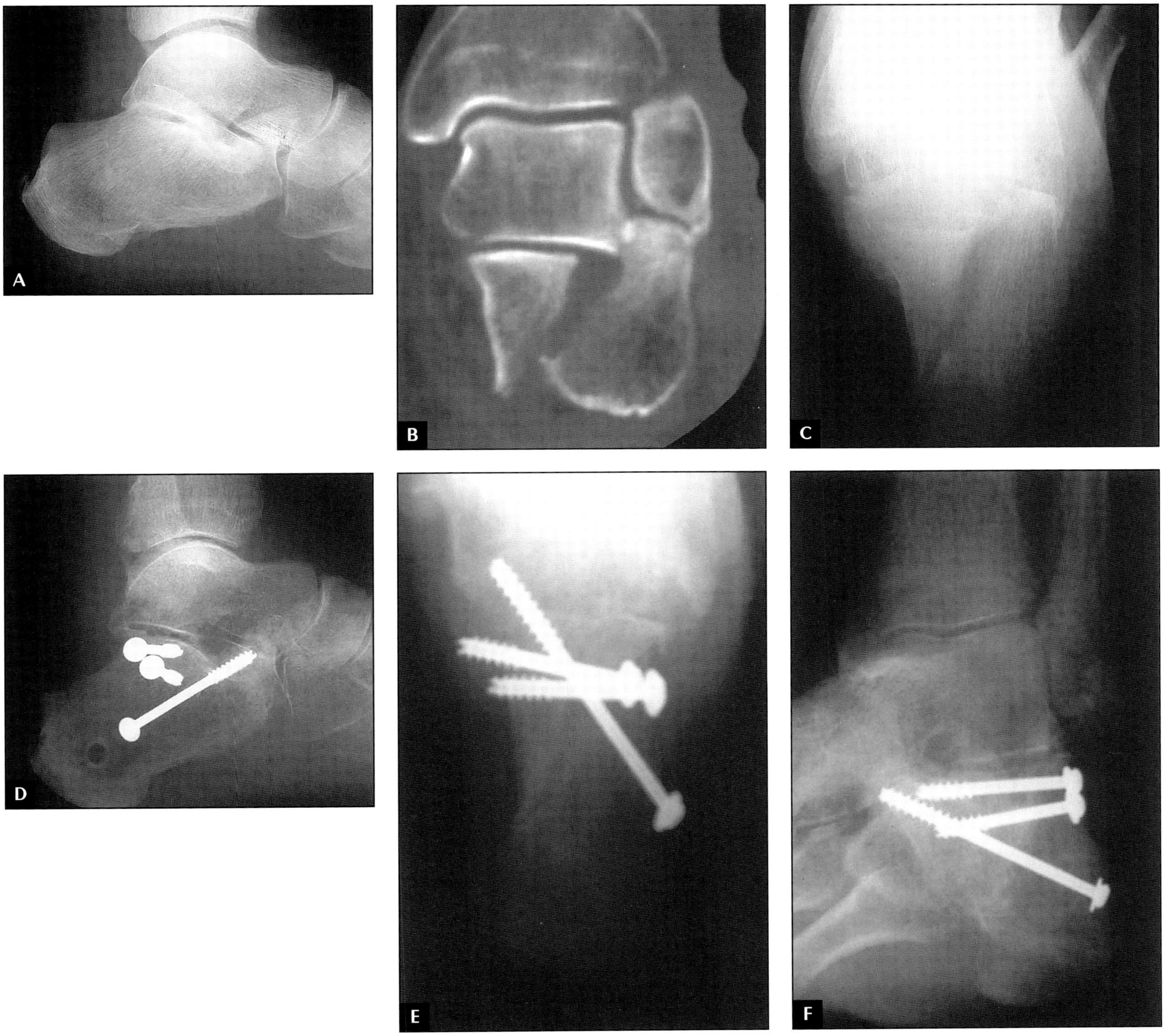

FIGURE 19-1. A, Lateral radiograph of a woman aged 87 years demonstrating a fracture-dislocation of the posterior talocalcaneal articular facet following a fall from a height. **B**, Axial radiograph and **C**, computed tomography (CT) scan demonstrating fracture-dislocation of the lateral third of the posterior talocalcaneal facet. **D**, Postoperative lateral radiograph demonstrating reduction of fracture-dislocation using "limited" internal fixation placed percutaneously. **E**, Postoperative axial radiograph demonstrating reduction of fracture-dislocation. **F**, Postoperative Broden's radiograph demonstrating "near-anatomic" reduction of the posterior talocalcaneal articular facet.

Fractures of the posteromedial process of the talus may involve a significant portion of the tibiotalar and talocalcaneal articulations. Open reduction through a posteromedial approach provides improved exposure for low-profile minifragment screw or plate fixation.

MIDFOOT FRACTURES

Because of multiple articulations and the anatomic uniqueness of the small bones of the midfoot, these injuries may often be overlooked. Unfortunately, they can result in considerable disability if left untreated. The midfoot functions as a rigid segment transmitting body weight from the flexible hindfoot articulations forward to the metatarsophalangeal joint for effective propulsion. If excessive motion exists in this ordinarily rigid segment, arthrosis and dysfunction soon predominate. Careful scrutiny of anteroposterior, oblique, and lateral radiographs is needed to avoid overlooking a midfoot injury. CT scanning is often helpful in evaluating the swollen, painful midfoot following trauma.

Chopart's joint (the transverse tarsal articulation), includes the talonavicular and the calcaneocuboid articulations. Traumatic injury at this level often produces a characteristic abduction deformity. Combined osseous and soft tissue injury is often present. The osseous injuries may include a crush to either the anterior process of the calcaneus, the cuboid, or a combination of these injuries. As a result, the lateral column cannot maintain its length and "falls" into abduction as a result of this compression. The clinician must carefully examine the soft tissue integrity of the medial column. If sufficient energy was involved in the injury, the posterior tibial tendon may be avulsed from its insertion and the talonavicular capsule may have been stripped from its bony origins. Healing in this deformed position greatly alters the mechanics of the foot and leads to further deformity, arthrosis, and dysfunction.

After such an injury has been noted on plain radiographs, CT and magnetic resonance imaging (MRI) scanning can further delineate the extent of bony and soft tissue injury, respectively. The mainstay of treatment is the restoration and maintenance of lateral column length. Cast treatment is routinely less than satisfactory because the lateral column shortens once swelling diminishes and the cast no longer effectively resists the abduction moment. Surgical intervention, in our experience, has proven effective with little morbidity. A small external fixator spans the zone of bony injury with small Schanz pins placed into the base of the fifth metatarsal and the anterior process of the calcaneus. Distraction provides sufficient ligamentotaxis such that internal fixation with small plate and screw constructs is possible, effectively restoring the stability of the lateral column. Occasionally, however, such comminution exists that internal fixation is not possible. In this case, the external fixator is maintained for 6 to 8 weeks. Cancellous autografting is a useful adjunct in this case to assist with the restoration of osseous stability.

Based on results of the physical examination and additional radiographic studies, exploration of the medial aspect of the midfoot may be warranted. Avulsion of the posterior tibial tendon must be treated with reapproximation and, occasionally, with tendon augmentation using the flexor digitorum longus. Capsular stripping is imbricated using a nonabsorbable suture. Early hindfoot range-of-motion is encouraged, however, weight bearing is delayed for approximately 8 to 10 weeks.

Fractures of the navicular uncommonly result from a fall from a height or from an MVA. They are seen more commonly with associated injuries to the ipsilateral foot than as isolated injuries. CT scanning often augments plain radiography and reveals significant plantar comminution. The navicular makes up an integral portion of the medial column of the foot. As in the case of lateral column injury, loss of medial column length results in deformity (typically adduction and varus) that alters the normal kinematics of the foot and subsequently causes pain and limited function.

Sangeorzan *et al.* [7] classified navicular fractures into three types based on the orientation of the fracture line and the degree of comminution. Nondisplaced or dorsal lip fractures may be treated nonoperatively in a short leg cast for 6 weeks. Displaced fractures of the navicular body are best treated with open reduction and internal fixation. A small distractor is used medially to regain length of the medial column. Reduction and fixation can be accomplished through medial and lateral incisions. Alternatively, a single longitudinal incision directly over the fracture line can be supplemented by percutaneous stab incisions for implant placement. Early hindfoot motion is encouraged; however, weight bearing is delayed for 8 to 10 weeks.

Fractures of the cuneiform occur infrequently. Both direct and indirect mechanisms have been described. The clinician should carefully scrutinize the surrounding osseous structures and their relationships to one another because such fractures may be associated with a tarsometatarsal fracture-dislocation. The three cuneiform bases (the navicular, cuboid, and metatarsal) function as a unit providing a rigid, stable midfoot segment. Disruption of either the osseous or ligamentous integrity of the midfoot can impart excessive motion, thus resulting in painful limitation of function. Plain radiography is usually sufficient to identify the pathology. Typically, shortening of the medial column of the foot is noted. Relative dorsiflexion or plantarflexion of the medial column should not be overlooked. If present, such a deformity must be corrected.

Management is determined by whether displacement and deformity are present. Nondisplaced fractures may be treated nonoperatively in a short leg cast for 6 weeks. Displaced fractures should be treated operatively with restoration of length of the medial column and restoration of articular congruity. A medial utility incision is made between the tibialis anterior and posterior tendons. A second longitudinal incision is made dorsally over the second metatarsal base. Internal fixation with lag screws placed perpendicular to the fracture lines is preferred.

Occasionally, a purely ligamentous injury to the navicular–cuneiform or intercuneiform articulations is noted. Because of the less predictable healing of ligamentous injuries in the foot, we are more frequently performing primary midfoot arthrodeses in these selected cases.

Postoperative management includes non–weight bearing for 8 to 10 weeks. If the stability of the internal fixation is certain, early aggressive hindfoot motion is encouraged.

LISFRANC FRACTURE-DISLOCATIONS

Injuries of the tarsal–metatarsal joint articulation (Lisfranc's joint) have been extensively studied. Direct and indirect mechanisms may result in various injury patterns. It is now widely recognized that significant functional limitation and disability may occur if such an injury is missed and treatment is delayed.

The tarsometatarsal articulation links the inflexible midfoot and the flexible forefoot. The osseous anatomy centers around the second metatarsal base. Its recessed position among the three cuneiform as well as its position as the apex of the transverse arch of the foot define its position as the keystone of Lisfranc's joint. The strong plantar interosseous ligaments that interconnect the multiple cuneiform and metatarsal–cuneiform articulations add considerably to the stability of the foot at this level.

Multiple classification systems have been used to describe such injuries, including that of Quenu and Kuss [8], which defines isolated, homolateral, or divergent patterns and is used most frequently. AP, oblique, and lateral weight-bearing radiographs are obtained if possible. A fracture of the base of the second metatarsal is pathognomonic of a Lisfranc injury. Frequently, osseous injury may be quite subtle. Various constant bony relationships have been described on plain radiographs [9]. On the AP radiograph, the medial border of the second metatarsal should line up with the medial border of the middle cuneiform. On the oblique radiograph, the medial border of the fourth metatarsal should align with the medial border of the cuboid. Failure of either of these two relationships is consistent with an injury to Lisfranc's articulation. Strong suspicion of an injury to Lisfranc's articulation despite negative radiographs is an indication for stress radiographs. Abduction, adduction, and dorsiflexion stress radiographs are helpful in cases of subtle ligamentous injury.

Nondisplaced fractures without deformity are treated in a non–weight-bearing short leg cast for 6 weeks. Displacement and deformity are strong indications for surgical intervention. After the initial swelling has subsided, a dorsal longitudinal incision is used to approach the first and second tarsometatarsal joints. A longitudinal incision in the third interspace is used to visualize the third through the fifth tarsometatarsal articulations. Lag screws providing interfragmental compression provide the best method of fixation and restoration of the regional anatomy. Neutralization screws traversing the numerous midfoot articulations provide increased stability while osseous and ligamentous healing occur. The fourth and fifth tarsometatarsal articulations have considerable motion under normal circumstances. As such, rigid internal fixation may be avoided and use of K-wires may be used instead (Figure 19-2).

As mentioned previously, purely ligamentous injuries at Lisfranc's articulation do occur. Perhaps with a heightened awareness of the importance of these injuries, fewer are being overlooked and thus their number appears to be increasing. We perform a primary midfoot arthrodesis at the first through third tarsometatarsal joints in such a setting. Given that healing of ligamentous injury is typically less reliable than osseous healing, arthrodesis of these nonessential articulations provides a reliable and more expeditious return of function without sacrificing the normal function of the hindfoot.

Postoperatively, non–weight-bearing status is maintained for 8 to 10 weeks in a short leg cast. Early range-of-motion is begun at 2 weeks in a reliable patient with secure internal fixation.

METATARSAL FRACTURES

Fractures of the metatarsals occur commonly through direct (crush) and indirect (MVA) mechanisms. Fractures of the metatarsals should be treated based not only on the location of the fracture (*eg*, base, neck, and head) but also based on which metatarsal bone is fractured.

Fractures of the first metatarsal occur infrequently. They are often the result of a direct crush injury or a high-energy injury (MVA). Given the importance of the alignment of the first metatarsal in the normal weight-bearing function of the foot, all but the nondisplaced fracture are treated surgically. Rigid internal fixation employing low-profile plate and screw constructs are used whenever possible. Again, restoration of the normal weight-bearing role of the first metatarsal in the sagittal plane must be verified intraoperatively both clinically and radiographically.

Fractures of the base of the fifth metatarsal occur frequently, most commonly as a result of an indirect mechanism. Unexpected inversion of the hindfoot can result in the base of the fifth metatarsal being avulsed outward due to the pull of the lateral band of the plantar fascia. Often nondisplaced or minimally displaced, these injuries can be treated with 3 weeks of partial weight bearing in a walking cast followed by an additional 3 weeks in a removable cast boot.

Fractures of the internal (second through fourth) metatarsals are frequent. They may occur in isolation or together. In isolation, the neighboring metatarsals often maintain the fracture fragments closely aligned through the intact intermetatarsal ligaments. On the contrary, in the presence of multiple metatarsal fractures, greater displacement, shortening, and malrotation may be seen. Management is based on the degree of malalignment, that of the sagittal plane being most important. Excessive plantarflexion of the metatarsal results in overload of the metatarsal during future weight bearing, whereas excessive dorsiflexion of the metatarsal results in transfer metatarsalgia to its neighboring metatarsals. As a result, an isolated metatarsal fracture without malalignment may be treated nonoperatively in a removable cast boot. Multiple internal metatarsal fractures, especially in the polytraumatized patient, should be treated with surgical stabilization. K-wire fixation is used most frequently for metatarsal shaft and neck fractures, either placed percutaneously or through limited dorsal longitudinal exposure. Fractures with joint involvement require rigid internal fixation using plates and screws, thus restoring articular congruity and allowing early motion. Non–weight bearing for 6 weeks in a removable cast boot is usually sufficient. In cases in which nonoperative management is chosen, weekly radiographs should be obtained to identify sagittal plane displacement prior to osseous union.

PHALANGEAL FRACTURES

Like fractures of the metatarsals, phalangeal fractures occur commonly. Often the result of a direct blow or an indirect force, the management depends on the location and which phalanx is affected. Fractures of the hallux deserve special consideration. Fractures of the hallux proximal phalanx have a characteristic apex posterior angulation owing to the pull of the extensor hallucis longus and flexor hallucis brevis tendons. Restoration of normal alignment is important to avoid difficulty with footwear. Percutaneous K-wire fixation or plate and screw constructs are routinely employed for these diaphyseal fractures. Intra-articular fractures of the proximal phalanx should be treated surgically. Newer low-profile implants can reliably and effectively restore articular congruity and allow immediate motion. Distal phalangeal fractures of the hallux are typically crush fractures of the distal tuft. These fractures are treated with generous irrigation and débridement (when open); however, the closed osseous injury is usually treated nonoperatively. Intra-articular fractures are treated with low-profile screws to provide interfragmental compression.

Fractures of the lesser phalanges are treated individually. Most frequently, minimally displaced metaphyseal or diaphyseal fractures are treated with splinting (usually buddy-taping the injured

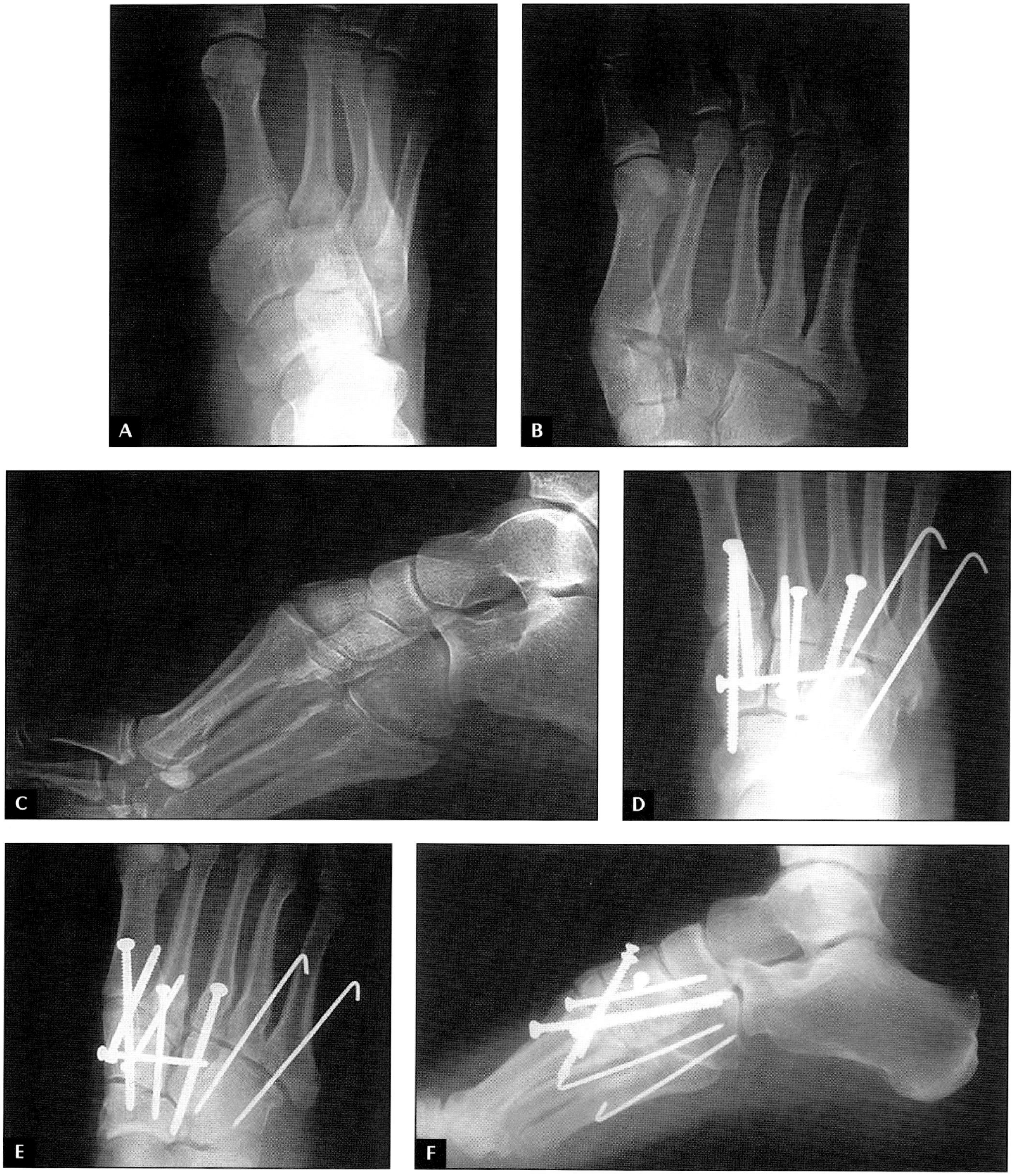

FIGURE 19-2. Anteroposterior (A), oblique (B), and lateral (C) radiographs of a woman aged 37 years demonstrating a displaced tarsometatarsal fracture-dislocation of the homolateral type following a motor vehicle accident. D–F, Postoperative radiographs demonstrating reduction using compression screw fixation of the medial column and Kirschner-wire fixation of the lateral column.

digit to its neighbor). Displaced extra-articular fractures are treated with reduction and splinting. Displaced intra-articular fractures may be treated operatively with low-profile screws or K-wire fixation. Limited weight bearing in a postoperative shoe is usually sufficient.

CONCLUSIONS

An increase in complex foot trauma can be attributed to advances in "prehospital" health-care delivery and improved automobile safety systems. Recent evidence suggests that foot fractures can result in considerable disability and significantly limit functional outcome in the multiply injured patient. The application of well-established principles of articular and periarticular fracture management has resulted in an aggressive, early, proactive approach to complex foot injuries. Our experience suggests that such an approach can result in improved restoration of function. Prospective controlled studies employing these concepts to evaluate the functional outcome of such injuries are few and will require careful comparison to series in the existing literature.

REFERENCES AND RECOMMENDED READING

Recently published papers of particular interest have been highlighted as:
- • Of interest
- •• Of outstanding interest

1. Trace R: While airbags save lives, MVA victims' fractures pose challenges. *Orthopedics Today* 1997:16–21.
2. Turchin DC, Schemitsch EH, McKee MD, *et al.*: Do foot injuries significantly affect the functional outcome of multiply injured patients? *J Orthop Trauma* 1999, 1:1–4.
3. Sanders R: Intra-articular fractures of the calcaneus: present state of the art. *J Orthop Trauma* 1992, 6:252–265.
4. Letournel E: Open reduction and internal fixation of calcaneal fractures. In *Topics in Orthopedic Surgery.* Edited by Spiegel P. Baltimore: Aspen Publishers; 1984:173–192.
5. Benirschke SK, Sangeorzan BJ: Extensive intra-articular fractures of the foot: surgical management of calcaneal fractures. *Clin Orthop Rel Res* 1993, 292:128–134.
6. Canale ST, Kelly FB: Fractures of the neck of the talus. *J Bone Joint Surg Am* 1978, 60A:143–156.
7. Sangeorzan BJ, Benirschke SK, Mosca V, *et al.*: Displaced intra-articular fractures of the tarsal navicular. *J Bone Joint Surg Am* 1989, 71:1504–10.
8. Quenu E, Kuss G: Etude sur les luxations du metatarse. *Rev Chir* 1909, 39:1.
9. Stein RE: Radiological aspects of the tarsometatarsal joints. *Foot Ankle* 1983, 3:286–289.

Section VI

Fractures of the Upper Extremities

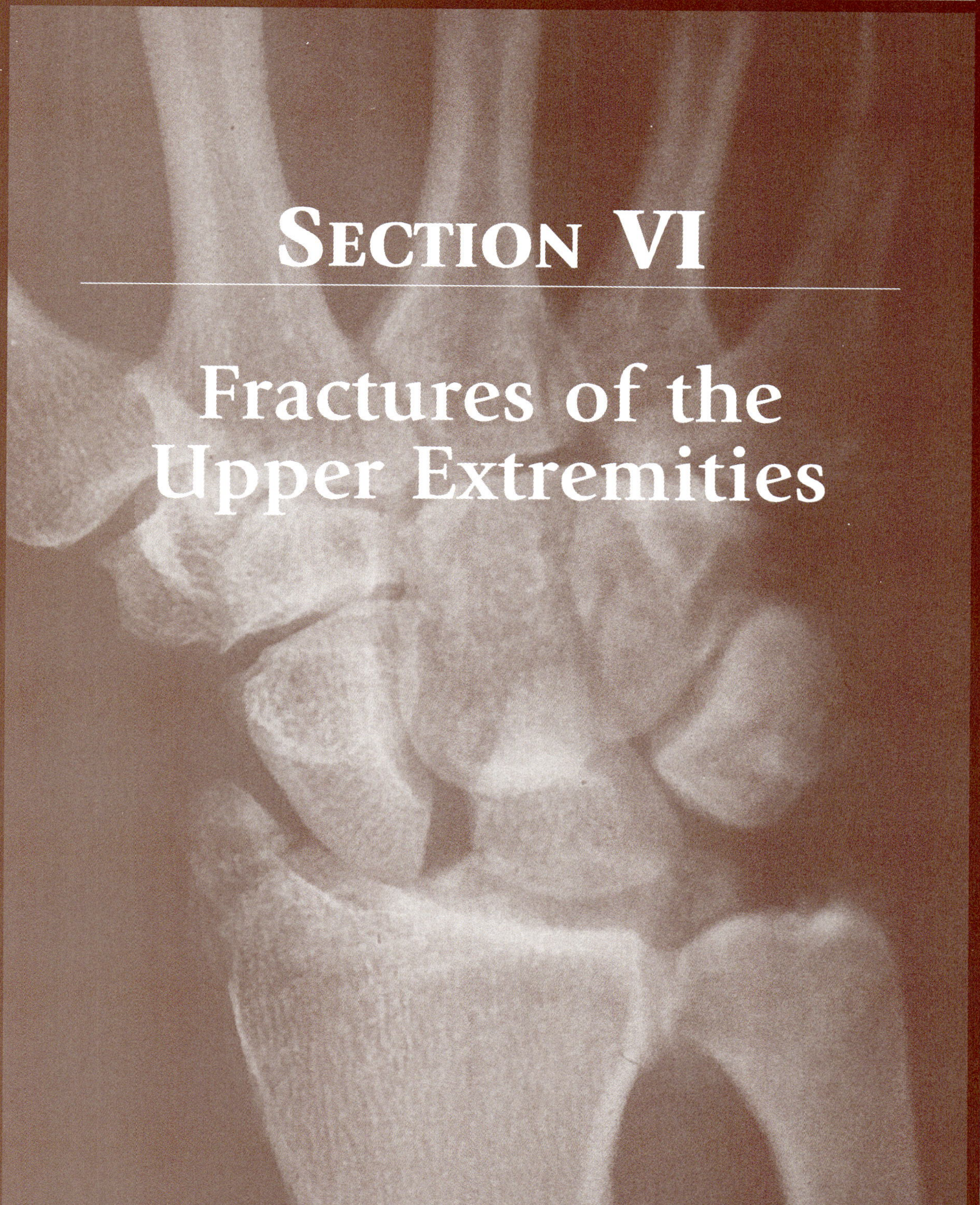

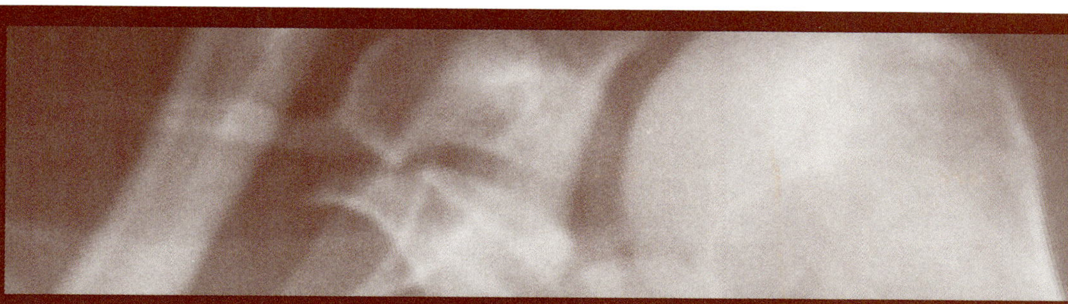

20

Fractures of the Scapula

Thomas P. Goss

Fractures of the scapula are uncommon and generally managed nonoperatively. These injuries involve a major articulation, however, and when significantly displaced are capable of causing considerable morbidity. Consequently, these fractures have recently received more consideration in the literature. This review will deal with the current evaluation and treatment of these challenging injuries.

INCIDENCE AND MECHANISMS OF INJURY

Scapular fractures constitute only 1% of all fractures, 3% of shoulder-girdle injuries, and 5% of all shoulder fractures. Most scapular fractures involve the body and spine (approximately 50%) [1–3]. Fractures of the glenoid neck constitute approximately 25% of the total, whereas fractures of the glenoid cavity (the glenoid rim and the glenoid fossa) make up approximately 10%. About 8% of these injuries involve the acromial process, and approximately 7% involve the coracoid process (Figure 20-1).

Scapular fractures are usually caused by high-energy trauma. Direct forces are most common, but indirect mechanisms can also be responsible (*eg,* a fall on the outstretched arm that causes the humeral head to produce an impact on the glenoid cavity). As a result, between 80% and 95% of these fractures are associated with other injuries that may be major, multiple, and even life-threatening. Consequently, scapular fractures are often diagnosed late and definitive treatment is often delayed. This, combined with the possibility of injury to adjacent osseous and soft tissue structures, may compromise the patient's final outcome.

DIAGNOSIS AND NONOPERATIVE TREATMENT

Injuries involving the scapula are often missed initially or detected incidentally on the patient's admission chest radiograph. If a scapular fracture is noted or suspected, true anteroposterior (AP) and lateral views of the scapula (Figure 20-2) as well as a true glenohumeral axillary projection make up the "scapula trauma" series. The clinician must be able to visualize and evaluate the scapular body and spine as well as its three processes: glenoid, acromial, and the coracoid. The scapula also takes part in three articulations (the acromioclavicular [AC] joint, the glenohumeral joint, and the scapulothoracic articulation) each of which must be carefully evaluated. The clinician should also look for associated shoulder girdle injuries including those involving the clavicle, the proximal humerus, and the sternoclavicular joint.

If an injury to the linkage between the clavicle and the scapula (*eg*, a disruption of the coracoclavicular or acromioclavicular ligaments) is suspected, a weight-bearing AP radiograph of the shoulder should be obtained (Figure 20-2). The scapula trauma series should suffice for most injuries but if the fracture pattern appears to be complex, computed tomography (CT) scanning is necessary. In certain clinical situations, reconstructed views may be of great value. Finally, three-dimensional scanning can be extremely helpful in evaluating the most complex fracture patterns. The proximal humerus can be eliminated for optimal visu-

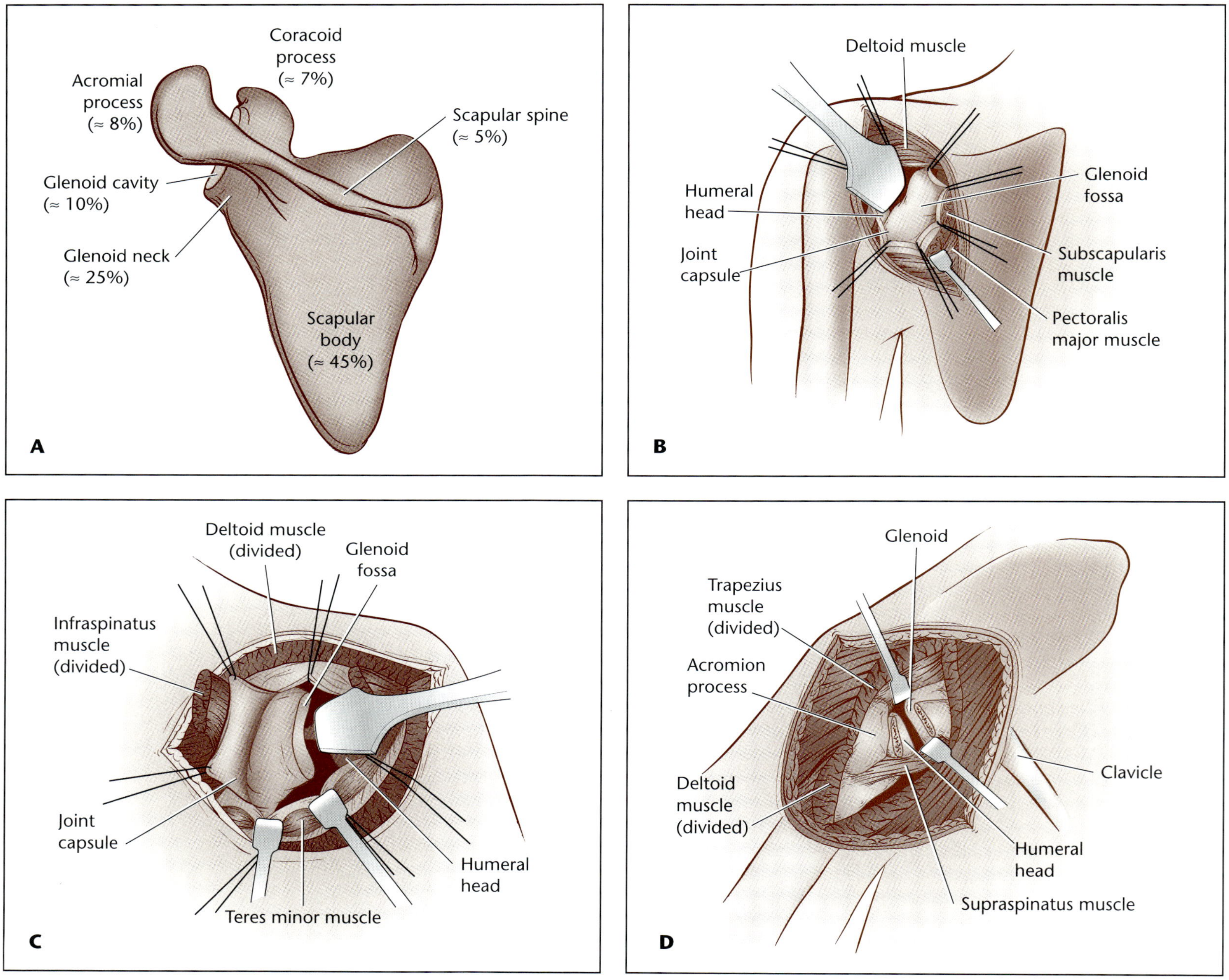

FIGURE 20-1. A, Incidence of scapular fractures according to region: the body (approximately 45%); the scapular spine (approximately 5%); the glenoid neck (approximately 25%); the glenoid cavity (approximately 10%); the acromial process (approximately 8%); and the coracoid process (approximately 7%). **B**, Anterior surgical approach to the glenoid cavity. **C**, Posterior surgical approach to the glenoid cavity with development of the infraspinatus–teres minor interval to expose the posteroinferior glenoid cavity and lateral scapular border. **D**, Superior surgical approach to the glenoid cavity. (Panel A *adapted from* Goss [4]. Panels B–D *adapted from* Goss [5].)

alization of the glenoid cavity and other reconstructed images are possible.

More than 90% of scapular fractures and virtually all that involve the scapular body and spine are minimally displaced or acceptably displaced. Treatment therefore is nonoperative and symptomatic.

OPERATIVE INDICATIONS

Although most scapular fractures are managed successfully without surgery, most physicians agree that surgical management should be considered for severely displaced injuries. Significantly displaced fractures of the glenoid cavity (glenoid rim and glenoid fossa) or glenoid neck and double disruptions of the superior shoulder suspensory complex (SSSC)—in which one or more elements of the scapula are significantly displaced—occur with enough frequency to merit discussion.

FRACTURES OF THE GLENOID PROCESS

The glenoid process includes the glenoid neck and the glenoid cavity, which, in turn, is composed of the glenoid rim and the glenoid fossa. Depending on the clinical situation, the glenoid process may be surgically approached anteriorly, posteriorly, superiorly, or combinations thereof (Figure 20-1). Thick, solid bone for fixation is at a premium because much of the scapula is paper thin. However, four satisfactory areas exist—the glenoid neck, the lateral scapular border, the base of the scapular spine, and the coracoid process (Figure 20-3). Fixation can be achieved with various devices; however, the most useful are Kirschner (K)-wires, which can be used for temporary as well as permanent fixation, malleable reconstruction plates, and cannulated interfragmentary compression screws. These devices can be used alone or in combination, depending on the clinical situation and taking into account the available bone stock as well as the surgeon's preference and experience.

SIGNIFICANTLY DISPLACED FRACTURES OF THE GLENOID CAVITY (RIM AND FOSSA)

Fractures of the glenoid cavity make up 10% of scapular fractures and fewer than 10% are significantly displaced [8–11]. Figure 20-4 offers a classification scheme. Type I fractures involve the glenoid rim: Type IA, the anterior glenoid rim and Type IB, the posterior rim. Fractures of the glenoid fossa make up Types II through V, and Type VI fractures include all comminuted (*ie*, more than two glenoid cavity fragments) injuries.

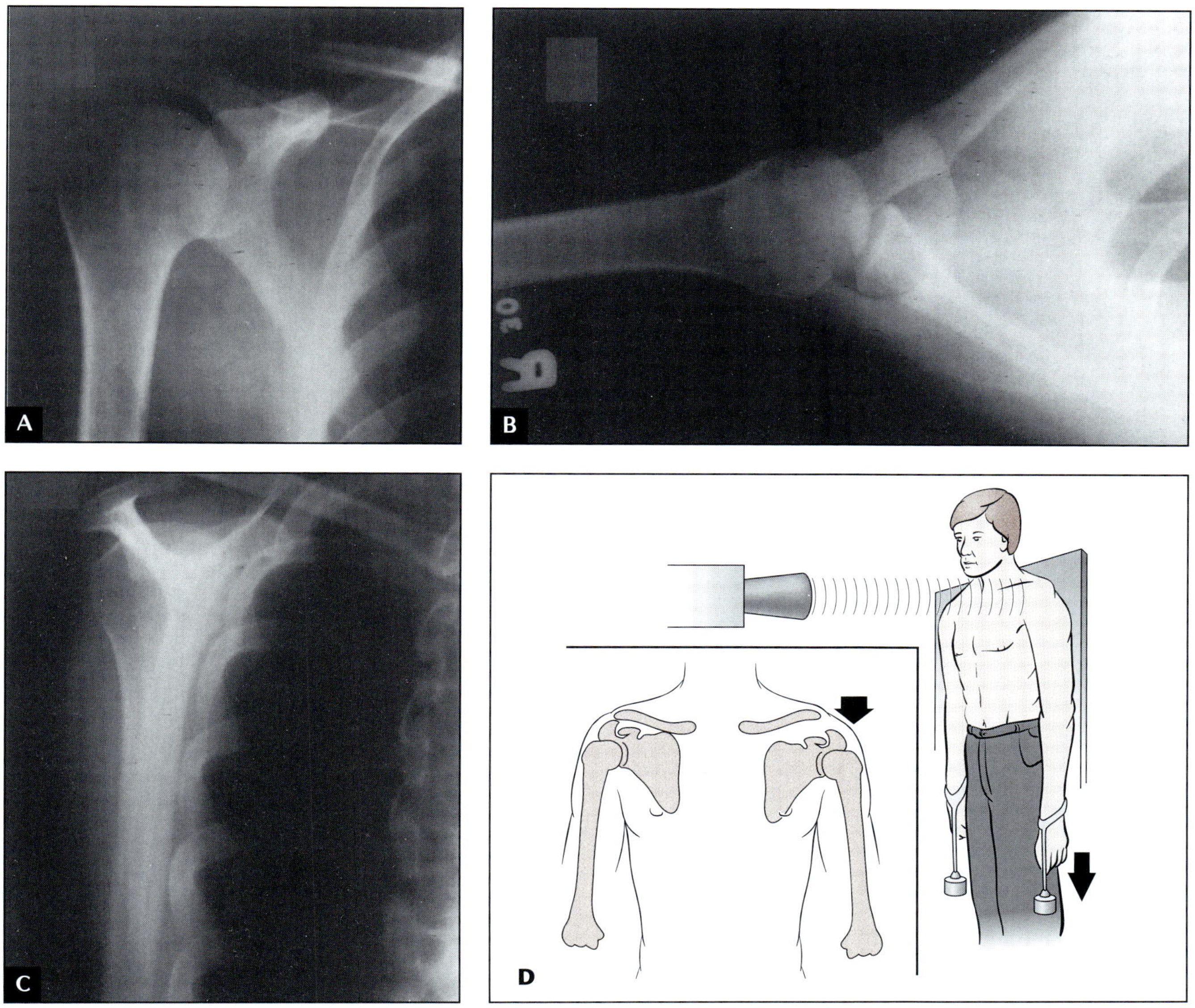

FIGURE 20-2. The "scapula trauma" series. **A**, True anteroposterior projection of the scapula. **B**, True axillary projection of the glenohumeral joint and scapula. **C**, True lateral projection of the scapula. **D**, Weight-bearing projection of the shoulder complex designed to evaluate the integrity of the clavicular-scapular linkage (optional and depending on the clinical situation). (*From* Goss [6]; with permission.)

Fractures of the glenoid rim (*ie,* Type I fractures) occur when the humeral head strikes the periphery of the glenoid cavity with considerable violence. These are true fractures, distinct from the small avulsion injuries that occur when a dislocating humeral head applies a tensile force on the periarticular soft tissues. Surgical management is indicated if the fracture results in persistent subluxation of the humeral head (failure of the humeral head to lie concentrically within the glenoid cavity) or if the reduction of the fracture or humeral head is unstable. Instability should be expected if the fracture is displaced 10 mm or more and if one quarter or more of the glenoid cavity anteriorly or one third or more of the glenoid cavity posteriorly is involved. A true axillary view of the glenohumeral joints, CT images (routine and reconstructive) and, if necessary, three-dimensional scanning allow the clinician to determine the size and displacement of the rim fragment, whether persistent subluxation of the humeral head is present, and therefore whether stability of the glenohumeral articulation is significantly compromised. Surgery, if necessary, is designed to restore articular stability and prevent posttraumatic degenerative disease. Type IA fractures are approached anteriorly. The displaced fragment is mobilized, reduced anatomically, and fixed in position with cannulated interfragmentary compression screws (ideally two screws are used to provide rotational stability). Type IB fractures are approached posteriorly and reduced and stabilized in the same manner (Figure 20-5). If the fracture is comminuted, the fragments are excised and a tricortical graft harvested from the iliac crest is placed intra-articularly, filling the defect.

Fractures of the glenoid fossa (Types II through V) occur when the humeral head is driven with sufficient force into the center of the glenoid concavity. The fracture generally begins as a transverse disruption (or a slightly oblique one) and then propagates in various directions depending on the exact direction of the humeral head force. An AP projection of the glenohumeral joint, reconstructed CT images in the coronal plane, and even three-dimensional CT scanning may be necessary to determine accurately whether and to what degree articular incongruity or separation, alone or in combination, is present. The goals of operative intervention are to prevent posttraumatic glenohumeral osteoarthritis, chronic glenohumeral instability, and nonunion at the fracture site from occurring.

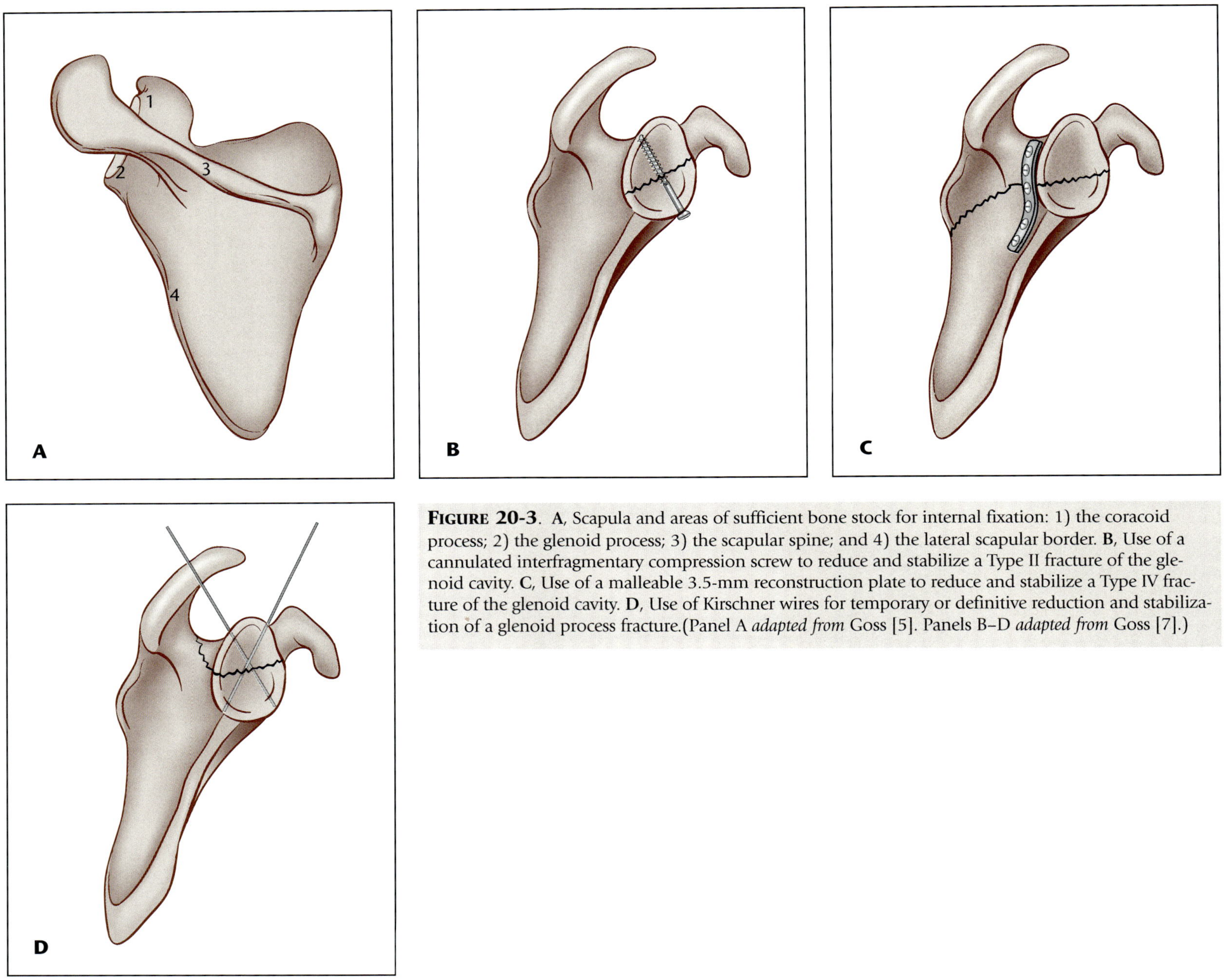

FIGURE 20-3. **A**, Scapula and areas of sufficient bone stock for internal fixation: 1) the coracoid process; 2) the glenoid process; 3) the scapular spine; and 4) the lateral scapular border. **B**, Use of a cannulated interfragmentary compression screw to reduce and stabilize a Type II fracture of the glenoid cavity. **C**, Use of a malleable 3.5-mm reconstruction plate to reduce and stabilize a Type IV fracture of the glenoid cavity. **D**, Use of Kirschner wires for temporary or definitive reduction and stabilization of a glenoid process fracture.(Panel A *adapted from* Goss [5]. Panels B–D *adapted from* Goss [7].)

Type II Fractures

With these injuries, the humeral head is driven inferiorly, which creates an inferior glenoid fragment. Surgery is indicated if there is an articular step-off of 5 mm or more and if the fragment displaces inferiorly, carrying with it the humeral head such that the humeral head fails to lie in the center of the glenoid cavity. These injuries can result in posttraumatic degenerative joint disease and glenohumeral instability. Type II fractures are approached posteriorly. The infraspinatus/teres minor interval is developed, exposing the displaced inferior glenoid fragment and the lateral scapular border. The fragment is reduced as nearly anatomically as possible and stabilized, generally with two cannulated interfragmentary compression screws passed posteroinferiorly to anterosuperiorly or with a contoured reconstruction plate placed along the posterior aspect of the glenoid process and the lateral scapular border.

Type III Fractures

These injuries occur when the force of the humeral head is directed superiorly causing the transverse disruption to propagate upward, generally exiting through the superior scapular border in the vicinity of the suprascapular notch. One might question whether this is a fracture of the glenoid cavity or a proximal fracture of the coracoid process because the superior third of the glenoid cavity and the base of the coracoid process are formed from the same ossification center. Surgical management is indicated if an articular step-off exists of 5 mm or more with superior fragment displaced laterally or in the presence of a significantly displaced associated disruption of the superior shoulder suspensory complex (the clavicular–coracoclavicular ligamentous–coracoid [C-4] linkage or the clavicular–AC joint–acromial strut). These injuries can result in posttraumatic degenerative joint disease and severe functional impairment. A posterosuperior surgical exposure (or an anterior approach through the rotator interval without taking down the subscapularis musculotendinous unit) is used. The fragment is reduced as anatomically as possible and stabilized with a cannulated interfragmentary compression screw placed superiorly to inferiorly. Associated disruptions of the superior shoulder suspensory complex may need to be addressed as well.

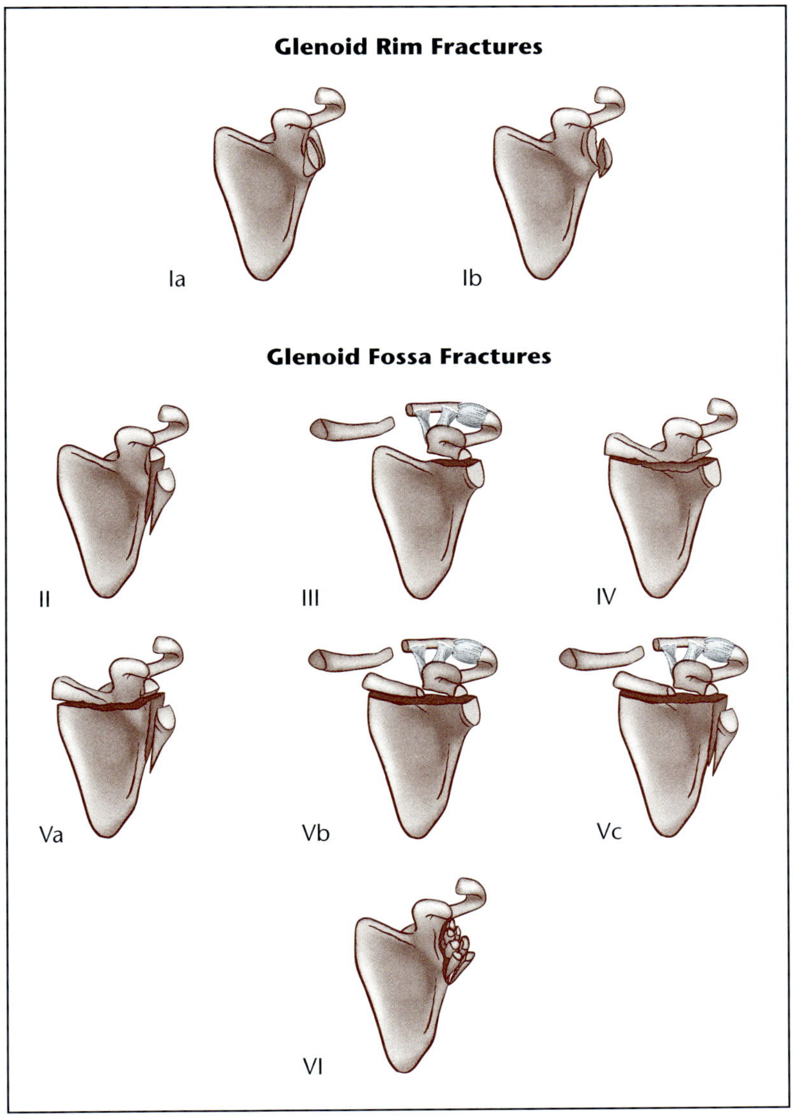

Figure 20-4. Classification scheme for fractures of the glenoid cavity.(*Adapted from* Goss [8].)

Type IV Fractures

These injuries result when the humeral head is driven directly into the center of the glenoid fossa. The fracture created courses transversely across the entire scapula exiting along its vertebral border. If there is an articular step-off of 5 mm or more with the superior fragment displaced laterally or if the superior and inferior fragments are severely separated, open reduction and internal fixation is indicated to avoid symptomatic degenerative joint disease, nonunion at the fracture site, and instability of the glenohumeral joint. These fractures are approached posterosuperiorly. The superior glenoid-scapular segment is reduced relative to the inferior segment while directly visualizing the reduction through the posterior exposure. A cannulated interfragmentary compression screw is then placed superiorly to inferiorly. A cerclage wire or cerclage suture passed around the glenoid neck has also been used for fixation.

Type V Fractures

Types Va, Vb, and Vc fractures are combinations of Types II, III, and IV injuries and are caused by more violent and complex forces. The same clinical concerns, operative indications, and surgical principles detailed with Types II, III, and IV fractures apply.

Type VI Fractures

These injuries include all disruptions of the glenoid cavity in which more than two articular fragments are present; they are caused by the most violent forces. Operative treatment is contraindicated because exposing these injuries surgically disrupts what little soft tissue support remains, thus rendering the fragments even more unstable and making a bad situation worse. An associated disruption of the superior shoulder suspensory complex may warrant operative correction, however, and this may indirectly improve glenoid articular congruity. These injuries obviously have the highest potential for posttraumatic degenerative joint disease and glenohumeral instability.

Significantly Displaced Fractures of the Glenoid Neck

Fractures of the glenoid neck make up 25% of scapular fractures and fewer than 10% are significantly displaced [9,12]. Figure 20-

6 offers a classification scheme based on whether these injuries are minimally or significantly displaced. If significant displacement occurs, it may be in either the translational or the rotatory plane.

Fractures of the glenoid neck may be caused by a direct blow over the anterior or the posterior aspect of the shoulder, a fall on an outstretched arm with impaction of the humeral head against the glenoid process, or force applied over the superior aspect of the shoulder complex.

The glenoid neck is that portion of the glenoid process that lies between the scapular body and the glenoid cavity. The coracoid process arises from its superior aspect. To be a glenoid neck fracture, the disruption must be complete, that is, exiting along the lateral scapular border and the superior scapular margin, either just lateral or just medial to the coracoid process. Displacement may then occur. If, in addition, its secondary support is compromised (*ie*, its attachment superiorly to the clavicular–AC joint–acromial strut through the clavicular–coracoclavicular ligamentous–coracoid [C-4] linkage and the coracoacromial ligament) (*eg*, a coracoid process fracture), there is a potential for severe displacement.

Type I fractures include all insignificantly displaced injuries and constitute 90% and more of the total. Management is nonoperative and a good-to-excellent functional result can be anticipated.

Type II fractures include all significantly displaced injuries; significant displacement is defined as translational displacement of the glenoid fragment greater than or equal to 1 cm alone or combined with angulatory displacement of the fragment greater than or equal to 40° in either the coronal or the sagittal plane. Significant translational displacement changes the normal relationships between the glenohumeral articulation and the undersurface of the distal clavicle, AC joint, and acromial process, thereby altering the mechanics of nearby musculotendinous units (especially the rotator cuff), which results in a functional imbalance of the shoulder complex as a whole with resultant shoulder discomfort and dysfunction. Significant angulatory displacement also results in adversely altered bony relationships and musculotendinous dynamics as well as shoulder pain and dysfunction related to gleno-humeral instability.

Basic radiographs necessary to detect and define these fractures include true AP and lateral views of the scapula and a true axillary view of the glenohumeral joint. However, CT scanning is usually also necessary to determine whether a complete fracture of the glenoid neck is present, to define the degree of translational and angulatory displacement, and to reveal injury to adjacent osseous structures. The clinician must not confuse these injuries with the more common fractures that course through the inferior glenoid neck and scapular body and do quite nicely with nonoperative care.

If surgical management is indicated (*ie*, with Type II fractures), the glenoid neck is approached posteriorly and the interval

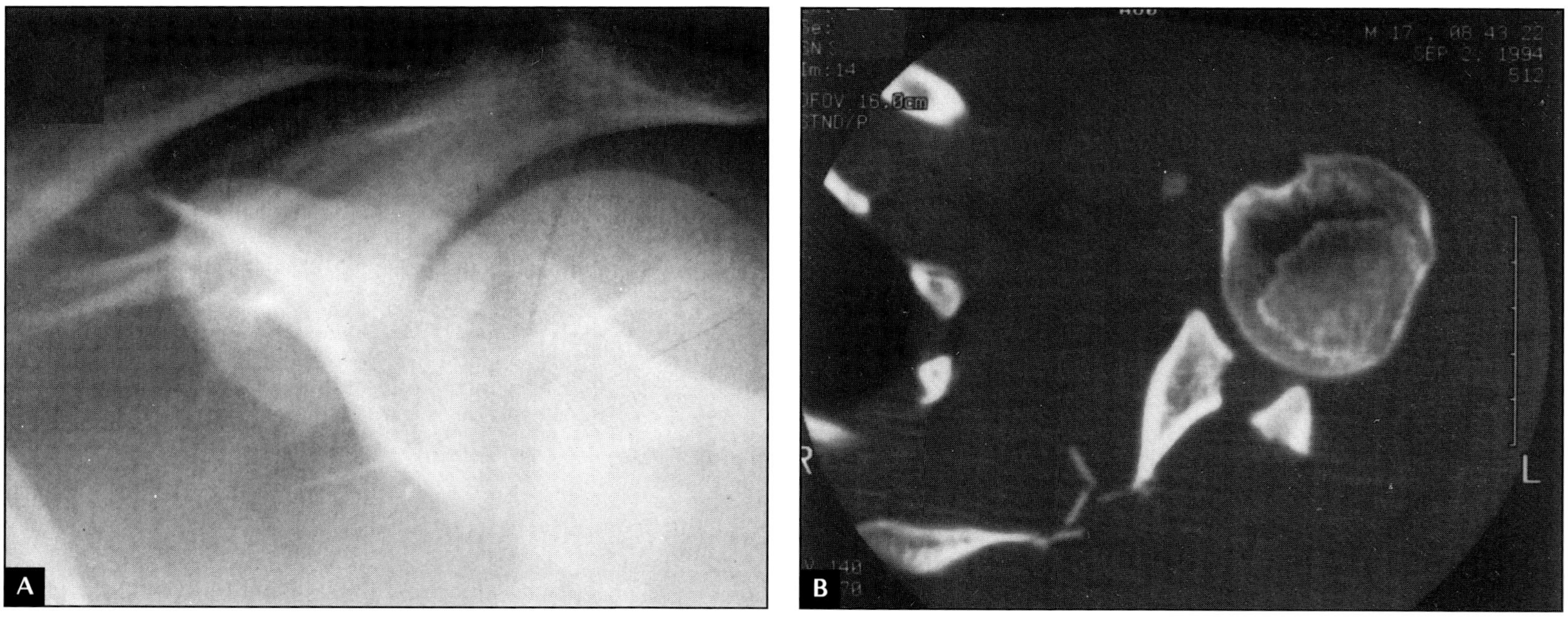

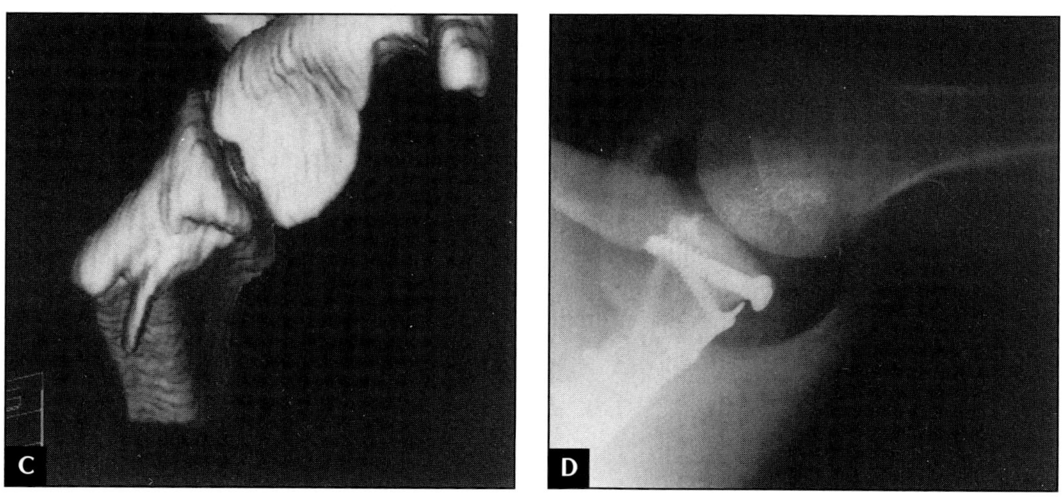

FIGURE 20-5. Radiographs of an individual who sustained a Type Ib fracture of the glenoid cavity. **A**, Preoperative lateral scapular radiograph showing what appears to be a fracture of the glenoid cavity with significant posterior involvement. **B**, Axial computed tomography (CT) image showing a severely displaced fracture of the posterior glenoid rim with posterior subluxation of the humeral head. **C**, Three-dimensional CT image of the glenoid cavity with the humeral head subtracted showing the severely displaced and rotated posteroinferior glenoid rim fragment. **D**, Postoperative axillary radiograph showing anatomic reduction and stabilization of the posterior glenoid rim fragment, with restoration of articular congruity. (*From* Goss [6]; with permission.)

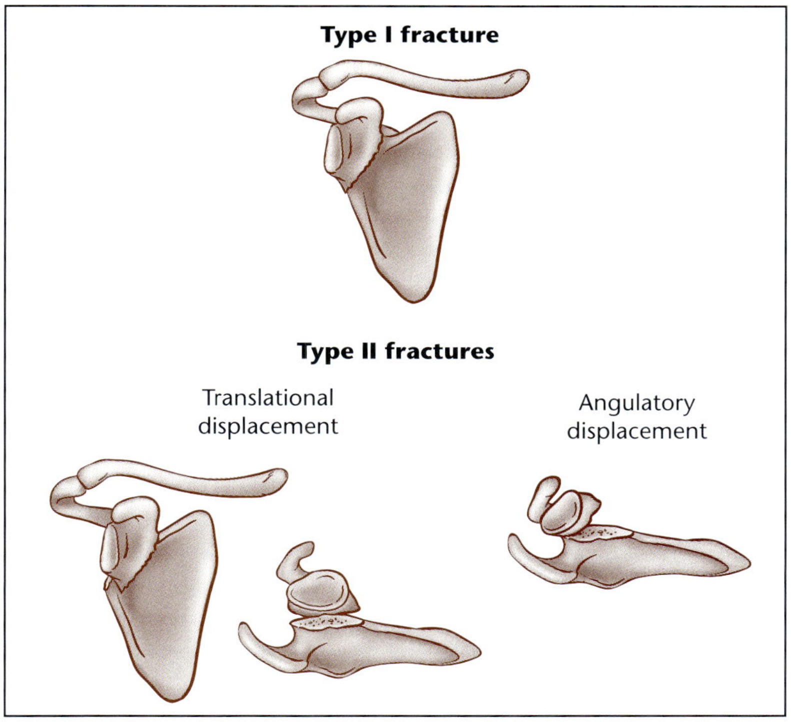

FIGURE 20-6. Classification scheme for fractures of the glenoid neck. (*Adapted from* Goss [12].)

between the infraspinatus and teres minor muscles is developed to expose the inferior glenoid process and the lateral scapular border. A superior extension can be added to gain access to the superior aspect of the glenoid process. After reduction of the fracture, fixation is generally achieved with a 3.5-mm contoured reconstruction plate applied along the posterior aspect of the glenoid fragment and the lateral scapular border (Figure 20-7). Temporary or supplemental fixation can be provided by K-wires or interfragmentary screws passed between the glenoid fragment and adjacent osseous structures.

Occasionally, comminution of the scapular body or spine may be so severe or the size of the glenoid fragment so small as to preclude plate fixation. In these cases, K-wire or interfragmentary screw fixation can be used to secure the reduced glenoid fragment to adjacent osseous structures, including the acromial process and the distal clavicle. In those rare instances in which the scapular body and spine, the acromial process, and the distal clavicle are all severely comminuted, either overhead olecranon pin traction must be considered or displacement of the glenoid neck fracture must be accepted.

If a disruption of the clavicular–AC joint–acromial strut is also present, it may need to be addressed as well. Disruptions of the coracoid process–coracoclavicular ligamentous–clavicular (C-4) linkage are managed indirectly by reducing and stabilizing the glenoid neck fracture and restoring the integrity of the clavicular–AC joint–acromial strut.

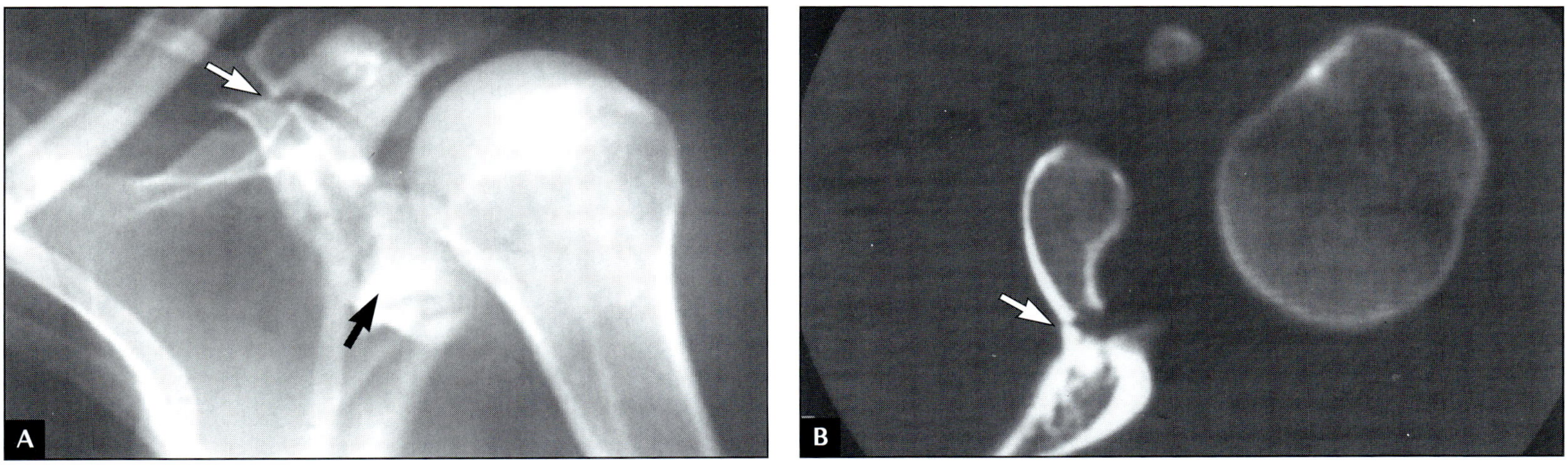

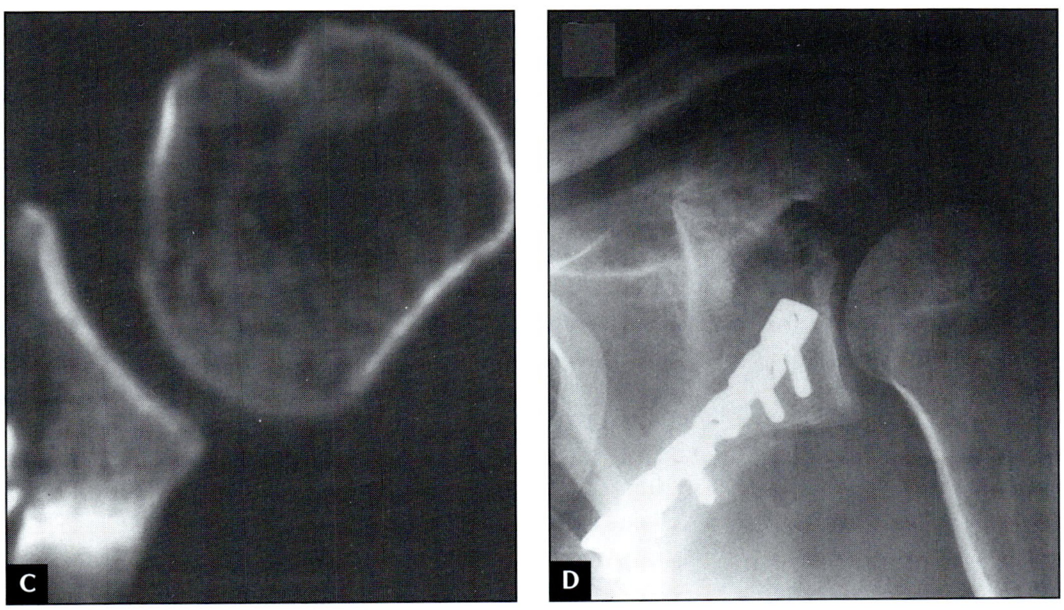

FIGURE 20-7. Patient who sustained a Type II fracture of the glenoid neck with significant angulatory displacement of the glenoid fragment. **A**, Preoperative anteroposterior radiograph showing the glenoid neck fracture with severe angulation of the glenoid fragment (*black arrow*) and a fractured coracoid process (*white arrow*). **B**, Preoperative axillary computed tomography (CT) projection showing the coracoid process fracture (*arrow*; a violation of the C-4 linkage) that further destabilized the glenoid fragment and allowed severe angulatory displacement (a double disruption of the superior shoulder suspensory complex). **C**, Preoperative axillary CT projection showing the glenoid neck fracture. **D**, Postoperative amteroposterior radiograph showing the glenoid fragment reduced and stabilized with a contoured reconstruction plate (the coracoid process fracture was allowed to heal spontaneously). (*From* Goss [12]; with permission.)

DOUBLE DISRUPTIONS OF THE SUPERIOR SHOULDER SUSPENSORY COMPLEX WITH SIGNIFICANT DISPLACEMENT OF ONE OR MORE SCAPULAR ELEMENTS

The SSSC is a bony soft-tissue ring at the end of a superior and an inferior bony strut (Figure 20-8) [9,13,14]. The ring is composed of the glenoid process, the coracoid process, the coracoclavicular ligaments, the distal clavicle, the AC joint, and the acromial process. The superior strut is the middle third of the clavicle. The inferior strut is the junction of the most lateral portion of the scapular body and the most medial portion of the glenoid neck. The complex can be subdivided into three units: the clavicular–AC joint–acromial strut; the three process–scapular body junction; and the clavicular–CC ligamentous–coracoid (C-4) linkage with additional support provided by the coracoacromial ligament. Each individual structure has its own particular function(s). The complex as a whole maintains a normal, stable relationship between the scapula/upper extremity and the axial skeleton, allows limited motion to occur through the AC joint and the coracoclavicular ligaments, and provides a firm point of attachment for several soft tissue structures. The "double-disruption" concept is a biomechanical principle that underlies, unites, and allows the clinician to understand various difficult-to-treat injuries involving the shoulder complex that have previously been described in isolation. This double-disruption concept also has a predictive value in terms of certain injuries that are only rarely encountered.

Disruptions of one of the components of the SSSC are common. These are anatomically stable situations, however, because the overall integrity of the complex is not significantly violated and nonoperative management generally yields a good-to-excellent functional result. If the complex is disrupted in two places, however (*ie,* a double disruption), the integrity of the SSSC is clearly compromised, creating a potentially unstable anatomic situation. Significant displacement can then occur at either or both sites, resulting in bony healing problems (delayed unions, malunions, and nonunions) as well as adverse long-term functional difficulties (subacromial impingement, decreased strength and muscle fatigue discomfort, neurovascular compromise due to a "drooping shoulder," and degenerative joint disease) depending on the particular injury. Double disruptions may take various forms: two fractures of the bony soft-tissue ring; two ligamentous disruptions of the ring; a fracture and a ligamentous disruption of the ring; fractures of both bony struts; or a fracture of one strut combined with a ring disruption (either a fracture or a ligamentous disruption).

If a single disruption is noted on routine radiographs (true AP and lateral views of the shoulder, a true axillary view of the glenohumeral joint, and a weight-bearing AP view of the shoulder to evaluate the integrity of the clavicular-scapular linkage), the clinician should look carefully for a second disruption (CT scanning is often necessary because of the complex bony anatomy in the area). If unacceptable displacement is present, surgical reduction and stabilization of one or both of the injury sites are necessary. Frequently, operative management of one of the injury sites satisfactorily reduces and stabilizes the second disruption indirectly. If not, both disruptions may need to be addressed. The glenoid, acromial, and coracoid processes are all components of the SSSC. Consequently, many double-disruption injuries involve the scapula. Conversely, many, if not most, significantly displaced coracoid and acromial fractures are part of a double disruption.

Significantly displaced fractures of the coracoid process are generally approached anteriorly, splitting the deltoid and opening the rotator interval for exposure. After reduction, the fracture is usually stabilized with a cannulated interfragmentary screw (Figure 20-9, panels *A* and *B*). Significantly displaced fractures of the distal acromion are generally stabilized using the tension band technique while disruptions of the proximal acromion are more amenable to plate fixation (Figure 20-9, panels *C* and *D*).

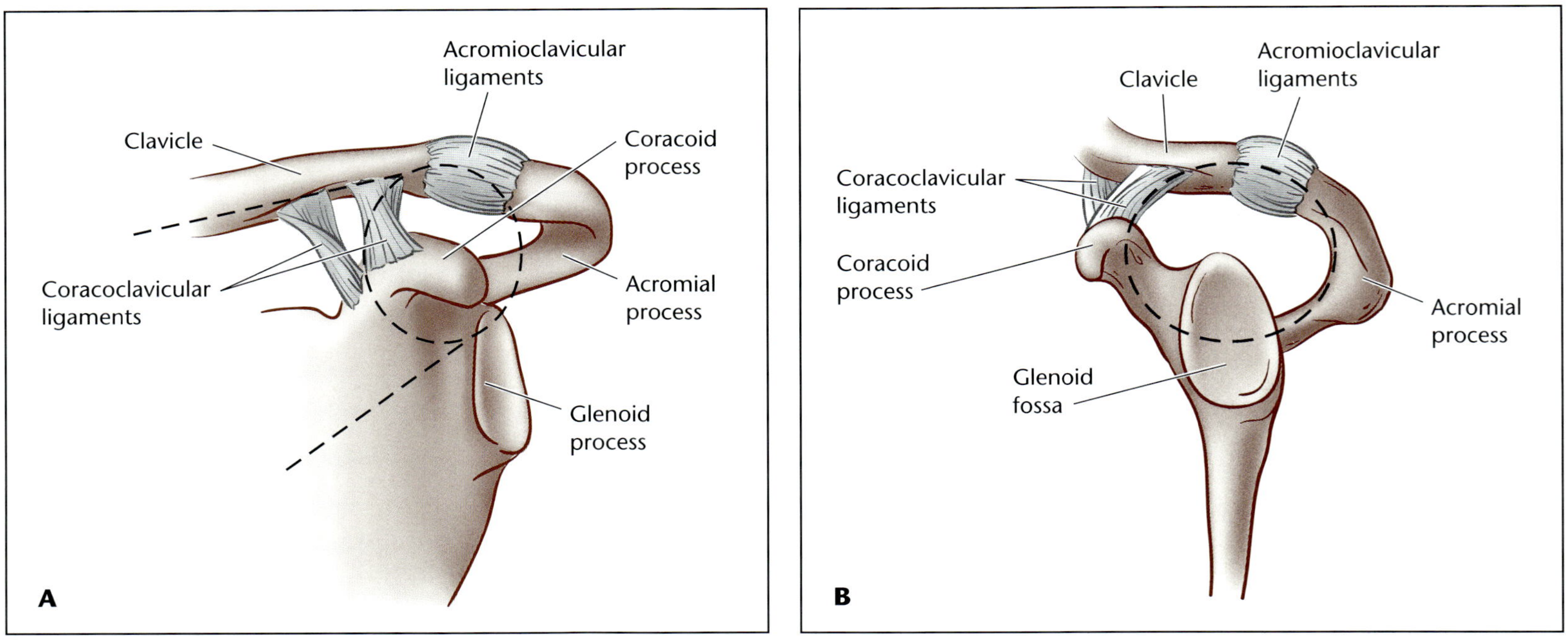

FIGURE 20-8. Superior shoulder suspensory complex. A, Anteroposterior view of the bony soft tissue ring and the superior and inferior bony struts. B, Lateral view of the bony soft-tissue ring. (*Adapted from* Goss [12].)

POSTOPERATIVE MANAGEMENT AND REHABILITATION

Postoperative care of surgically-treated scapular fractures depends on the degree of stability achieved. Immobilization in a sling and swathe bandage is usually prescribed during the first 24 to 48 hours following surgery. If fixation is rigid, progressive range-of-motion exercises and functional use of the shoulder out of the sling within clearly defined limits are then begun. If surgical fixation is less than rigid, the shoulder may need to be protected in a sling and swathe immobilizer, an abduction brace, or even overhead olecranon pin traction for 7 to 14 days (depending on the clinical situation). The patient is followed clinically and radiographically every 2 weeks to ensure that displacement does not occur at the fracture site and also to monitor and update the rehabilitation program. At 6 weeks, healing is sufficient to discontinue all external support and encourage unprotected progressive functional use of the extremity. Physiotherapy continues to focus on regaining range of motion until satisfactory, at which time progressive strengthening exercises are added. The patient's rehabilitation program continues until range of motion, strength, and overall function are maximized. Light use of the shoulder is emphasized through postoperative week 12. Heavy, physical use of the shoulder, including athletic activities, is prohibited for 4 to 6 months. The patient is encouraged to work diligently on his or her rehabilitation program because range of motion and strength can improve and a true end result is often not achieved for approximately 6 months to 1 year after injury.

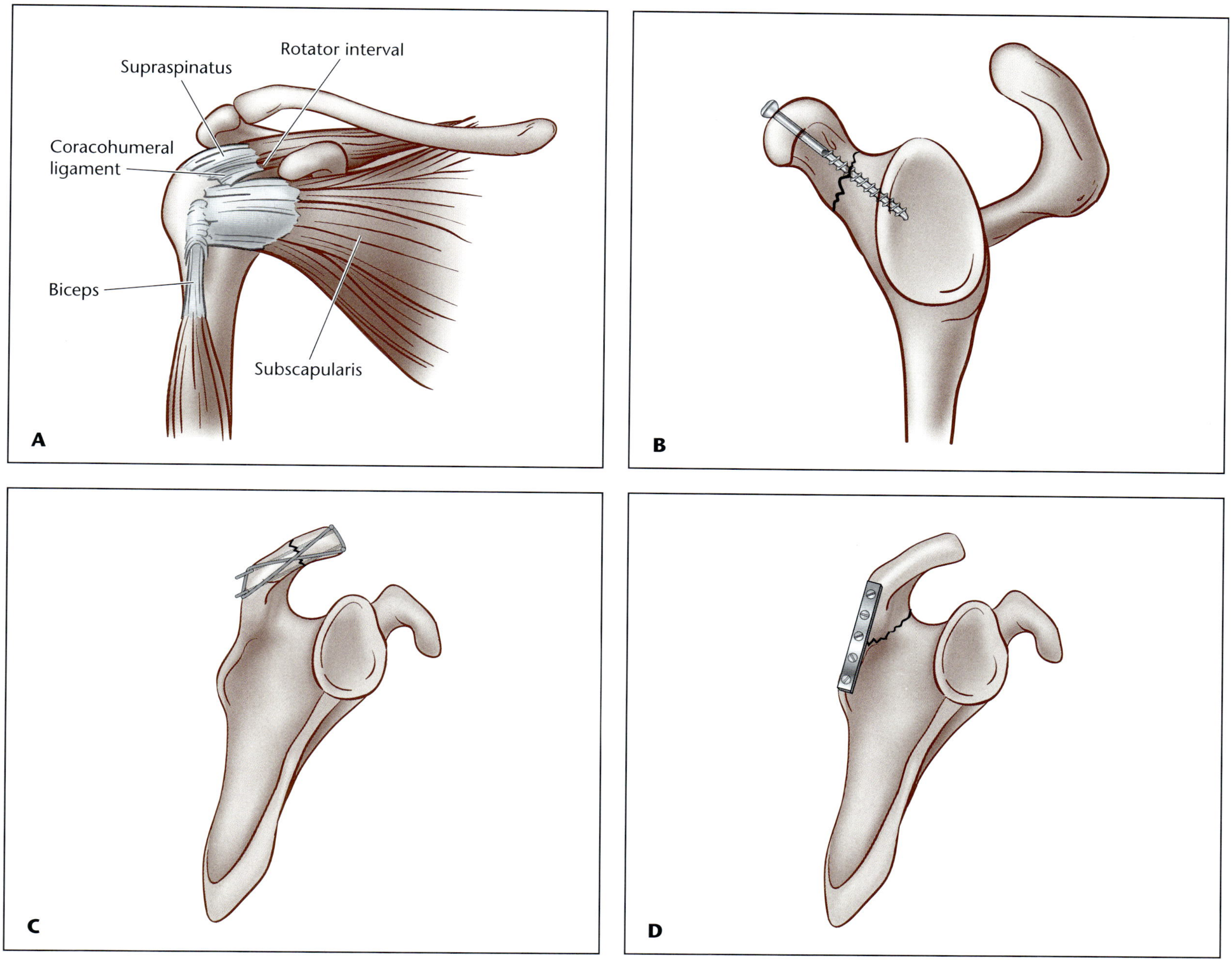

FIGURE 20-9. Surgical principles and techniques used for managing fractures of the coracoid and acromial processes. **A**, Rotator interval, which can be incised and the surrounding soft tissues retracted to expose the coracoid process including its junction with the glenoid process. **B**, Coracoid process fracture reduced and stabilized with an interfragmentary compression screw. **C**, Tension-band construct to reduce and stabilize a fracture through the distal portion of the acromion. **D**, Screw plate fixation for reduction and stabilization of proximal acromial fractures. (*Adapted from* Goss [6].)

REFERENCES AND RECOMMENDED READING

Recently published papers of particular interest are highlighted as:
- • Of interest
- •• Of outstanding interest

1. DePalma AF: *Surgery of the Shoulder* edn 3. Philadelphia: JB Lippincott; 1983.
2. Miller ME, Ada JR: Injuries to the shoulder girdle. In *Skeletal Trauma: Fractures, Dislocations, Ligamentous Injuries*. Philadelphia: WB Saunders; 1992:1291–1310.
3. Rockwood CA Jr, Matsen FA III: *The Shoulder*. Philadelphia: WB Saunders; 1990.
4. Goss TP: The shoulder and upper arm. In *Orthopedics in Primary Care*. Philadelphia: Lippincott Williams & Wilkins; 1999:30–69.
5. Goss TP: Fractures of the glenoid cavity: operative principles and techniques. In *Techniques in Orthopedics* vol 8. Edited by McPherson EJ. New York: Raven Press; 1994:119–204.
6. Goss TP: Fractures of the scapula: diagnosis and treatment. In *Disorders of the Shoulder: Diagnosis and Management*. Edited by Iannotti JP, Williams GR. Philadelphia: Lippincott Williams & Wilkins; 1999:597–637.
7. Goss TP: Glenoid fractures: open reduction and internal fixation. In *Master Techniques in Orthopedic Surgery: Fractures*. Edited by Wiss DA. Philadelphia: Lippincott Williams & Wilkins, 1999:3–17.
8. Goss TP: Fractures of the glenoid cavity. *J Bone Joint Surg Am* 1992, 74:299–305.
9. Goss TP: Scapular fractures and dislocations: diagnosis and treatment. *J Am Acad Orthop Surg* 1995, 3:22–33.
10. Ideberg R: Fractures of the scapula involving the glenoid fossa. In *Surgery of the Shoulder*. Edited by Bateman JE, Welsh RP. Philadelphia: BC Decker; 1984:63–66.
11. Kavanagh BF, Bradway JK, Cofield RH: Open reduction and internal fixation of displaced intra-articular fractures of the glenoid fossa. *J Bone Joint Surg Am* 1993, 75:479–484.
12. Goss TP: Fractures of the glenoid neck. *J Shoulder Elbow Surg* 1994, 3:42–52.
13. Goss TP: Double disruptions of the superior shoulder suspensory complex. *J Orthop Trauma* 1993, 7:99–106.
14. Goss T: The scapula: coracoid, acromial and avulsion fractures. *Am J Orthop* 1996, 25:106–115.

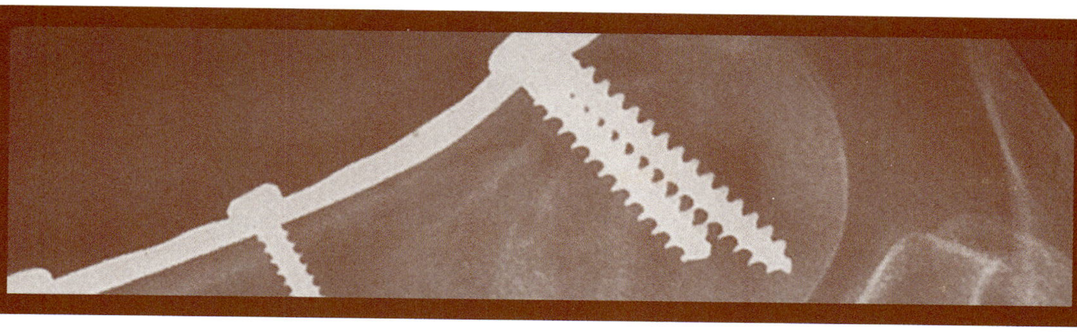

21

Fractures of the Humeral Head and Neck

Michael E. Torchia

Despite recent advances in imaging and fixation techniques, the treatment of displaced fractures affecting the proximal humerus remains a challenge. Many such fractures occur in elderly patients with poor general health, poor bone quality, and poor post-operative compliance. The remainder occur in younger patients with better bone quality who have experienced high-energy trauma that may cause associated severe soft tissue injuries. Specifically, the labrum, capsule, rotator cuff, brachial plexus, peripheral nerves, and blood vessels can be injured in situations of high-energy trauma. As with the treatment of almost any fracture, the goal is to obtain and maintain acceptable reduction while healing progresses. Although this goal can often be achieved with limited internal fixation and a period of prolonged immobilization, the subsequent stiffness can be disabling. Optimal treatment involves providing fixation that will withstand the stress of early passive movement. In practice, this ideal cannot always be achieved.

SURGICAL INDICATIONS

Most fractures of the proximal humerus (approximately 80%) are minimally displaced, impacted, relatively stable, and can be treated symptomatically [1].

Displaced, unstable fracture patterns are typically reduced (closed versus open) and fixed with various types of implants [2]. Although Neer's [3,4] classification system is well known, the importance of displacement has been underemphasized in the literature. Determining whether individual fractured bone segments are displaced to a significant degree requires high-quality radiographs: these films can be difficult to obtain in the acutely injured patient. Often, it is helpful for operating surgeon to assist the radiology technician in supporting the arm, positioning the patient, and confirming appropriate trajectory of the x-ray beam (Figure 21-1). In most cases, high-quality radiographs allow the fracture pattern to be understood. If not, thin-cut computed tomography (CT) scanning can be done. This modality allows the option of three-dimensional reformatting, which can be particularly helpful in the evaluation of complex fractures and malunions.

Provided the necessary radiographs are obtained, Neer's [3,4] classification is a practical and useful guide to treatment, particularly when applied to fractures of the surgical neck. Fractures with less than 1 cm of displacement or 45° of angulation of the head fragment (relative to the shaft) can generally be treated in a closed manner. It is worth noting that these guidelines may not apply to the greater tuberosity. Others have suggested that displacement between 5 and 10 mm may be significant in selected patients [5–7]. This relatively small degree of displacement can be difficult to determine given the variability in individual anatomy; therefore, comparison views of the opposite shoulder with the arm held in a similar degree of external rotation can be useful. The clinician must be aware of the so-called valgus impacted four-part pattern (Figure 21-2) [8–10]. Subtle impaction of the lateral aspect of the head may often mimic greater tuberosity displacement. If this fracture pattern is not appreciated before surgery, the greater tuberosity will be found to be irreducible. Although all four segments are fractured, the displacements in this pattern are not typically sufficient to qualify as a true four-part pattern according to Neer's [3,4] criteria. This lack of severe displacement is thought to lessen the chance of posttraumatic avascular necrosis in this fracture pattern.

The most common patterns requiring surgical treatment are the two-part with shaft displacement (displaced surgical neck fracture), three-part with shaft and tuberosity displacement, and four-part fracture-dislocation typically occurring in elderly patients. Less common patterns involve the isolated two-part greater tuberosity fracture, the two-part anatomic neck fracture (displacement of the head segment alone), and the so-called valgus impacted pattern.

ANATOMIC CONSIDERATIONS

The blood supply to the humeral head has been well described and should be respected during internal fixation [11,12]. During surgery, this means avoiding soft tissue disruption in the region of the arcuate artery that runs near the lateral aspect of the bicipital groove. Equally important is an awareness of the course of the axillary nerve and its vulnerability during exposure and fixation of fractures that involve displacement of the greater tuberosity. Exposure can be safely accomplished by abducting the arm to relax the deltoid muscle and working within the subacromial bursa. Such maneuvers become particularly important in cases that are treated late or in revision surgery, in which the anatomical planes are obscured by extensive callus or scar tissue.

The points available for fixation in the proximal humerus include the shaft, head fragment, and tuberosities. The shaft is characterized by its hollow tubular structure and constant availability for fixation with plates (screws), intramedullary devices, and prosthetic stems (bone cement). The tuberosities are characterized by their fragility, fragmentation, and the consistency of rotator cuff tendon attachment. These tendon attachments serve as a second point of reliable fixation.

The quality of the humeral head fragment varies with the age of the patient and the evident fracture pattern. In elderly patients this is most often a thin, hollow shell of bone that precludes rigid fixation but may be supported by bone graft or a fixed angle device such as a blade plate (Figure 21-3) [13]. Alternatively, in younger patients, ample high-quality cancellous bone is often available in the head to allow adequate purchase and fixation with standard bone screws (Figure 21-4).

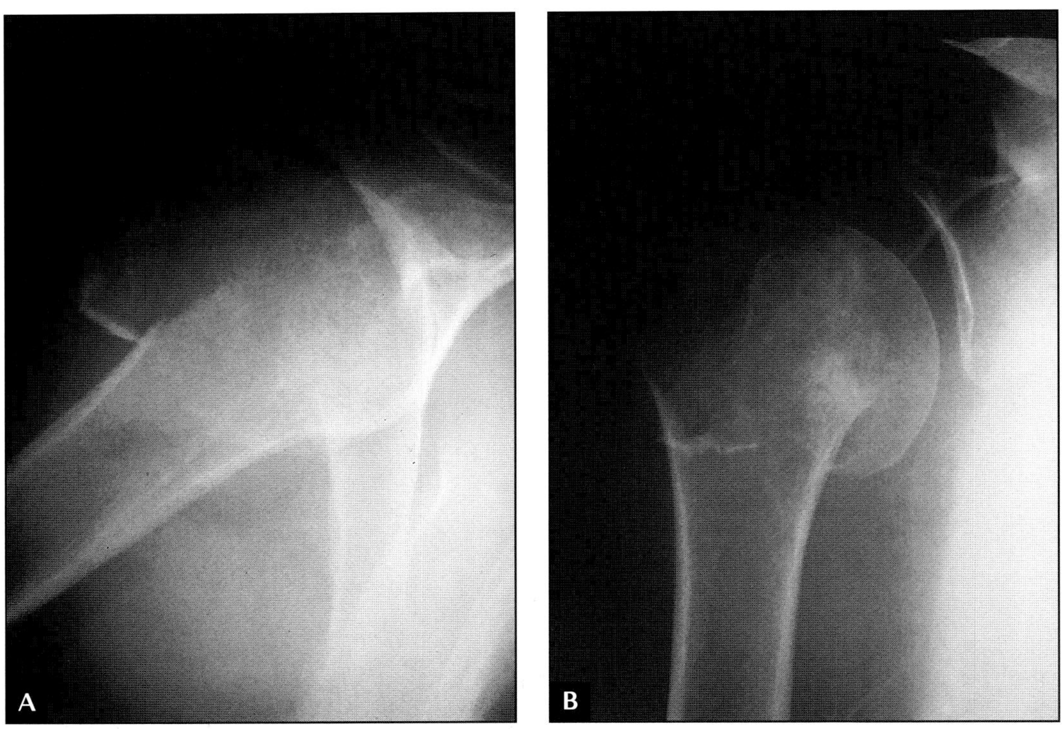

FIGURE 21-1. A, Proximal humerus fracture imaged with a radiograph oblique to the plane of the scapula. It is not possible to classify the fracture or determine the degree of displacement. **B**, Same fracture imaged perpendicular to the plane of the scapula with the arm in neutral position. This is a stable, impacted surgical neck fracture that was treated conservatively.

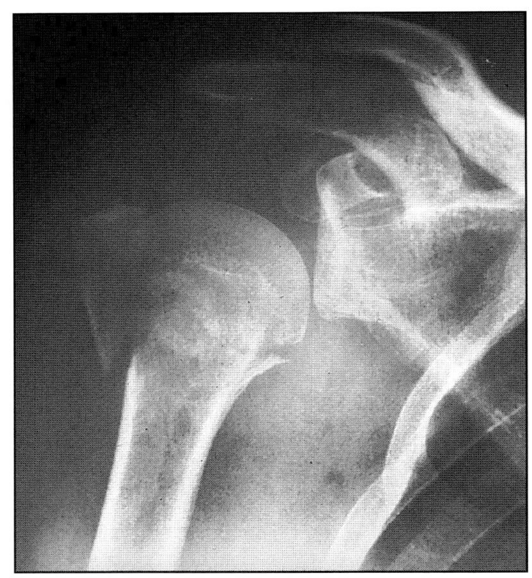

FIGURE 21-2. Example of a valgus impacted fracture pattern. Although four fractured segments are displaced, none is displaced sufficiently to qualify as a true four-part fracture according to Neer's [3,4] system of classification. Greater tuberosity is minimally displaced relative to the shaft. The head has been impacted into a valgus position relative to the shaft.

Patient Characteristics

In addition to bone quality, other patient characteristics associated with age influence decision making in the management of proximal humeral fractures. Specifically, younger patients tend to experience high-energy trauma that often results in associated dislocations and soft tissue trauma. In this population, a high propensity exists for postoperative stiffness, thus the goal of achieving stable fixation becomes paramount. Fortunately, this can be achieved consistently due to adequate bone quality and typically good postoperative compliance with passive exercises. In contrast, older patients are often subjected to low-energy trauma (falls), typically have poorer bone quality, and often have limitations of mental capacity and lack the social support necessary to protect the fixation by avoiding active use of the arm during the early postoperative period. These considerations also apply to proximal humeral replacement. As with any fracture fixation, postoperative protection is required to allow the opportunity for healing between the greater tuberosity and shaft. Thus, it is not surprising that the results of hemiarthroplasty for trauma have been only fair at best.

Intraoperative Set-Up and Positioning

Regardless of the planned procedure (internal fixation versus hemiarthroplasty), intraoperative set-up and positioning are the same. The key features include neutral positioning of the cervical spine and lateral positioning of the shoulder to allow access to the humeral canal (Figure 21-5). It is helpful to confirm that fluoroscopic images of the entire humeral head can be obtained before prepping and draping to confirm that similar images will be available as needed during the process of internal fixation. Particular attention should be directed to cleansing the skin. Many operations on fractures occur several days following the injury and most patients find maintenance of axillary hygiene impossible during this time interval. Subsequently, the bacterial growth in this region can become substantial and theoretically may contribute to a postoperative deep infection [14].

SURGICAL APPROACH

Percutaneous

In selected cases, a percutaneous approach is valuable. Typically, 2.5-mm terminally threaded wires are used as described by Jaberg *et al.* [15] (Figure 21-6). Although it is possible to apply other devices, such as cannulated screws, nails, rods, or pins, in a percutaneous fashion, the guidelines recently set forth by Gerber [16] still apply. The technique is well suited for fractures with minimal communion that can be reduced by closed means in patients with good bone quality who accept postoperative immobilization. Following preliminary reduction and fixation, the stability of the construct must be tested under fluoroscopy. If stability to passive

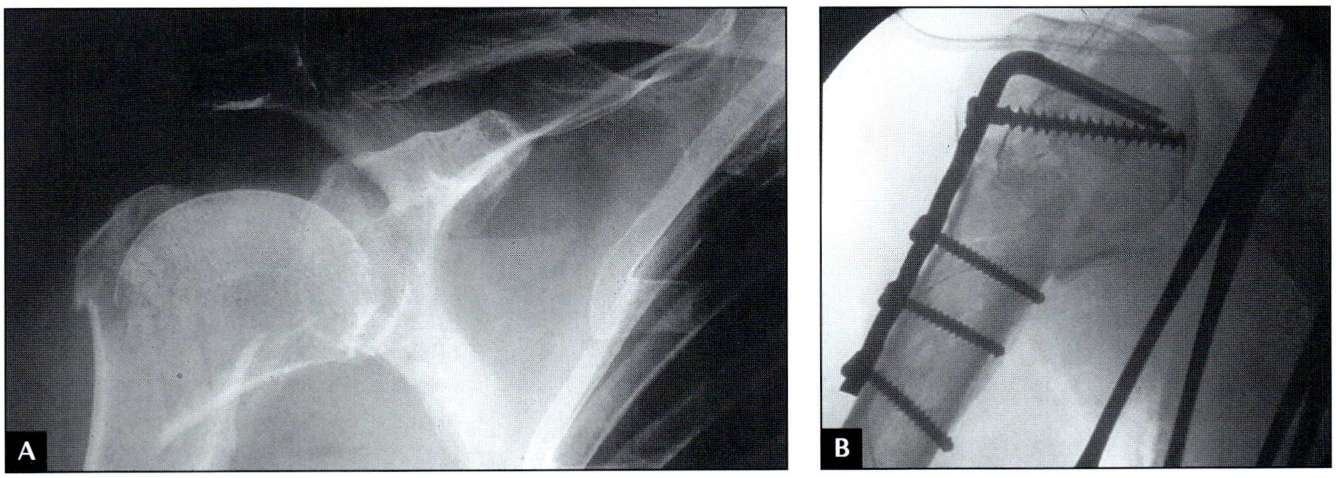

Figure 21-3. A and B, Humeral head supported with a fixed-angle device and bone graft. In this case, the plate was implanted in the neutral mode.

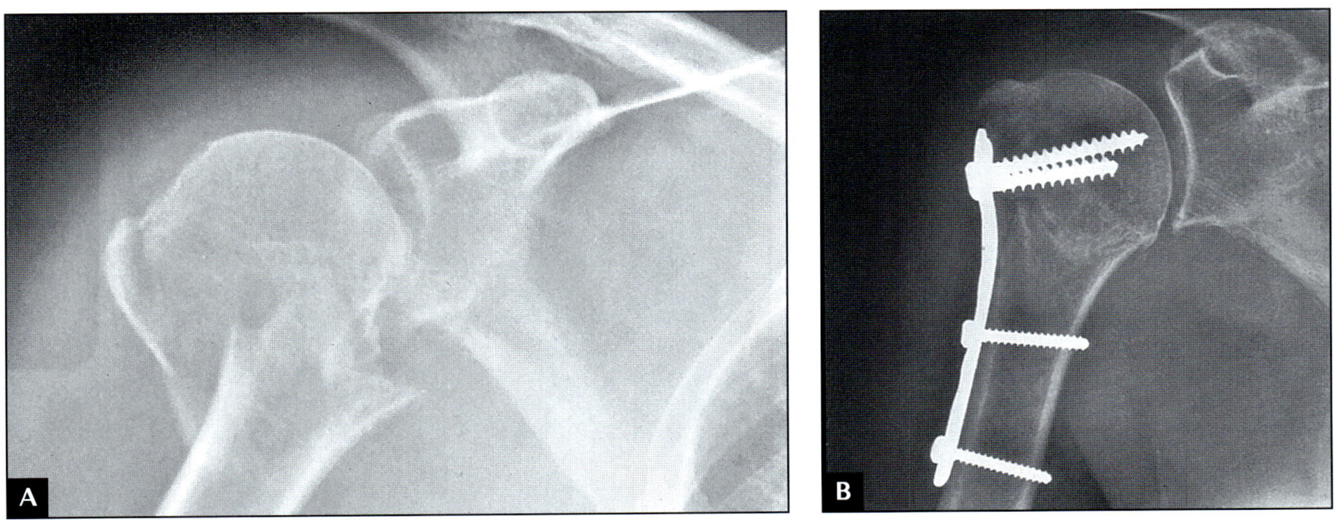

Figure 21-4. A and B, Humeral head fixed rigidly with screws in a case in which bone quality is good and comminution absent. Use of a precontoured anatomic bone plate is shown.

motion is not present, an alternative approach must be selected. If the bone quality is poor, as in the elderly, percutaneous fixation may still be possible with a long, prestressed stainless-steel staple (Figure 21-7) [17]. This implant provides good rotational stability by gaining purchase in the subchondral bone of the humeral head and endosteal surface of the humeral shaft.

Although arthroscopically assisted techniques have been applied in the treatment of these fractures, no reports of large series have been published in the peer-reviewed literature.

Anterosuperior Approach

Depending on the fracture pattern and complexity, a deltoid-splitting incision or even a formal anterosuperior approach with removal of a portion of the deltoid origin from the acromion can be applied. If this approach is selected for the treatment of greater tuberosity fractures, as always, care should be taken to avoid excessive distal propagation of the split and subsequent injury to the axillary nerve from overzealous retraction.

Long Deltopectoral Approach

Almost all fractures of the proximal humerus can be addressed through this approach. The following modifications allow extensile exposure to be achieved with complete preservation of the deltoid origin (Figure 21-8). First, the incision is placed slightly lateral to the deltopectoral interval and extends from the clavicle to the deltoid origin. A medial subcutaneous flap is raised to the level of the cephalic vein. Second, the deltopectoral interval is developed in its entirety from origin (clavicle) to insertion (deltoid tuberosity). Third, the plane between the deltoid and the coracoacromial ligament is developed. This maneuver allows greater mobility of the anterior deltoid. Fourth, a transbursal exposure is made with complete release of adhesions that may limit mobility of the rotator cuff, proximal humeral fracture fragments, and humeral shaft. Fifth, a large blunt Brown's retractor is used to effectively displace the deltoid muscle mass posteriorly and lever the proximal humerus forward. Sixth, retention sutures are placed in the supraspinatus, infraspinatus, and subscapularis, which allows the fractured tuberosity to be controlled and reduced.

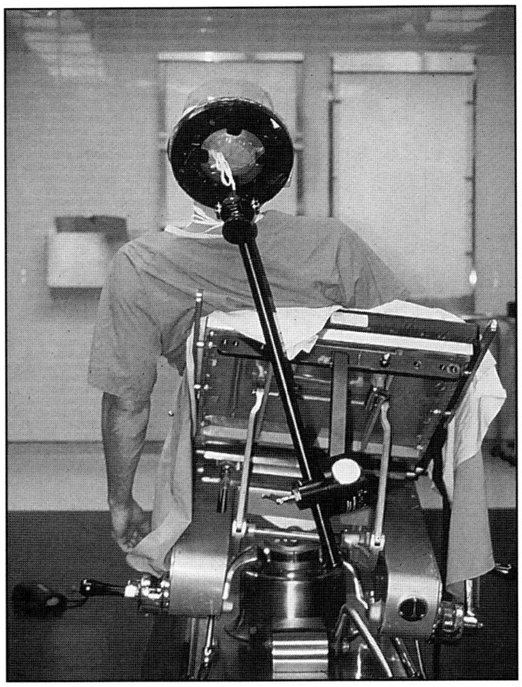

Figure 21-5. View from behind the operating table demonstrating the important features of patient postioning—access to the intramedullary canal of the humerus and neutral postioning of the cervical spine.

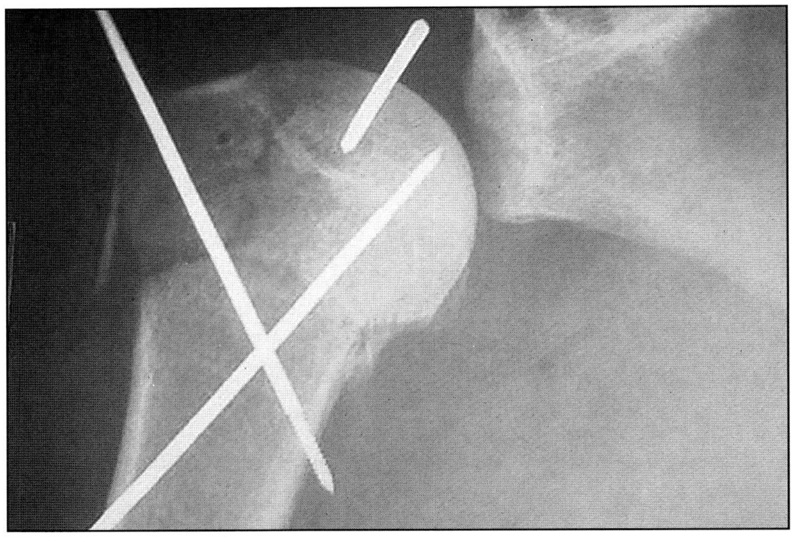

Figure 21-6. Use of 2.5-mm terminally threaded pins placed percutaneously.

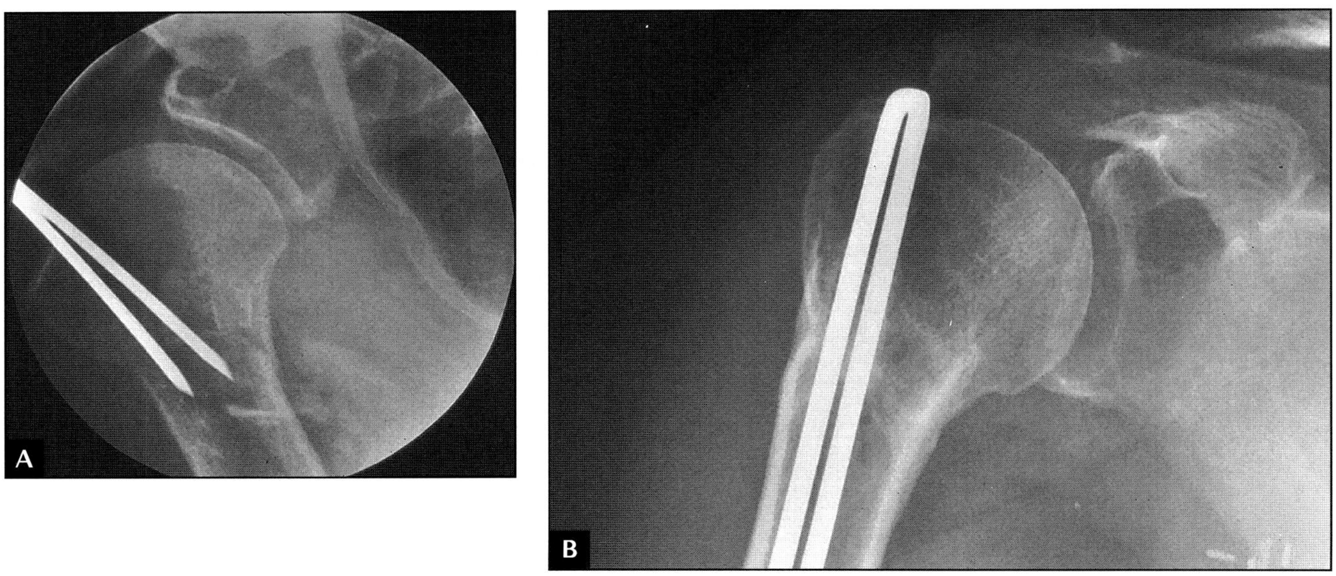

Figure 21-7. **A** and **B**, Use of a prestressed intramedullary staple inserted percutaneously to treat an unstable surgical neck fracture.

Implants

Various implants are available, including sutures, flexible wires, rigid pins, screws, intramedullary devices, and plates. In fact, combinations of these devices are often used to achieve stable fixation.

Sutures have the desirable qualities of simplicity of use, softness of texture, and radiolucency. Heavy suture material is perhaps the method of choice for fixation of the tuberosities with or without prosthesis. This is particularly effective when the tuberosities are comminuted and the suture is placed at the bone–tendon junction. Suture fixation alone typically does not provide adequate rigidity to control larger segments of bone, such as the head relative to the shaft as seen in surgical neck fractures. In these situations, tension band wiring as described by Hawkins *et al.* [18] (with or without additional intramedullary fixation) has proven effective. This method is particularly useful in elderly patients with poor bone quality in whom the only available points of fixation are the shaft and the rotator cuff (Figure 21-9) [17,19].

Nails can be effective but have the distinctive disadvantages of violating the rotator cuff and of becoming prominent (Figure 21-10).

Plate fixation has a definite role in the treatment of proximal humeral fractures. Some indications include fixation of fractures extending distally into the diaphysis (Figure 21-11), severe metaphyseal comminution, and support of a fragile head segment, particularly after elevation from a valgus impacted position (*see* Figure 21-3).

It has been suggested that plate fixation of the proximal humeral may cause avascular necrosis [20]. This potential complication may be related more to iatrogenic injury to the arcuate artery (blood supply to the humeral head) than the implants. Esser [21] reported a low incidence of avascular necrosis after open reduction and modified cloverleaf fixation of three- and four-part fractures. Posttraumatic avascular necrosis can and does occur in the absence of surgical treatment (Figure 21-12). If plates are used, they must be positioned low on the tuberosity to avoid subacromial impinge-

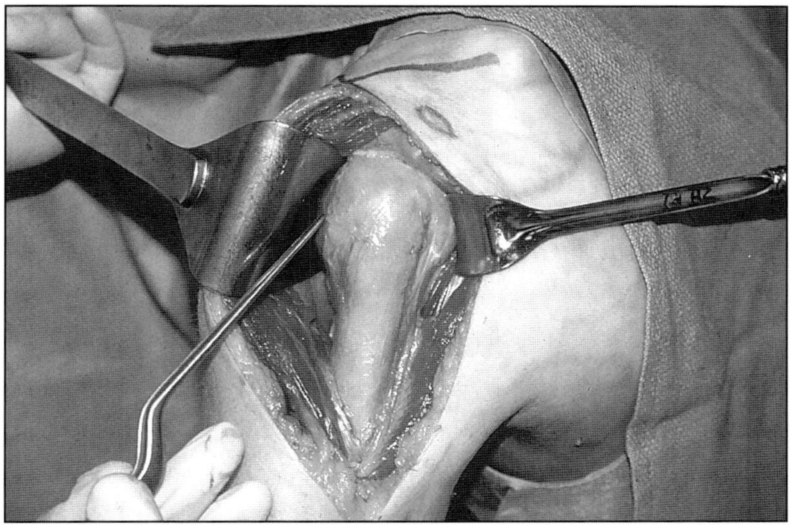

Figure 21-8. Dissection in a fresh cadaver specimen demonstrating how the entire proximal humerus (including the posterior aspect of the greater tuberosity) can be exposed with a modified extensile deltopectoral approach. The deltoid origin is preserved in its entirety.

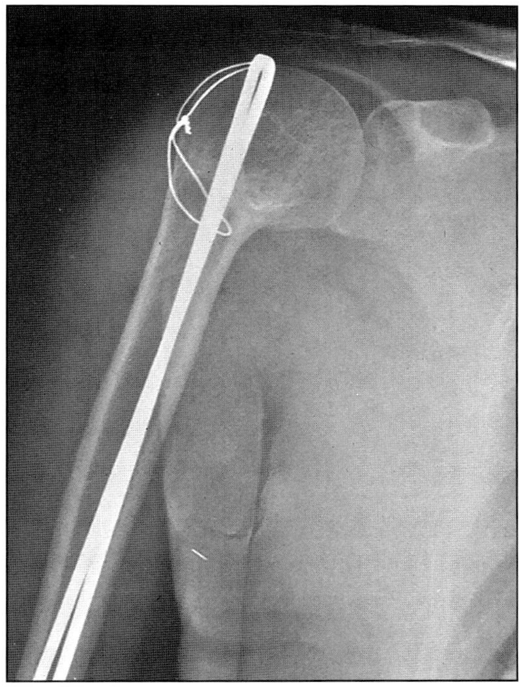

Figure 21-9. Combined intramedullary fixation and tension band wiring.

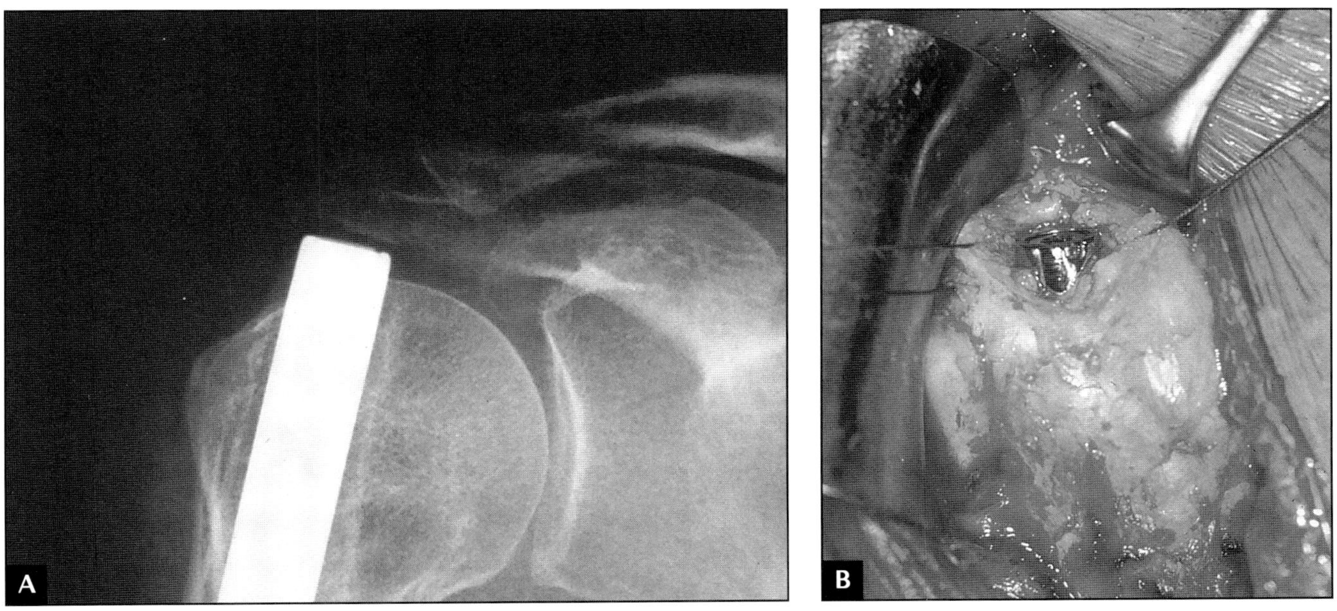

Figure 21-10. A and B, Iatrogenic subacromial impingement and rotator cuff tear resulting from the use of an intramedallary nail.

ment (Figure 21-13). Plates can also serve as a point of attachment for multiple tension band sutures. This additional fixation can neutralize the pull of the rotator cuff and can prevent varus deformity.

Proximal Humeral Replacement

When true four-part fractures and fracture dislocations occur in the elderly (Figure 21-14), primary prosthetic replacement of the humeral head may be indicated. Although Neer [3,4] reported good results with this operation, others have not been able to reproduce the degree of function he described. Residual pain is typically absent; however, motion and strength are usually only fair [14,22,23].

Certain technical details are critical to the success of the arthroplasty. Exposure is most often achieved by working through the fractured greater tuberosity. Displaced fractures often do not occur in the hard bone in the bicipital groove between the greater and lesser tuberosities but rather through the greater tuberosity just posterior to the groove. Frequently, a small longitudinal tear exists in the supraspinatus tendon at this level. The tear can be surgically lengthened (medially) to allow wide separation of the fractured tuberosity and access to the intramedullary canal. This "transtuberosity" approach leaves the rotator interval capsule and long-head biceps tendon undisturbed and may reduce the incidence of late anterosuperior migration.

Humeral length and retroversion must be recreated with the implant. When the humeral head is positioned too low, permanent inferior subluxation can occur. If the implant is too high, the tuberosity and rotator cuff repair come under excessive tension and may fail. Boileau and Walch [24] have pointed out the negative impact of excessive retroversion. If the greater tuberosity is reduced and repaired under a prosthetic head placed in too much retroversion, the repair experiences excessive tension when the arm is brought into internal rotation against the abdomen. The

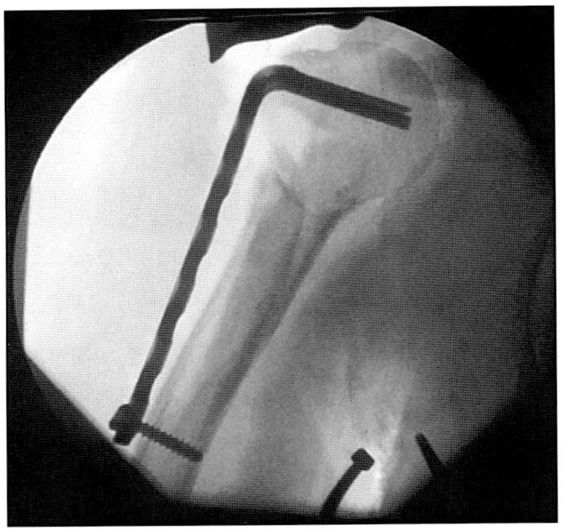

Figure 21-11. View of a plate that spans metaphyseal comminution.

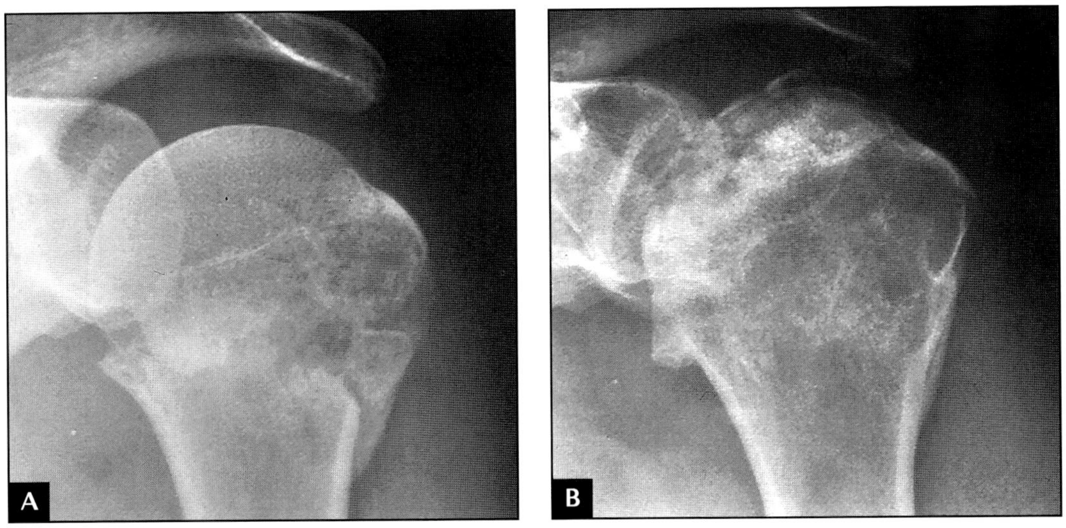

Figure 21-12. A and B, Avascular necrosis in the absence of surgery.

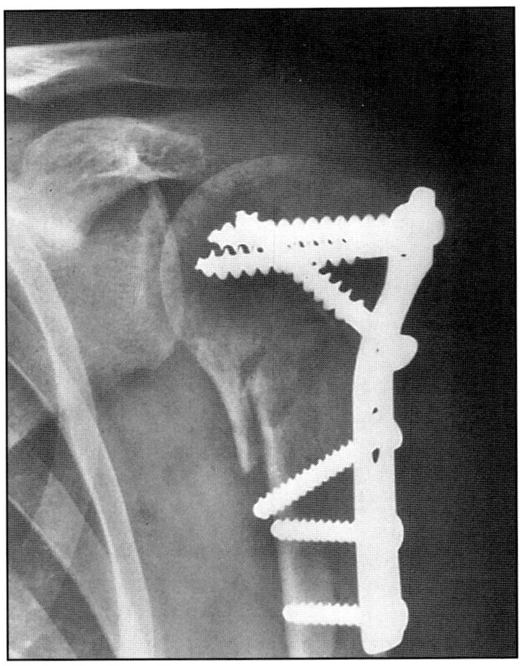

Figure 21-13. Large plate positioned too high on the greater tuberosity.

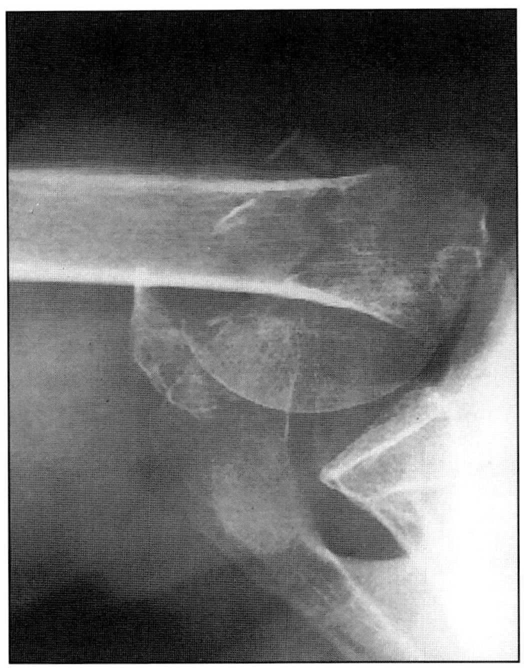

Figure 21-14. Axillary view demonstrating a true four-part fracture in an elderly patient.

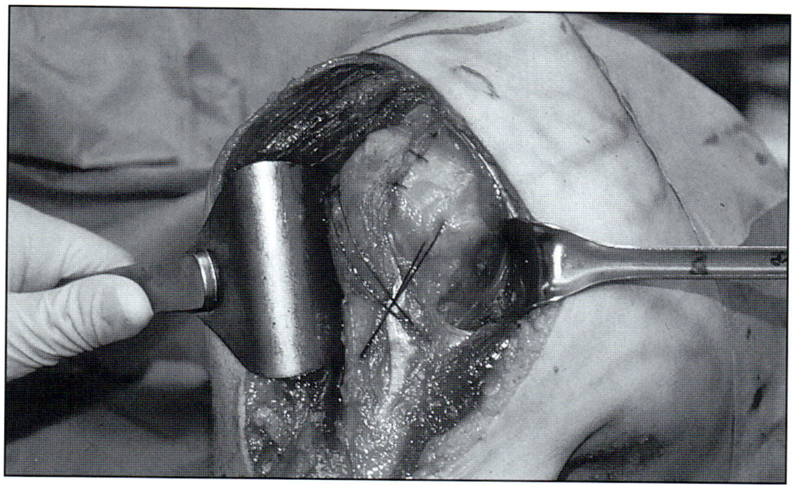

FIGURE 21-15. Tension band suturing of the tuberosities. We now routinely add cerclage sutures to compress the tuberosities.

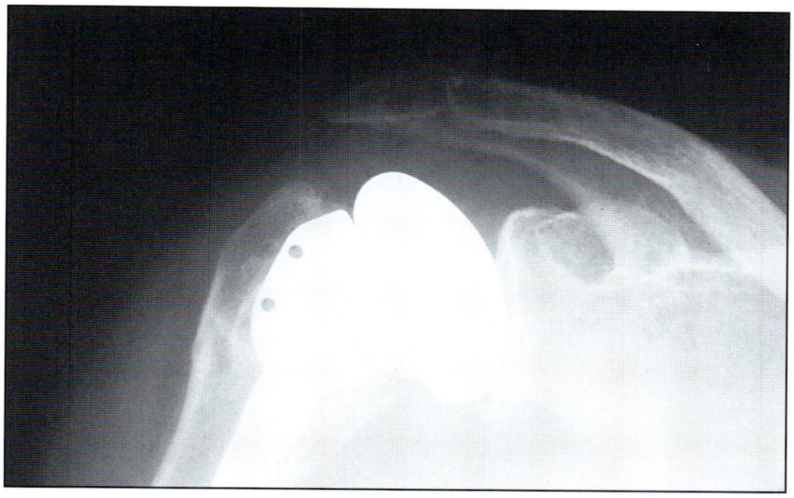

FIGURE 21-16. A well-healed greater tuberosity following hemiarthroplasty.

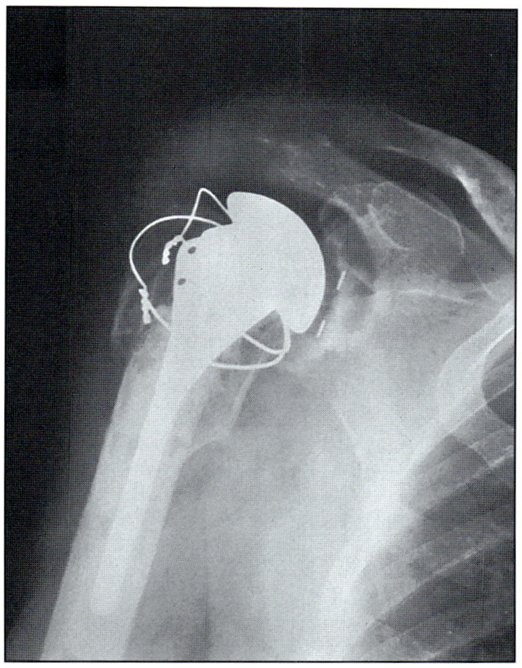

FIGURE 21-17. Fixation of a large, noncomminuted tuberosity fragment with cerclage wires.

posterior tuberosity displacement cannot always be appreciated on plain radiographs and may be one cause of "tuberosity resorption." Perhaps a more common cause of tuberosity migration is nonunion. Conditions for healing may be optimized by avoiding the tendency to trim or thin the tuberosity too much, not filling the metaphysis with metal and cement, and selecting a humeral head size similar to the fractured head or opposite side. Cancellous bone grafting from the resected humeral head is advisable, and secure repair of the tuberosities is essential. Heavy #5 nonabsorbable suture placed in the configuration described by Hawkins *et al.* [18] is typically supplemented with fixation in compression by placing "cerclage" sutures or wires around the medial neck of the implant and the tuberosities (Figures 21-15 and 21-16). Wires can be used most effectively when the greater tuberosity fragment is large and without comminution (Figure 21-17). In summary, the principles of tuberosity fixation involve preservation of periosteal attachments (if possible) sufficient bony apposition, secure fixation in compression, and rehabilitation based on passive movements determined intraoperatively.

REFERENCES AND RECOMMENDED READING

Recently published papers of particular interest have been highlighted as:
- • Of interest
- •• Of outstanding interest

1. Young TB, Wallace WA: Conservative treatment of fractures and fracture-dislocations of the upper end of the humerus. *J Bone Joint Surg Br* 1985, 67:373–377.
2. Tile M: *Fracture of the Proximal Humerus in the Rationale of Operative Fracture Care.* New York: Springer-Verlag; 1996.
3. Neer CS: Displaced proximal humeral fractures, part I: classification and evaluation. *J Bone Joint Surg Am* 1970, 52:1077–1089.
4. Neer CS: Displaced proximal humeral fractures, part II: treatment of three-part and four-part displacement. *J Bone Joint Surg Am* 1970, 52:1090–1103.
5. McLaughlin HL: Dislocation of the shoulder with tuberosity fracture. *Surg Clin North Am* 1963, 43:1615–1620.
6. Weber SC: The ten millimeter rule revisited: nonoperative treatment of the displaced greater tuberosity fractures. Presented at the 14th Annual Meeting of the American Shoulder and Elbow Surgeons, San Francisco, CA, February, 1997.
7. Rodosky MW, Puraldi X, Pollock R, *et al.*: Operative treatment of malunions of the proximal humerus. Presented at the 13th Annual Meeting of the Minnesota Orthopedic Society, Minneapolis, MN, May, 1997.
8. Jakob RP, Miniaci A, Anson PS, *et al.*: Four-part valgus impacted fractures of the proximal humerus. *J Bone Joint Surg Br* 1991, 73:295–298.
9. Resch H, Beck E, Bayley I: Reconstruction of the valgus-impacted humeral head fracture. *J Shoulder Elbow Surg* 1995, 4:73–80.
10. Resch H, Povacz P, Fröhlich R, *et al.*: Percutaneous fixation of three- and four-part fractures of the proximal humerus. *J Bone Joint Surg Br* 1997, 79:295–300.
11. Gerber C, Scheneeberger AG, Vingh TS: The arterial vascularization of the humeral head. *J Bone Joint Surg Am* 1990, 72:1486.
12. Brooks CH, Revell WJ, Heatley FW: Vascularity of the humeral head after proximal humeral fractures: an anatomical cadaver study. *J Bone Joint Surg Br* 1992, 75:132–136.
13. Jupiter JB, Mullaji AB: Blade plate fixation of proximal humeral nonunions. *Injury* 1994, 25:301–303.
14. Muldoon MP, Cofield RH: Complications of humeral head replacement for proximal humeral fractures. *Instruct Course Lect* 1997, 46:15–24.

15. Jaberg H, Warner JJP, Jakob RP: Percutaneous stabilization of unstable fractures of the humerus. *J Bone Joint Surg Am* 1992, 74:508–515.
16. Gerber C: Alternatives to hemiarthroplasty for complex proximal humeral fractures. In *Complex and Revision Shoulder Surgery.* Edited by Warner JP, Inonotti JP, Gerber C. Philadelphia: Lippincott-Raven; 1997.
17. Evans DC, Katz I: Prestressed humeral staple for fully displaced surgical neck fractures (poster). Presented at the American Association of Orthopaedic Surgeons' Annual Meeting, Las Vegas, NV, February, 1989.
18. Hawkins RJ, Bell RH, Gurr K: The three-part fracture of the proximal part of the humerus. *J Bone Joint Surg Am* 1986, 68:1410–1414.
19. Flatow EL, Cuomo F, Maday MG, *et al.*: Open reduction and internal fixation of two-part displaced fractures of the greater tuberosity of the proximal part of the humerus. *J Bone Joint Surg Am* 1991, 73:1213–1218.
20. Sturzenegger M, Fornaro E, Jakob RP: Results of surgical treatment of multifragmented fractures of the humeral head. *Arch Orthop Trauma Surg* 1982, 100:249–259.
21. Esser RD: Treatment of three- and four-part fractures of the proximal humerus with a modified cloverleaf plate. *J Orthop Trauma* 1994, 8:15–22.
22. Goldman RT, Koval KJ, Cuomo F, *et al.*: Functional outcome after humeral head replacement for acute three- and four-part proximal humeral fractures. *J Shoulder Elbow Surg* 1995, 4:81–86.
23. Green A, Lippitt S, Wirth M: Humeral head replacement for acute proximal humerus fracture: a multicenter prospective functional outcomes study. Presented at the 14th Open Meeting of the American Shoulder and Elbow Surgeons, New Orleans, LA, March 22, 1998.
24. Boileau P, Walch G: The shoulder prosthesis in four-part fractures: problems and solutions. *Orthop Spec Ed* 1998, 4:27–32.

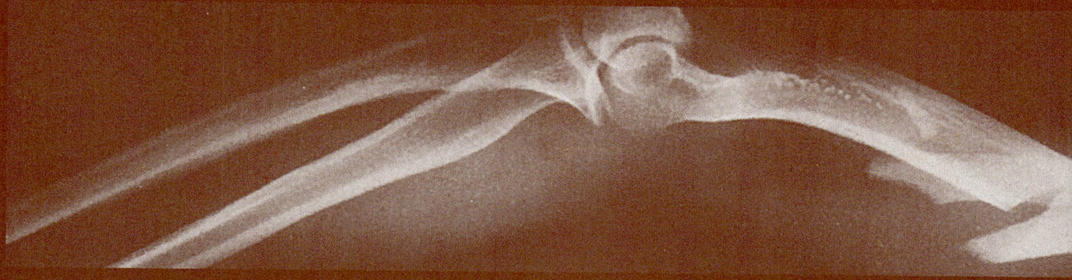

22

Functional Bracing of Diaphyseal Humeral Fractures and Operative Management of Humeral Shaft Fractures

Augusto Sarmiento
J. Tracy Watson

Until recently, the nonoperative management of diaphyseal fractures of the humerus has been considered a safe and effective method of treatment. Its high union rate and satisfactory functional results have given credence to this method [1–5]. Plating has been associated with a relatively high complication rate. More recently, several reports have been published suggesting that intramedullary nailing has also earned a place in the armamentarium of the orthopedic surgeon [6–8].

RATIONALE

Immobilization of joints above and below diaphyseal fractures has proven to be unnecessary. Success obtained over the years with hanging casts, coaptation splints, and braces in the management of humeral fractures has eloquently proven this [1–5,9–11]. Stabilization of bony structures provided by the compression of the rigid wall of the brace against the soft tissue seems to provide sufficient stability to allow uninterrupted fracture repair. In addition, the compression of the tissues by the adjustable sleeve plus the weight of the extremity during the patient's erect position provide restoration of adequate alignment of the fracture fragments in most instances.

Nonsurgical treatment of diaphyseal humeral fractures with functional braces does not ensure anatomic reduction of fragments. In fact, perfect restoration of anatomy should not be expected. However, experiences have indicated that in most instances, final angulatory deformities are cosmetically and functionally satisfactory.

Early passive and subsequent active exercises, which the brace permits, create motion between the bony fragments and the early formation of peripheral callus. Motion at the fracture site, if physiologically induced, appears to be one of the most important factors in osteogenesis [10,11]. Bracing does not immobilize joints above and below the fracture, thus ensuring that permanent limitation of motion of the shoulder and elbow is precluded in most instances.

The cost of care of humeral fractures treated by nonsurgical means is an important factor and should be considered, especially now when health-care expenditures have become a subject of increased attention on the part of third-party payers. Because hospitalization and surgery are not necessary, the nonunion rate is low, and corrective surgical measures are seen rarely, if ever, this methodology should be favorably supported.

INDICATIONS

Not all diaphyseal humeral fractures should be treated with functional braces. Patients who, for one reason or another, cannot assume an erect position and therefore allow the extremity to hang to the side of the body are best treated by other methods, such as Velpeau slings or fixation with external fixators, plates, or intramedullary nailing. Polytraumatized patients, particularly those with injuries involving multiple organs, are often best managed by the methods mentioned. Patients suffering from spastic disorders are difficult to manage with functional bracing because unsightly deformities can occur. Type II and III open fractures that require débridement of the wound should not be braced early, if at all. This is particularly true when associated nerve or vascular injuries have been identified.

The presence of a major angular deformity at the fracture site after the application of the initial hanging cast often requires discontinuation of nonsurgical treatment and, most likely, internal fixation of the fragments. Distraction between the fragments in a longitudinal direction suggests major soft tissue damage. These fractures are most likely to experience delayed union or nonunion.

MANAGEMENT PROTOCOL

Closed diaphyseal humeral fractures as well as Type I open fractures are the best indications for functional bracing. The presence of an associated radial palsy that develops immediately after the injury does not preclude functional treatment. In the case of closed fractures and following appropriate sedation, a hanging cast or a coaptation splint is applied. This must be accompanied by a sling or a collar and cuff. During application of the cast, care must be exercised to allow the extremity to hang to the side of the body in a relaxed position. If the patient's shoulder is shrugged as a result of apprehension, this must be eliminated before application of the sling or collar and cuff or an angular deformity will occur on relaxation of the elevators of the shoulder. Following the cast application, the patient should be instructed on the conduct of pendulum exercises that, at first, might require assistance from the uninjured hand. As symptoms subside, range of motion can be increased. Active exercises of the hand should also be conducted in an attempt to reduce distal swelling.

We prefer the hanging cast because swelling of the forearm is better controlled. In most instances, the cast can be discontinued and replaced with a functional brace at the end of the first week or at the beginning of the second week following the initial insult. If the patient's extremity remains very swollen with significant discomfort, an additional week of exercises is preferred. However, in most patients the functional brace may be applied at the end of 1 week of passive exercises in the cast. The brace should be applied while the patient is standing up or sitting on a high table with the arm hanging loosely over the side of the body. The procedure should not be painful because manipulation of the extremity is not necessary.

BRACE

The functional brace or "sleeve" must be adjustable to maintain compression of the soft tissues throughout (Figure 22-1). A circular nonadjustable cast or sleeve rapidly loosens and slips distally, running the risk of irritating the anticubital space and thus failing to maintain the necessary compression of the tissues. The sleeve should extend from just below the axilla to slightly above the epicondyles of the humerus (Figure 22-2). Extension of the

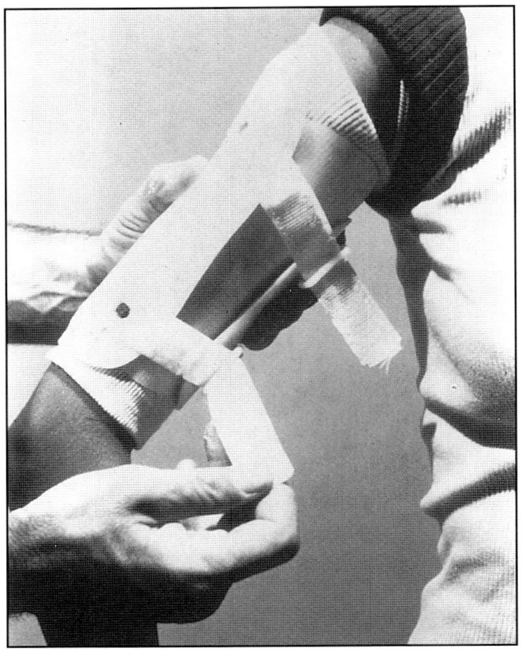

FIGURE 22-1. The functional brace must be adjustable with straps to maintain a snug fit at all times.

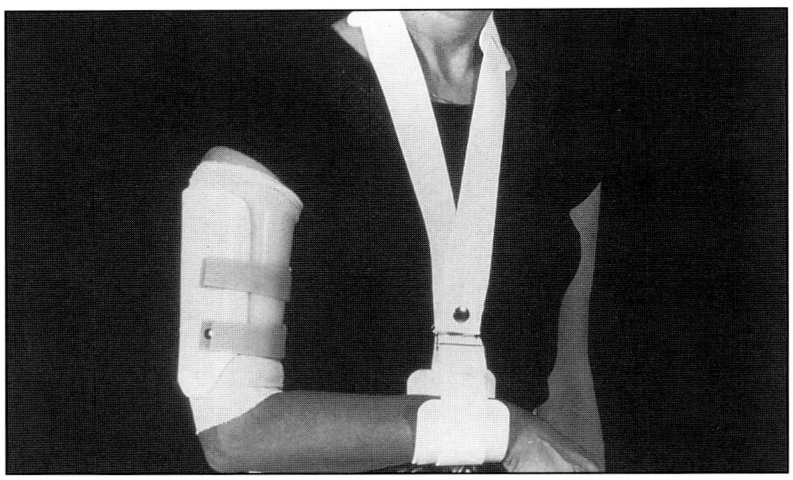

FIGURE 22-2. The sleeve should extend from about 1 in below the axilla to slightly above the humeral condyles.

brace over the acromion or condylar humeral bony prominence is not necessary. Quite to the contrary, it is uncomfortable and misleading. To depend on extension of the brace over the acromion as a means of suspension is wrong. The brace does not need suspension other than that provided by its firm compression over the soft tissues. If the brace extends too far distally, it precludes full flexion of the elbow.

As in application of the cast and to prevent angular deformities, the shoulder should not be shrugged during brace application and, more particularly, when the collar and cuff are added (Figure 22-3). Before application of the brace, a thin sock should be placed over the upper arm to prevent contact of the plastic brace with the skin because such contact might increase the possibility of excessive perspiration, particularly during warm weather.

Prefabricated braces are widely used and typically come in three sizes: large, medium, and small. The proximal and distal ends of the brace should prevent impingement on the axilla and proximal forearm. Custom-made braces composed of plastic material or soft cast are equally effective. However, they must be adjustable and the snugness of the brace must be maintained with velcro straps.

Manipulation of humeral fractures is not necessary with functional bracing treatment because dependency of the extremity and compression of the soft tissues around the humerus restore adequate alignment of the fragments in most instances. Only 2% of the fractures heal with deformities higher than 25°. Manipulation of humeral fractures should be strongly discouraged because of the associated high incidence of nerve palsy.

Postbrace Application

After application of the brace and the collar and cuff, patients should be instructed to continue the pendulum exercises as well as anteroposterior and medial-lateral swing exercises. These exercises should be conducted with the patient leaning forward to allow maximum range of motion. Within 2 or 3 days after application of the brace, most patients find it possible to remove the collar and cuff and begin passive range-of-motion exercises of the elbow with the assistance of the uninjured hand. Emphasis should be placed on regaining extension of the elbow in the hope that full extension of this joint can be achieved by the end of the second week. Passive exercises of the elbow can gradually be combined with active muscular assistance to be determined by the degree of symptoms. Under no circumstances should patients be told to carry out active exercises associated with significant pain.

Active abduction and elevation of the shoulders should not be undertaken because of the strong possibility that angular deformities may develop. The weight of the arm represents a long lever against the short proximal fragment, which leads to angular deformities. Under no circumstances should active abduction and elevation of the shoulder be instituted until intrinsic stability has been demonstrated clinically and radiologically.

Patients should be instructed not to lean on the elbow at any time and to allow the arm to hang to the side of the body at all times. Leaning on the elbow may produce angular deformities, especially if the fracture is transverse and the fragments are in close contact with one another. As time passes, changes in the girth of the extremity occur more slowly as muscle atrophy is arrested and the fluids in the extremity become stable. Therefore, adjustments become less frequent. After the brace has been applied, instructions are given concerning the frequent readjustment of the brace during the first few days, because as the swelling of the extremity decreases, the brace loses its snug contact with the underlying soft tissue structures. Patients should receive instructions on putting on and removing the brace for hygienic purposes.

Full extension of the elbow within the first 2 weeks is desirable. This allows the patient to ambulate without needing the sling. The patient's arm swing becomes normal. The weight of the extremity further assists in improving alignment (Figure 22-4). The active contraction of the flexors and extensors of the elbow correct major rotary deformities that might have been present from the outset. This correction occurs because the triceps, brachialis, and biceps have insertions on the humeral diaphysis and any malrotation of the bony fragments can be corrected by these muscles' contraction. The coiled muscle fibers uncoil during active contraction, bringing about a parallel uncoiling of the bony fragments.

It is not uncommon to see subluxation of the shoulder following fractures of the humerus, particularly in those located in its proximal third. Correction of the subluxation is easily accomplished by active contraction of the flexors and extensors of the elbow because these muscles have origins on the scapula. Contracture of the muscles brings the humeral diaphysis superiorly and, in doing so, relocates the subluxated joint.

Active abduction and elevation of the shoulder should not be initiated until clinical and radiologic evidence of early bony stability has been documented. After such stability has developed, elevation and abduction exercises can be carried out without the risk of developing angular deformities. After full extension of the elbow has been obtained, patients can ambulate without the sling. This has significant benefits, particularly in a women with large breasts, because the hanging arm falls behind the breast, thus eliminating the fulcrum effect that often leads to varus deformity.

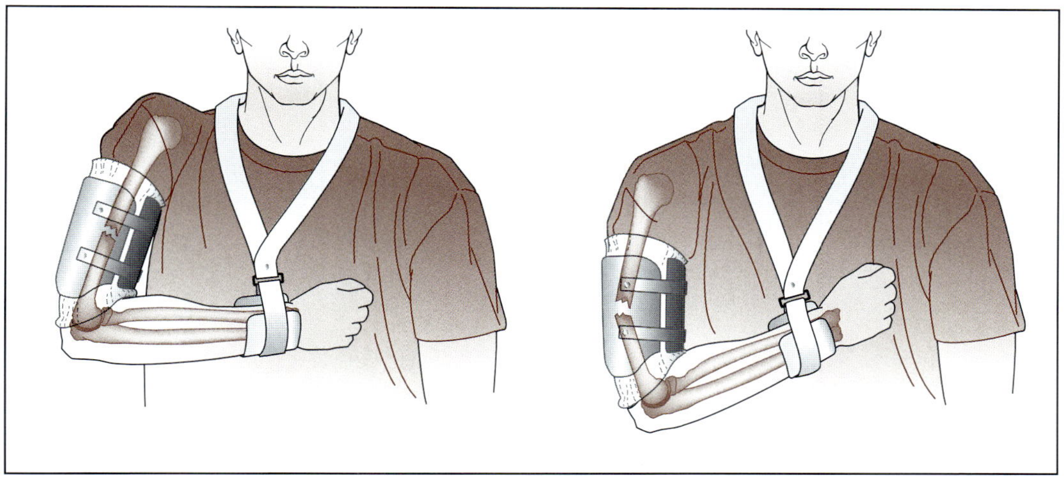

Figure 22-3. The shoulder must not be shrugged during fitting of the brace to prevent the development of a varus deformity.

Patients do not need to sleep in a sitting position, but it is recommended that the sling be used at night until early intrinsic bony stability has been demonstrated. Radiographs of the extremity should be obtained immediately after the application of the brace and repeated 1 week later. After that, radiographs are desirable every 4 weeks until union is complete. Large peripheral callus often forms because of physiologically induced motion at the fracture site. On removal of the brace, it is best for patients to continue to actively build up the musculature of the arm and gradually increase physical demands. Sporting activities should be postponed, however, until solid radiologic union has been confirmed because some degree of osteoporosis is inevitable following a fracture, regardless of the treatment used.

The presence of a radial palsy does not mitigate good results. Palsy that occurs in closed fractures immediately following the accident has a good prognosis and most palsies recover spontaneously.

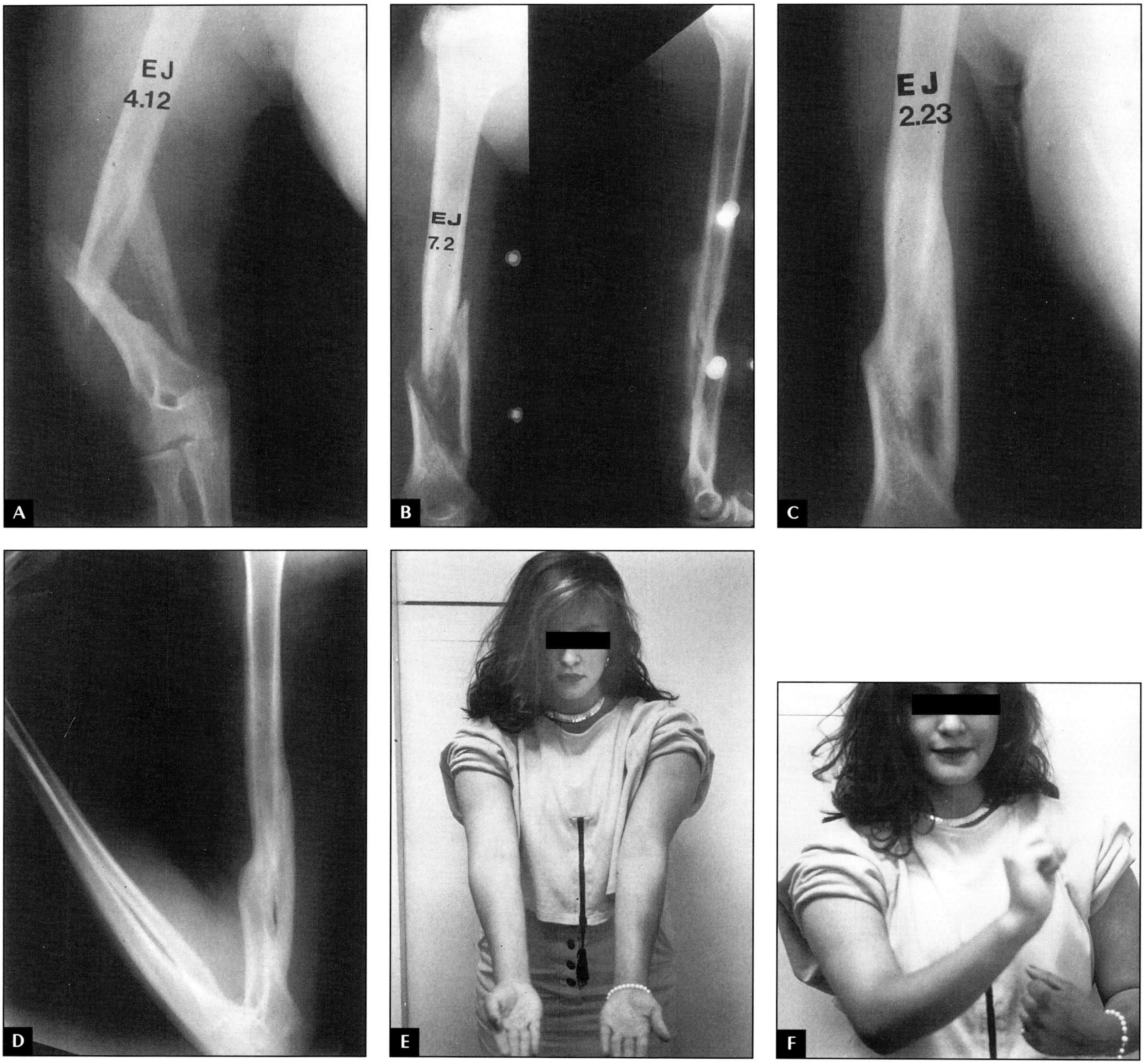

FIGURE 22-4. A, Anteroposterior (AP) radiograph of a comminuted extra-articular fracture of the distal humerus. B, Correction of original deformity accomplished by compression of the soft tissues by the brace and forces of gravity. C, AP radiograph of the healed fracture. Notice loss of carrying angle. D, Lateral radiograph demonstrating good alignment of the fragments. E, Very acceptable cosmetic appearance of the fractured arm. F, Patient demonstrates recovery from initial radial palsy.

Because the arm is allowed to hang over the side of the body with the elbow extended, beginning 2 weeks after the initial injury a cock-up splint for the wrist is unnecessary. This splint is designed to prevent the development of flexion contractions of the wrist, but the danger of a contracture is eliminated after the elbow has been extended and the wrist has assumed the neutral position. Patients should, however, use the hand as much as possible and passively abduct the thumb on a regular basis to prevent a possible adduction contraction.

Electromyographic studies and other tests should be carried out if, after approximately 6 weeks, there are no signs of return of function. Because nerve injuries recover proximally to distally, it is logical to assume that the brachioradialis should be the first muscle to experience improvement. The extensors of the fingers are the last ones to do so.

The humeral shaft tolerates angular deformities of 15° to 20° very well without unsightly appearance. In patients with muscular or flabby arms, greater deformities are well camouflaged (Figure 22-5). Loss of the carrying angle in itself is of no consequence and patients find it difficult to recognize the deformity. Their function is not compromised.

RESULTS

Sarmiento *et al.* [9] described the original brace for fractures of the humerus in 1977 and documented the clinical and radiologic findings on several occasions [2,9,11]. Others have also done so [1,8,9,12,13]. From a joint review of experiences at the Universities of Miami and Southern California with 922 patients [14], the following conclusions were drawn. In all, 33% of patients were lost to follow-up, apparently because on disappearance of symptoms, patients assumed that further visits to the treating physicians were unnecessary. Overall healing time took place at 11.5 weeks. Closed fractures healed at a median time of 9.5 weeks and open fractures at a median time of 14 weeks. Transverse fractures healed at a median of 12, oblique fractures at a median time of 10, comminuted fractures at median time of 10.5, and segmental fractures at a median time of 11.5 weeks. Fractures located on the proximal third of the humeral diaphysis healed at a median time of 9.5, those on the middle third at a median time of 10, those on the distal third at a median time of 9, and segmental fractures at a median time of 11.5 weeks.

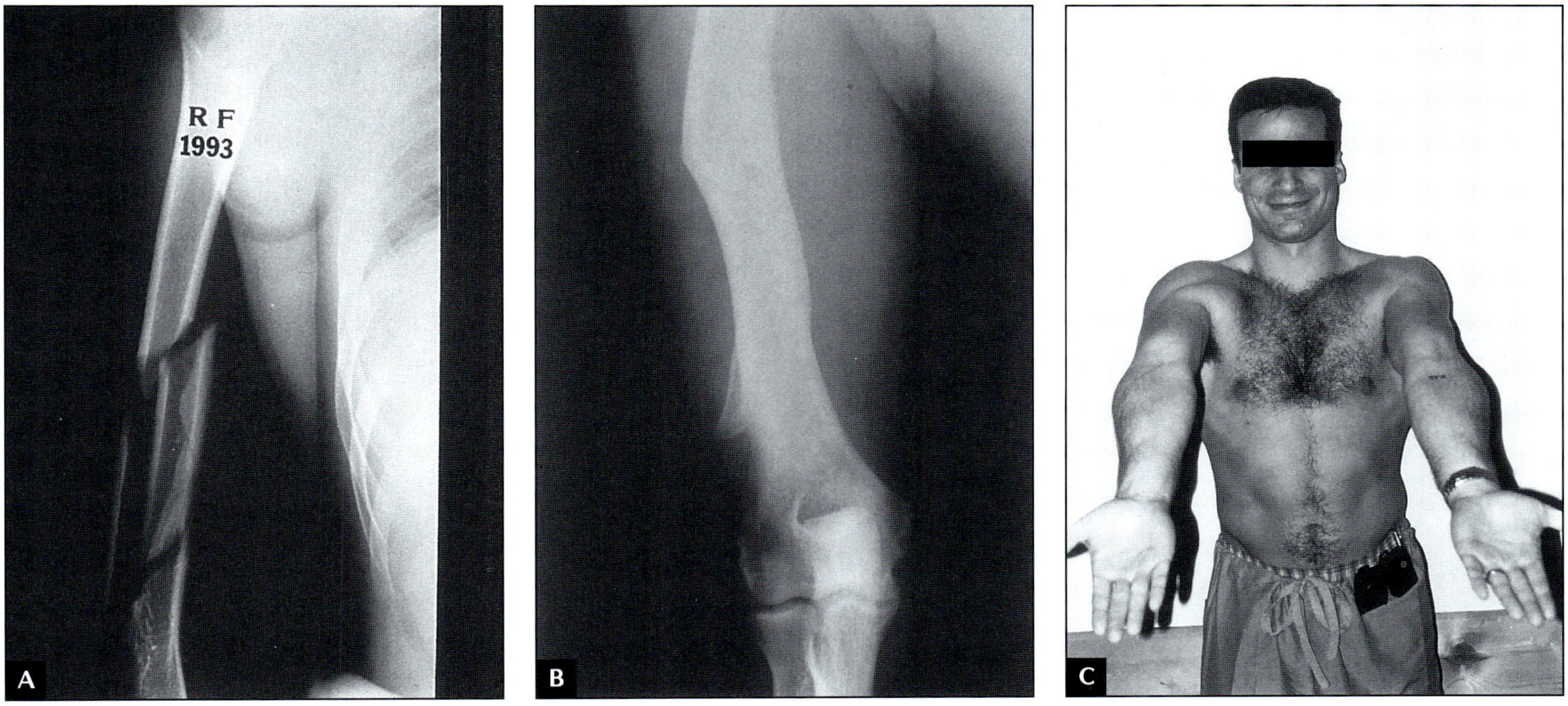

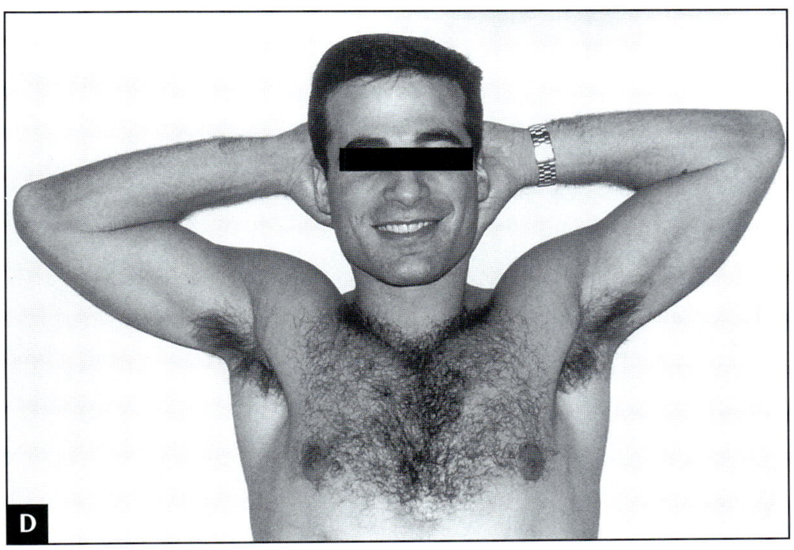

FIGURE 22-5. **A**, Initial radiograph of segmental fracture of the humerus. **B**, Anteroposterior radiograph of healed fracture. Notice the varus angulation. **C**, Acceptable cosmetic appearance of the fractured arm. **D**, Patient demonstrates range of motion of his shoulders and elbows.

In the same study, 16 (2.6%) fractures developed nonunion and required an operation; nine (5.8%) occurred in open fractures and seven (1.5%) in closed fractures. The mechanism of injury for the 16 nonunions were falls to the ground in four (25%) patients, vehicular accidents in nine (56%) patients, and low-velocity gunshot wounds in three (18%) patients. Four (0.6%) refractures occurred between the second and eighth weeks following removal of the brace: two from a fall, one from a sporting activity, and one from an unknown mechanism. All four refractures healed following reapplication of the brace.

Radiologic measurement of angulation was possible in 90% of the patients. Of these, 546 (88%) lateral radiographs were available for measurement of angulation. The average final varus angulation was 9° in transverse fractures, 4° in oblique fractures, and 8° in comminuted fractures. Among those studied, 87% of the fractures healed with less than 15° of varus angulation and 1.9% had a permanent varus angular deformity of 25°—degrees of angulation considered by most to be aesthetically acceptable [1,2,4,5,9,12]. Because functional bracing does not restore anatomic alignment of the fractures, it is not surprising that 87.2% had equal to or less than 15° and 95.8% had equal to or less than 25° of varus angulation. These deviations are cosmetically and physiologically well tolerated [1–5] and should not be considered complications, simply minor deviations from the norm.

Of the 67 (11.1%) patients with closed fractures associated with radial nerve palsy, 0.2% failed to show signs of appreciable recovery of function. Our follow-up was relatively short and consquently we are in no position to determine the degree of ultimate recovery. The 12 patients (2%) who had inferior shoulder subluxation demonstrated spontaneous correction of that subluxation. Range of motion of the shoulder was recorded in 396 (63.8%) patients. Lack of elbow motion was minimal and it was recorded in 301 (48%) patients.

In this series, 59% of the patients had full range of motion of the shoulder on the day the brace was discontinued. In all, 97% of the patients had 25° or less limitation of shoulder motion on permanent removal of the brace. For the 301 patients who had range of motion recorded, 230 (76%) had full range of motion on removal of the brace and 97.9% had limitation of motion of 25° or less at that time.

A nonunion rate of 1.5% in closed fractures and 5.8% in open fractures was found. The high incidence of union in this large group of diaphyseal humeral fractures gives credence to the long-held hypothesis that motion at the fracture site is the most important factor in osteogenesis [10,11]. The exact mechanism through which motion encourages fracture healing is not known, but it is suspected that pain and the subsequent irritation created by motion between the fragments results in a cascade of favorable events, such as increased vascularity, piezoelectrical potentials, and local chemical and thermal changes.

OPERATIVE MANAGEMENT OF HUMERAL SHAFT FRACTURES

As previously discussed, most humeral shaft fractures do not require surgery and are commonly treated with a functional orthosis. Two earlier epidemiologic studies demonstrated that humeral shaft fractures occur predominantly in a bimodal age distribution. One peak occurs between the ages of 16 and 35 years. These fractures reflect a more violent mechanism of injury: 43% are caused by motor-vehicle accidents and 17% occur as a result of gunshot wounds. Of these patients, 94% had other associated fractures or multiple trauma. Fractures that occur as a result of high-energy fracture patterns are more likely to warrant operative treatment [15,16].

The second peak occurs in patients in their 70s. Over 75% of shaft fractures occurring in women are the result of falls from a standing height. These are primarily simple fracture patterns in patients who are likely to be osteoporotic [16].

INDICATIONS FOR SURGERY

Open fractures with or without a nerve injury are an absolute indication for surgical management. In general, radial nerve palsy occurs in association with an open fracture approximately 18% of the time. Surgical management is directed toward the open wound in terms of irrigation, débridement, and stabilization of the bone for soft tissue stabilization. The nerve is usually explored in these situations. Patients with open fractures that present with radial nerve palsy had the nerve entrapped within the fracture site 60% of the time [17].

Progressive or new-onset radial nerve palsy following closed manipulation and initiation of conservative management is an indication for operative stabilization of the fracture with concomitant nerve exploration [18–20]. Shaft fractures, whether open or closed, that occur in concert with a vascular injury should also be surgically stabilized to facilitate and protect the vascular repair [15]. The humerus is the most mobile of the long bones. Although the freely movable scapulohumeral articulation minimizes torsional stresses on the intact humeral shaft, a shaft fracture transfers those rotational stresses to the region of the fracture, which may disrupt the vascular repair if the shaft is not stabilized.

RELATIVE INDICATIONS FOR SURGERY

Relative indications for surgery have developed as a result of the difficulties encountered when attempting to treat complex fractures in a conservative fashion. It has been shown that failure of closed treatment can be predicted early if the fracture is not clinically united or is not showing progressive consolidation on radiographs by 6 to 10 weeks postinjury. Klinerman has demonstrated that up to 30° of anterior angulation, 30° of varus, and 3 cm of shorting represent an acceptable reduction [21]. Therefore, perfect alignment and apposition are not essential. The soft-tissue sleeve and the mobility associated with the shoulder and elbow joints help to conceal any cosmetic deformity. However, excessive distraction or angulation at the fracture gap may indicate interposed muscle; unacceptable alignment following closed treatment can occur in many instances.

Other relative indications for surgery include obese patients (it may be difficult to avoid varus angulation due to distal fragment angulation over the increased chest girth, breast mass, or other bodily features, and substantial adipose tissue in the upper arm may make fracture brace fitting problematic) [22]; athletes who throw an object (those that fracture secondary to muscular contraction may be candidates for surgery to facilitate early shoulder and elbow rehabilitation) [23]; segmental shaft fractures; distal fractures with articular extension or distal extra-articular shaft fractures that would necessitate prolonged immobilization of the elbow in order to maintain acceptable alignment; pathologic fractures [24,25]; bilateral humeral shaft fractures; humeral fractures in association with polytrauma patients; ipsilateral shoulder dislocations with shaft fractures [26]; floating elbows; and fractures in association with a spinal cord or brachial plexus injury.

SURGICAL ANATOMY

When considering surgical management, the complex anatomy of the humerus should be fully appreciated. Many important anatomic considerations particular to the type of treatment methodology and type of fixation selected must be made. Plate fixation, intramedullary nailing, or external fixation each has its own specific concerns with regard to humeral osteology.

OSTEOLOGY

Proximal and distal portions of the humerus terminate in the shoulder and elbow joints. The medullary canals are located in direct axial alignment with these respective joint surfaces. This means that a direct, in-line approach to the medullary canal for intramedullary nailing would have to broach either articular surface. Because of this arrangement, eccentric portals have been developed to achieve access to the medullary canal. An axial approach for antegrade nailing of the humeral shaft, although it may allow near-direct access to the canal, necessitates splitting or cutting through the proximal rotator cuff and placing the nail just lateral to the superior articular surface of the humeral head. To avoid splitting the cuff, alternative approaches have been used, such as placing the entry portal more laterally or anteriorly through the greater tuberosity. This eccentric starting location has demanded a change in nail design from a straight rigid nail design to one that incorporates a lateral bend in the proximal nail segment.

This eccentric location also means that the nail will contact the proximal medial cortex and then slide distally as nail insertion progresses. Proximal humeral fractures have occurred in this location during nail placement, especially in weakened osteoporotic bone. The nail should be flexible enough to slide past this medial cortex without fracture (Figure 22-6).

The proximal 80% of the humeral shaft is cylindrical in cross-section and accommodates all nail designs easily. The distal 20% of the shaft becomes triangular in cross-section with the flat base oriented posteriorly. This area further narrows to approximate a fishtail cross-section area just above and below the olecranon fossa. This triangular narrowing makes distal seating of any nail type problematic, especially if distal fractures are to be fixed in an antegrade fashion. This apical anterior canal configuration makes distal interlocking difficult because of the inability to maintain a drill point on this narrow ridge of bone when using interlocking techniques that place locking screws in an anterior to posterior direction (Figure 22-6).

When viewed from the lateral aspect, the distal humeral medullary canal curves anteriorly (*ie,* comma-shaped) and this also limits the distal extent of antegrade rigid nail placement. Retrograde nailing techniques have been developed to take into account the supracondylar curve and canal narrowing configuration. This has been done to avoid nail-insertion site fractures in the supracondylar region when a retrograde nailing method is selected (Figure 22-7). The posterior aspect of the humeral surface is relatively flat, extending from the olecranon fossa distally to the proximal third of

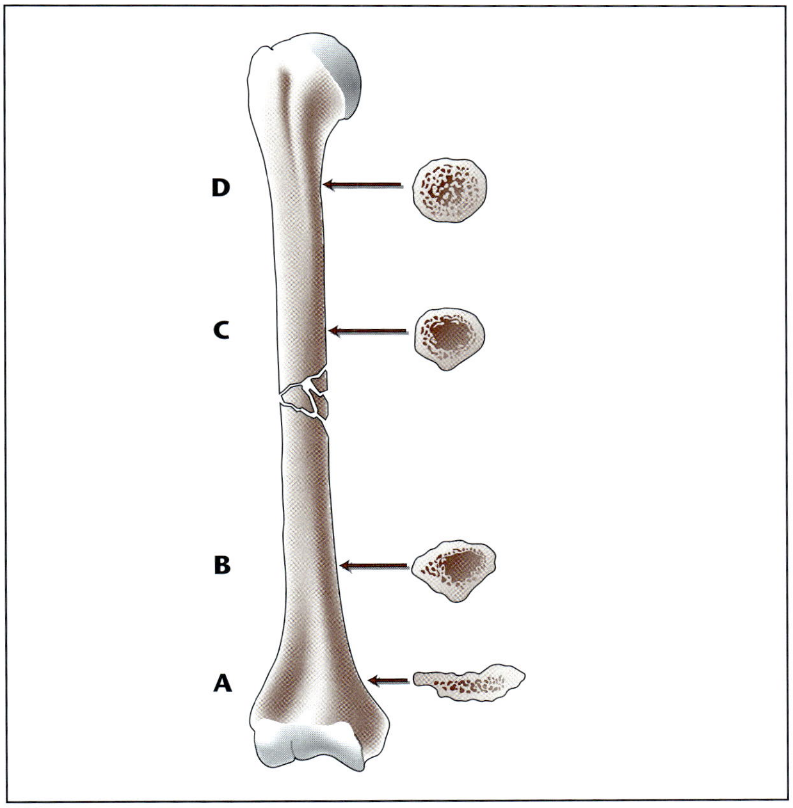

FIGURE 22-6. Cross-sectional osteology of the entire humeral shaft. **A**, The distal segment shows the narrowing of the distal condylar flair at the olecranon and coronoid fossa. **B**, The distal third of the humeral shaft is triangular in cross-section and thus makes anterior plating approaches somewhat problematic. This finding may also complicate the ability to place an anterior-to-posterior interlocking screw in this region. The flat posterior surface of the humerus in this location is ideal for plating. Because of narrowing in this region, clinicians using antegrade or retrograde nailing must ensure that incarceration of the nail does not occur here. **C**, The mid- and proximal-shaft portions of the humerus are roughly circular in cross-sectional area and is amenable to anterior or posterior plating. **D**, The proximal cortex may be very thin and atrophic in some elderly individuals and may fracture when placing antegrade or retrograde nails in this region.

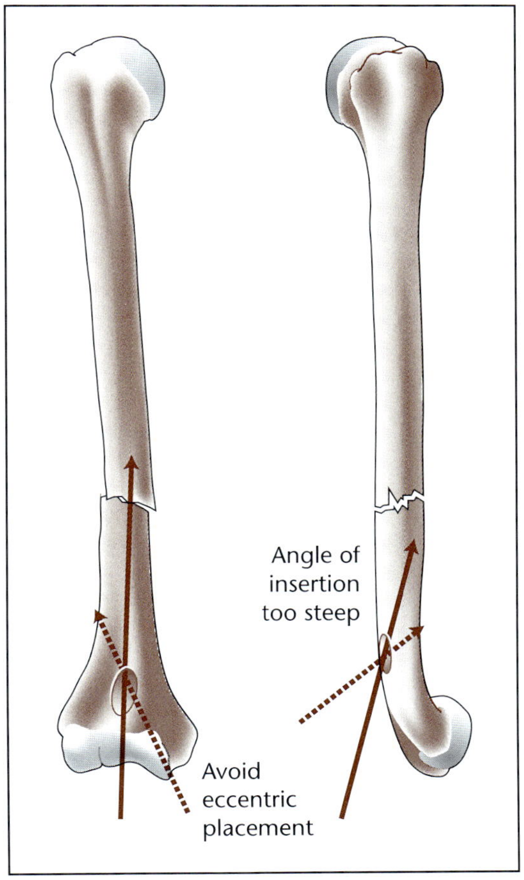

FIGURE 22-7. The distal aspect of the humeral medullary canal curves anteriorly (*ie,* comma shaped), which is important when considering retrograde or antegrade intramedullary nailing techniques. The entry portal for retrograde nailing is located 1.5 cm superior to the olecranon fossa. Care should be taken to fashion an oval window using a high-speed burr to avoid fracture through this region. Angle of nail entry should be closely monitored to avoid protrusion of the anterior cortex or medial or lateral walls.

the shaft. This flat surface makes it an ideal location for easy plate application. The distal anterior surface is triangular with the apex anterior configuration noted distally and only slightly flattened in the midshaft portion, but it becomes cylindrical in the proximal aspect. Plate application is problematic from an anterior or lateral approach because of these triangular surfaces (Figure 22-8) [27].

The biggest complication with plate fixation is radial nerve palsy [17,21,28–33]. The radial nerve is accompanied by the profundus brachialis artery and lies posteriorly in the area of the spiral radial groove. The proximal portion of the medial head of the triceps separates the nerve from the bone and serves as a useful landmark posteriorly to identify the nerve location. Posterior plating may require the nerve to be mobilized and positioned over the plate. The nerve then courses laterally and pierces the lateral intramuscular septum and enters the anterior compartment. It passes anteriorly to the surface of the brachialis muscle. The radial nerve is then in direct contact with the lateral cortex of the humerus in this epicondylar area and is more susceptible to trauma in this region. Lateral insertion of external fixator pins or interlocking screws must be done carefully in this distal area because of the midposition of the nerve in this location. The nerve then courses between the brachioradialis and brachialis muscles as it crosses the elbow joint [34]. Anterior and lateral approaches to the humerus must therefore note the location of the nerve and the clinician must be aware that the intramuscular septum tethers the nerve in this area, further adding to its susceptibility in this distal region [34].

SURGICAL APPROACHES

Operative treatment of humeral shaft fractures has generally used the anterior, anterolateral, and posterior approaches [34]. Most authors advocate posterior plating for fractures located in the distal half to distal third of the humerus. In addition, they recommend that this posterior approach be used when exploration or repair of the radial nerve is indicated or necessary [21,29,30,33,35–37]. The disadvantage of this approach is that it requires that the patient be placed prone or in a lateral decubitus position, which may be problematic when dealing with a multiply injured patient. The anterior and lateral approaches may be performed with the patient in a supine position, which may be advantageous when treating a multiply injured patient.

ANTERIOR APPROACH

This approach can be used to expose the entire humeral shaft, if necessary, by using the extensile exposure as described by Henry [38]. The incision begins at the tip of the coracoid process and runs obliquely in line with the deltopectoral groove to the deltoid insertion on the anterolateral aspect of the humeral shaft. The incision then runs distally along the lateral border of the biceps and stops approximately 4 cm proximal to the antecubital fossa. The incision can be extended into the forearm if necessary (Figure 22-9).

The deltopectoral groove is identified using the cephalic vein as a guide, and the interval between the anterior portion of the deltoid and the pectoralis major is developed down to the deltoid tuberosity. The deltoid can be retracted laterally to expose the bicipital groove, greater tuberosity, and proximal humerus.

Insertion of the pectoralis major can be released from the lateral aspect of the bicipital groove. The anterior portion of the deltoid insertion can also be elevated from the deltoid tuberosity to expose the lateral and anterior portions of the shaft. Distal extension is achieved by identifying the biceps muscle and developing the interval between the biceps and brachialis muscles. The biceps muscle is retracted medially and the brachialis is split longitudinally down

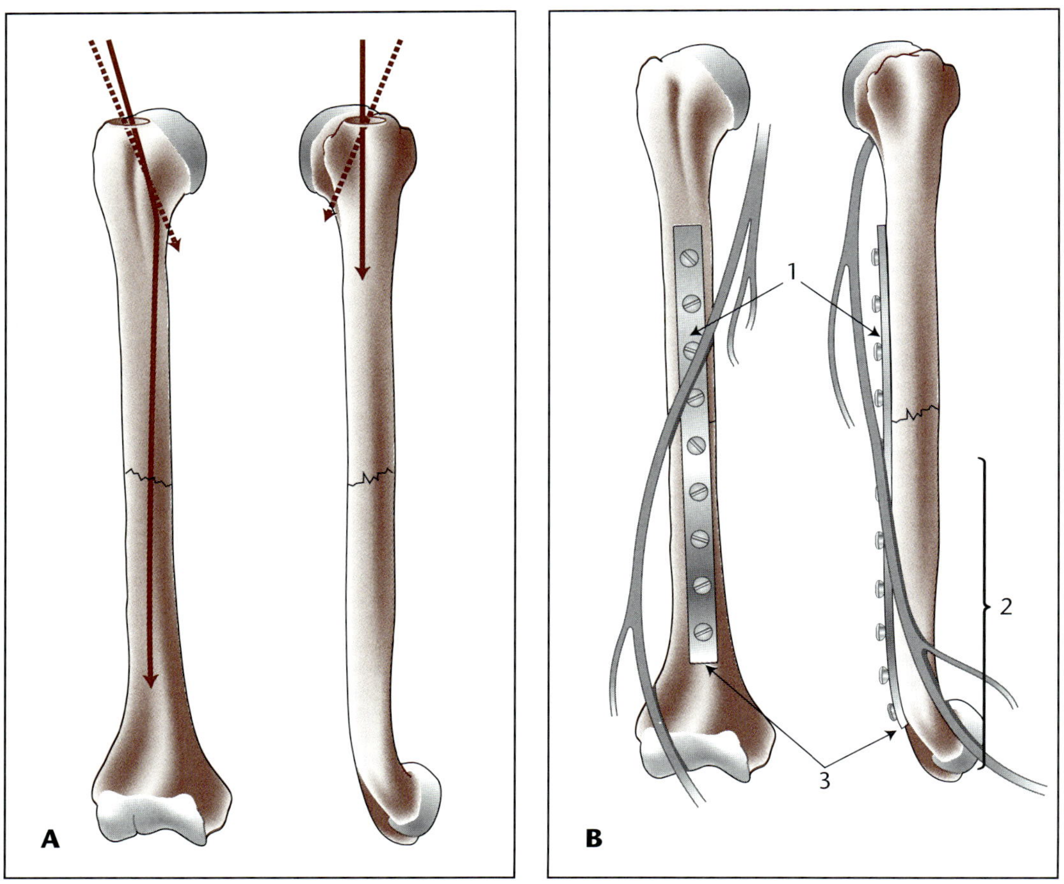

FIGURE 22-8. **A,** The portal for antegrade intramedullary nailing lies just lateral to the proximal humeral articular surface. Care must be taken to ensure that the insertion point is in line with the humeral canal on both anteroposterior and lateral images. The entry portal for antegrade nail insertion is not in direct line with the medullary canal. This eccentric location means that the nail contacts the proximal medial cortex and glides down the canal medially before centralizing in the distal segments of the canal. The nail (guide wire) *must* be centered on the lateral view to avoid anterior/posterior cortical protrusion. **B,** The posterior surface of the humerus is ideal for application of a dynamic compression plate. *1,* The radial nerve may lie directly over the plate in some proximal fracture patterns. *2,* In this location, the nerve is susceptible to injury with the use of laterally placed external fixation pins or interlocking screws. *3,* The plate may be contoured and placed into the olecranon fossa to achieve adequate cortical purchase for distal fractures.

the anterior aspect of the shaft. By reflecting a lateral portion of the brachialis muscle, the radial nerve is also reflected laterally with this cuff of tissue. By staying in a true subperiosteal plane, the anterior and lateral aspects of the distal humerus can be safely exposed with the radial nerve protected by this cuff of brachialis muscle.

Posterior Approach

The incision runs from the tip of the olecranon process proximally toward the acromion process on the posterior aspect of the humerus. The extreme proximal portion of the posterior humerus is covered by the posterior deltoid and thus limits the proximal extent of this incision, which is carried down to the overlying triceps fascia and incised in line with the skin incision. The key to this approach is identifying the two layers of the triceps. The outer layer is composed of a confluence of fibers from the lateral head (which arises from the infraglenoid tubercle of the scapula) and the long head (which arises from the lateral lip of the spiral groove). From above, the interval between these two muscles can be identified bluntly following the fascial split. Confluence of these heads can be separated in the midline, progressing distally by sharp dissection. After the superficial layer has been separated, the (deep) medial head can be identified. This arises from the whole width of the posterior humerus at the inferior portion of the spiral groove. This finding helps identify the radial nerve. When the nerve at the top of the deep head is identified, the deep head can thus be split longitudinally directly to bone. The nerve can be traced laterally out the lateral intramuscular septum. If necessary, the nerve can be elevated and placed over a plate if the fracture is in a more proximal location.

Lateral Approach

Mills *et al.* [26] have described a lateral approach to expose the distal two thirds of the humeral shaft through a plane developed between the triceps and anterior musculature; this exposure also facilitates identification of the radial nerve. This incision begins 1 cm proximal to the lateral epicondyle and proceeds proximally to the deltoid insertion. The overlying fascia is identified and the fascial incision is intentionally located posterior to the lateral intramuscular septum, thus placing the dissection in the posterior humeral compartment. The triceps is dissected from its investing fascia until the posterior aspect of the intramuscular septum is identified. This interval between the lateral intramuscular septum and the triceps is developed distally to proximally. As the dissection proceeds proximally, the loose areolar tissue is encountered with the nerve in the middle third of the arm. When most of the nerve has been identified and protected, the lateral intramuscular septum can be incised and the nerve followed distally. The triceps is retracted posteriorly and the brachioradialis retracted anteriorly. The anterolateral and posterior surfaces are now available for instrumentation.

Anterolateral Approach

This approach can be used for most fractures in the distal half of the shaft. It avoids the brachialis (muscle-splitting) incision that the anterior approach requires. It also has an advantage over the anterior approach in that it can be extended distally. The incision is extended distally along the lateral border of the biceps beginning approximately 12 cm above the antecubital fossa. The deep fascia is incised and the biceps retracted medially to identify the brachialis and brachioradialis. The interval between these muscles is defined and the radial nerved identified distally at the elbow. The nerve is then traced proximally to the lateral intramuscular septum. The brachialis is then retracted medially and the anterior aspect of the shaft is now accessible (Figure 22-10). Proximal extension can be accomplished by incising the periosteum between the brachialis and lateral triceps. The brachialis can be retracted medially and can then incorporate the deltopectoral approach proximally.

SURGICAL TREATMENT

Various options exist for the operative treatment of shaft fractures. Three primary treatment categories exist: 1) plate fixation;

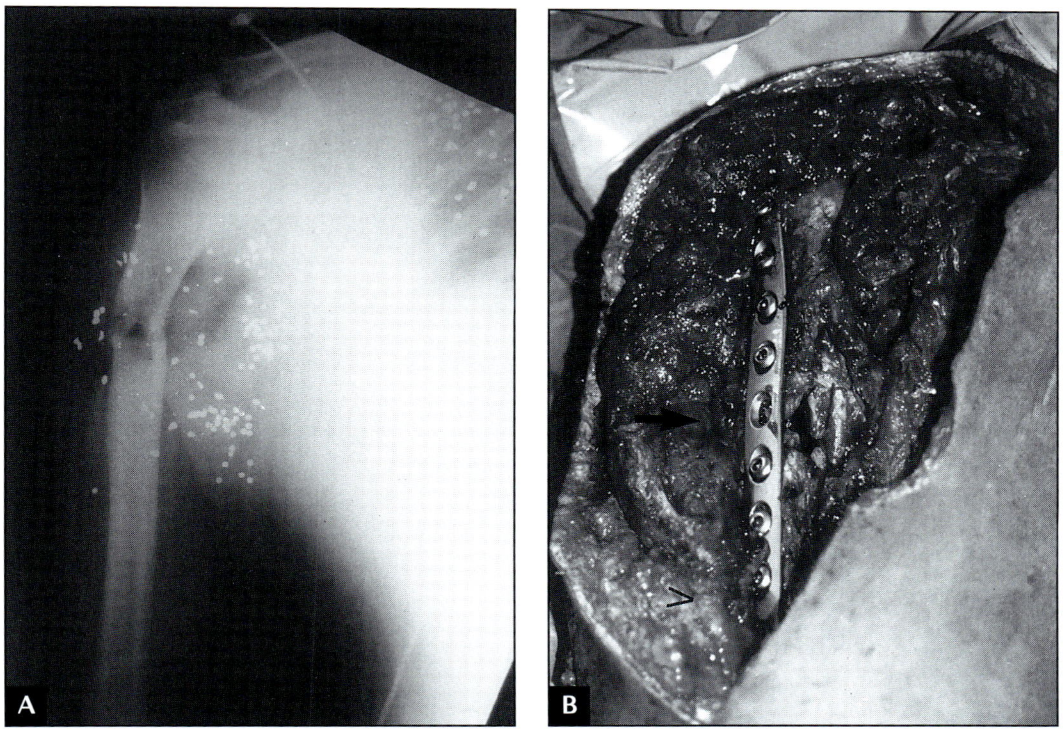

Figure 22-9. **A**, Anteroposterior radiograph of proximal humeral shaft fracture, secondary to a gunshot wound. **B**, The proximal exposure has been accomplished using Henry's [38] extensile approach. Note the oblique incision beginning from the tip of the coracoid process and running in line obliquely with the deltopectoral groove to the deltoid insertion (*black arrow*).

2) intramedullary nailing using both rigid and flexible nails; and 3) external fixation.

Before the availability of contemporary instrumentation and design-specific interlocking nails, plate fixation was the primary treatment option for these injuries. Many surgeons, however, are reluctant to pursue this option because of the concern for iatrogenic radial nerve injury and the tedious dissection necessary to apply a plate.

The humerus is accessible by many approaches as previously discussed. Considerations for patient positioning (*ie,* supine or prone) and location of the fracture as well as the necessity for simultaneous radial nerve exploration should be reviewed before selecting the appropriate surgical approach.

In most men, a broad 4.5-mm dynamic compression plate should be applied. This plate uses staggered holes that were designed to reduce torsional stresses to the bone [20]. Theoretically, these alternating holes may avoid a longitudinal stress fracture that can occur with high torsional stresses. Application of this broad plate may be problematic in smaller people. As noted previously, the distal humeral region becomes triangular in cross-sectional area and anterior plating with large plates may be difficult. Likewise, lateral plating becomes tedious because of the contouring necessary to avoid eccentric plate locations. It may be necessary in these instances to use a narrower plate for these anterior or anterolateral locations. Alternatively, the surgeon could choose the posterior approach, which has an ideal broad, flat surface for fractures in this distal region.

As the fracture becomes more distal, concern exists about the ability to achieve enough cortical purchase with screws below the fracture. For fractures located far distal, the plate can be precontoured to fit into the olecranon fossa. In this fashion, the last screw hole actually lies within the olecranon fossa. In this position, six cortices below the fracture may be achieved. The tip of the olecranon process may be safely excised to avoid impingement of the tip onto the plate and to allow for elbow extension (Figure 22-11).

In smaller individuals, it may be necessary to use 3.5-mm dynamic compression plates. Because of the shorter distance between the screw holes, this procedure may allow the capture of at least six cortices below the fracture, whereas a 4.5-mm plate may only allow two holes, or four cortices of purchase, below the fracture site.

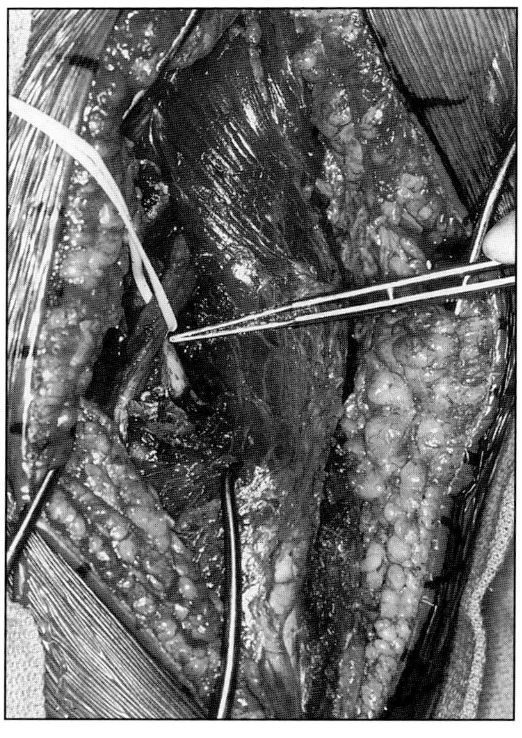

FIGURE 22-10. The biceps and brachialis have been retracted medially. The interval between these muscles and the brachoradialis is located and the radial nerve identified (vessel loop) distally above the elbow.

Indirect reduction techniques should be employed to minimize the extent of periosteal stripping and hematoma disturbance. Interfragmentary compression should be achieved through the use of a lag screw through the plate; otherwise, dynamic compression, using the plate itself, should be accomplished [21]. Bone grafting may be necessary in cases where less than 50% of cortical apposition has been achieved, or if segmental bone loss of more than 1 cm prevents compression across the fracture site. This occurs most often following open fractures; delayed bone grafting is recommended following complete healing of the soft-tissue sleeve (Figure 22-12).

Contemporary results using strict AO techniques have been excellent. Rates of union are high (92% to 100%) with most series reporting an average 97% union rate [30–33]. The most common complication appears to be iatrogenic nerve palsy [36], which ranges from 0% in two studies (Rodrigez-Merchán [39] and Foster *et al.* [35]) to as high as 10% (as reported by Nast-Kolb *et al.* [32]) and 12.8% in a prospective AO multicenter study of humeral shaft fractures treated operatively (Rommens *et al.* [40]). These authors attribute the high rate of nerve palsy to surgeon inexperience. The location of the fracture had a high correlation to the development of the nerve injury, with all palsies occurring in spiral fractures of the middle and distal thirds of the shaft [32,40].

Infection is an infrequent complication; no infections were reported by several authors (Dabezies *et al.* [29], Hegelmaier and von Aprath [36], Rommens *et al.* [40]) to as high as 6% reported by others (Vander Griend *et al.* [33]). However, all infections reported in this series occurred in open fractures. When infection statistics in other series are further stratified, infection appears to be an infrequent complication when primarily treating closed humeral shaft fractures with rates reported from none to only 1% to 2% for these injuries [28–31,35,37,39,41].

Most studies document function following plate fixation as excellent with regard to shoulder and elbow function and ability to return to "normal activity" for isolated fractures. Most patients who documented a decrease in functional outcome had a high percentage of associated local injuries or concomitant injuries to other organ systems.

Compression-plate fixation has demonstrated a consistently high rate of union and excellent functional outcome. For surgeons inexperienced in the surgical approaches to the middle and distal humerus, iatrogenic nerve palsy is the biggest complication to be avoided. However, in experienced hands this is a rare occurrence.

INTRAMEDULLARY NAILING

Intramedullary nailing has theoretical advantages over plating techniques [42]. However, before the development of interlocking nails, fixation was often not sufficiently rigid and external splinting was usually necessary to facilitate union [43]. Two primary implant types have been offered: flexible solid nails (*eg,* Ender nails, Rush pins, Hackethal nails) and more contemporary reamed interlocking nail systems.

Flexible nails are inserted in a nonreamed fashion. Fixation is accomplished using a three-point fixation through slight bending of the rods (either Ender or Rush pins) or by filling the endosteal canal and packing as many small nails as possible to confer rotational stability using a "stacked nailing" method (Hackethal). The overall goal is to achieve an internal splint, which provides only limited axial and rotational control, and thus external splinting support is necessary (Figure 22-13).

Brumback *et al.* [44] used Rush pins or Ender nails in 61 patients with 63 fractures. Treatment with immediate closed stabilization resulted in a 94% union rate and 62% rate of excellent results. Patients in this particular study group, however, were primarily polytrauma patients; the authors' technique was particularly applicable in this patient population because it minimized loss of blood and risk to neurovascular structures (no nerve injury was reported). In this review of patients, as with all application of flexible nonreamed devices, the surgeons had a choice as to whether the nails were inserted in an antegrade, retrograde, or epicondylar approach. The authors found that stabilization by antegrade insertion gave excellent results if the entry portal did not violate the rotator cuff. Symptoms of impingement in the shoulder and pain associated with an incorrect entry portal required early removal of the hardware. Fractures treated through the epicondylar approach had a poor result, and thus this technique is not recommended. Retrograde insertion with the entry portal proximal to the olecranon fossa yielded excellent results. However, the hardware must be prevented from encroaching into the olecranon fossa. If this complication occurs, it can produce an extension block to the elbow, and early hardware removal is then indicated.

All retrograde insertions, using either flexible or interlocking nails, require an entry slot rather than a hole (Figure 22-7) [45]. The gentle anterior curve of the distal humerus (which is shaped like a comma) requires that the entry portal be positioned as parallel with the humeral shaft as possible to avoid fracture during nail insertion. Although the elbow is not mechanically altered by retrograde insertion, prominent hardware can block extension; dissection in the olecranon fossa has lead to heterotopic ossification with an accompanying flexion contracture of the elbow [46,47]. A secondary study by Shazar *et al.* [48], in which a retrograde insertion with Ender nails was used exclusively, demonstrated a 91.5% union rate. Functional results were good in over 81% of the patients, and only one iatrogenic radial nerve palsy was identified. The reoperation rate, including nonunion, was 19%. This included eventual hardware removal. Even so, the authors continued to recommend this approach to humeral shaft fractures in the polytrau-

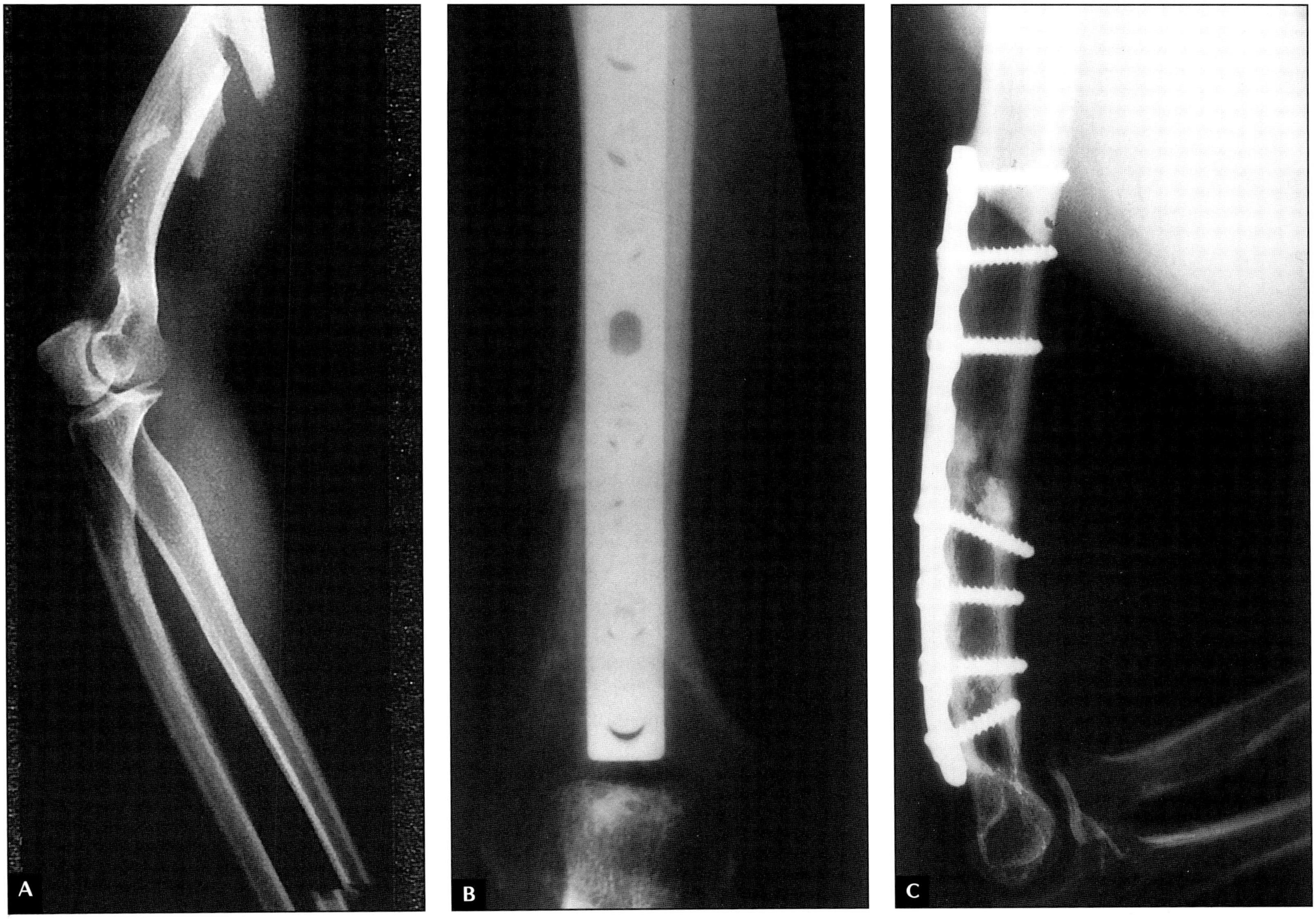

FIGURE 22-11. A, Distal humeral shaft fracture with concomitant both-bone forearm fracture. **B** and **C**, Anteroposterior and lateral views of the distal humerus showing fixation using a narrow 4.5-mm direct compression plate. The distal aspect of the plate has been curved to lie in the olecranon fossa. The tip of the olecranon has been excised to avoid impingement of the tip of the olecranon in this region.

matized patient. Other authors evaluated antegrade techniques and found similarly questionable results [49]. Stern *et al.* [50] reported on 70 fractures that had been treated with Rush pins inserted primarily in an antegrade fashion. They experienced complications in 67% of fractures, with 64% of patients requiring at least one additional operation. The rates of delayed union and nonunion seen were unacceptable. Painful adhesive capsulitis developed in over half of these patients [50]. Hall [51] also noted shoulder dysfunction in 10% of cases treated with antegrade Ender nails, of which the discomfort persisted following hardware removal.

Henley *et al.* [47], using retrograde insertion of stacked Hackethal nails, demonstrated a high rate of union (97%) with minimal rates of nonunion and infection and with no nerve palsies. One infection did occur in an open fracture [47]. These results rival those for plate fixation. Normal shoulder motion was demonstrated in all patients, although they did demonstrate an average 5° decrease in elbow extension loss, and heterotopic ossification occurred in three patients at the supraolecranon insertion site. However, in two patients, complications related to the smooth nail migration required a second operation at the olecranon fossa. These excellent results were echoed by other contemporary series using flexible nails (*ie,* Ender and Hackethal) through retrograde starting points. These studies have also shown results similar to those found in plate fixation. Rates of nonunion range from 2% to 9%, with 0% to 2% rates of infection. Radial nerve palsy associated with this technique is infrequent (less than 3%) and is usually temporary. Distal nail migration has been the most common complication, but it has been prevented somewhat by locking the Ender nails together by applying a small loop of wire or small screws through the eyelets [21,39,42,48,52–55].

Retrograde nail insertion techniques may be performed with the patient either supine or prone. A small triceps-splitting incision is centered over the olecranon fossa and the triceps is bluntly dissected in its midline directly down to bone. The olecranon fossa is identified, and the canal is opened approximately 1 cm proximal to olecranon fossa. Multiple small drill holes are made in an oval shape and then these are connected with a high-speed burr. Ideally, the nail should be prebent to achieve three-point fixation and a wide, divergent spread into the proximal humeral head. In this fashion, some degree of rotational stability is given to the fracture construct. The nail should always be passed with care and not forced if resistance is met. If resistance is encountered, the fracture site and location of nail incarceration should be thoroughly visualized with fluoroscopic views to determine whether the radial nerve is blocking the canal. If any doubt exists, the fracture site should be opened and the nerve explored.

Because these devices do not confer axial stability, long oblique spiral fractures or those with significant comminution are not ideal fracture patterns for these techniques. Rather, ideal fractures are those that occur with a transverse or short oblique fracture pattern. As noted, the biggest disadvantage to using these nails for retrograde insertion techniques is that implant removal may be neces-

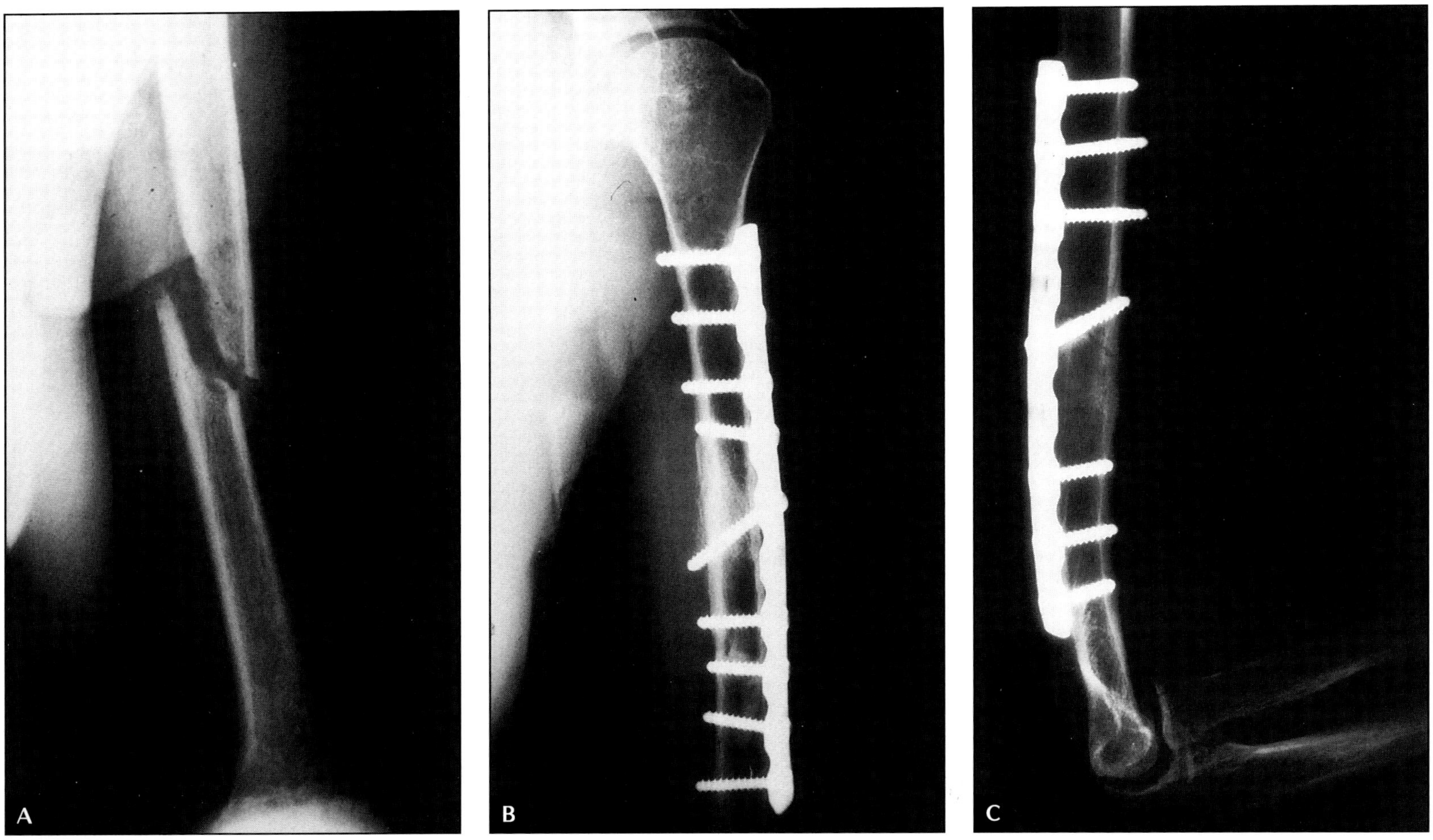

FIGURE 22-12. A and B, Midshaft humerus fracture treated unsuccessfully in a brace, necessitating open reduction and internal fixation using a broad dynamic compression plate. Note the interfragmentary lag screw. An anterolateral approach was used for this procedure. C, Distal one third humeral shaft fracture treated with a dynamic compression plate. Note the interfragmentary lag screw. This plate was applied through a posterior triceps-splitting approach.

sary because of nail migration, despite locking the Ender nail eyelets with a screw or a single wire loop. In general, antegrade flexible nail techniques are not the method of choice at this time.

INTERLOCKING NAILS

Because of the perceived limitations with the use of flexible nails (*ie*, lack of axial and rotational stability with coexistent hardware complications), rigid interlocking nails with design-specific instrumentation have been developed.

Biomechanically, interlocking nail constructs are stiffer in anteroposterior and lateral bending and torsional testing when compared with flexible nails (Ender and Hackethal). Compared with an intact humerus, interlocking nails are stiffer in torsion, but in bending, they more closely simulated the stiffness of bone [56]. Rigid nails, like flexible nails, can be inserted either through an antegrade or retrograde approach. Mechanical studies have determined that for distal-third shaft fractures, retrograde interlocking nails, with both proximal and distal locking screws, showed significantly more initial stability and higher bending and torsional stiffness than a similar fracture treated in antegrade fashion. In addition, for proximal fractures, antegrade nailing showed similar superior properties when compared with retrograde approaches for this particular fracture. For middle-to-distal diaphyseal junction fractures, the surgical approach had no effect on fracture stability. Finally, the defect created for retrograde nail insertion at the supraolecranon region reduced bone strength only 11.1% so long as the bone defect for nail entry was less than 2.5 cm long and 1 cm wide. Mechanical advantages were obtained by passing the nail from the short segment to the long segment provided 5 cm of nail/bone contact can be achieved in the short segment [57].

Using an antegrade approach for interlocking nails requires an entry site in proximity to the greater tuberosity near the rotator cuff insertion. Numerous techniques for proximal insertion have

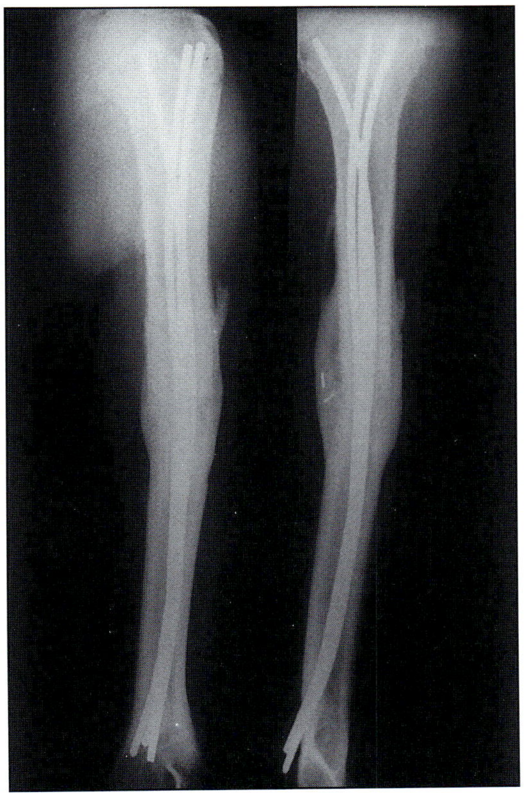

FIGURE 22-13. Comminuted midshaft fracture treated with the application of three Hackethal nails. These were applied through a supracondylar retrograde approach. The three nails were used to obtain a "stacked nailing" technique. The goal is to achieve an internal splint that provides rotational control, however, this requires external splinting and support because of limited axial control.

been described. Placing the nail through the greater tuberosity at the lateral edge of the cuff has been performed most often versus direct incision of the cuff just lateral to the articular surface of the humeral head. Neither method has been shown to be superior in terms of late shoulder pain and dysfunction [7,8,42,58,59].

During the 1980s, Seidel developed a thick, rigid nail inserted antegrade following reaming of the medullary canal [13,58]. The proximal aspect of this nail type has conventional interlocking-screw mechanisms, whereas distal stability is obtained by a spreading screw, which results in an interference fit distally. The outcomes, however, with this early design were mixed. Robinson *et al.* [8] reported a complication rate (operative or postoperative) of 87%, including a 70% reoperation rate. Most attendant complications were related to the failure of the locking mechanism distally, which resulted in axial collapse or angular malalignment. Poor shoulder function was apparent in another 66% of patients in this series. The large entry portal required for reaming and splitting of the rotator cuff was implicated in these poor functional results. Some investigators have reported favorable results with this device; however, most authors continued to report a high rate of complications, including nonunion, shoulder pain, compromised shoulder function, iatrogenic comminution, and proximal nail migration [45,58].

Other "locking" nail types have been used that have modified interlocking capabilities (interference-fit screw mechanisms or fins that can wedge the narrow distal canal). These have also demonstrated similar complications with rates of nonunion as high as 30% [60,61].

With the introduction of locking nails that had both proximal and distal interlocking screws, the problems with nail migration and malunion/nonunion have been reduced. Additionally, because of concerns about radial nerve damage with reaming, these new implants are of a sufficiently small diameter that they can be inserted without reaming. When placing these nails without reaming, it is important to avoid distraction at the fracture site. Acute distraction is deleterious to fracture healing and may cause nerve injury. This occurs most often in fractures in which the medullary canal is very narrow and the surgeon fails to recognize that the nail becomes incarcerated distally because of the anatomic peculiarities previously discussed. Further proximal impaction will not seat the nail deeper within the distal humeral canal but simply distract the fracture by pushing the entire segment distally. Additionally, forceful nail impaction in these circumstances can result in fractures at the distal aspect of the nail [62,63].

Results with the Russell-Taylor nail have demonstrated excellent results using both antegrade and retrograde approaches [62,63]. Crates and White [64] demonstrated a 94.5% rate of primary union, with two additional fractures uniting after bone grafting. Incidence of iatrogenic radial nerve palsy was only 2.7%, and only one patient demonstrated shoulder symptoms attributed to a prominent nail. All patients without full retention of elbow and shoulder function had other associated injuries or multiple trauma (Figure 22-14) [65].

Rommens *et al.* [62] also used this nail through a retrograde approach and noted similar rates of union (94.9%). Only one iatrogenic nerve palsy occurred. After healing, shoulder function was excellent in 92.3% and elbow function in 87.2%. Their conclusions were that retrograde locked nailing was a better choice of treatment than antegrade nailing or plate and screw fixation [62]. Other authors have noted the advantages of the retrograde approach for interlocking nailing, including faster rehabilitation with respect to regaining shoulder and elbow function [7].

Hems and Bhullar [59], however, did report a significant rate of nonunion (33% with a 26% rate of shoulder discomfort) related to

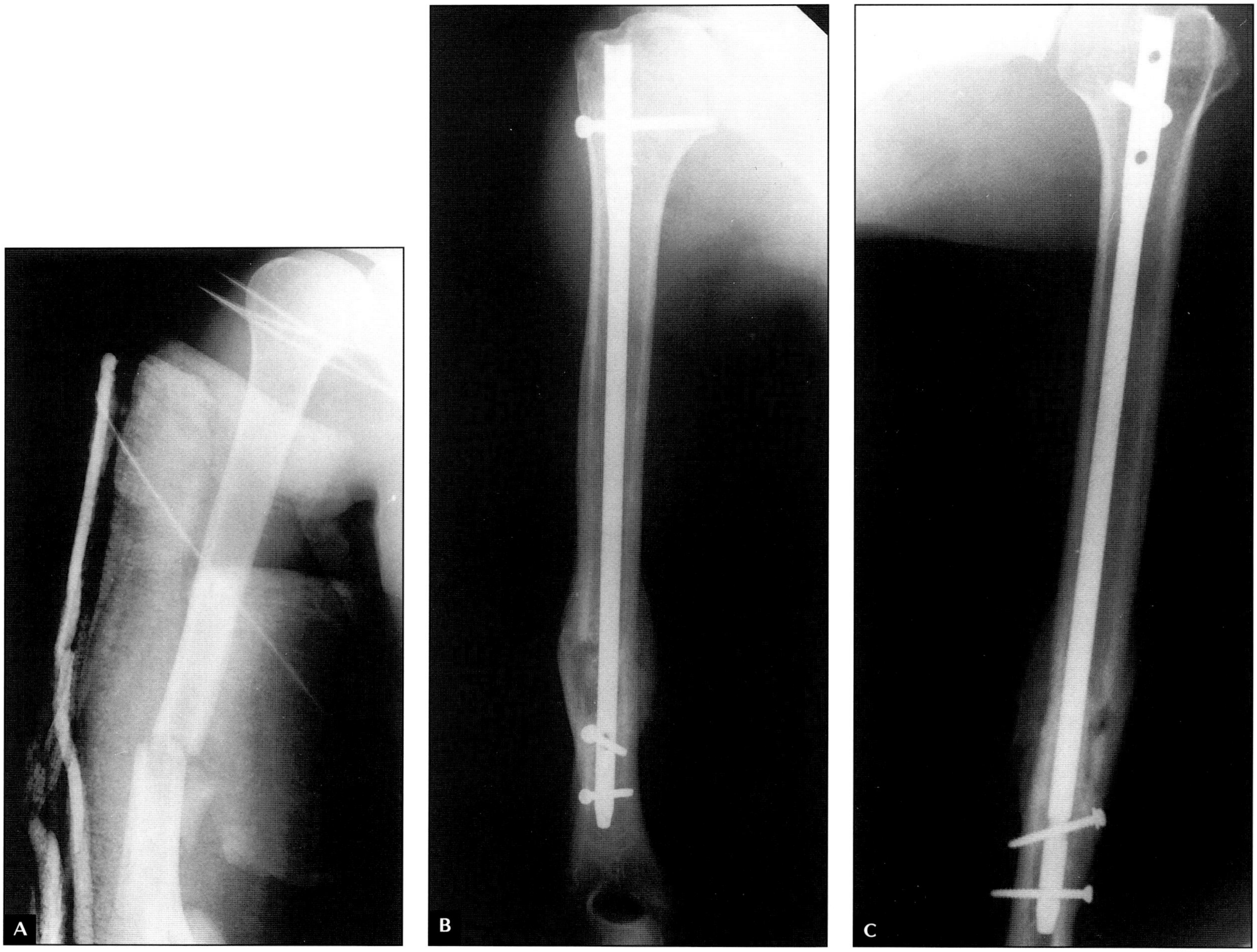

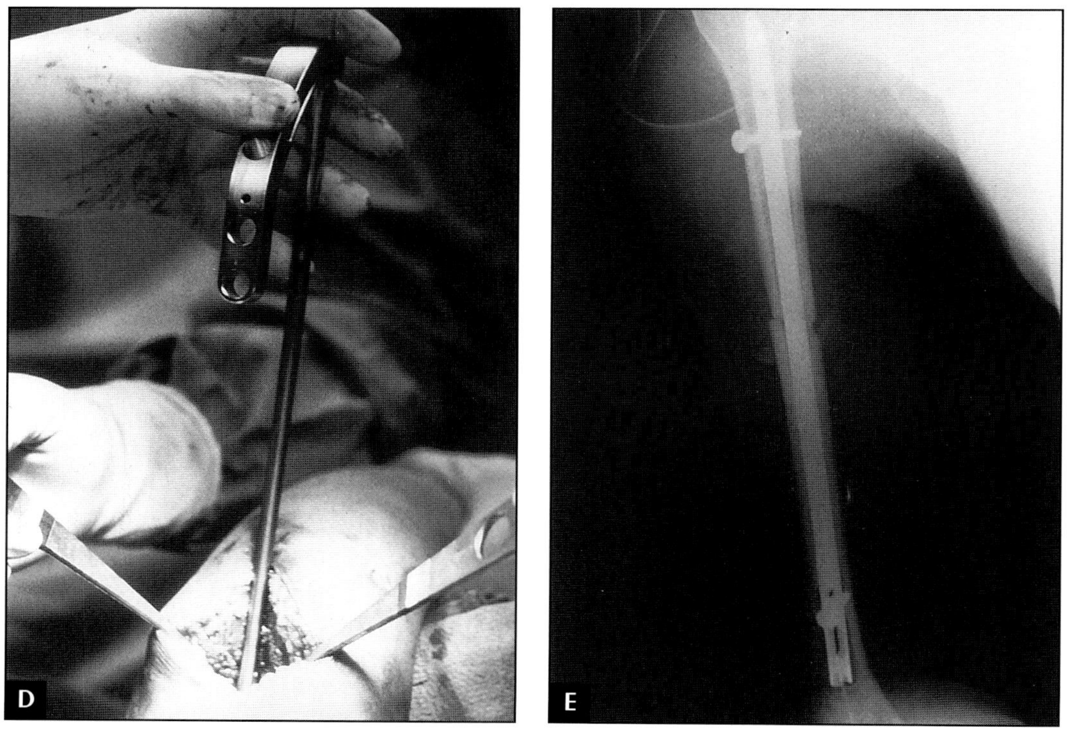

FIGURE 22-14. A–C, Midshaft comminuted fracture in a polytraumatized patient. This fracture underwent antegrade interlocking nailing. Note the correct location of the proximal insertion portal on both the anteroposterior and lateral images. The nail was statically locked to achieve both rotational and axial control. Because of the narrowing of the canal in the distal supracondylar region, care must be taken to avoid vigorous impaction of the nail, which can result in distraction at the fracture site or iatrogenic fracture at the tip of the nail. **D** and **E**, Retrograde interlocking nailing using a supracondylar approach with a statically locking retrograde intramedullary nail.

the antegrade approach used in their series of interlocking nails. Additional proximal shaft comminution occurred during nail insertion. This was attributed to improper entry portals too lateral in the tuberosity that caused the nail to impinge onto the medial cortex with nail insertion, thus fracturing osteoporotic bone (Figure 22-15).

In a series of 190 retrograde nailings performed in a prospective multicenter study using the AO-designed nails, a 92.6% rate of union was demonstrated. The most frequent intraoperative problems were fissure or avulsion at the supraolecranon entry portal. This occurred in 4.2% of patients. Iatrogenic nerve palsy also occurred in the same percentage of patients. Additionally, 5.9% encountered difficulty with the proximal freehand locking technique at the tip of the nail in the vicinity of the proximal humeral head. No untoward side effects were noted from this locking difficulty, however. The functional results of shoulder and elbow mobility were excellent in over 90% of the patients in this series [46].

Intramedullary stabilization, with and without methyl methacrylate augmentation, appears to be the treatment of choice for pathologic fractures. This technique has demonstrated excellent relief from pain and few, if any, implant-related complications. This treatment option provides immediate stability and can be accomplished with a closed technique, brief operative time, and an early functional return for these compromised patients [24,25].

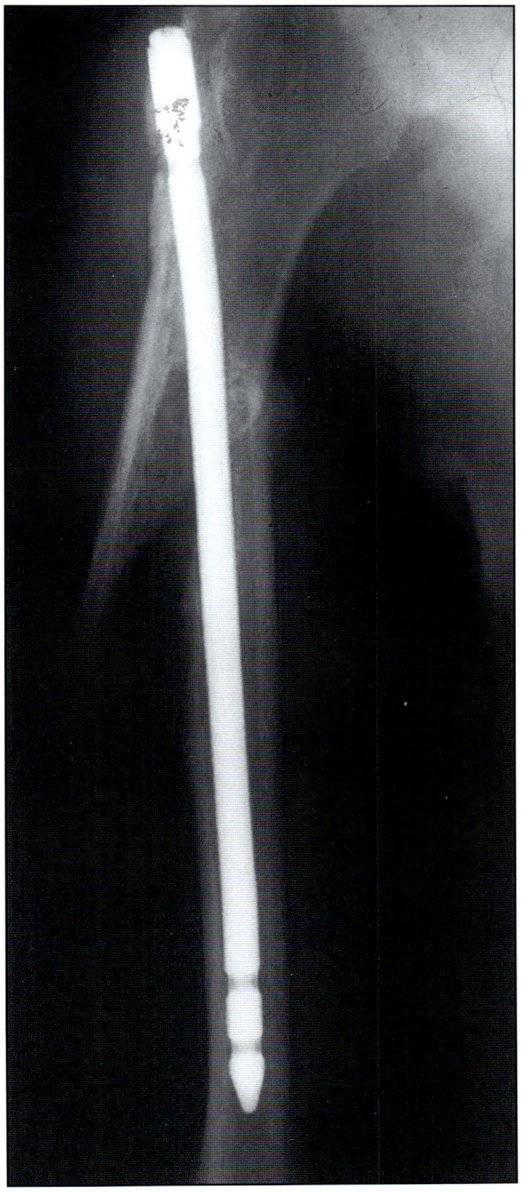

FIGURE 22-15. Improperly positioned antegrade nail-insertion site. The entry portal is placed too far laterally along the base of the greater tuberosity. The nail was placed without interlocking fashion, thus causing extension and malrotation of the proximal fragment.

Three recent studies have directly compared the modalities of plate fixation, flexible intramedullary nailing, and rigid interlocking nails. Rodriguez-Merchán [39] reported on a prospective series of humeral fractures treated with retrograde Hackethal nails compared with compression plating. In both groups, the rate of healing was similar (95%) as was the functional outcome. However, approximately 95% of patients in the nail group required hardware removal because of nail protrusion. No other differences were noted [39].

Two other groups of authors [66,67] have published abstracts comparing antegrade locked intramedullary nails versus compression plating for humeral shaft fractures. Their results mimic what has been demonstrated for retrospective series evaluating similar techniques individually. Both research teams noted a similar rate of union for both the nail and plates. They also noted a similar rate of complications in terms of nerve injury and infection. However, antegrade intramedullary nailing demonstrated an increased incidence of shoulder symptoms (42% and 31%) in comparison with those in patients treated with humeral plating. In contrast, the functional outcome after compression plating in both series was consistently good [66,67].

EXTERNAL FIXATION

External fixation is an infrequent treatment option for management of acute humeral shaft fractures. Indications for external fixation include open fractures, secondary fracture displacement following closed reduction, and multiple trauma.

Unlike the tibia, in which external fixator pins can be placed perpendicular to the subcutaneous medial tibial face, external fixation in the humerus often involves the transfixion of musculotendinous units. This has several deleterious side effects: patient discomfort, pin-tract sequelae, and hindrance in free-shoulder and elbow function due to deltoid and triceps tethering. Therefore, external fixation as a routine treatment method has not been universally embraced.

At this time, the most frequent indication for this method appears to be in the stabilization of severely contaminated open fractures or in gunshot wounds that occur in association with vascular disruption (Figure 22-16) [68–71]. This technique allows rapid skeletal stabilization to occur prior to revascularization or massive débridement procedures. Its use, together with radical débridement, has reduced the incidence of chronic infection and improved the prognosis for the vascular repairs. In addition, secondary surgical procedures for soft-tissue or bony reconstruction are easily facilitated.

CONCLUSIONS

Nonoperative management continues to be the standard of care for isolated humeral shaft fractures. Operative management, however, is indicated in specific situations. Contemporary compression plate fixation has demonstrated excellent rates of union with low rates of complications and excellent functional outcomes. However, enthusiasm for this technique must be tempered with the realization that if the surgeon is not familiar with the often tedious soft-tissue dissection, inferior results and a high rate of complications will occur. Definitive evidence does not exist with respect to technical ease to support the use of one procedure over the other when comparing plate fixation versus intramedullary nailing.

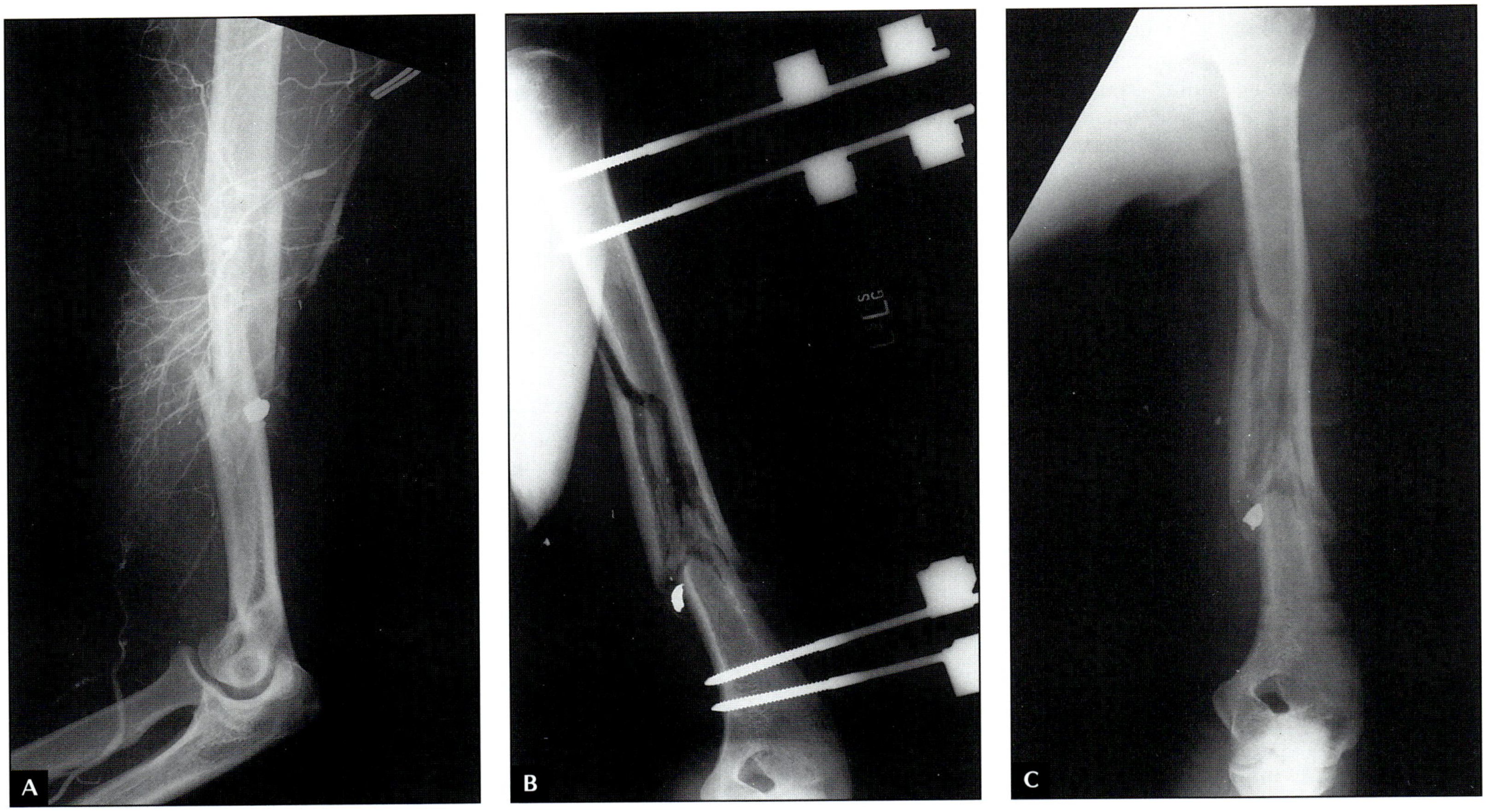

FIGURE 22-16. **A**, Comminuted midshaft fracture secondary to a gunshot wound. Also note the angiogram shows an arterial injury which required repair. **B**, Following emergent application of a spanning four-pin external fixator, the artery was repaired uneventfully. The fixator remained in place until healing was apparent at approximately 12 weeks. **C**, Excellent alignment has been maintained following removal of the external fixation device.

Intramedullary nailing has its own technical peculiarities and the surgeon must be generally comfortable with intramedullary nailing techniques. Special care should be undertaken with antegrade approaches to avoid undue damage to the rotator cuff. Flexible intramedullary nails give good functional results but lack the ability to maintain axial and rotational alignment.

Interlocking nails using proximal and distal interlocking screws have demonstrated rates of union and complications comparable with those for plate fixation. It does appear at this time that the retrograde approach to nailing has improved the functional outcomes in terms of shoulder and elbow motion when compared with antegrade techniques.

External fixation has limited indications and its use is now primarily confined to treatment of severe contaminated open fractures or those fractures that occur in association with gunshot wounds and arterial disruption.

REFERENCES AND RECOMMENDED READING

Recently published papers of particular interest have been highlighted as:
- • Of interest
- •• Of outstanding interest

1. Osterman PAW, Ekkernkamp A, Muhr G: Functional bracing of fractures of the shaft of the humerus: an analysis of 195 cases. *Proc Am Acad Orthop Surg* 1993:69.
2. Sarmiento A, Horowitch A, Abulafia A, Vangsness CT: Functional bracing of comminuted extra-articular fractures of the distal third of the humerus. *J Bone Joint Surg* 1990, 72B:283.
3. Sharme VK, Jain AK, Gupa RK, *et al.*: Nonoperative treatment of humeral shaft: a comparative study. *J Indian Med Assoc* 1991, 89:157.
4. Zagorski JB, Latta LL, Zych GA, Finnieston AR: Diaphyseal fractures of the humerus: treatment with prefabricated braces. *J Bone Joint Surg* 1988, 70A:607.
5. Zych GA, Zagorski JB, Latta LL: Current concepts in fracture bracing, part one: upper extremity. *Orthop Surg Update* 1986, 4:18.
6. Habernek H, Orthner E: A locking nail for fractures of the humerus. *J Bone Joint Surg* 1991, 73B:651–653.
7. Ingman AM, Waters DA: Locked intramedullary nailing of humeral shaft fractures. *J Bone Joint Surg* 1994, 76B:23–29.
8. Robinson CM, Bell KM, Court-Brown CM, McQueen MM: Locked nailing of humeral shaft fractures. *J Bone Joint Surg* 1992, 74B:558–562.
9. Sarmiento A, Kinman PB, Galvin EG, *et al.*: Functional bracing of fractures of the shaft of the humerus. *J Bone Joint Surg* 1977, 59A:596.
10. Sarmiento A, Latta LL, Tarr R: The effects of function on fracture healing and stability. *AAOS Instructional Course* vol 33. St. Louis: Mosby; 1994.
11. Sarmiento A, Latta LL: *Functional Fracture Bracing*. Berlin: Springer-Verlag; 1995.
12. Klestil T, Rangger C, Kathrein B, *et al.*: Sarmiento bracing of humeral shaft fractures: a comparative study. *SOT* 1997, 20:2.
13. Reimer BL, Bell KM, Burke JV III, Butterfield SL: Complications of Seidel intramedullary nailing of narrow diameter humeral diaphyseal fractures. *Orthopaedics* 1994, 17:19–29.
14. Sarmiento A: Diaphyseal humeral fractures: treatment options. Presented at the 66th meeting of the American Academy of Orthopedic Surgeons, 1999.

15. Mast JW, Spiegel PG, Harvey JP Jr, Harrison C: Fractures of the humeral shaft: a retrospective study of 240 adult fractures. *Clin Orthop* 1975, 112:254–262.
16. Tytherleigh-Strong G, Walls N, McQueen MM: The epidemiology of humeral shaft fractures. *J Bone Joint Surg* 1998, 80B:249–253.
17. Foster RJ, Swiontkowski MF, Bach AW, Sack JT: Radial nerve palsy caused by open humeral shaft fractures. *J Hand Surg* 1993,18:121–124.
18. Bostman O, Bakalim G, Vainionpaa S, *et al.*: Immediate radial nerve palsy complicating fracture of the shaft of the humerus: when is early exploration justified? *Injury* 1985,16:499–502.
19. Sonneveld GJ, Patka P, van Mourik JC, Broere G: Treatment of fractures of the shaft of the humerus accompanied by paralysis of the radial nerve. *Injury* 1987, 18:404–406.
20. Vansteenkiste FP, Rommens PM, Broos PL: Is een nervus radialis paralyse bij een humerus schaft fractuur een indicatie tot operatie? Indikationen. *Acta Chir Belg* 1989, 89:215–220.
21. Gregory PR, Sanders RW: Compression plating versus intramedullary fixation of humeral shaft fractures. *J Am Acad Orthop Surg* 1997,5:215–223.
22. Jensen AT, Rasmussen S: Being overweight and multiple fractures are indications for operative treatment of humeral shaft fractures. *Injury* 1995, 26:263–264.
23. Di Cicco JD, Mehlman CT, Urse JS: Fracture of the shaft of the humerus secondary to muscular violence. *J Orthop Trauma* 1993, 7:90–93.
24. Redmond BJ, Biermann JS, Blasier RB: Interlocking intramedullary nailing of pathological fractures of the shaft of the humerus. *J Bone Joint Surg* 1996, 78A:891–896.
25. Vandeweyer E, Gebhart M: Treatment of humeral pathological fractures by internal fixation and methylmethacrylate injection. *Eur J Surg Oncol* 1997, 23:238–242.
26. Calderone RR, Ghobadi F, McInerney V: Treatment of shoulder dislocation with ipsilateral humeral shaft fracture. *Am J Orthop* 1995, 24:173–176.
27. Mills WJ, Hanel DP, Smith DG: Lateral approach to the humeral shaft: an alternative approach for fracture treatment. *J Orthop Trauma* 1996, 10:81–86.
28. Bell MJ, Beauchamp CG, Kellam JK, McMurtry RY: The results of plating humeral shaft fractures in patients with multiple injuries: the Sunnybrook experience. *J Bone Joint Surg* 1985, 67B:293–296.
29. Dabezies EJ, Banta CJ II, Murphy CP, d'Ambrosia RD: Plate fixation of the humeral shaft for acute fractures, with and without radial nerve injuries. *J Orthop Trauma* 1992, 6:10–13.
30. Heim D, Herkert F, Hess P, Regazzoni P: Surgical treatment of humeral shaft fractures: the Basel experience. *J Trauma* 1993, 35:226–232.
31. Leutenegger A, Bereiter H, Endrizzi D, Ruedi T: Plattenosteosynthese bei humerusschaftfrakturen: indikationen und resultate. *Helv Chir Acta* 1989, 56:245–248.
32. Nast-Kolb D, Knoefel WT, Schweiberer L: Die Behandlung der Oberarmschaftfraktur: ergebnisse einer prospektiven AO-Sammelstudie. *Unfallchirurg* 1991, 94:447–454.
33. Vander Griend R, Tomasin J, Ward EF: Open reduction and internal fixation of humeral shaft fractures: results using AO plating techniques. *J Bone Joint Surg* 1986, 68A:430–433.
34. Blum J, Rommens PM: Surgical approaches to the humeral shaft. *Acta Chir Belg* 1997, 97:237–243.
35. Foster RJ, Dixon GL Jr, Bach AW, *et al.*: Internal fixation of fractures and non-unions of the humeral shaft: indications and results in a multicenter study. *J Bone Joint Surg* 1985, 67A:857–864.
36. Hegelmaier C, von Aprath B: Die Plattenosteosynthese am diaphysaren oberarmschaft: indikation—risiken—ergebnisse. *Aktuelle Traumatol* 1993, 23:36–42.
37. Modabber MR, Jupiter JB: Operative management of diaphyseal fractures of the humerus: plate versus nail. *Clin Orthop* 1998, 347:93–104.
38. Henry AK: *Extensile Exposure*. New York: Churchill Livingstone; 1945.
39. Rodriguez-Merchan EC: Compression plating versus Hackethal nailing in closed humeral shaft fractures failing nonoperative reduction. *J Orthop Trauma* 1995, 9:194–197.
40. Rommens PM, Vansteenkiste F, Stappaerts KH, Broos PL: Indikationen, gefahren und ergenbnisse der operativen behandlung von oberarmschaftfrakturen. *Unfallchirurg* 1989, 92:565–570.
41. Michiels I, Broos P, Gruwez JA: The operative treatment of humeral shaft fractures. *Acta Chir Belg* 1986, 86:147–152.
42. Brumback RJ: The rationales of interlocking nailing of the femur, tibia, and humerus. *Clin Orthop* 1996, 324:292–320.
43. Vander Griend RA, Ward EF, Tomasin J: Closed Kuntscher nailing of humeral shaft fractures. *J Trauma* 1985, 25:1167–1169.
44. Brumback RJ, Bosse MJ, Poka A, Burgess AR: Intramedullary stabilization of humeral shaft fractures in patients with multiple trauma. *J Bone Joint Surg* 1986, 68A:960–970.
45. Lin J, Hou SM, Hang YS, Chao EY: Treatment of humeral shaft fractures by retrograde locking nailing. *Clin Orthop* 1997, 342:147–155.
46. Blum J, Rommens PM, Janzing H, Langendorff HS: Retrograde nagelung von humerusschaftfrakturen mit dem UHN: Eine internationale multizentrische studie. *Unfallchirurg* 1998, 101:342–352.
47. Henley MB, Chapman JR, Claudi BF: Closed retrograde Hackethal nail stabilization of humeral shaft fractures. *J Orthop Trauma* 1992, 6:18–24.
48. Shazar N, Brumback RJ, Vanco B: Treatment of humeral fractures by closed reduction and retrograde intramedullary Ender nails. *Orthopedics* 1998, 21:641–646.
49. Mackay I: Closed Rush pinning of fractures of the humeral shaft. *Injury* 1984, 16:178–181.
50. Stern PJ, Mattingly DA, Pomeroy DL, *et al.*: Intramedullary fixation of humeral shaft fractures. *J Bone Joint Surg* 1984, 66A:639–646.
51. Hall RF Jr: Closed intramedullary fixation of humeral shaft fractures. *Instr Course Lect* 1987, 36:349–358.
52. Durbin RA, Gottesman MJ, Saunders KC: Hackethal stacked nailing of humeral shaft fractures: experience with 30 patients. *Clin Orthop* 1983, 179:168–174.
53. Neumann HS, Holmenschlager F, Winckler S, Brug E: Bundle nailing of diaphyseal fractures of the humerus. *Acta Orthop Belg* 1995, 61:159–161.
54. Peter RE, Hoffmeyer P, Henley MB: Treatment of humeral diaphyseal fractures with Hackethal stacked nailing: a report of 33 cases. *J Orthop Trauma* 1992, 6:14–17.
55. Rodriguez-Merchan EC: Hackethal nailing in closed transverse humeral shaft fractures after failed manipulation. *Int Orthop* 1996, 20:134–136.
56. Henley MB, Monroe M, Tencer AF: Biomechanical comparison of methods of fixation of a midshaft osteotomy of the humerus. *J Orthop Trauma* 1991, 5:14–20.
57. Lin J, Inoue N, Valdevit A, *et al.*: Biomechanical comparison of antegrade and retrograde nailing of humeral shaft fracture. *Clin Orthop* 1998, 351:203–213.
58. Bain GI, Sandow MJ, Howie DW: Treatment of humeral shaft fractures with the Seidel intramedullary nail. *Aust N Z J Surg* 1996, 66:156–158.
59. Hems TE, Bhullar TP: Interlocking nailing of humeral shaft fractures: the Oxford experience, 1991 to 1994. *Injury* 1996, 27:485–489.
60. Garnavos C, Seaton J, Lunn PG: The treatment of selected fractures of the humeral shaft with the True-Flex nail. *Injury* 1998, 29:269–275.
61. Watanabe RS: Intramedullary fixation of complicated fractures of the humeral shaft. *Clin Orthop* 1993, 292:255–263.
62. Rommens PM, Verbruggen J, Broos PL: Retrograde locked nailing of humeral shaft fractures: a review of 39 patients. *J Bone Joint Surg* 1995, 77B:84–89.
63. McKee MD, Pedlow FX, Cheney PJ, Schemitsch EH: Fractures below the end of locking humeral nails: a report of three cases. *J Orthop Trauma* 1996, 10:500–504.
64. Crates J, Whittle AP: Antegrade interlocking nailing of acute humeral shaft fractures. *Clin Orthop* 1998, 350:40–50.

65. Rommens PM, Verbruggen J, Broos PL: Retrograde Verriegelungsnagelung der humerusschaftfraktur: eine klinische studie. *Unfallchirurg* 1995, 98:133–138.
66. Chapman J, Weber TG, Henley MB, Benca PJ: Randomized prospective study of humerus fixation: nails vs. plates. Presented at the Annual Meeting of the Orthopaedic Trauma Association, Tampa, FL, September, 1995.
67. Wagner MS, Patterson BM, Wilber JH, Sontich JK: Comparison of outcomes for humeral diaphyseal fractures treated with either closed intramedullary nailing or open reduction internal fixation using a dynamic compression plate in the multiple trauma patient. Presented at the Annual Meeting of the Orthopaedic Trauma Association, Tampa, FL, September 1995.
68. Karas EH, Strauss E, Sohail S: Surgical stabilization of humeral shaft fractures due to gunshot wounds. *Orthop Clin North Am* 1995, 26:65–73.
69. Lenoble E, Terracher R, Kessi H, Goutallier D: Traitement des fractures diaphysaires de l'humerus par fixateur externe de Hoffman. *Rev Chir Orthop Reparatrice Appar Mot* 1993, 79:606–614.
70. Wisniewski TG, Radziejowski MJ: Gunshot fractures of the humeral shaft treated external fixation. *J Orthop Trauma* 1996, 10:273–278.
71. Zinman C, Norman D, Hamoud K, Reis ND: External fixation for severe open fractures of the humerus caused by missiles. *J Orthop Trauma* 1997, 11:536–539.

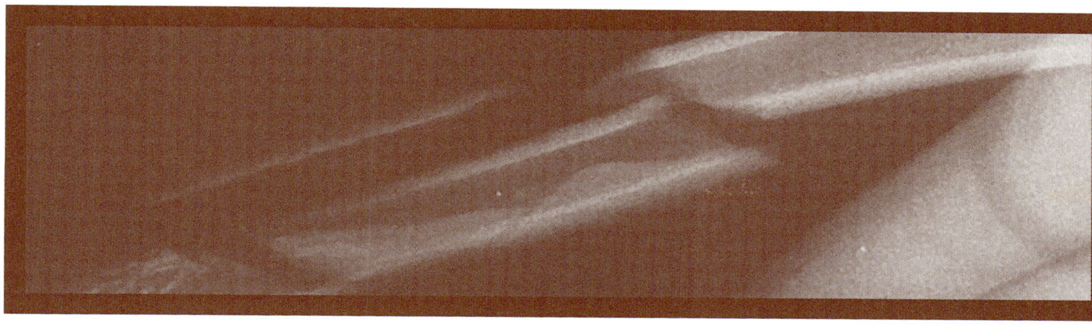

23

Supracondylar Fractures of the Humerus

Mark S. Vrahas
Michael J. Leddy, III

Fractures to the distal humerus provide some of the most challenging and complex cases for today's orthopedic surgeon. Treatment options have ranged from nonoperative care to surgical reduction and fixation. Today, with the understanding of documented cases and results of new techniques developed over the past 15 years, open reduction and internal fixation is recognized as the standard of care for these fractures [1–5]. Even so, the high complication rate associated with distal humerus fractures warrants concern.

The purposes of this chapter are to review the anatomy and classification of distal humerus fractures and to review techniques for open reduction and internal fixation.

ANATOMY

The distal humerus is one of three bones that make up the articulating surface of the elbow. Its components create the shape of a triangle (Figure 23-1). The distal humerus comprises two columns, a medial and a lateral, that terminate with their respective condyles. The condyles are linked together by the trochlea, which acts as a bridge between the two columns. Within the triangle lies the olecranon fossa where the proximal tip of the olecranon resides during full extension. Also within the fossa is the posterior fat pad. Swelling resulting from intra-articular trauma frequently displaces this fat pad. This displacement is visible on radiographs as the posterior fat-pad sign.

The trochlea is the key to the range of motion of the elbow joint. Mehne and Jupiter [6] described the trochlea as a spool held between the thumb and index finger of an examiner's hand (representing the two columns). This best describes the function of the trochlea as the articulating axis of the joint [6]. It is almost completely encased in articular cartilage, leaving a smooth range on which the olecranon glides. The trochlea has medial and lateral ridges with a groove between. These ridges lend to elbow joint stability.

When fracture occurs in the distal humerus, the construct of the triangle is disrupted, thus leading to dysfunction of the joint. It is imperative that with any fracture of the distal humerus, the articulating surface and the bony anatomy should be restored as anatomically as possible to prevent complications [7,8]. Special attention must be paid to the trochlea to avoid loss of its width or alteration of its alignment to prevent uneven tracking of the olecranon or instability of the joint as a whole.

MECHANISM OF INJURY AND ASSOCIATED INJURIES

It has been reported that fractures near the elbow make up as much as 7% of all fractures treated, and that one third of these fractures involve the distal humerus [9]. These injuries can be attributed to both penetrating and blunt trauma. Fractures from blunt trauma can occur either from a direct blow, such as from a baseball bat, or from indirect torque. Torque placed on the distal humerus can lead to fracture with extension to the supracondylar or intracondylar area. Penetrating trauma from a missile can cause extensive bone and soft tissue damage as well as neurovascular compromise secondary to the high energy of the insult and the associated blast injury.

When dealing with fractures of the distal humerus, the clinician must be alert for associated injuries. Neurovascular elements travel in close association to the distal humerus. This puts the patient at risk, so that a careful neurovascular assessment is critical when evaluating a patient with such a fracture. With open fractures, particularly Type C, a slightly higher incidence of minor nerve injury has been reported [10]. This could reflect the greater degree of trauma associated with the original injury. Comminuted fractures about the elbow with displacement of fragments can contuse, lacerate, or completely sever any of the arteries at the fracture level [11].

Postoperative ulnar neuropathy has also been reported in treating intra-articular fractures of the distal humerus [5,12,13]. Manipulation of the nerve intraoperatively, inadequate release of the fascia over the flexor carpi ulnaris, and prolonged postoperative immobilization can all lead to this neuropathy. Substantial functional improvement in the ulnar nerve can be obtained following neurolysis and mobilization of the nerve [6].

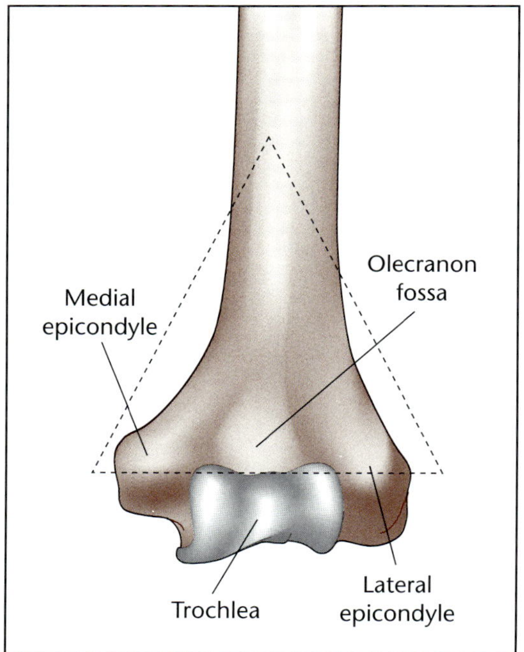

FIGURE 23-1. Posterior view of distal radius (*Adapted from* Mehne and Jupiter [6].)

CLASSIFICATION

Currently, the two most widely used classifications are those by Mehne and Matta [14] and by Müller *et al.* [15], which is a more comprehensive classification.

Müller *et al.*'s [15] classification is a detailed staging of fractures that helps evaluate the projected outcome of treatment. Numeric codes are used to detail the anatomy and severity of the fracture (Figure 23-2). Type A fractures are extra-articular, Type B are fractures partially articular, and Type C are completely articular. Each of these types is divided into three groups, and each group into three subgroups. Further qualifications have been made for each subgroup. Combining all the qualifications, approximately 66 unique distal humerus fractures have been defined. In clinical practice, it is usually adequate to identify the fracture by its type, group, and subgroup.

Mehne and Matta's [14] classification divides fractures into categories based on the columnar concept of the distal humerus. The classification includes three main categories with multiple subtypes (Table 23-1). Extracapsular fractures denote isolated injuries to the epicondyles. Extra-articular/intracapsular fractures involve

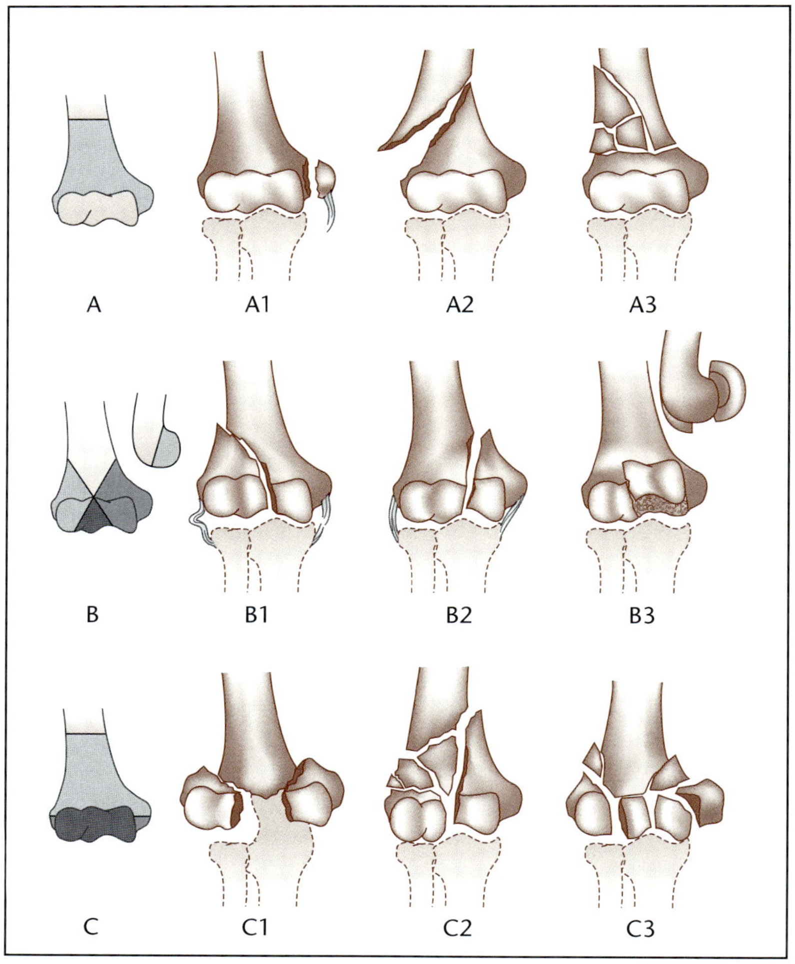

FIGURE 23-2. The AO classification of fractures of the distal humerus. (*Adapted from* Müller *et al.* [15].)

the supracondylar region but do not extend into the joint. Intra-articular fractures extend through the articular surface. The subtypes to these categories further clarify the extent and location of these injuries and help determine proper treatment procedures.

Extracapsular Fractures

Extracapsular fractures are those involving the medial and lateral condyles. These fractures are much more common in children and are associated with epiphyseal separation secondary to avulsion. Isolated fractures of these are not commonly seen in adults [16].

Fractures of the lateral condyle are extremely rare. Treatment involves simple immobilization with range-of-motion exercises after pain has subsided [17,18]. Medial epicondyle fractures are more common than lateral types. Fusion of the ossification center of the medial epicondyle with the distal humerus does not occur until about the 20th year and in some adults never occurs [16]. This could explain the higher incidence. Smith [18], in his series of 143 patients with medial epicondyle fractures, found only 2 cases of an isolated medial epicondyle fracture with no other fracture or dislocation to the affected elbow. Because of its prominence, the medial epicondyle is susceptible to trauma from direct blows.

Treatment of fractures of the medial epicondyle are based on the degree of displacement of the fracture. Minimally displaced fractures can be treated with immobilization and early range-of-motion exercises. Fragments produced in fractions of the joint warrant surgical exploration and removal. Sisk's [19] indication for open reduction and internal fixation is displacement of greater than 1 cm. This was done to avoid weakness of grip, ulnar nerve dysfunction, and instability [20,21]. However, Bernstein *et al.* [22] demonstrated no ulnar nerve symptoms or wrist weakness in displaced fractures treated nonoperatively. With either treatment, early range of motion is the key to avoid stiffness.

TABLE 23-1. FRACTURE CATEGORIZATION BASED ON THE COLUMNAR CONCEPT OF THE DISTAL HUMERUS

Intra-articular fractures	Extraarticular intracapsular fractures
Single-column fractures	Transcolumnar fractures
Medial	High
High	Extension
Low	Flexion
Lateral	Abduction
High	Adduction
Low	Low
Divergent	Extension
Bicolumnar fractures	Flexion
T pattern	Extracapsular fractures
High	Medial epicondyle
Low	Lateral epicondyle
Y pattern	
H pattern	
Lambda pattern	
Medial	
Lateral	
Multiplanar	
Capitellum fractures	
Trochlear fractures	

Adapted from Mehne and Matta [14].

Extra-articular Intracapsular Fractures.

Extra-articular fractures are transcolumnar fractures that present with increasing swelling and exquisite tenderness in the area of the elbow joint. The fracture line spans both columns and does not involve the articulating surface of the joint. The most common location of the fracture is the thin bone that runs between the medial and lateral columns. The fractures occur in four patterns: high, low, abduction, or adduction. Displacement position is the result of the forces that cause the injury. Fracture lines that extend proximal posterior to distal anterior with posterior displacement reflect a high extension force, whereas fractures that extend proximally anterior to distal posterior with anterior displacement occur with a high flexion force. Low fractures are more transverse; extension injuries are posteriorly displaced and flexion injuries are anteriorly displaced. Abduction injuries show lateral proximal to medial fracture lines with lateral displacement and adduction injuries the exact opposite.

The mechanism of injury also often determines the type of fracture sustained. Extension injuries are thought to result from falls on outstretched hands, but direct trauma can also cause these. Flexion injuries are rarer and thought to be caused by direct blows to the posterior aspect of the flexed elbow. Abduction and adduction fractures are the result of direct trauma or axial loading with an incorporated varus-valgus stress. With an adequate history, the clinician could make a preliminary diagnosis before taking radiographs.

High extension and flexion extra-articular fractures that are nondisplaced or minimally displaced can be treated with immobilization in plaster for 1 to 2 weeks and then undergo gentle range-of-motion exercises. Percutaneous pinning, though used as the treatment of choice in pediatric patients, has not been widely implemented as treatment in adults [23]. Open reduction and internal fixation should be considered in cases with an inability to obtain adequate closed reduction, in cases with associated vascular injury, and in cases with associated ipsilateral humerus and forearm fractures [13,14].

Low extension and flexion extra-articular fractures are managed using roughly the same parameters as high fractures. Bryan and Bickel [12] recommend closed reduction and immobilization for nondisplaced and minimally displaced fractures. Grantham and Tiejen [24] report difficulties in obtaining and maintaining closed reduction and support open reduction and internal fixation in these cases as well as in complex fracture dislocation.

Intra-articular Fractures

Intra-articular fractures occur in multiple varieties, as indicated by Mehne's classification (Table 23-1). However, in all types, some component extends through the articular surface. These fractures probably result from impaction of the ulna into the trochlea and can occur in flexion and extension [25]. Comminution at the fracture site is not uncommon. In flexion-type fractures, the condyles are found anterior to the humeral shaft, whereas in extension injuries, the ulna is directed anteriorly against the posterior aspect of the trochlea, thus separating the condyles at the same time as the supracondyle portion is fractured [16]. These fractures are seen mostly in high-energy trauma such as motor vehicle accidents, falls, and penetration wounds [3]. The management of these fractures is operative, unless some extenuating factor makes surgery impossible [6].

APPROACHES TO THE DISTAL HUMERUS

Isolated fractures of the condyle can be addressed either through a medial or a lateral approach. However, most fractures are best attended posteriorly through a triceps-splitting approach, or posteriorly with an olecranon osteotomy so that the joint can be easily visualized. The same approach should be used for low extra-articular intracapsular fractures to achieve appropriate stabilization of the condyles.

For either approach, the patient is placed in the lateral decubitus position. The upper arm is supported on a large roll to position the humerus parallel to the floor and to allow the elbow to flex 90°. The entire upper extremity is draped into the field. A tourniquet can be used if the fracture does not extend up the shaft, but if the fracture is high or if the patient's arm is extremely large, the clinician ought consider using a sterile tourniquet.

For the triceps-splitting approach, begin the incision 4 cm distal to the tip of the olecranon, and extend it up the back of the arm as necessary. Center the incision just ulnar to the tip of the olecranon to decrease chances of the incision's breaking down. Split the triceps in the midline to expose the bone. Subperiosteal dissection can be carried proximally; however, if it is necessary to expose beyond the distal third of the humerus, the radial nerve should be identified. Split the triceps tendon in its midline. This split should be extended onto the ulna and distal for 3 cm. The triceps insertion can then be reflected medially and laterally as continuous flaps. This allows exposure of the entire distal humerus but does not allow visualization of the joint.

A similar incision is made for the posterior approach with olecranon osteotomy. Opening the skin and subcutaneous tissue exposes the width of the triceps. The ulnar nerve is identified and protected. The medial and lateral borders of the triceps tendon distally are identified. The soft tissues are incised along these borders down to the bone of the ulna. The periosteum on the ulnar side of the olecranon is reflected to expose the joint. An osteotomy at the level of the zenith of the joint is made, and the olecranon is reflected proximally (Figure 23-3).

FRACTURE STABILIZATION

The principles of stabilization and its priorities are the same regardless of fracture type: 1) the joint should be reduced anatomically and stabilized with interfragmental compression; 2) the condylar segment should be reduced and stabilized to the shaft with proper alignment; and 3) stabilization should be adequate to allow early motion when possible.

Careful preoperative planning is necessary to accomplish these goals. The surgeon should first plan the joint reconstruction. In most cases, the condyles break into two or three relatively large fragments. The fragments can be reduced and held in place with large bone clamps. They can then be stabilized using a standard cancellous lag-screw technique (Figure 23-4). Alternatively, the fragments can be reduced and held in place with Kirschner wires. Cannulated lag screws can then be placed over the wires. It is essential to replace missing articular segments with bone graft from the iliac crest to ensure the dimensions of the trochlear grove. Lag screws provide the best stabilization and should be used whenever possible. However, when it is necessary to replace an articular segment, it is frequently necessary to use fully threaded positioning screws rather than lag screws (Figure 23-5).

Next, the surgeon should make a plan for attaching the condylar segment to the shaft. Biomechanically, the best construct is to place two plates at 90° angles. Ideally, a 3.5-mm reconstruction plate is placed posteriorly along the radial column, and either a one-third tubular plate or a second reconstruction plate is placed on the lateral border of the ulnar column (Figure 23-6). The exact technique depends on the type of stability the surgeon would like to achieve. Absolute stability requires anatomic reduction interfragmental compression. Relative stability is achieved by simply bridging the fractured segment. In either case, stability must be adequate to move the elbow. The decision should be made based on the degree of comminution. Absolute stability is ideal in the presence of two or three large fragments. With multiple fragments, it is usually impossible to achieve anatomic reduction and interfragmental compression without excessive fragment devitalization. For these fractures, it is better simply to bridge the comminuted segment taking great care not to detach the comminuted fragments from their muscular attachments (Figure 23-7). It is not necessary to reduce the fragments in the comminuted area anatomically. The key is to reduce the joint anatomically and to use the bridge plates to fix alignment and length. It is better to leave the comminuted segments unreduced than to remove them

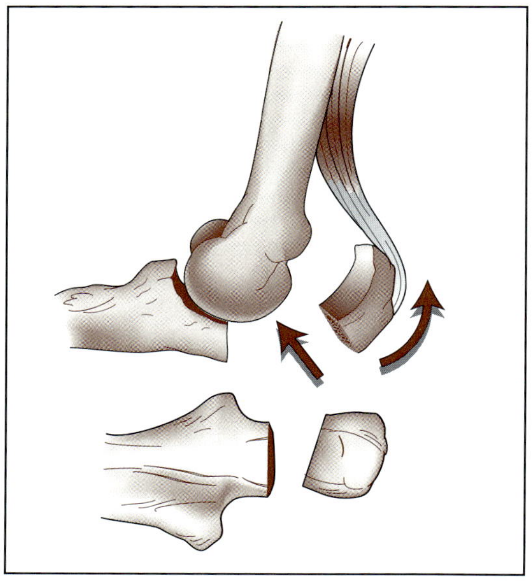

FIGURE 23-3. Olecranon osteotomy.

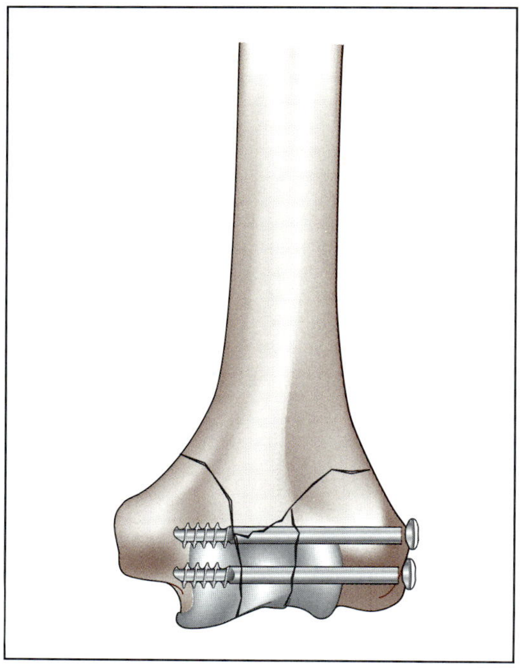

FIGURE 23-4. Standard lag screw technique for large fragment fixation.

from their soft tissue attachments. In any case, the surgeon should decide on the desired type of stability before beginning the case.

The radial column plate can be extended distally to the cartilage of the capitulum. This helps to improve fixation for extremely distal fractures. If the fracture is so far distal that only one screw can be placed through the plate into the distal fragment, fixation may be better achieved by placing a lag screw along the column (Figure 23-8). The same technique can be used for low fractures on the ulnar side.

It can be difficult to stabilize very distal fractures (*see* earlier discussion of low extra-articular intracapsular fractures). Usually, these fractures occur in pronouncedly osteopenic bone. In such cases, it is helpful to capture the distal fragment with three one-third tubular plates. One plate is placed on the radial border of the radial column, one posteriorly, and one on the lateral border of the ulnar column (Figure 23-9).

In a relatively small number of cases, it may be impossible to achieve stability adequate to allow elbow movement due to extreme comminution. In these cases, it is best to use a limited approach to reduce and stabilize the articular segment and to bridge the elbow and the remainder of the fracture with an external fixator.

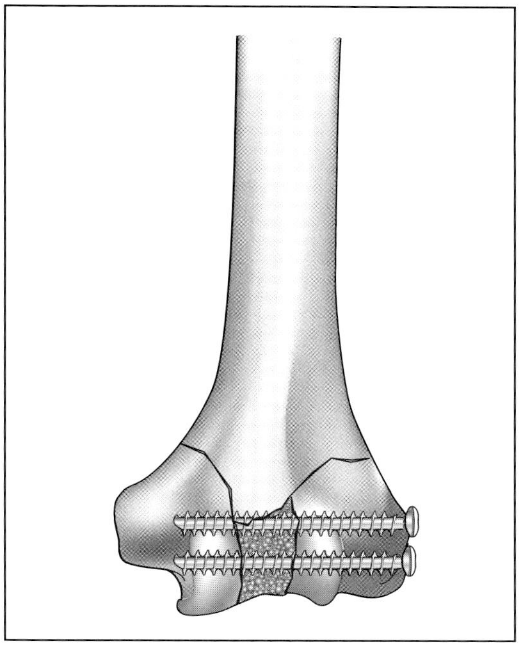

FIGURE 23-5. Use of bone graft for repair of articular surface with fully threaded screws.

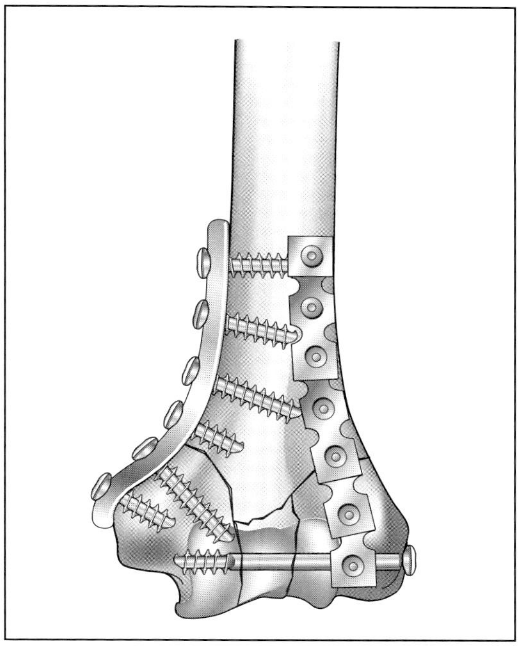

FIGURE 23-6. 90°-90° plating for attachment of condylar segments to shaft with 3.4-mm reconstruction plate posteriorly and one-third tubular plate laterally.

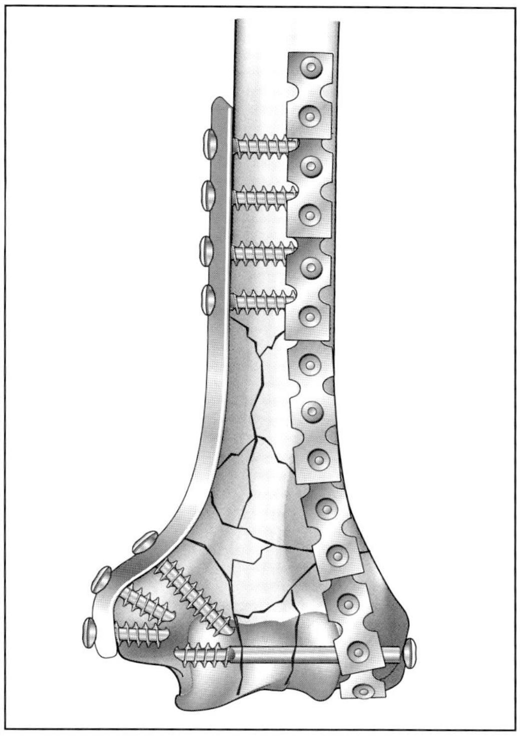

FIGURE 23-7. Bridge plate construct for comminuted fractures.

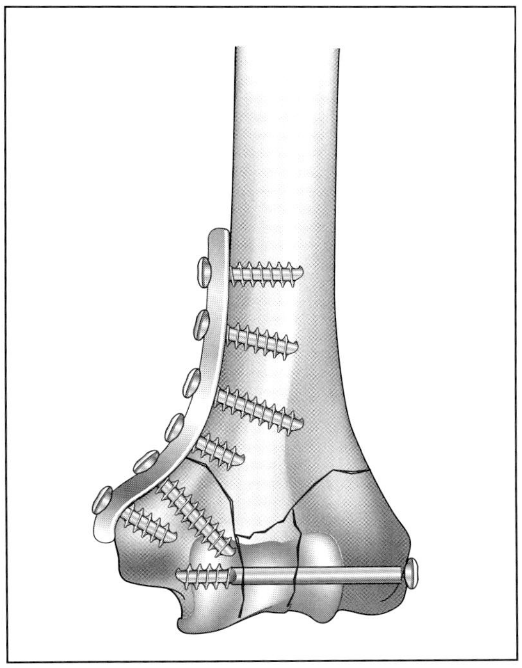

FIGURE 23-8. Lag screw with semitubular plate construct.

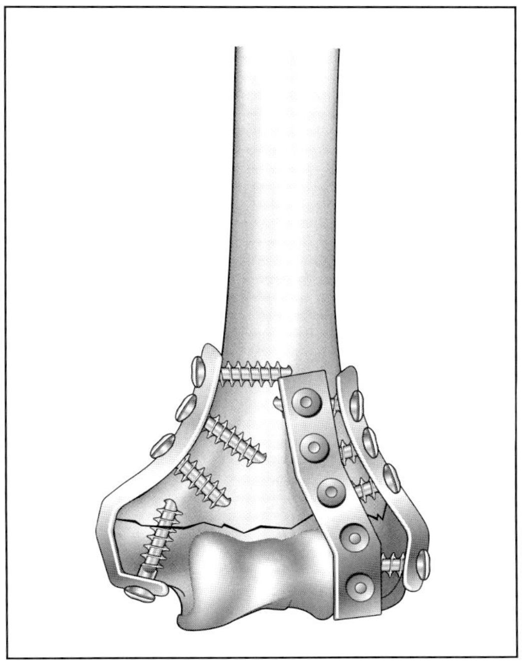

FIGURE 23-9. Use of one-third tubular plate to capture distal fragment.

CONCLUSIONS

Supracondylar fractures of the humerus provide a challenging and difficult presentation. Treatment of such fractures is related to the surgeon's understanding the personality of the injury. The classification systems just reviewed, along with a well developed preoperative plan, aid in the understanding them and the techniques that can be used for definitive treatment.

REFERENCES AND RECOMMENDED READING

Recently published papers of particular interest have been highlighted as:
- • Of interest
- •• Of outstanding interest

1. Aitken GK, Rorabeck CH: Distal humerus fractures. *Clin Orthop* 1986, 207:191–197.
2. Gabel GT, Hanson G, Bennett JB, *et al.*: Intra-articular fractures of distal humerus in the adult. *Clin Orthop* 1987, 216:99–108.
3. Henley MB, Bone LB, Parker B: Operative management of intra-articular fractures of the distal radius. *J Orthop Trauma* 1987, 1:24–35.
4. Pereles TR, Koval KJ, Gallagher M, *et al.*: Open reduction and internal fixation of the distal humerus: functional outcome in the elderly. *J Trauma* 1997, 43:578–584.
5. Waddell J, Hatch J, Richards R: Supracondylar fractures of the humerus: results of surgical treatment. *J Trauma* 1988, 28:1615–1621.
6. Mehne DK, Jupiter JB: Fractures of the distal humerus. In *Skeletal Trauma: Fractures, Dislocations, Ligamentous Injuries*. Edited by Browner BD, Jupiter JB, Levine AM, *et al.* Philadelphia: WB Saunders; 1992:1146–1176.
7. Sanders AS, Sackett JR: Open reduction and internal fixation of delayed union and nonunion of the distal humerus. *J Orthop Trauma* 1990, 4:254–259.
8. Thompson HC, Garcia A: Myositis ossificans: aftermath of elbow injuries. *Clin Orthop* 1967, 50:129–134.
9. Jupiter JB, Morrey BF: Fractures of the distal humerus in adults. In *The Elbow and Its Disorders.* Edited by Morrey BF. Philadelphia: WB Saunders; 1993:328–366.
10. Aitken GK, Rorabeck CH: Distal humerus fractures in the adult. *Clin Orthop* 1986, 207:191–197.
11. Ashbel, TS, Kleinert HE, Kutz JE: Vascular injuries about the elbow. *Clin Orthop* 1967, 50:107–127.
12. Bryan RS, Bickel WH: "T" condylar fractures of the distal humerus. *J Trauma* 1971, 11:830–835.
13. Jupiter JB, Neff U, Jolzach P, *et al.*: Intercondylar fractures of the humerus: an operative approach. *J Bone Joint Surg Am* 1985, 67:226–239.
14. Jupiter JB: Complex fractures of the distal part of the humerus and associated complications. *J Bone Joint Surg Am* 1994, 76: 1252–1264.
15. Müller ME, Nazarian S, Koch P, *et al.*: *The Comprehensive Classification of Fractures in Long Bones.* Berlin:, Springer-Verlag; 1990:74–85.
16. Hotchkiss RN: Fractures and dislocations of the elbow. In *Rockwood and Green's Fractures in Adults.* Edited by Rockwood CA, Green DP, Bucholz RW *et al.* Philadelphia: Lippincott-Raven; 1996.
17. Keon-Cohen BT: Fractures at the elbow. *J Bone Joint Surg Am* 1966, 48:1623–1639.
18. Smith FM: Medial epicondyle injuries. *JAMA* 1950, 142:396–402.
19. Sisk TD: Fractures. In *Campbell's Operative Orthopaedics.* Edited by Crenshaw AH. St. Louis: CV Mosby; 1980:508–713.
20. Milch H: Fractures and fracture dislocatons of the humeral condyles. *J Trauma* 1964, 4:592–607.
21. Linscheid RL, Wheeler D: Elbow dislocations. *JAMA* 1965, 194:1171.
22. Bernstein SM, King JD, Sanderson RA: Fractures of the medial epicondyles of the humerus. *Contemp Orthop* 1981, 3:637–642.
23. Perry CR: Transcondylar fractures of the distal humerus. *J Orthop Trauma* 1989, 3:98–106.
24. Grantham SA, Tiejen R: Transcondylar fracture-dislocation of the elbow. *J Bone Joint Surg Am* 1976, 58:1030–1031.
25. Bicknel WE, Perry RE: Comminuted fractures of the distal humerus. *JAMA* 1963, 84:553–557.

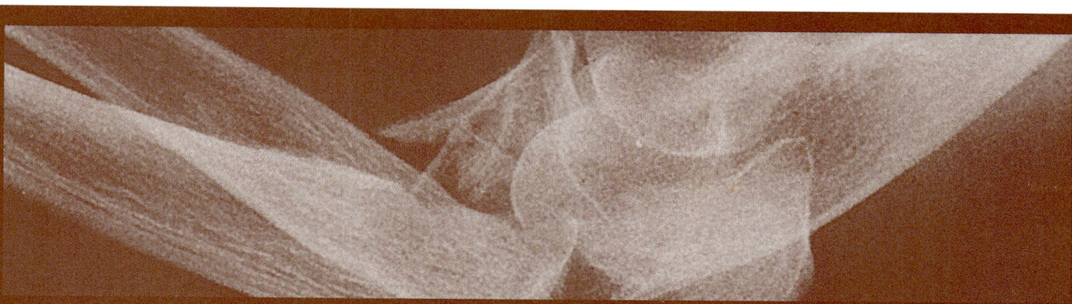

24

Fracture-Dislocations of the Elbow

David Ring
Jesse B. Jupiter

This is a time of substantial transition in concepts of traumatic elbow instability. Interest has turned from the medial to the lateral side of the elbow; from emphasis on the ligamentous to the osseous-articular stabilizers of the elbow; and from the component parts of the injury to the identification of overall patterns of injury. A better understanding of traumatic elbow instability has led to more rational treatment algorithms; however, the operative exposures and internal fixation of small articular fractures continue to evolve and are unfamiliar to many orthopedic surgeons. It may be best to refer a difficult fracture-dislocation of the elbow to a surgeon with interest and experience in the care of these injuries.

ANATOMY AND MECHANICS

Management of traumatic elbow instability requires a good understanding of the anatomy and mechanics of the elbow. It is useful to divide the stabilizing structures of the elbow into four columns: medial, lateral, anterior, and posterior. These columns overlap somewhat, blending into a ring concept of elbow stability similar to that encountered at other anatomic sites such as the shoulder, pelvis, and ankle (Figure 24-1) [1].

Medial Column

The anterior band of the medial collateral ligament originates on the inferior surface of the medial epicondyle and inserts on the base of the coronoid process of the ulna [2]. A displaced fracture of the medial epicondyle or the coronoid process at its base represents an alternative means of disrupting the function of the medial collateral ligament. The former is nearly unique to pediatric patients, and the latter to adults. If failure of the ligament occurs through bone, it is unlikely that the ligament substance is also torn.

The medial collateral ligament complex heals after simple elbow dislocations [3,4] and most acute isolated medial collateral ligament tears (a rare injury) [5]. Chronic isolated medial collateral ligament insufficiency is a problem largely encountered in athletes who use a throwing motion [6,7]. Such patients have an attenuated medial collateral ligament that will no longer support repetitive forceful throwing. Most daily activities are not affected, however, and a reconstructive procedure is necessary only if the patient desires to return to competitive athletics [6,7].

In patients with chronic attenuation of the medial collateral ligament complex, the intact radial head provides sufficient stability against valgus force to support most activities. Conversely, excision of the radial head has little effect on elbow stability if the medial collateral ligament remains competent [8]. Therefore, it is probably better to consider the valgus constraints of the elbow as overlapping and complementary rather than hierarchical. When both the radial head and medial collateral ligament are incompetent, the elbow is severely unstable [1,9,10]. This is an example of the usefulness of the ring theory of elbow instability—the greater the number of breaks in the ring, the greater the resulting instability.

Lateral Column

The foundation of the lateral column of elbow stability is radiocapitellar contact. Its importance with respect to elbow stability has already been reviewed in the context of concomitant medial column disruption. Moreover, cadaveric studies suggest that silicone implants are not sufficiently stiff to restore lateral column stability, and that metal implants are a better choice [10–12]. Although it is best to repair the radial head in the management of acute injury, this is usually not an option for chronic instability because fragments are often missing or avascular.

The stability of the lateral column also depends on an intact lateral collateral ligament complex [13,14]. This complex maintains appropriate contact in the radiocapitellar articulation and is also an important stabilizer of the ulnohumeral joint.

Osbourne and Cotteril [15], among others, emphasized the importance of lateral collateral ligament incompetence in chronic elbow instability. As recent advocates of this view, O'Driscoll *et al.* [16] have demonstrated that it is possible to dislocate the ulnohumeral articulation with the anterior band of the medial collateral ligament intact and have attributed most recurrent simple elbow dislocations to attenuation of the lateral collateral ligament complex [13,17].

The Mayo group has implicated a structure that they have labeled the lateral ulnar collateral ligament [13,17]. The cadaveric investigations performed by Cohen and Hastings [18] suggest that the situation may be more complex. They found that several lateral structures contributed to varus and rotatory stability of the elbow, including the ulnar and annular insertions of the lateral collateral ligament complex and the annular ligament itself. Musculotendinous contributions include the supinator tendon, a fascial band of the extensor carpi ulnaris, and the conjoined extensor origin reinforced by its intramuscular septae [18].

Anterior Column

The schematic anterior column consists of the bony buttress provided by the coronoid process and radial head along with the anterior capsule. In addition, the elbow flexor musculature, in conjunction with the posterior extensor muscles, provides an important dynamic stabilizing effect by compressing the trochlea into the trochlear notch of the ulna; however, the brachialis inserts quite distally on the ulna (the insertion blending with the base of the coronoid) and is unlikely to provide much static constraint [2].

The bad reputation of the so-called terrible triad lesion (posterior dislocation of the elbow with fractures of the radial head and coronoid) is a testament to the importance of the anterior column of elbow stability. These injuries are among the most difficult to

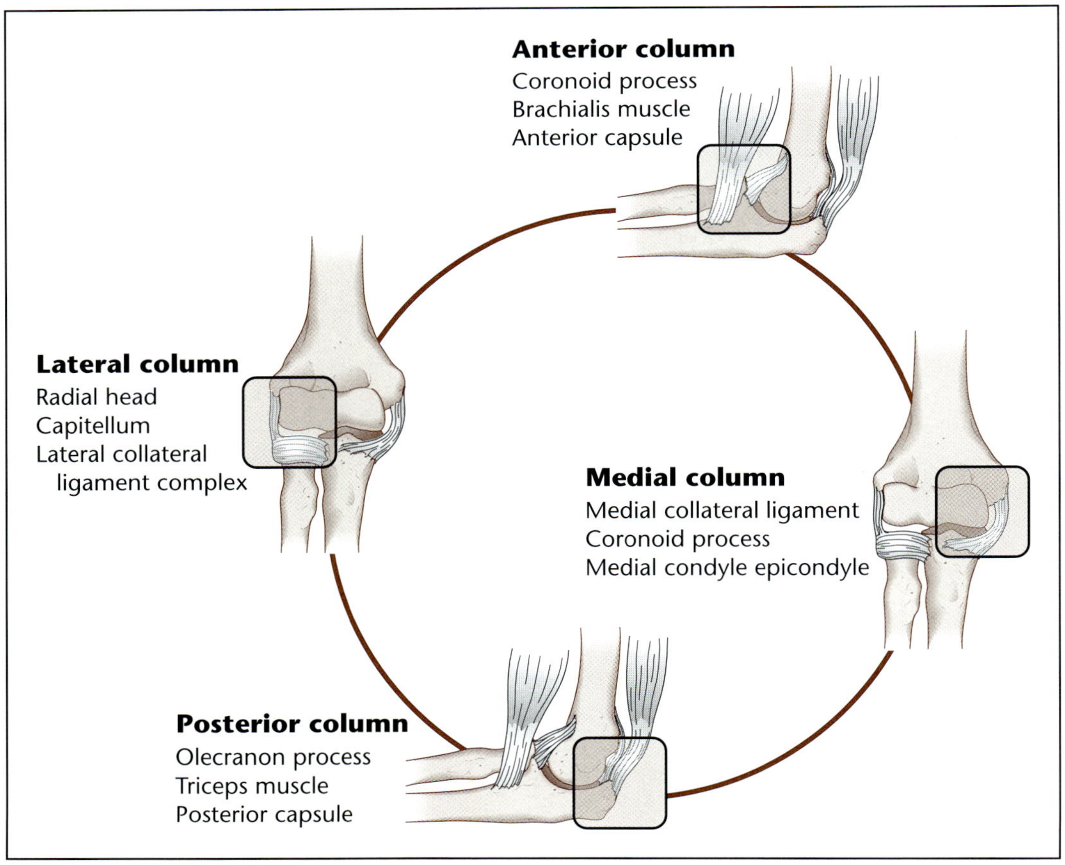

Figure 24-1. It is useful to consider the stabilizers of the elbow in four separate columns. Each of these overlaps and interrelates somewhat, forming a schematic ring. (*Adapted from* Ring and Jupiter [1].)

treat in the elbow, with recurrent dislocation and subluxation commonplace [19,20].

A fracture of the coronoid process near its base, even as an isolated injury, is sufficient to allow anterior subluxation of the ulnohumeral articulation [21]. This may result from the combined loss of an anterior bony buttress in addition to the incompetence of the medial collateral ligament.

Posterior Column

The posterior column consists of the olecranon process of the ulna, the posterior capsule, and the dynamic contribution of the triceps. Given that excision of comminuted olecranon fractures is an accepted practice [22], this column might seem at first to be of relatively little importance. However, the inherent stability of the elbow after posterior dislocation without associated fractures is largely a result of the nearly 180° envelopment of the trochlea by the trochlear notch of the ulna in conjunction with the interdigitation of the trochlear ridge of the ulnar articular surface with the trochlear groove [23]. Such simple dislocations can be mobilized immediately with little risk of recurrent dislocation [3,4]. Fracture of the olecranon process disrupts the trochlear notch of the ulna—the keystone of this inherent stability of the elbow.

PATTERNS OF INJURY

One important yet underemphasized facet of traumatic elbow instability is the pattern of injury. Ulnohumeral dislocations without fracture can occur with disruption of both the medial and lateral collateral ligament complexes or with lateral-sided disruption alone [16]. There are four common patterns of fracture-dislocation: 1) anterior and 2) posterior fracture-dislocation of the olecranon, and posterior dislocation of the ulnohumeral articulation with 3) fracture of the radial head alone or 4) fracture of both the radial head and coronoid process (Figure 24-2). Each pattern is associated with injury to specific structures, leading to distinct patterns of acute and chronic instability. Identifying the pattern of the original injury is helpful in selecting appropriate management.

Anterior Fracture-Dislocation of the Olecranon

Anterior and posterior fracture-dislocations of the olecranon represent disruptions rather than true dislocations of the ulnohumeral joint. The articular surfaces usually remain apposed, and there is at least partial sparing of the collateral ligaments. Anterior pat-

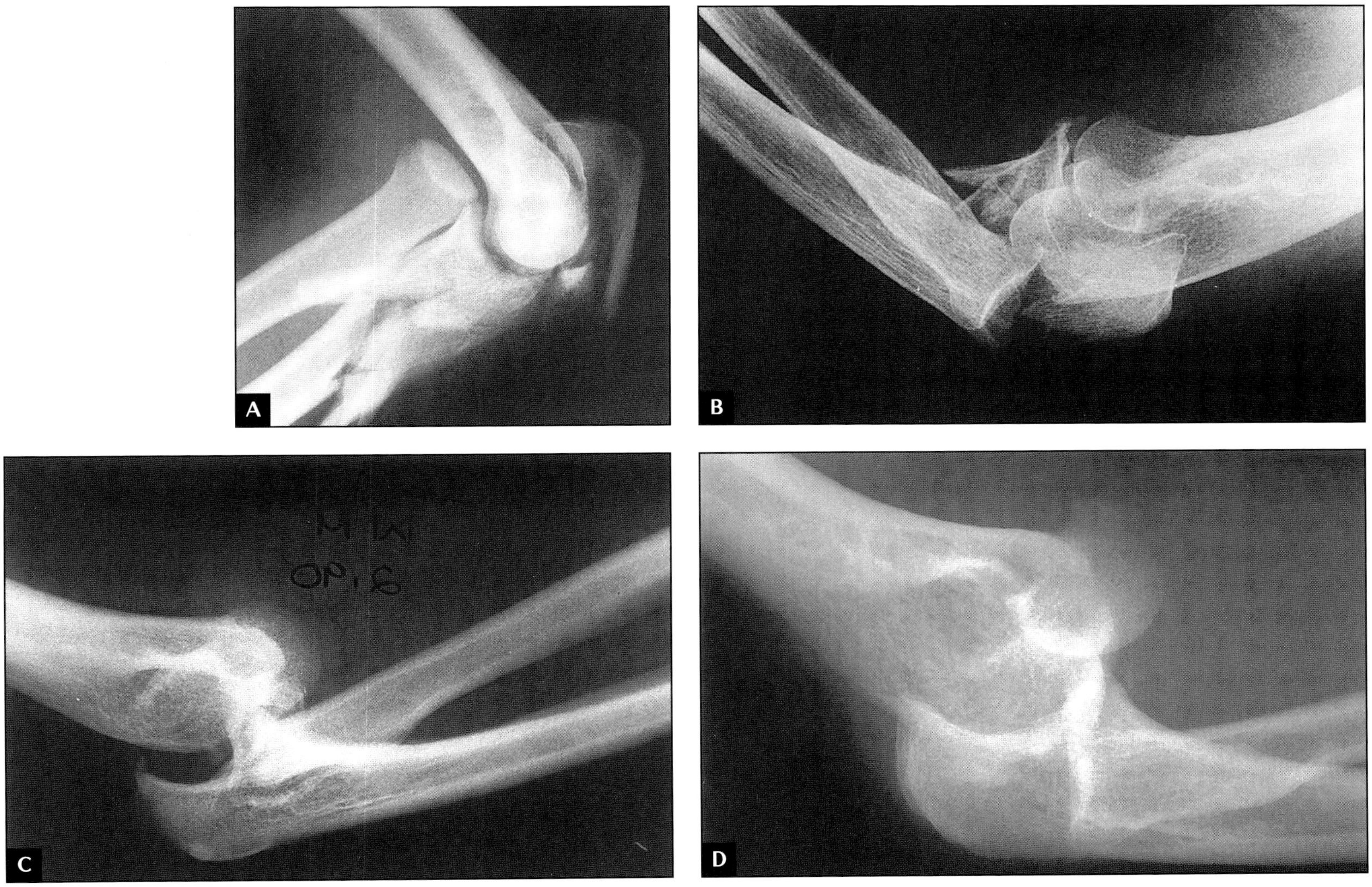

Figure 24-2. Most elbow fracture-dislocations fit one of four common patterns. **A**, Anterior or transolecranon fracture-dislocation. **B**, Posterior Monteggia pattern fracture-dislocation. **C**, Posterior dislocation of the ulnohumeral joint with fracture of the radial head. **D**, Posterior dislocation with fractures of the radial head and coronoid. A small fracture of the coronoid may not always be apparent on initial radiographs. (Panels A–C *from* Ring and Jupiter [1]; with permission.)

tern injuries have been referred to as transolecranon fracture-dislocations of the elbow [24,25]. Although they are frequently misidentified as anterior Monteggia lesions, the radioulnar relationship is not affected; the entire forearm dislocates anteriorly as the trochlea passes through the disrupted trochlear notch of the ulna (Figure 24-2) [25]. The medial and lateral collateral ligament complexes are likely to be at least partially spared in this injury pattern; the failure of the articulation occurs largely through bone. Large coronoid fractures (representing between 50% and 100% of the height of the coronoid—Type III according to the system of Regan and Morrey [26]) occur in slightly more than half of the injuries, and fragmentation of the region between the coronoid and olecranon facets of the trochlear notch occurs in most of the injuries [25].

Chronic instability has been rare in these injuries when appropriate initial treatment with a dorsally applied contoured plate and screws and stable anatomic fixation of the coronoid fracture is rendered [25]. Persistent instability usually reflects nonunion or malunion of the coronoid process or narrowing of the trochlear notch.

Posterior Fracture-Dislocation of the Olecranon

Posterior fracture-dislocation of the olecranon resembles a posterior Monteggia pattern injury and may represent the most proximal form of this injury pattern [27,28]. An apex posterior fracture of the ulna occurs through the olecranon process. The coronoid process is usually also fractured. The radial head dislocates posteriorly from the proximal radioulnar joint and is often fractured [27–30]. The lateral collateral ligament complex is likely to be injured as the radial head dislocates posteriorly [31].

Although the ulnohumeral articulation is usually disrupted rather than dislocated by the initial injury force, instability or dislocation of the ulnohumeral articulation represents a common form of chronic elbow instability after this injury [28]. Ulnohumeral instability can result from a number of factors, including residual apex posterior angulation of the ulnar fracture contributing to diminished anterior column support by the coronoid process and radial head; malalignment of a coronoid fracture with similar consequences; fracture of the radial head with loss of lateral column support; and damage of the lateral collateral ligament complex leading to posterolateral rotatory instability (Figure 24-3).

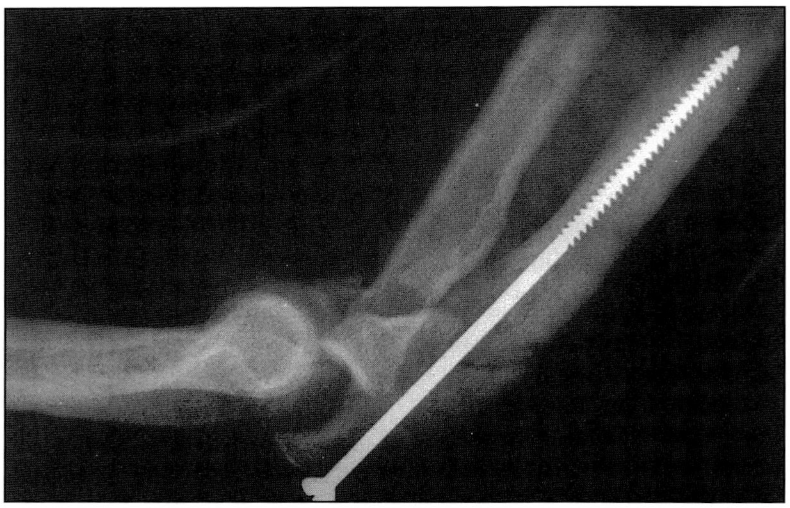

FIGURE 24-3. Although most posterior Monteggia type fracture-dislocations of the elbow present with disruption (but not true dislocation) of the ulnohumeral joint, true ulnohumeral instability can occur postoperatively and may be related to residual angulation of the ulna, fracture of the radial head and coronoid, and injury to the lateral collateral ligament complex.

Posterior Dislocation with Fracture of the Radial Head

Posterior dislocation of the ulnohumeral articulation with associated fracture of the radial head is more difficult to manage than a simple dislocation [1,32,33]. These injuries often require cast immobilization to maintain reduction; even rigid external immobilization is sometimes not sufficient to prevent redislocation [19,34]. Current recommendations for treatment of the acute injury include repair or replacement of the radial head and reattachment of the origin of the lateral collateral ligament complex to the lateral epicondyle [1]. Routine operative treatment is appropriate to allow mobilization of the elbow and limit the risk of posttraumatic arthrosis.

This injury pattern has been associated with the development of ulnohumeral arthrosis within 10 to 15 years of the injury [19,35]. This is likely to be related to slight and often asymptomatic chronic ulnohumeral instability. In one series, 12 of 19 patients who had radial head excision without replacement developed severe arthrosis at an average follow-up of 14 years [19]. In another, arthrosis was noted in 22 of 24 patients (92%) evaluated an average of 10 years after fracture-dislocation of the elbow treated without radial head repair or replacement [34]. Although only seven patients were rated as having moderate or severe arthrosis, a correlation was observed between a longer duration of follow-up and more severe radiographic changes [34].

Posterior Dislocation with Fractures of the Radial Head and Coronoid Process (Terrible Triad)

The most infamous source of chronic elbow instability is the previously mentioned terrible triad fracture-dislocation of the elbow consisting of posterior dislocation, fracture of the radial head, and fracture of the coronoid process [20]. In addition to the extensive capsuloligamentous disruption associated with most ulnohumeral dislocations, the osseous-articular contributions to the anterior and lateral columns are disrupted. It can be difficult to maintain a closed reduction of these injuries even with cast immobilization (Figure 24-4) [19]. Temporary Steinmann pin fixation of the ulnohumeral articulation or dynamic hinged fixation have been used to maintain reduction while the ligaments heal. Current treatment recommendations are evolving but include, at a minimum, repair or replacement of the radial head and repair of the lateral collateral ligament complex [1]. The fracture of the coronoid is an extremely important element of the loss of stability of this lesion, but it is not clear whether fixation of the coronoid is necessary to restore adequate stability. Some recent biomechanical work has suggested that even small fractures of the coronoid (less than 50% of the coronoid height) cause substantial loss of stability [36,37]; however, the operative exposure and fixation of small coronoid fractures is unfamiliar to most surgeons, even elbow experts. Exposure of the coronoid is easier to perform before reconstruction of the radial head and lateral collateral ligament complex. The surgeon must therefore make a preoperative judgment regarding the need for fixation or reconstruction of the coronoid process rather than testing the stability of the joint after the radial head and lateral ligament have been repaired.

OPERATIVE TACTICS

The goal in the treatment of fracture-dislocation of the elbow is to restore sufficient stability to the elbow to allow early active mobilization safely. This can usually be achieved by providing stable anatomic fixation of all osseous-articular elements of the injury, thereby reducing the injury to a capsuloligamentous disruption resembling a simple posterior dislocation [38]. When repair of the osseous-articular elements alone does not restore stability, the possibility that a soft tissue structure or osteocartilaginous fragment is trapped within the joint should be considered [20]. Next, repair or reconstruction of the collateral ligaments is considered. Hinged elbow distraction represents a last resort when all measures fail to restore sufficient stability to allow active mobilization of the elbow [39–41].

Fracture of the Radial Head

Hotchkiss [42] has modified Mason's [43] classification of radial head fractures to reflect management options: Type I includes small marginal fractures that do not contribute appreciably to stability and minimally (*ie,* less than 2-mm) displaced fractures that do not restrict forearm rotation; Type II includes larger, displaced (*ie,* 2-mm) two-part fractures, any fracture that restricts forearm rotation, and relatively simple comminuted fractures that are amenable to operative fixation; Type III fractures are limited to those that are so comminuted that operative fixation is not possible [20,43]. This scheme proves particularly useful in directing the management of fracture-dislocations of the elbow: Type I fractures rarely require operative intervention, whereas Type II fractures should be repaired and Type III fractures should be resected and replaced with a prosthesis to restore the stabilizing influence of an intact lateral column.

Various operative techniques are used for exposure of the radial head. A midline posterior skin incision is advised when repair of the medial collateral ligament, coronoid, or olecranon may be considered [44,45]. Exposure of nearly the entire elbow can be gained through separate intermuscular intervals by the elevation of large medial and lateral skin flaps while at the same time limiting the risk to cutaneous nerves [44]. Recent emphasis has been placed on the need to minimize the risk of operative disruption of the lateral collateral ligament complex. [13,17,18] If Kocher's [46] exposure through the interval between the extensor carpi ulnaris and the anconeus is used, the capsular incision must remain anterior to the anterior margin of the anconeus and parallel to the fascial limit of the extensor carpi ulnaris [18]. Hotchkiss [42] has described an alternative exposure in which the elbow joint is first entered by elevating the capsule off the anterior aspect of the lateral humerus in a safe area anterior to the origin of the lateral collateral ligament complex. This allows visualization of the articular surface of the radial head. More distal exposure is accomplished by incising the capsule longitudinally along a line that bisects the anteroposterior diameter of the radial head. The lateral collateral ligament complex and annular ligament can be elevated anteriorly, but not posteriorly to this line. More distal exposure of the neck requires entrance into the common extensor muscle compartment, mobilization of the muscle fibers anteriorly, and incision of the facial floor of the compartment [42]. This will expose the supinator muscle that is incised at its posterior margin and swept anteriorly with the forearm in full pronation to protect the posterior interosseous nerve. Long right-angled retractors rather than Bennett or Hohmann retractors should be used to avoid injury to the posterior interosseous nerve. If a long plate will be used, it is

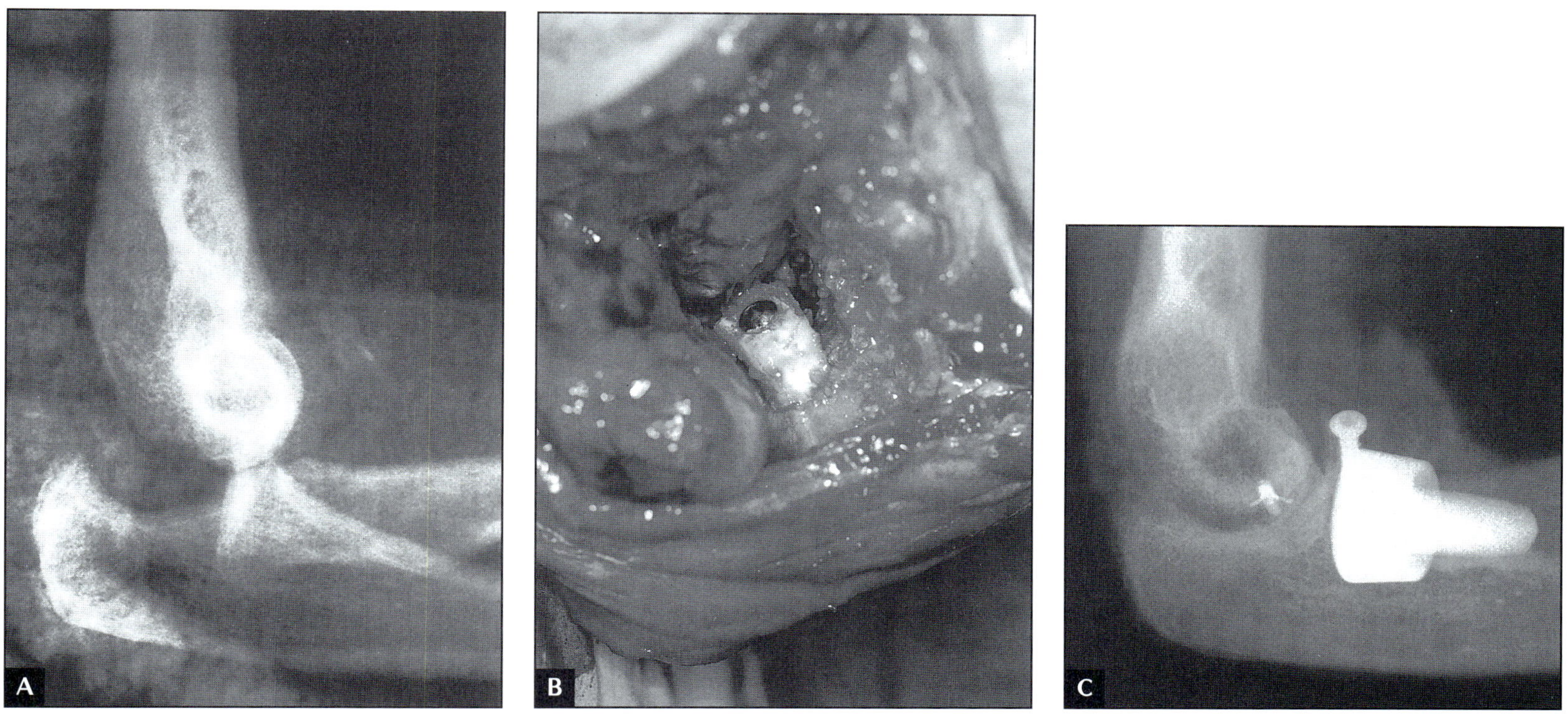

FIGURE 24-4. The injury depicted in Figure 24-2, *panel D* was reduced and splinted. **A**, Redislocation in a cast was not recognized for 4 weeks. By this time, the coronoid had been further eroded. **B**, Exposure of the coronoid was possible through a lateral exposure because the origin of the lateral collateral ligament was avulsed from the lateral epiconydle and the fractured radial head had been excised. Part of the excised radial head was secured with a screw to restore an anterior buttress. **C**, The radial head could not be repaired and was replaced with a titantium prosthesis. The origin of the lateral collateral ligament complex was reattached to the lateral epicondyle.

advisable to expose and protect the posterior interosseous nerve to ensure its protection [42].

Radial head exposure following fracture-dislocation of the elbow must take into account that the origin of the lateral collateral ligament complex is often avulsed from the lateral condyle of the distal humerus and the fractured radial head may not be useful as an anatomic landmark. Repair of the avulsed origin of the lateral collateral ligament with sutures anchored to bone—using either drill holes or suture anchors—should be performed at the time of closure. Optimal tension is restored by repair with the forearm in pronation [18].

Operative repair of radial head fractures has been facilitated by development of improved implants for the fixation of small fractures [47–52]. Minifragment screws can provide stable fixation of articular fragments when interfragmentary compression is applied [48].

Provided that the screw is inserted through the nonarticular peripheral surface of the radial head, the implant will not block rotation of the forearm. A "safe-zone" for the application of screws and plates to the radial head and neck without interference with forearm rotation has been described by Smith and Hotchkiss [53]. It is defined intraoperatively using three reference marks chosen as the bisecting point of the anteroposterior diameter of the radial head in full supination, neutral rotation, and full pronation. The anterior limit for fixation is a point two thirds of the distance from the neutral mark to the mark made in full supination and the posterior limit is a point halfway between marks made in neutral rotation and full pronation. In the presence of articular impaction or comminution of the radial neck, minifragment plates should be used to buttress the repair [47,48]. The defects created by repositioning of the fracture fragments should be filled with autogenous cancellous bone graft to provide further support and enhance healing.

When fixation of articular fragments requires insertion of the implant through an articular surface, options include self-compressing screws that can be sunk beneath the chondral surface (Herbert screws and variants) or small threaded Kirschner wires [47,50–52]. The development of bioabsorbable pins may also prove useful in this regard [54].

The goal of operative fixation is a stable radial head. Healing may be delayed and osteonecrosis can occur due to the often tenuous blood supply to this entirely intra-articular epiphysis, which is analogous to that of the femoral head. Fixation must therefore be sufficiently secure to maintain the lateral columnar support of the elbow until the ligaments heal, at which time a delayed resection of the radial head can more safely be performed.

Replacement of the radial head represents a viable option in the setting of traumatic instability of the elbow or forearm associated with Hotchkiss Type III fractures in which the fracture comminution precludes operative repair (Figure 24-4). The first radial-head prostheses were implanted over half a century ago [55–57] and were initially intended to prevent proximal migration of the radius, cubitus valgus, and heterotopic ossification after resection of the radial head. Although the need for replacement of the radial head after delayed resection has been challenged [8,35,58], several studies have demonstrated the advantages of prosthetic replacement for fracture-dislocations of the elbow or forearm [32,33,59]. For a time, the most widely available prosthesis was made of silicone rubber [60]. Although several cadaveric investigations have suggested that the silicone rubber prosthesis is not sufficiently rigid to restore lateral column support to the elbow [8,11,12,61], clinical experience suggests an advantage over simple resection in the treatment of fracture-dislocation of the elbow [59]. Prostheses made of silicone rubber, as with previous designs made of acrylic [57], are prone to breakage and may induce particulate synovitis [58,62].

The use of prostheses made of various types of metals has been evaluated [32,33,55,56], and their effectiveness in the treatment of fracture-dislocations of the elbow is well documented [32,33]. Harrington and Tountas [32] reported the results of treatment of 17 patients with complex traumatic elbow instability involving fracture of the radial head requiring excision. Eight patients had posterior dislocation of the elbow and four also had coronoid fractures, five had complete rupture of the medial collateral ligament, and four had fractures of the proximal ulna, one with an associated fracture of the coronoid. Radial head replacement was performed with a metallic prosthesis in 15 patients and a silicone rubber prosthesis in two. Using a strict rating scale that weighted residual pain heavily, good or excellent results were recorded in all but three patients at an average follow-up of 6.9 years [32]. Knight *et al.* [33] reviewed 31 patients with comminuted fractures of the radial head and 21 patients with associated dislocation or ulnar fracture, all treated with resection of the radial head and replacement with a prosthesis composed of Vitallium [33]. At an average of 4.9 years' follow-up, no residual instability or limited loss of motion occurred, aching pain with activity was present in only six patients (19%), and pain at rest was found in only one patient [33].

Replacement of the radial head with an osteoarticular allograft has been suggested [63,64]. This might prove most useful when comminution extends down into the radial neck and this portion must also be resected. Currently available prosthetics may not provide adequate length in this situation.

Following repair or replacement of the radial head, the stability of the elbow is checked through a full range of motion. If the elbow redislocates at greater than 30° flexion, stability should be reevaluated following repair of the lateral collateral ligament complex. In the face of persistent instability, consideration should be given to exposure and repair of the medial collateral ligament complex. In the unusual event that excessive instability persists after repair or replacement of the radial head and repair of both ligaments, a hinged distractor can be applied to allow active mobilization while ensuring that the ligaments heal with physiologic tension [40].

Fracture of the Coronoid

Little discussion of these injuries is found in the literature, particularly with regard to patterns of injury, management decisions, operative tactics, and outcome [19,26,65,66].

It is difficult to decide whether to internally fix a coronoid fracture based on the size of the fragment alone. Morrey [63] contends that the ulnohumeral joint will remain functional with loss of up to 50% of the height of the coronoid. Similar recommendations are made in the German-language literature, which states that a fragment representing greater than one sixth of the circumference of the trochlear notch should be fixed [65,66]. We recommend that each patient be evaluated individually, because we have encountered cases in which the elbow remained unstable until a small coronoid fracture was realigned and secured.

Indirect reduction and interfragmentary screw fixation of the coronoid, although useful for larger fractures, is rarely possible for smaller fractures. Through a posterior skin incision, the coronoid can be exposed from the medial side of the elbow after raising a medial skin flap and mobilizing and transposing the ulnar nerve anteriorly into the subcutaneous tissues. Medial exposure is obtained by mobilizing the forearm flexor musculature either by osteotomizing the medial epicondyle [48] or by elevating the flexor carpi ulnaris from its ulnar origin, thus leaving the humeral origin of the flexor-pronator musculature and the medial collateral ligament intact [45]. Alternatively, in the presence of a fracture of the radial head, it is usually possible to gain exposure of the coronoid from the lateral side prior to fixing or replacing the radial head (Figure 24-4). This is facilitated by hinging the unstable elbow open. Fixation of the coronoid is achieved either with a small screw or a wire or stout, braided nonabsorbable suture passed through drill holes in the fragment. Again, a hinged distractor is applied only in the uncommon circumstance that repair of the radial head and of the coronoid and ligamentous structures fails to restore stability sufficient to allow active mobilization of the elbow.

Fracture of the Olecranon

Large fractures of the coronoid are usually associated with fracture of the olecranon. On occasion, it may be possible to reduce and secure the coronoid fracture through direct visualization through the olecranon fracture [67]. The interval created by the fracture allows for direct visualization and manipulative reduction while fixation is achieved with interfragmentary screws entering through the dorsal surface of the ulna. Alternatively, realignment of the coronoid is often achieved indirectly when distraction is applied. A distractor is useful for repair of complex proximal ulna fractures with comminution in the depths of the trochlear notch between the olecranon and coronoid processes [25,68]. Temporary fixation of the olecranon fragment in anatomic position with respect to the distal humerus can be achieved using a large, smooth Kirschner wire passed through the olecranon fragment and into the distal humerus. Distraction applied between this wire and a second pin (2.5- or 4.0-mm Schantz screw) placed in the ulnar diaphysis restores the length of the ulna and the dimensions of the trochlear notch and maintains the reduction while fixation is applied. The distal humerus is used as a template to restore the contour of the notch. Definitive fixation is achieved using a 3.5-mm plate contoured around the proximal ulna and extending to the tip of the olecranon process (Figure 24-5) [25,27]. This provides for the placement of numerous screws in the often small and osteopenic proximal (olecranon) fragment, with large screws directed down the ulnar shaft inserted through the most proximal screw holes, and directed at a 90° angle to more distal screws, thereby creating an interlocking construct. Dorsal placement of the plate and reconstitution of the anterior ulnar cortex by rigid fixation of separate anterior fracture fragments will help to resist displacement as a result of active muscle forces about the elbow.

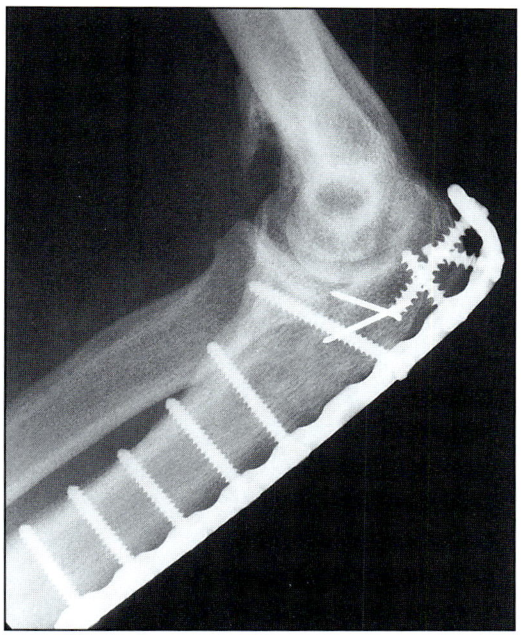

Figure 24-5. Complex fractures of the olecranon and proximal ulna are best fixed with a plate applied to the dorsal surface of the ulna. The plate is contoured so that a greater number of screws can be placed in the proximal fragment and the most proximal screws are oriented and 90° to more distal screws. (*From* Ring and Jupiter [1]; with permission.)

References and Recommended Reading

Recently published papers of particular interest have been highlighted as:
- • Of interest
- •• Of outstanding interest

1. Ring D, Jupiter JB: Fracture-dislocation of the elbow. *J Bone Joint Surg* 1998, 80A:566–580.
2. Cage DJN, Abrams RA, Callahan JJ, *et al.*: Soft tissue attachments of the ulnar coronoid process. *Clin Orthop* 1995, 320:154–158.
3. Melhoff TL, Noble PC, Bennet JB, *et al.*: Simple dislocation of the elbow in the adult: results after closed treatment. *J Bone Joint Surg* 1988, 70A:244–249.
4. Protzman RR: Dislocation of the elbow joint. *J Bone Joint Surg* 1978, 60:539–541.
5. Kuroda S, Sakamaki K: Ulnar collateral ligament tears of the elbow joint. *Clin Orthop* 1986, 208:266–271.
6. Jobe FW, Stark H, Lombardo SJ: Reconstruction of the ulnar collateral ligament in athletes. *J Bone Joint Surg* 1986, 68:1158–1163.
7. Conway JE, Jobe FW, Glousman RE, *et al.*: Medial instability of the elbow in throwing athletes. *J Bone Joint Surg* 1992, 74:67–83.
8. Morrey BF, Chao EY, Hui FC: Biomechanical study of the elbow following excision of the radial head. *J Bone Joint Surg* 1979, 61:63–68.
9. Morrey BF, Tanaka S, An KN: Valgus stability of the elbow: a definition of primary and secondary constraints. *Clin Orthop* 1991, 265:187–195.
10. Hotchkiss RN, Weiland AJ: Valgus stability of the elbow. *J Orthop Res* 1987, 15:327–333.
11. Gupta GG, Lucas G, Hahn DL: Biomechanical and computer analysis of radial head prostheses. *J Shoulder Elbow Surg* 1997, 6:37–48.
12. Carn RM, Medige J, Curtain D, *et al.*: Silicone rubber replacement of the severely fractured radial head. *Clin Orthop* 1986, 209:259–269.
13. O'Driscoll SW, Bell DF, Morrey BF: Posterolateral rotatory instability of the elbow. *J Bone Joint Surg* 1991, 73:440–446.
14. Sojberg JO, Ovesen J, Gundorf CE: The stability of the elbow following excision of the radial head and transection of the annular ligament. *Arch Orthop Trauma Surg* 1987, 106:248–250.
15. Osbourne G, Cotterill P: Recurrent dislocations of the elbow. *J Bone Joint Surg* 1966, 48:340–346.
16. O'Driscoll SW, Morrey BF, Korinek S, An KN: Elbow subluxation and dislocation: a spectrum of instability. *Clin Orthop* 1992, 280:186–197.
17. Nestor BJ, O'Driscoll SW, Morrey BF: Ligamentous reconstruction for posterolateral rotatory instability of the elbow. *J Bone Joint Surg* 1992, 74:1235–1241.
18. Cohen MS, Hastings H: Rotatory instability of the elbow: the anatomy and role of the lateral stabilizers. *J Bone Joint Surg* 1997, 79:225–233.
19. Josefsson PO, Gentz CF, Johnell O, *et al.*: Dislocations of the elbow and intraarticular fractures. *Clin Orthop* 1989, 246:126–130.
20. Hotchkiss RN: Fractures and dislocations of the elbow. In *Rockwood and Green's Fractures in Adults* vol 1, edn 4. Edited by Rockwood CA, Green DP, Bucholz RW, *et al.* Philadelphia: Lippincott-Raven, 1996:924–1024.
21. Hanks GA, Kottmeier SA: Isolated fracture of the coronoid process of the ulna: a case report and review of the literature. *J Orthop Trauma* 1990, 4:193–196.
22. Gartsman GM, Scales JC, Otis JC: Operative treatment of olecranon fractures. *J Bone Joint Surg* 1981, 63: 718–721.
23. Morrey BF: Anatomy of the elbow joint. In *The Elbow and Its Disorders* edn 2. Edited by Morrey BF. Philadelphia: WB Saunders; 1995:16–52.
24. Biga N, Thomine JM: La luxation trans-olécranienne du coude. *Rev Chir Orthop* 1974, 60:557–567.

25. Ring D, Jupiter JB, Sanders RW, *et al.*: Trans-olecranon fracture-dislocation of the elbow. *J Orthop Trauma* 1997, 11:545–550.
26. Regan W, Morrey BF: Fractures of the coronoid process of the ulna. *J Bone Joint Surg* 1990, 71:1348–1354.
27. Jupiter JB, Leibovic SJ, Ribbans W, *et al.*: The posterior Monteggia lesion. *J Orthop Trauma* 1991, 5:395–402.
28. Ring D, Jupiter JB, Simpson NS: Monteggia fractures in adults. *J Bone Joint Surg* 1998, 80:1733–1744.
29. Penrose JH: The Monteggia fracture with posterior dislocation of the radial head. *J Bone Joint Surg* 1951, 33:65–73.
30. Pavel A, Pittman JM, Lance EM, *et al.*: The posterior Monteggia fracture: a clinical study. *J Trauma* 1965, 5:185–199.
31. Johansson O: Capsular and ligament injuries of the elbow joint. *Acta Chir Scand Suppl* 1962, 287:1–159.
32. Harrington IJ, Tountas AA: Replacement of the radial head in the treatment of unstable elbow fractures. *Injury* 1980, 12:405–412.
33. Knight DJ, Rymaszewski LA, Amis AA, *et al.*: Primary replacement of the fractured radial head with a metal prosthesis. *J Bone Joint Surg* 1993, 75:572–576.
34. Broberg MA, Morrey BF: Results of treatment of fracture-dislocations of the elbow. *Clin Orthop* 1987, 216:109–119.
35. Broberg MA, Morrey BF: Results of delayed excision of the radial head after fracture. *J Bone Joint Surg* 1986, 68:669–674.
36. Beredjiklian PK, Miskovsky C, Hotchkiss RN: Effects of bony and ligamentous reconstructions in complex elbow dislocations. 53rd annual meeting of American Society for Surgery of the Hand. Minneapolis, MN, 1998.
37. O'Driscoll SW, Cheng S, Morrey B, *et al.*: Biomechanics of coronoid in complex elbow fracture–dislocations. 14th Open Meeting of the American Shoulder and Elbow Surgeons. New Orleans, LA, 1998.
38. O'Driscoll SW: Elbow instability. *Hand Clin North Am* 1994, 10:405–415.
39. Cobb TK, Morrey BF: Use of distraction arthroplasty in unstable fracture dislocations of the elbow. *Clin Orthop* 1995, 312:201–210.
40. McKee MD, Bowden SH, King GJ, *et al.*: Management of recurrent, complex instability of the elbow with a hinged external fixator. *J Bone Joint Surg* 1998, 80:1031–1036.
41. Simpson NS, Jupiter JB: Post-traumatic reconstruction of the elbow: the role of hinged distraction. *Orthop Trans* 1995, 19:145.
42. Hotchkiss RN: Displaced fractures of the radial head: internal fixation or excision. *J Amer Acad Orthop Surg* 1997, 5:1–10.
43. Mason ML: Some observations on fractures of the head of the radius with a review of one hundred cases. *Br J Surg* 1959, 42:123–132.
44. Dowdy PA, Bain GI, King GJW, *et al.*: The midline posterior elbow incision. *J Bone Joint Surg* 1995, 77B:696–699.
45. Patterson SD, King GJ, Bain GI: A posterior global approach to the elbow [abstract]. *J Bone Joint Surg* 1995, 77(suppl):316.
46. Kocher T: *Textbook of Operative Surgery* edn 3. London: Adam and Charles Black; 1911.
47. Geel CW, Palmer AK, Rüedi T, *et al.*: Internal fixation of proximal radial head fractures. *J Orthop Trauma* 1990, 4:270–274.
48. Heim U, Pfeiffer KM: *Internal Fixation of Small Fractures* edn 3. Berlin: Springer-Verlag; 1988.
49. Müller ME, Allgower M, Schneider R, *et al.*: *Manual of Internal Fixation: Techniques Recommended by the AO-ASIF Group*. Berlin: Springer-Verlag; 1991.
50. Odenheimer K, Harvey JP: Internal fixation of fracture of the radial head: two case reports. *J Bone Joint Surg* 1979, 61:785–787.
51. Sanders RA, Sackett JR: Operative treatment of bicondylar intraarticular fractures of the distal humerus. *J Orthop Trauma* 1990, 4:254–259.
52. Shmueli G, Herold HZ: Compression screwing of displaced fractures of the head of the radius. *J Bone Joint Surg* 1981, 63:535–538.
53. Smith GR, Hotchkiss RN: Radial head and neck fractures: anatomic guidelines for proper placement of internal fixation. *J Shoulder Elbow Surg* 1996, 5:113–117.
54. Hirvensalo E, Böstman O, Rokkanen P: Absorbable polyglycolide pins in fixation of displaced fractures of the radial head. *Arch Orthop Trauma Surg* 1990, 109:258–261.
55. Speed K: Ferrule caps for the head of the radius. *Surg Gyn Obst* 1941, 73:845–850.
56. Carr CR, Howard JW: Metallic prosthesis for replacement of the radial head following fractures. *West J Surg* 1951, 59:539–546.
57. Cherry JC: Use of acrylic prosthesis in the treatment of fracture of the head of the radius. *J Bone Joint Surg* 1953, 35:70–71.
58. Morrey BF, Askew L, Chao EY: Silastic prosthetic replacement for radial head. *J Bone Joint Surg* 1981, 63:454–458.
59. MacKay I, Fitzgerald B, Miller JH: Silastic replacement of the head of the radius in trauma. *J Bone Joint Surg* 1979, 61:494–497.
60. Swanson AB, Jaeger SH, La Rochelle D: Comminuted fractures of the radial head. *J Bone Joint Surg* 1981, 63:1039–1049.
61. Pribyl CR, Kester MA, Cook SD, *et al.*: The effect of radial head and prosthetic replacement on resisting valgus stress at the elbow. *Orthopedics* 1986, 9:723–726.
62. Mayhall WST, Tiley FT, Paluska DJ: Fracture of silastic radial-head prosthesis: case report. *J Bone Joint Surg* 1981, 63:459–460.
63. Morrey BF: Complex instability of the elbow. *J Bone Joint Surg* 1997, 79:460–469.
64. Szabo RM, Hotchkiss RN, Slater RR: The use of frozen-allograft radial head replacement for treatment of established symptomatic proximal translation of the radius: preliminary experience in five cases. *J Hand Surg* 1997, 22A:269–278.
65. Copf F, Holz U, Schauwecker HH: Biomechanische probleme bei ellenbogenluxationen mit frakturen am processus coronoideus und radiusköpfchen. *Langenbecks Arch Chir* 1980, 350:249–254.
66. König S, Kilga M, Kwasny O: Ergebnisse nach Plattenosteosynthese bei der Olekranontümmerfraktur. *Unfallchirurg* 1990, 93:216–220.
67. O'Driscoll SW: Technique for unstable olecranon fracture–subluxations. *Op Tech Orthop* 1994, 4:49–53.
68. Mast J, Jakob RP, Ganz R: *Planning and Reduction Techniques in Fracture Surgery*. Heidelberg: Springer-Verlag; 1979.

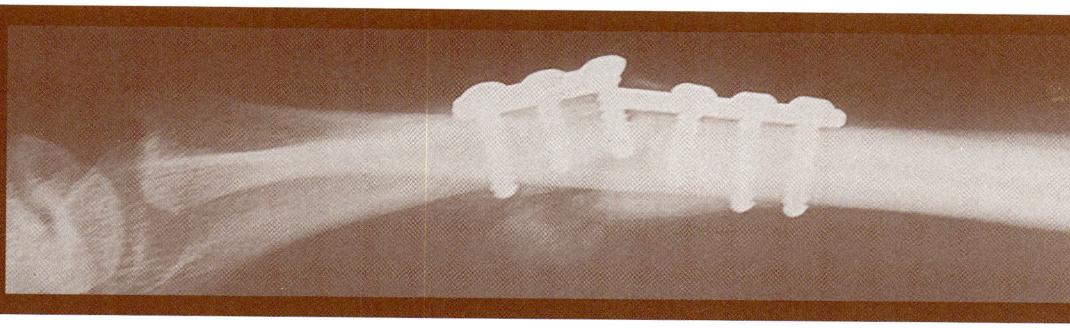

25

Fractures of the Radius and Ulna

Lawrence E. Weiss
A. Lee Osterman

The forearm serves an important role in spatial positioning of the hand. It effectively links the elbow and wrist, which allows for mobility and integrated function. Pronation and supination are tightly controlled through the proximal and distal radioulnar joints. The shafts of the radius and ulna connect these joints, so fractures of these bones adversely affect forearm rotation unless meticulous technique is used in their management.

EVALUATION

The radius and ulna are linked through the interosseous membrane and the proximal and distal radioulnar joints. These structures result in a well-constrained system such that mechanism of injury directly determines fracture patterns. Direct-blow injuries or gunshot wounds may result in isolated or combined fractures of the radius or ulna (*ie,* "night-stick" fractures or "both-bones" fractures). Alternatively, isolated fractures of the radius or ulna can occur in combination with dislocation of the proximal or distal radioulnar joints through energy transmission through the interosseous membrane (*eg,* Monteggia fractures, Galeazzi fractures, or Essex-Lopresti fractures).

Not infrequently, when a fracture of the forearm occurs, the possibility exists of an associated injury to the wrist alone or with elbow involvement. Therefore, the clinician must effectively examine these joints and obtain quality radiographs to rule out these injuries. At least two views of the elbow, forearm, and wrist are therefore necessary in all suspected fractures of the forearm. It can be difficult to evaluate rotational alignment of the forearm, especially the radius. A useful principle is that, on the plain radiograph, the bicipital tuberosity should normally point opposite the thumb. In addition, variations exist with regard to normal radial bow as well as the ulnar variance at the wrist. Radiographs of the opposite forearm can be particularly useful for these measurements. They can also be valuable in the preoperative planning of the high-energy, comminuted fracture with associated loss of radial or ulnar length.

As exists with all fractures, the presence of an open forearm fracture must not be missed. It can even be seen with the low-energy injury. This may be obvious with a gunshot wound or exposed bone. However, it can be difficult to differentiate between a superficial laceration secondary to associated trauma and an open wound that directly communicates with the fracture site. If doubt exists, these injuries should be treated as open fractures.

Immediate débridement, antibiotic therapy, and tetanus prophylaxis are part of the initial management of all open forearm fractures. Specific concerns related to the Gustilo and Anderson soft tissue injury type are then addressed as appropriate [1]. The skin may be intact in a crush injury, but this can represent a significant soft-tissue injury.

A detailed neurologic examination must be performed in all fractures of the radius and ulna. If radiographs demonstrate what appears to be an isolated ulnar shaft fracture, but a posterior interosseous nerve palsy is present, this may suggest the presence of an occult radial head dislocation, which is a higher energy and more serious injury than an isolated ulnar shaft fracture. Gunshot injuries can cause a concussive effect on neural structures and are usually managed with observation and electromyographic follow-up [2]. Because most fractures of the forearm are treated with open reduction and internal fixation (ORIF), nerve lacerations are addressed at the time of operative intervention with decompression and nerve repair or grafting as indicated.

In addition to the neurologic evaluation, a detailed vascular examination is important. Doppler or arteriogram examination is obtained when any question about vascular injury is present. Fractures with vascular injury are more common with high velocity gunshot wounds. The surgeon should be prepared for possible repair and should obtain appropriate vascular surgery consultation if necessary.

Although uncommon, compartment syndrome of the forearm should be considered at the time of the initial examination. Significant crush injury of the forearm or blast injuries should raise concern about the potential of a compartment syndrome [3••]. Furthermore, a compartment syndrome may frequently occur in the interval between the time the emergency department physician initially evaluates the patient and the time the patient is seen by the specialist.

Diagnosis of compartment syndrome is made through a detailed clinical examination. Frequently, patients may complain of pain unresponsive to what ought to be adequate doses of narcotics. The volar compartment is most frequently involved and will be tense and swollen. Generally, compartment syndromes occur more commonly with the proximal fractures because more muscle is present in this region as compared with that seen distally, where the tendinous portion of the muscle lies. As the muscle is injured, bleeding into the compartment occurs. This leads to edema and the presence of high pressure in a contained space. The most reliable physical finding is pain with passive digital extension (the flexor digitorum profundus is closest to the interosseous membrane). Altered two-point discrimination can be seen as well. Measurement of compartment pressures with a Stryker monitor is used most often at our institution when the diagnosis is equivocal (*ie,* the unconscious or uncooperative patient). We perform early fasciotomies if questionable physical findings and borderline compartment pressure readings are found. Our volar incision always includes the carpal tunnel.

SURGICAL ANATOMY AND OPERATIVE APPROACHES

The radius and ulna are parallel and joined by the proximal or distal radioulnar joints and the interosseous membrane. The interosseous membrane acts to prevent separation of the radius from the ulna and allows force transfer with axial loading. More specifically, the central bands of the interosseous membrane and the triangular fibrocartilage complex (TFCC) are important to the axial stability of the forearm [4]. Transfer of load from the wrist through the forearm to the elbow also depends on varus-valgus alignment of the elbow [5]. Usually 150° of pronosupination exists through an axis, extending from the center of the radial head through the center of the ulnar head (Figure 25-1). The osteology of the radius and ulna changes from a relatively circular appearance in cross-section proximally to a cam-shaped appearance distally. Figure 25-2 demonstrates this and other pertinent cross-sectional anatomy. This becomes important in attempts to perform plate osteosynthesis with proper plate contour when a longer plate is necessary. Restoration of radial bow must also be factored into this equation.

The operative approach to the ulna is along its subcutaneous border on the posterior side. This is in the internervous plane between the extensor carpi ulnaris (ECU) or the anconeus (proximal) and the flexor carpi ulnaris (FCU) distally (Figure 25-3). We prefer to place the incision either volar or dorsal to the direct subcutaneous border, which keeps the incision off the weight-bearing area. We usually place the incision more dorsally except when a dorsal approach to the radius is necessary; the skin bridge is smaller compared with the volar approach to the radius.

The radius is often approached through the anterior or Henry approach (Figure 25-4). The dissection is through the internervous plane between the brachioradialis (radial nerve) and the flexor-pronator group (median nerve). Distally, the radius is approached through the tendon sheath of the flexor carpi radialis and the radial artery is retracted radially. The pronator teres must be elevated off the radius as the dissection proceeds proximally. To gain additional exposure proximally, the proximal fragment must be manipulated into full supination to move the proximal interosseous nerve posteriorly and laterally. This allows further dissection through the supinator without injuring the nerve, although the clinician must be cognizant of a potential aberrant course through this muscle. In the more proximal dissection, it is important to ligate the recurrent branch of the radial artery and its leash of vessels (leash of Henry) to allow improved medial retraction of the radial artery. When performing the Henry approach, the superficial branch of the radial nerve can be injured by excessive retraction of the brachioradialis because this nerve lies on the undersurface of this muscle. Generally speaking, we use this exposure most often for approaching the radius.

In addition, the radius can be approached through the posterior or Thompson approach (Figure 25-5). This involves the interval between the radial innervated mobile wad (brachioradialis, extensor carpi radialis longus, extensor carpi radialis brevis) and the proximal interosseous nerve-innervated ulnar wrist extensors and finger extensors. Proximally, the radius is exposed by dissecting out the proximal interosseous nerve as it exits the supinator and elevating this muscle off the posterior shaft. The proximal interosseous nerve exits at this level 4- to 7-cm distal to the radiocapitellar joint. Distally, the muscles of the first dorsal extensor compartment (abductor pollicis longus and extensor pollicis brevis) must be elevated and retracted proximally or distally to approach the radius. Because of the higher potential to harm the proximal interosseous nerve proximally, most surgeons have not used this approach as frequently as the volar Henry approach.

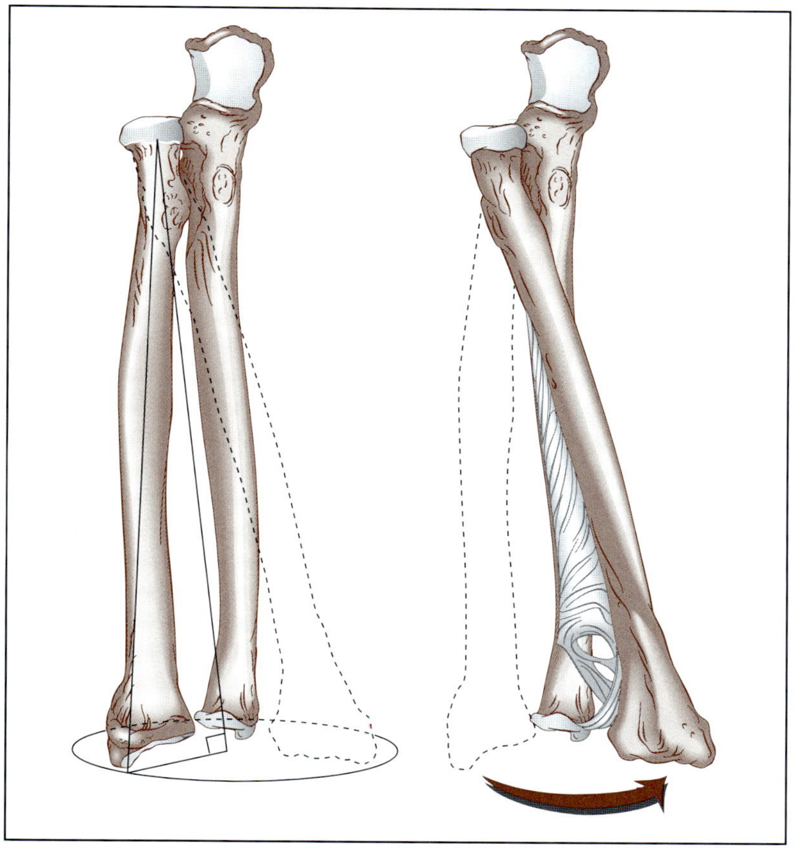

FIGURE 25-1. The axis of rotation of the forearm extends from the center of the radial head through the center of the ulnar head. (*Adapted from* Putnam and Fisher [3••].)

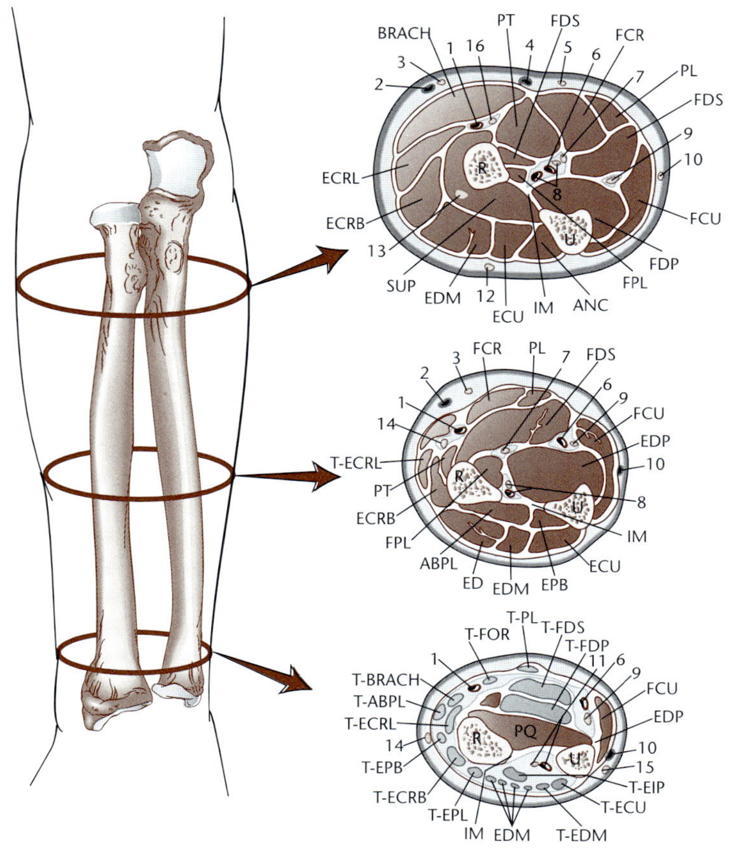

Key

1	Radial artery	IM	Interosseous membrane
2	Cephalic vein	T	Tendon
3	Lateral antebrachial cutaneous nerve	ANC	Anconeus
		ABPL	Abductor pollicis longus
4	Median antebrachial vein	BRACH	Brachialis
5	Anterior branch of medial antebrachial cutaneous nerve	ED	Extensor digitorum
		EDM	Extensor digiti minimi
		ECRB	Extensor carpi radialis brevis
6	Ulnar artery		
7	Median nerve	ECRL	Extensor carpi radialis longus
8	Anterior interosseous artery and nerve	ECU	Extensor carpi ulnaris
9	Ulnar nerve	EIP	Extensor indicis proprius
10	Basilic vein		
11	Posterior interosseous nerve and artery	EPB	Extensor pollicis brevis
		EPL	Extensor pollicis longus
12	Posterior antebrachial cutaneous nerve	FCR	Flexor carpi radialis
		FDS	Flexor digitorum superficialis
13	Radial nerve (deep branch)		
14	Radial sensory nerve	FCU	Flexor capri ulnaris
15	Ulnar nerve (dorsal branch)	FPL	Flexor pollicis longus
		PL	Palmaris longus
16	Radial nerve (superficial)	PQ	Pronator quadratus
R	Radius	PT	Pronator teres
U	Ulna	SUP	Supinator

FIGURE 25-2. Cross-sectional anatomy of the forearm. Note how the shape of the radius and ulna changes from a relatively circular appearance to a cam-shaped appearance distally. (*Adapted from* Putnam and Fisher [3••].)

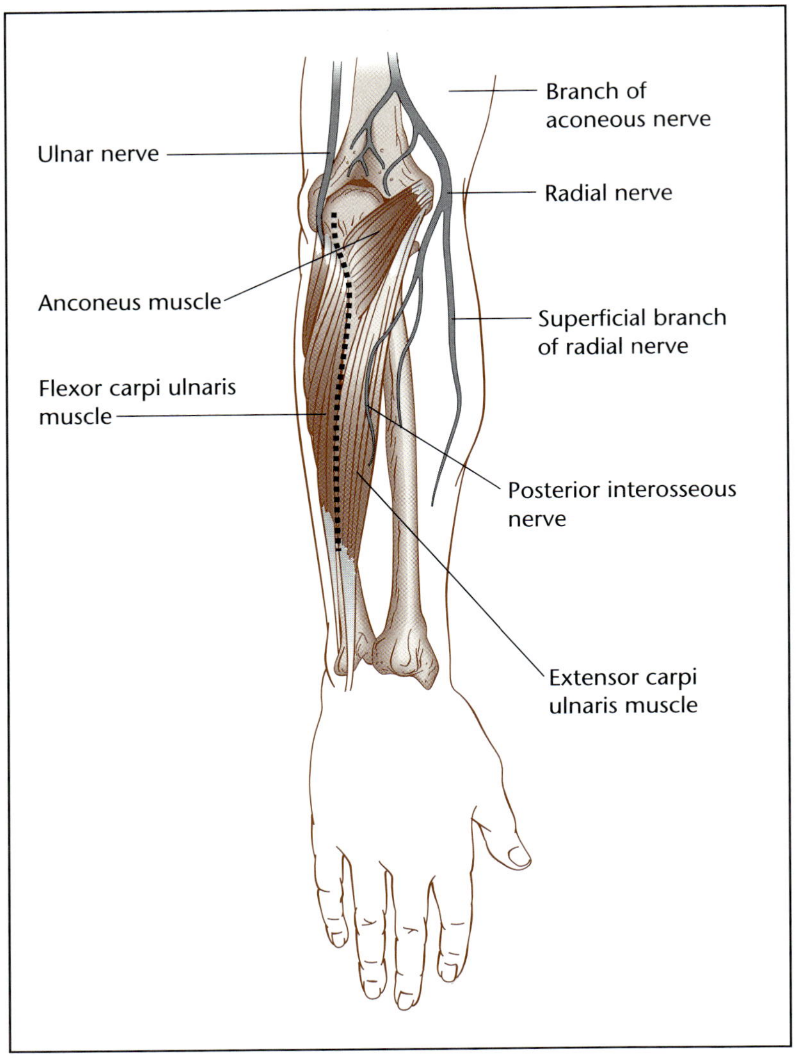

FIGURE 25-3. The operative approach to the ulna is along its subcutaneous border between the extensor carpi ulnaris, or anconeus proximally, and the flexor carpi ulnaris. (*Adapted from* Putnam and Fisher [3••].)

ISOLATED FRACTURES OF THE ULNA (NIGHT-STICK FRACTURES)

Isolated fractures of the ulnar shaft are common injuries frequently associated with a direct blow to the forearm. Frequently, they are nondisplaced or only minimally displaced. Fractures that are angulated less than 10° in any plane or displaced less than 50% of the diameter of the diaphysis are treated either a fracture brace or short arm cast with interosseous membrane molding (Figure 25-6). Because this bone is subcutaneous, it is paramount to rule out an open injury. For all open and clean injuries and fractures with significant angulation or displacement, our preferred technique is to perform an ORIF with 3.5-mm low-contact dynamic compression plate (LC-DCP) (Synthes, Paoli, PA). We attempt to obtain six to eight cortices on either side of the fracture site. If comminution is more than 50% of the shaft diameter, we recommend autogenous iliac crest bone grafting.

FRACTURES OF THE ULNA WITH DISLOCATION OF THE RADIAL HEAD (MONTEGGIA FRACTURES)

Fractures of the proximal third of the ulna with dislocation of the radial head were first described in 1814 by Monteggia. These fracture-dislocations have been classified as shown in Table 25-1 (Figure 25-7) [6•].

Injuries of Types I and IV are thought to occur as the result of a fall on a outstretched hand in forced pronation. Type II fracture is believed to be a variant of the posterior elbow dislocation where the ulnar shaft fails before the medial collateral ligament of the elbow. Type III fracture is speculated to occur secondary to a fall on an outstretched hand with an adduction force and the arm pronated; this causes varus angulation to the ulna and anterolateral dislocation of the radial head.

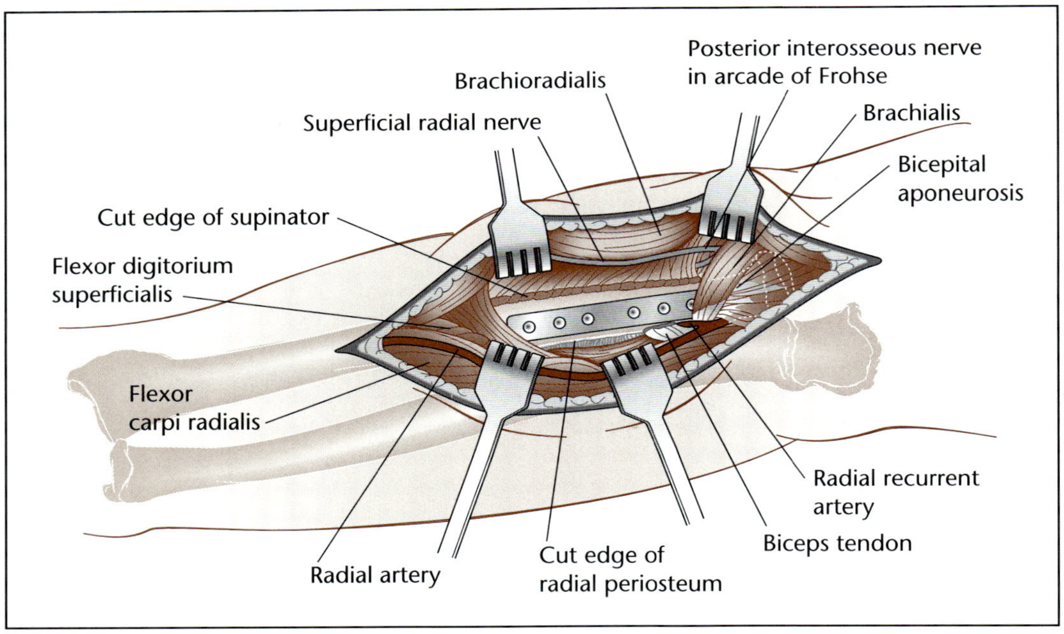

FIGURE 25-4. The anterior or Henry approach to the radius is between the radial-nerve innervated brachioradialis and the median nerve-innervated flexor-pronator group.(*Adapted from* Putnam and Fisher [3••].)

Anatomy of the proximal radioulnar joint is important to understand for successful management of the Type IV lesion. Normally, the anterior capsule and annular ligament are taut in supination, and the posterior capsule and annular ligament are taut in pronation (Figure 25-8). There is a 100° "safe-zone" centered through the coronal equator of the radial head, whereupon screws can be placed to achieve fixation of the proximal radius. For these lesions, we will restore length to the forearm and plate the ulna first. Usually, the radial head can be successfully reduced and radius can be fixed as well. We approach the radius through a second incision off the dorsum of the radius. Fixation is achieved using the Modular Hand Set (Synthes). We prefer to use 2.0- or 2.4-mm titanium T-plate (Figure 25-9).

Monteggia's fracture is associated with nerve injury more often than any other forearm fracture (up to 26%) [3••]. Most frequently, the radial nerve or proximal interosseous nerve is compromised through traction or entrapment. Anterior interosseus and ulnar nerve injuries have also been reported.

The difficulty with this fracture-dislocation is not usually in management, but rather in the initial clinical failure to diagnose the radial head dislocation. Additional concerns for this injury exist if the radial head is incompletely reduced or redislocates in the early postoperative period. A useful principle in evaluating these injuries radiographically is that a line drawn through the axis of the radial shaft should intersect the capitellum on all radiographs.

In the adult, we manage Monteggia's fractures with initial reduction of the radial head, followed by ORIF of the ulna. If the ulna is fixed before reduction of the radial head, the clinician may encounter a situation in which the radial head is irreducible. We prefer to use a 3.5-mm LC-DCP plate to fix the ulna. If the fracture is proximal and significant olecranon purchase will be necessary, we will use a 3.5-mm pelvic reconstruction plate. This can be bent along the dorsal, medial, or lateral surfaces. Augmentation with a tension band using 22-gauge steel wire may be necessary with proximal comminution and inadequate screw fixation.

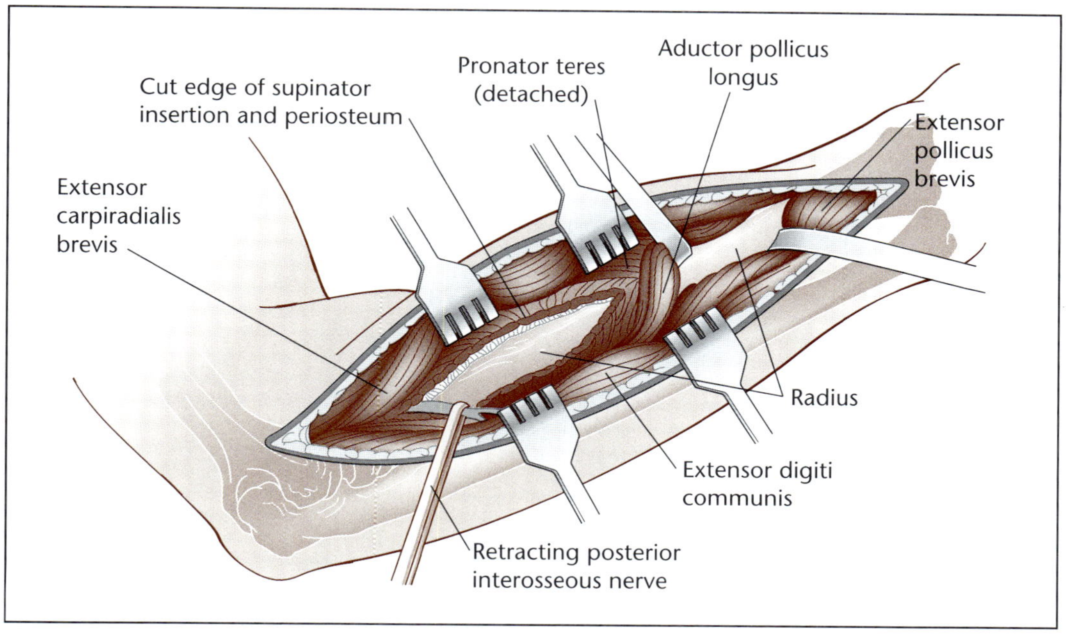

Figure 25-5. The posterior or Thompson approach to the radius is between the radial nerve-innervated mobile wad and the posterior interosseous nerve–innervated ulnar wrist and digital extensors.(*Adapted from* Putnam and Fisher [3••].)

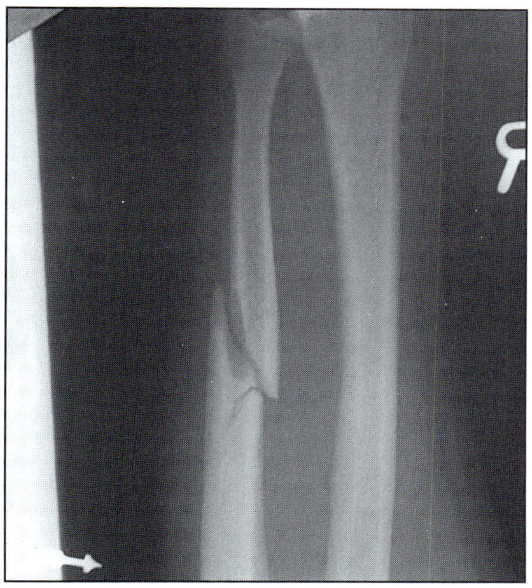

Figure 25-6. Nondisplaced night-stick fracture.

CLASSIFICATION OF MONTEGGIA FRACTURE-DISLOCATIONS

Type I: Fracture of the ulnar diaphysis with anterior angulation and an associated anterior radial head dislocation

Type II: Fracture of the ulnar diaphysis with posterior angulation and an associated posterior radial head dislocation

Type III: Fracture of the ulnar metaphysis with lateral/anterolateral radial head dislocation

Type IV: Similar to Type I with additional fracture of the proximal third of the radius

After restoration of length and plate fixation of the ulna, the radial head reduction is checked through a full range of elbow motion. Stable reductions can be managed with institution of a short arc motion program in a hinged elbow brace following resolution of swelling. If the radial head reduction is unstable, a malreduction of the ulna must be ruled out; revision of the ulnar fixation may be necessary if this condition is met. If the ulnar reduction is anatomic but the radial head redislocates, open reduction and annular ligament repair are necessary (Figure 25-10). We do not believe that radiocapitellar pinning should be performed.

If a preoperative radial or proximal interosseous nerve deficit exists, then we recommend observation for up to 3 months, because this usually is a neuropraxic lesion. If the deficit occurs after attempted radial head reduction, then open exploration should be performed. The possibility of nerve entrapment must be considered in this circumstance.

FRACTURES OF BOTH THE RADIUS AND ULNA (BOTH-BONES FRACTURES)

Both-bones fractures of the forearm most often result from a direct blow frequently related to motor vehicle accident trauma or to gunshot wounds. Occasionally, concomitant fractures of the humerus cause a floating elbow, and this situation must be ruled out with physical examination and radiographs.

Indications for nonoperative treatment are limited because many fractures are displaced. If the radius and ulna fractures are closed nondisplaced injuries, then long-arm casting is indicated with interosseous membrane molding. The clinician must be careful of the Type IV Monteggia injury because radial head dislocation can be overlooked even with nondisplaced fractures. As stated previ-

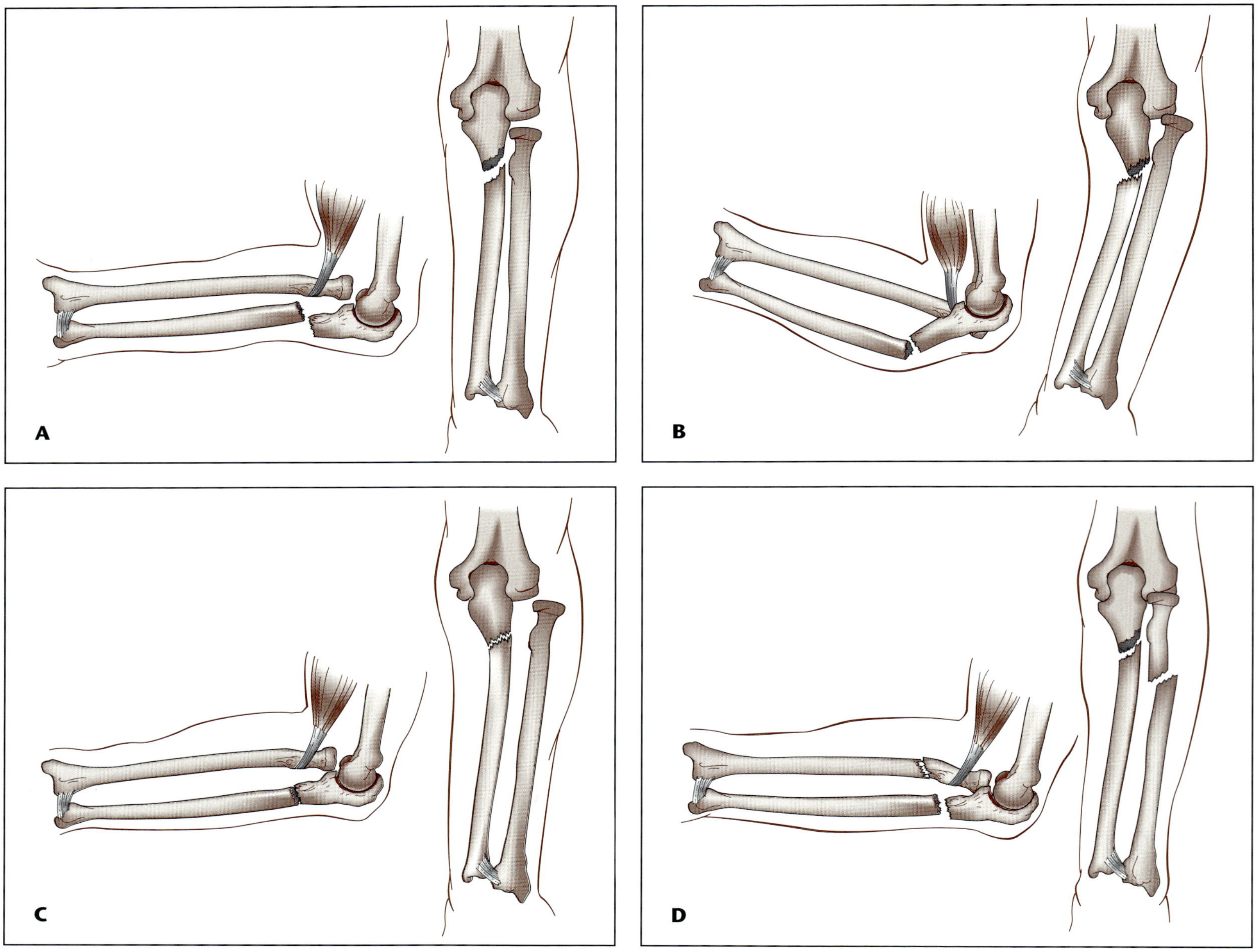

FIGURE 25-7. Monteggia fracture-dislocations. **A**, Type I; **B**, Type II; **C**, Type III; **D**, Type IV. (*Adapted from* Putnam and Fisher [3••].)

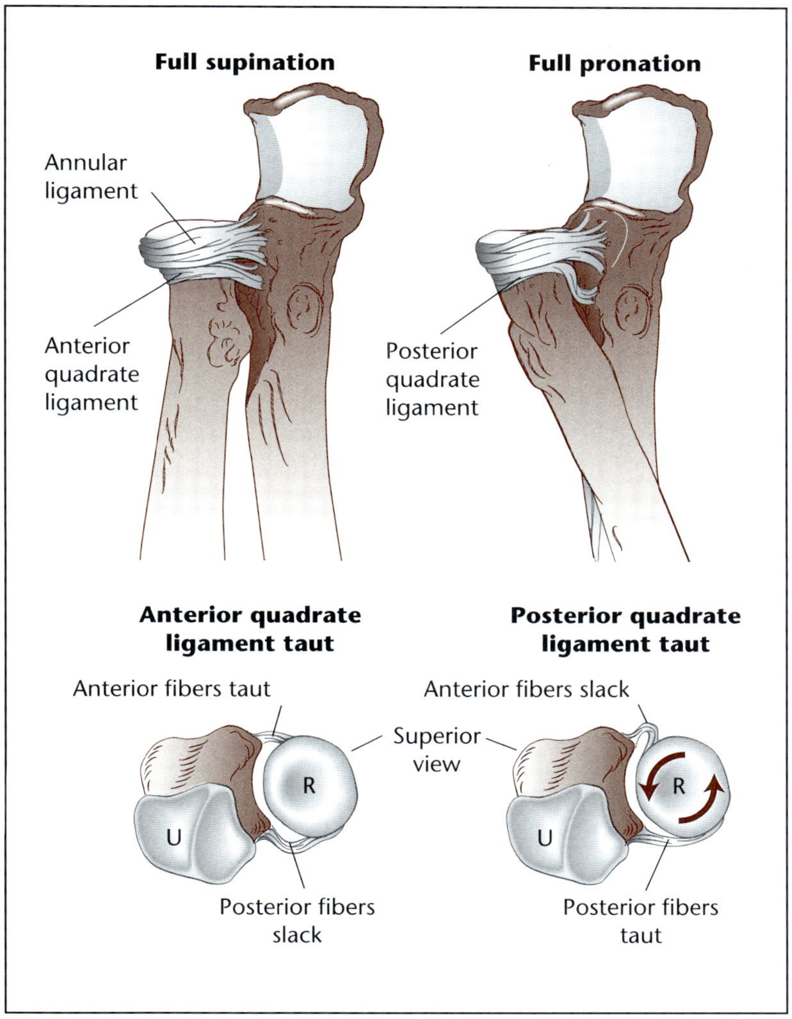

FIGURE 25-8. The proximal radioulnar joint. The anterior capsule and ligament are taut in supination and the posterior capsule and ligament are taut in pronation. (*Adapted from* Putnam and Fisher [3••].)

ously, the elbow and the wrist must be visualized on radiographs of all forearm fractures.

Severity of the soft tissue injury plays a key role in determining appropriate fixation [7]. Open fractures deserve soft-tissue management as mentioned previously. If the wound is severely contaminated or devitalized, staged débridement may be necessary, followed by local or free-flap coverage. Provisional external fixation may be more reasonable in this situation to provide skeletal stabilization. Delayed plate fixation can later be considered. We prefer to plate any open fracture that is not severely contaminated (even a Gustilo Grade IIIB or IIIC) [7]. This point, however, is controversial, and many authors argue for external fixation in the higher-grade open injury. However, we believe that more important than the fixation technique preferred is the use of aggressive and meticulous soft tissue débridement. Devitalized tissue and dead muscle or skin must be excised, and preparation for flap coverage or skin grafts must be considered. We consider the severely contaminated wound to be the only indication for external fixation in forearm fractures.

Most surgeons feel more comfortable handling fractures of the radius and ulna with plate fixation [8]. What is most important in achieving satisfactory fixation with these fractures is the restoration of forearm length and rotation. If the ulna is overlengthened, this may adversely affect not only the chance of success of its own healing, but also of that of the radius. This may result in the need for cancellous bone grafting, which can lead to the creation of a radioulnar synostosis if grafting is inappropriately performed [9,10•]. Additionally, a secondary ulnar abutment syndrome can occur at the wrist leading to TFCC perforation and lunate chondromalacia with ulnar-sided wrist pain.

Malrotation of the fracture may have significant functional consequences. We see more referrals because of failure to regain supination than because of pronation. This affects activities of daily living, such as using the toilet, as well as occupational capabilities, for example, assembly line work. This situation can be avoided by attention to detail in restoring proper rotation. Because of the deforming forces on the radius, proximal radius

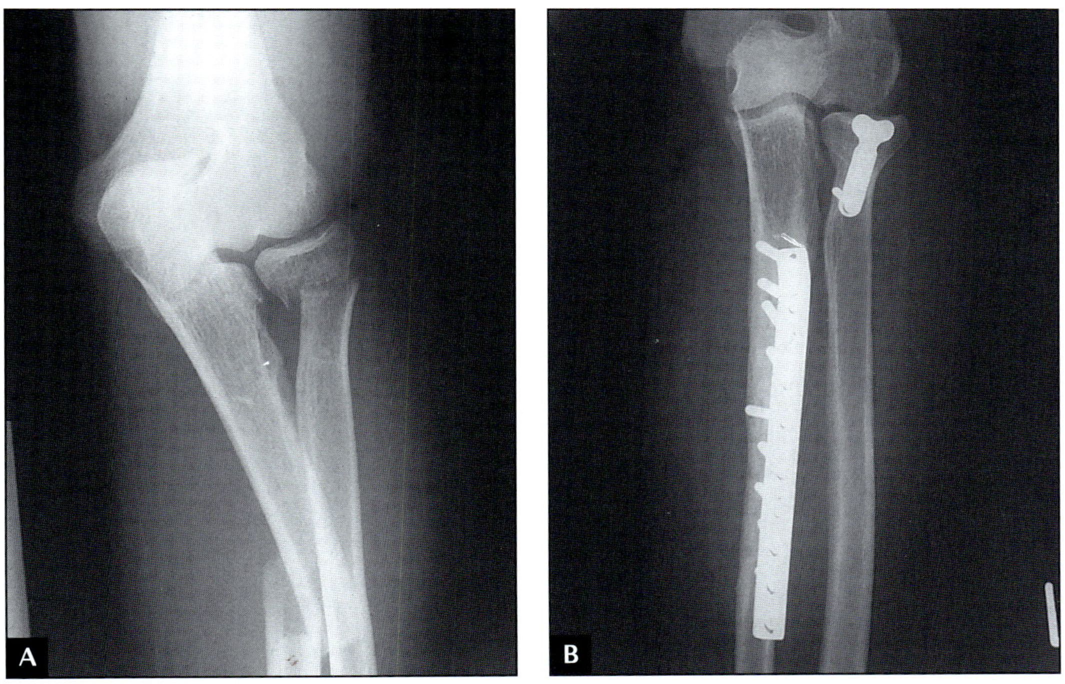

FIGURE 25-9. This Type IV Monteggia fracture-dislocation was managed by initial plating of the ulna followed by radial head reduction. The proximal radius fracture was then plated using a 2.4-mm titanium T-plate.

fractures (proximal to the pronator teres insertion) result in proximal fragment supination. Fractures of the middle or distal shaft fractures (distal to the pronator teres insertion) result in proximal fragment neutralization. Knowledge of the deforming properties of the attaching muscles is important in the success in restoration of forearm rotation (Figure 25-11).

Segmental fractures pose a particularly difficult problem. Restoration of forearm rotation is the paramount goal in the surgery, which can be difficult with two fracture sites. It can also be very challenging to contour and span both fractures with a single plate properly, so that using two plates is technically easier (Figure 25-12).

Bone graft is used in cases with more 50% cortical comminution and in segmental fractures. The operative surgeon must avoid placement of graft material at the interosseous membrane to prevent the development of radioulnar synostosis. However, routine use of bone grafting in comminuted forearm fractures has been debated recently [11]. In the case of large segmental defects (*ie,* larger than 7 cm), vascularized fibular autogenous grafting (with or without a skin pedicle), is an effective technique [7,12].

The usual type of plate selected a 3.5-mm titanium LC-DCP variety. The LC-DCP plate has the theoretical benefit of reduced periosteal ischemia, and the titanium has the benefit of less bone-stress shielding. We prefer six cortices on either side of the fracture site. In the presence of bone loss with attendant inability to achieve axial compression, we secure eight cortices on each side of the fracture. Provisional reduction of the ulna is achieved, before the radius is reduced. The ulna is usually plated first, and attempts are made to recess the plate dorsal to the direct subcutaneous border. Next the radius is plated; the plate is placed either radial or volar depending on whichever surface best accepts the plate or has the most comminution. Full-length intraoperative films should be obtained to assess both adequacies of reduction and alignment as well as screw lengths and position. Screws that penetrate extensively into the interosseous membrane can lead to the development of a radioulnar synostosis.

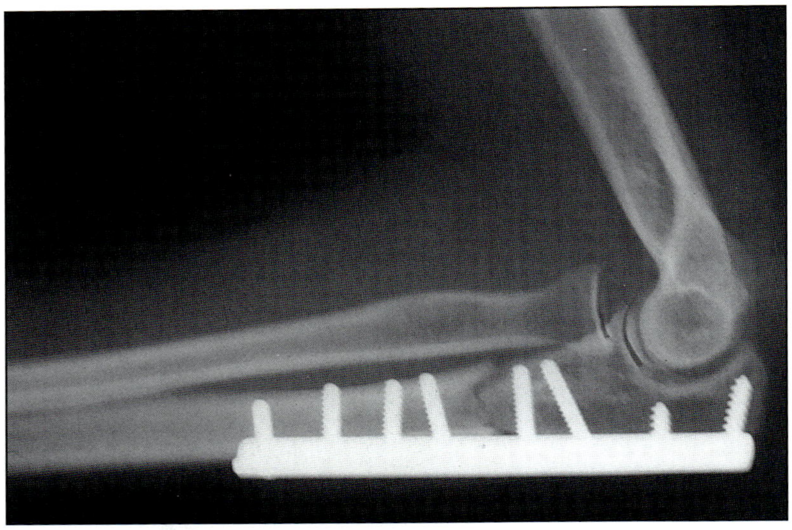

FIGURE 25-10. This Type I Monteggia fracture-dislocation required open reduction and annular ligament repair because of recurrent radial head dislocation in spite of anatomic ulnar fixation.

Postoperatively, the patient is maintained in a splint for 3 weeks to allow for subsidence of swelling and then motion is begun out of a protective splint. Light forearm loading with Theraband resistance is begun at 6 weeks, and repetitive motion is allowed at 3 months.

Alternatively, some authors have had success with intramedullary nailing of diaphyseal fractures of the forearm. This technique has the advantage of smaller incisions and limited exposures compared with those found with plate fixation. This method can even be used in gunshot wounds and segmental fractures with comminution. It is contraindicated in the skeletally immature and is best avoided in patients with small medullary canals or preexisting deformity. Intramedullary rods are weaker in torsion and compression compared with plates [13].

Nailing is performed through an incision over the olecranon for the ulna and on the dorsum of the wrist over Lister's tubercle for the radius. Guide wires and reamers are used. Intramuscular rodding systems are now available with proximal and distal locking bolts. The canal normally averages 3 to 7 mm in diameter at its narrowest point, and this determines the nail size. Alternatively, Rush's rods may be used but these do not provide the benefit of rotational control.

FRACTURES OF THE RADIUS WITH AND WITHOUT DISTAL RADIOULNAR JOINT DISLOCATION (GALEAZZI, ESSEX-LOPRESTI, AND ISOLATED RADIUS FRACTURES)

In 1934, Galeazzi called attention to the associated injuries of a fracture of the distal radial diaphysis with dislocation of the distal

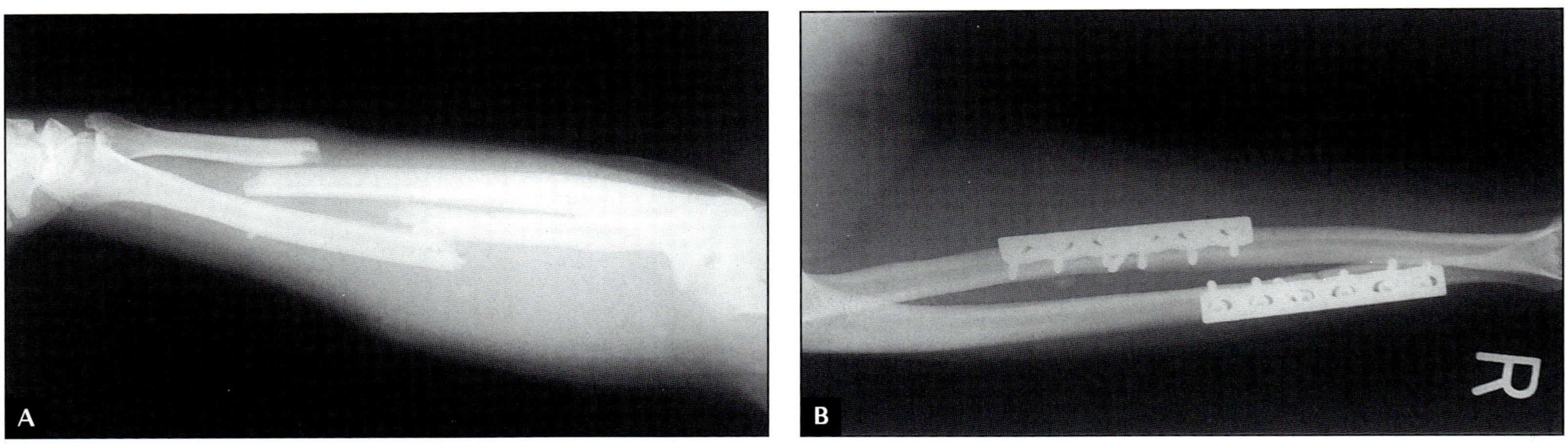

FIGURE 25-11. Exact restoration of length and rotation are important for success in managing both-bones forearm fractures.

radioulnar joint. Its true incidence is unknown because the distal radioulnar joint injury is commonly missed. The cause of this injury is felt to be secondary to a direct blow to the dorsolateral wrist in pronation. The ulna may be prominent, signaling the distal radioulnar joint injury. Radiographically, distal radioulnar joint dislocation is suspected when there is anteroposterior widening of the distal radioulnar joint, ulnar styloid fracture, dorsally subluxed/dislocated ulna on a true lateral, or more than 5-mm radial shortening. Obtaining contralateral views of the wrist and forearm assists in detecting asymmetry. The clinician should always consider the Galeazzi injury with any distal radius fracture.

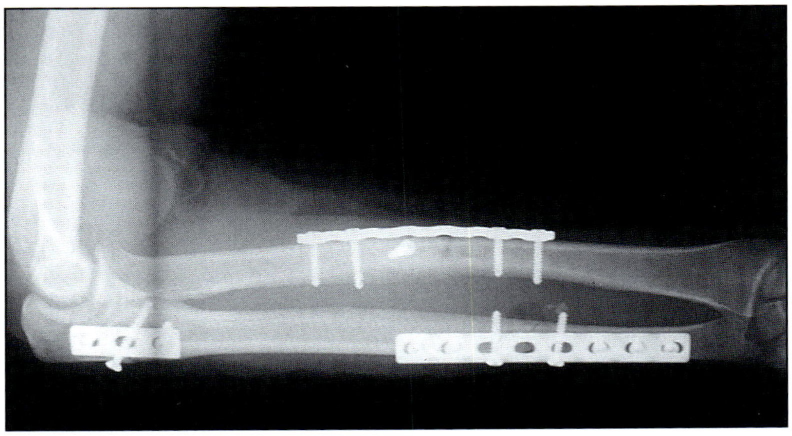

FIGURE 25-12. Segmental fractures of the radius or ulna can be managed using either a long plate to span both fracture sites or 2 plates to manage each fracture separately.

Galeazzi injuries with more proximal radius fractures should not be overlooked (Figure 25-13).

In addition, distal radioulnar joint dislocation is seen with even more proximal injuries, such as radial head fractures. When distal radioulnar joint dislocation is seen with a more proximal radius fracture (usually radial head), this injury is known as an Essex-Lopresti fracture (Figure 25-14) [4]. These injuries are often missed on initial evaluation. In this injury, the force necessary to cause a distal radioulnar joint dislocation is transferred up the interosseous membrane and a proximal radial fracture develops. Because the central band of the interosseous membrane is disrupted, axial instability can develop, which results in late distal migration of the ulna particularly with radial head excision.

When an Essex-Lopresti injury is suspected, care should be taken to reconstruct the fractured radial head. Retention of the radial length using a radial head implant or allograft radial head may be necessary when the radial head is not salvageable. Consideration should be given to repair the TFCC. It remains unclear whether the central band of the interosseous membrane can heal, but some authors would advocate cross-pinning the radius and ulna for 6 to 8 weeks [6•].

In the long-term situation in which axial migration has occurred, multiple options exist including titanium radial head implant or allograft radial head combined with ulnar shortening to restore neutral ulnar variance. We have had success with reconstruction of the interosseous membrane using bone-patellar ligament-bone autograft.

Galeazzi fractures are managed by plating of the radius using the volar Henry approach followed by reduction of the ulna. Restoration of the radial rotation is key as in all forearm fractures. With the usual dorsal distal radioulnar joint dislocation, the forearm is immobilized in supination (Figure 25-15). Volar disloca-

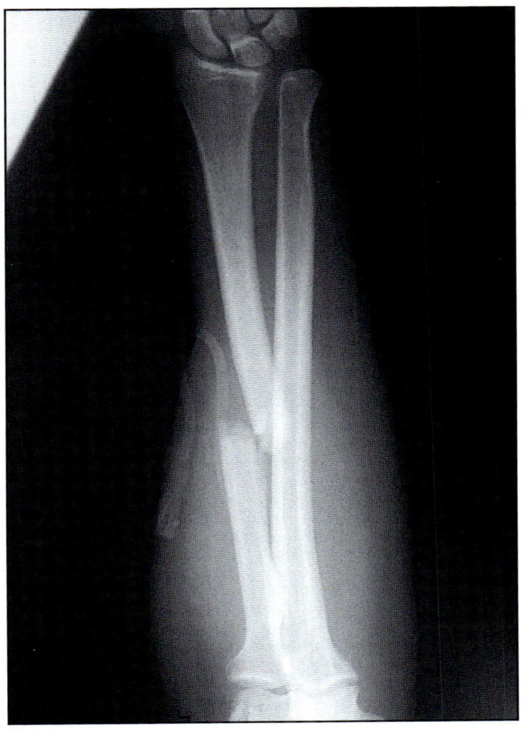

FIGURE 25-13. Galeazzi fracture-dislocations can be seen even with a more proximal radius fracture.

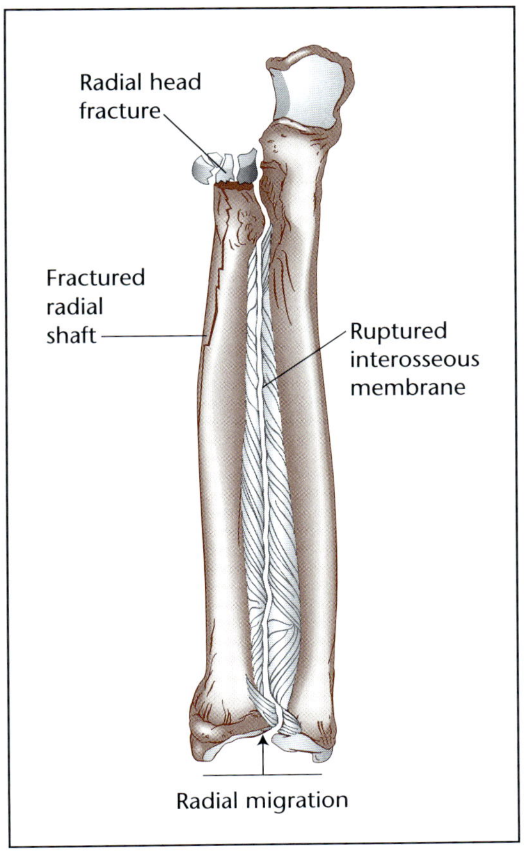

FIGURE 25-14. Essex-Lopresti fracture-dislocation.(*Adapted from* Putnam and Fisher [3••].)

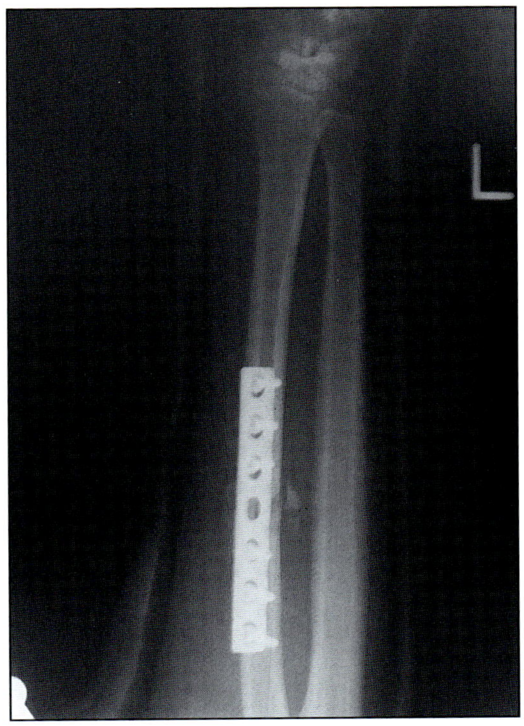

FIGURE 25-15. Galeazzi fracture-dislocation was plated and casted in supination.

tions are immobilized in pronation. If the distal radioulnar joint is irreducible, the surgeon must consider the possibility of ECU interposition. If the distal radioulnar joint is reducible but easily redislocates, we consider pinning the distal radioulnar joint with Kirschner wires; alternatively, we perform an ORIF of the TFCC if the ulnar styloid is fractured. Remember that the main stabilizer of the distal radioulnar joint is the TFCC. Postoperatively, the patient is immobilized for 4 weeks in a long-arm cast, followed by protected mobilization in a brace.

Isolated fractures of the radial shaft are uncommon. Once the possibility of a Galeazzi injury has been ruled out, it must be ruled out *again*. The displaced fracture is treated with ORIF using either Thompson's or Henry's approach. Because the ulna can act as a strut to prevent adequate axial compression of the radius, a potential to develop nonunion may be present (Figure 25-16).

SPECIFIC ISSUES

Plate Removal

We recommend plate removal not be done before 18 months after injury. The physician should not be cavalier about these "hardware-out" cases. The risk of nerve injury during plate removal is higher because of the scarring present and poor soft-tissue planes. The indication for plate removal is for the symptomatic case only. We do not remove plates to return athletes to contact sports. Moreover, the surgeon must always consider the possibility of nonunion or infection with painful hardware.

The forearm should be protected for 6 weeks following removal of hardware. Retained plates do not adversely affect forearm bone density and grip strength [14].

Complications

Nonunion of the radius or ulna can occur particularly with significant soft-tissue stripping or crush injury with associated disturbance of the blood supply. In addition, extensive fracture comminution or contamination as well as inadequate fracture fixation or distraction can lead to nonunion. Treatment of the hypertrophic nonunion involves compression plating and the use of autogenous bone graft. The atrophic nonunion should be treated with autogenous bone grafting with or without exogenous stimulation (electrical stimulation or ultrasound). Segmental defects or fractures with a devascularized bed require vascularized bone grafting [12].

Osteomyelitis is rare and is seen more often with high-energy injuries [7]. If osteomyelitis is present, curettage of necrotic bone and rigid osseous stabilization is necessary along with appropriate antibiotics.

Radioulnar synostosis can result in complete loss of supination and pronation of the forearm. Operative resection of the synostosis can restore rotational motion. In the past, use of adjuvant treatments such as low-dose irradiation or nonsteroidal anti-inflammatory medications along with the placement of interpositional materials (*eg*, fat, silicone sheeting, muscle) have been used. Recent data suggest that extensive excision alone may be sufficient [9].

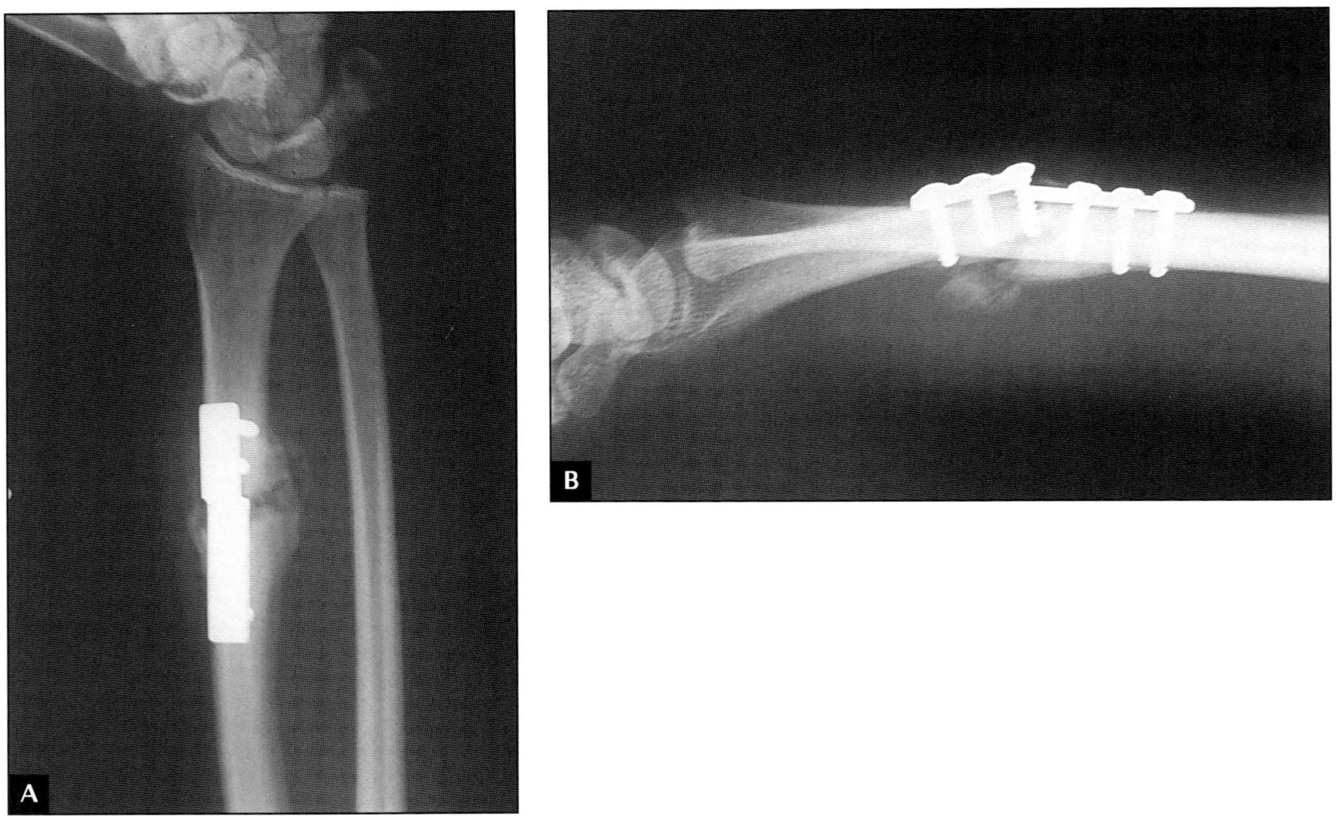

Figure 25-16. The ulna can act as a strut to prevent axial compression of the radius. This is seen with this hypertrophic nonunion of the radius, which eventually resulted in plate failure.

CONCLUSIONS

Fractures of the radius and ulna generally do not represent significant technical challenges for the managing surgeon who is vigilant about ruling out associated injuries and is meticulous with respect to restoration of length and rotation of these long bones. This can be easily overlooked, especially with multitrauma. A sound appreciation of the anatomy of the forearm, wrist, and elbow is the basis for the fund of knowledge necessary for successful treatment of these injuries.

REFERENCES AND RECOMMENDED READING

Recently published papers of particular interest have been highlighted as:
- • Of interest
- •• Of outstanding interest

1. Morgan WJ, Breen TF: Complex fractures of the forearm. *Hand Clin North Am* 1994, 10:375–390.
2. Hahn M, Strauss E, Yang EC: Gunshot wounds to the forearm. *Orthop Clin North Am* 1995, 26:85–93.
3.•• Putnam MD, Fischer M: Forearm fractures. In *Surgery of the Hand and Upper Extremity.* Edited by Peimer CA. New York: McGraw-Hill; 1996:599–635.

This is an outstanding chapter on forearm fractures with useful diagrams and algorithms.

4. Skahen JR III, Palmer AK, Werner FW, *et al.*: Reconstruction of the interosseous membrane of the forearm in cadavers. *J Hand Surg [Am]* 1997, 22:986–994.
5. Markolf KL, Lamey D, Yang S, *et al.*: Radioulnar load-sharing in the forearm. *J Bone Joint Surg Am* 1998, 80:879–888.
6.• Richards RR, Corley FG: Fractures of the shafts of the radius and ulna. In *Rockwood and Green's Fractures in Adults.* Edited by Rockwood CA, Green DP, Bucholz RW, *et al.* Philadelphia: Lippincott-Raven; 1996.

This chapter has an excellent section that emphasizes important principles in managing these fractures.

7. Shea KG, Fernandez DL, Casillas M: Fixation methods in contaminated wounds and massive crush injuries of the forearm. *Hand Clin North Am* 1997, 13:737–743.
8. McAuliffe JA: Forearm fixation. *Hand Clin North Am* 1997, 13:689–701.
9. Jupiter JB, Ring D: Operative treatment of posttraumatic proximal radioulnar synostosis. *J Bone Joint Surg Am* 1998, 80:248–257.
10.• Richards RR: Chronic disorders of the forearm. *J Bone Joint Surg Am* 1996, 78:916–930.

This is an excellent review that highlights salvage issues as related to forearm fractures and functional disorders.

11. Wright RR, Schmeling GJ, Schwab JP: The necessity of acute bone grafting in diaphyseal forearm fractures: a retrospective review. *J Orthop Trauma* 1997, 11:288–294.
12. Jupiter JB, Gerhard HJ, Guerrero J, *et al.*: Treatment of segmental defects of the radius with use of the vascularized osteoseptocutaneous fibular autogenous graft. *J Bone Joint Surg Am* 1997, 79:542–553.
13. Jones DJ, Henley MB, Schemitsch EH, *et al.*: A biomechanical comparison of two methods of fixation of fractures of the forearm. *J Orthop Trauma* 1995, 9:198–206.
14. Lindsey RW, Fenison AT, Doherty BJ, *et al.*: Effects of retained diaphyseal plates on forearm bone density and grip strength. *J Orthop Trauma* 1994, 8:462–467.

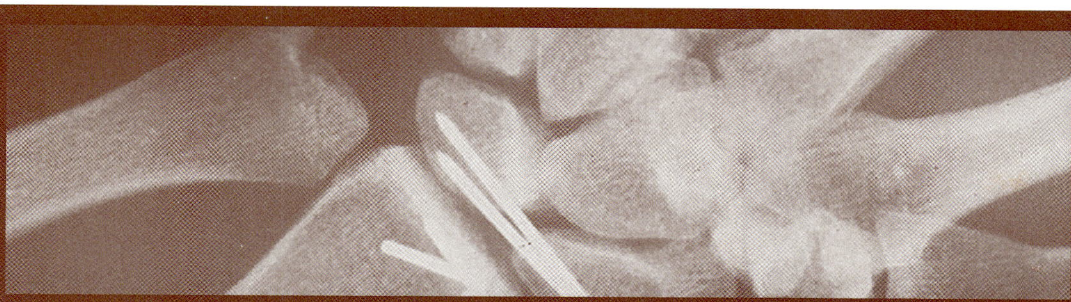

26

Distal Radius Fractures

Larry R. Padgett
Terry L. Whipple

Distal radius fractures are the most common of all skeletal injuries or fractures except finger fractures [1]. Physicians in the past thought distal radius fractures were a relatively homogenous group of injuries with excellent or good prognosis regardless of the treatment applied [2]. Recently, however, physicians have noted that distal radius fractures can be complex injuries and a variable prognosis is given depending on the nature of the fracture pattern. As more and more surgeons have become aware of the complexity of treatment, a steady change has taken place in the evaluation, interpretation, classification, and subsequent treatment of distal radius fractures. Today, with advancements in wrist arthroscopy, newer imaging techniques, and newer surgical fixation devices, the treatment of distal radius fractures has become much more advanced and beneficial to the patient population.

Incidence of distal radius fractures has been listed as high as 15% of all fractures [3]. Despite their frequency, the extent of anatomic disruption, associated soft tissue injuries, and eventual outcome has been difficult to assess and predict [4,5]. It has generally been accepted that restoration of anatomy, particularly joint congruency, is essential to ensure a satisfactory functional result [6–9]. Knirk and Jupiter [8] recognized that an articular offset larger than 1 mm was associated with a poor result.

Closed reduction and casting or closed reduction and external fixation as treatment options, based on the concept of ligamentotaxis, have suffered from the inability of clinicians to manipulate displaced or depressed articular fragments [7,9]. Percutaneous pinning has been recommended as an adjunct to reduce and maintain displaced articular fragments. Conventional open techniques and arthroscopic techniques have been proposed to correct some of these difficulties. This chapter summarizes the current available literature and information on distal radius fractures, including classification and anatomy. We address nonoperative or closed treatment as well as operative treatment (*eg,* external fixation, percutaneous pinning, open reduction and internal fixation techniques, the role of arthroscopy) and their respective indications.

ANATOMY

The distal end of the radius is the anatomic foundation of the wrist joint [10]. The wrist depends on both osseous and ligamentous integrity for its mobility as well as its capacity to support axial load.

The wrist joint in humans is distinguished from that in lower primates by having a well-developed radiocarpal joint [10]. The distal radius functions as a plateau on which the carpus rests, and from which the radially based supporting ligaments of the wrist arise [11]. The hand and radius, as a unit, articulate with and rotate about the ulnar head through the sigmoid notch of the radius [11]. This latter relationship is maintained primarily by the ulnar-based supporting ligaments of the wrist: the triangular fibrocartilage complex and the capsule of the distal radioulnar joint [11]. Development of the triangular fibrocartilage complex and the absence of a well-defined articulation between the ulna and the carpus enhances the ability to position the hand in space [11].

Three concave articular surfaces on the distal radius involve articulation with the carpus and the distal ulna. These include the scaphoid fossa, the lunate fossa, and the sigmoid notch. Any or all of these may be involved with distal radius fractures.

The metaphyseal flare of the distal radius begins approximately 2 cm proximal to the distal articular surface. As the radius flares, the thickness of the cortical bone decreases and the amount of cancellous bone increases [11]. Various studies have quantified the geometric positions of the articular surfaces and bone stock about the distal radius. Radial inclination is measured by an angle drawn between a tangential line to the distal radial articular surface on a posteroanterior (PA) radiograph and a line perpendicular to the shaft of the radius. The palmar tilt is measured by the angle between the plane of the distal articular surface as seen on lateral projection and a line perpendicular to the longitudinal axis of the radius. The radial inclination or slope of the distal radial articular surface has been estimated to be 22° and the palmar tilt is approximately 11° [11,12]. The palmar surface of the distal end of the radius is mostly flat but gently curves volarly [10]. The radioscaphoid ligament arises from a tubercle in the middle of the radial palmar surface. A smooth impression on the radial styloid process represents the origin of the stout radioscapholunate and radiotriquetral intracapsular ligaments [10]. As previously explained, the articular end of the radius slopes in an ulnar and palmar direction. The carpus therefore has a natural tendency to slide in an ulnar direction, resisted primarily by the intracapsular and interosseous carpal ligaments. These ligaments include the radial supporting ligaments of the wrist: the radiocollateral, radiocapitate, and radiotriquetral. At the palmar aspect of the anteroposterior (AP) midradial ridge is a tubercle for the origin of the important radioscapholunate ligament. Relatively weak and unimportant supporting ligaments, the radioscaphoid and radial triquetral, arise from the dorsoradial aspect of the radius. The triangular fibrocartilage complex arises at the ulnar aspect of the lunate facet of the distal radius and extends to the base of the ulnar styloid process, functioning as an important stabilizer of the distal radioulnar joint [10]. Its volar and dorsal margins are thickened, blending into the dorsal and volar radioulnar ligaments. It is therefore evident that stability and mobility are ensured by the design of the radius and its interactions with the carpal and ulnar articulations. Fractures of the distal end of the radius that heal with deformity or disruption of these articulations may have a significant effect on the function of the entire wrist joint.

MECHANISM OF INJURY

Jupiter [10] has divided the mechanism of injury of distal radius fractures into two categories: shearing and compression. He proposed that shearing marginal fractures have been attributed to an axial load imparted to the end of the radius by the carpal bones. King and Lovell [13] postulated that when impaction occurs with the hand and wrist in particular positions, the intrinsic ligamentous support of the lunate is injured sufficiently to permit it to migrate along the sheared articular fragment of the end of the radius. The radiocarpal ligaments or extrinsic support arising from the radius remain intact. This is in contrast to a true radiocarpal dislocation. Jupiter [10] explained that the resultant volar and dorsal marginal fractures are more common and are associated with injuries arising from vehicular trauma and high-velocity impact. Such compressive forces have been postulated to occur when the wrist is locked in palmar flexed position, such as gripping the handlebars of a motorcycle, or when the wrist is flexed in extension, as when holding onto an automobile's steering wheel. These forces are postulated to lead to volar and dorsal shearing fractures, respectively. The second type of fracture mechanism mentioned by Jupiter [10] is compression fracture. Scheck [14] described the *die punch* compression injury, named after a tool then commonly used in fabrication of products in steel. Scheck hypothesized that in some cases both compression and bending forces are exerted in the direction of the longitudinal axis of the radius.

Melone [15] further extended this analysis of the injury pattern and concluded that the medial aspect of the radius was most often affected. Melone used the term "medial complex" to describe the lunate facet as well as the ligamentous attachment with the proximal row of the carpal bones and the ulnar styloid. The lunate has been the nexus of direct compression injuries. It has been suggested that the injury occurs when the hand is flat on the ground and the wrist is extended, thus driving the lunate into the dorsal aspect of the distal radius [10]. This suggestion helps to explain why the dorsal aspect of the lunate facet has been more commonly involved than its palmar counterpart. With higher-velocity injuries, however, wider separation of the lunate facet was observed, which at times would result in a palmar medial facet fragment's becoming displaced and rotated [10].

CLASSIFICATION

Fracture classification schemes are intended to help the surgeon choose an appropriate method of treatment for every fracture in a particular anatomic area and to provide a reasonable estimation of outcome. Most classification schemes require radiographs as methods of measurement or observation, which are then compared with a published set of rules. It is generally thought that an orthopedic tool works if it produces the same results time and time again in the hands of anyone who uses it, therefore providing inter- and intraobserver reproducibility. Hastings [16] wrote that the two primary requirements of distal radius fracture schemes should be to dictate some manner of treatment and suggest or correlate long-term functional results.

Numerous classification schemes exist for distal radius fractures. In 1814, Abraham Colles [2] described the first scheme; since then, many descriptions have been published. To understand the classifications, some researchers began by assessing normal conditions. Friberg and Lundstrom [17] studied 50 normal patients' radiographs and defined the measurements of radial inclination, palmar slope, and radial length as discussed earlier in this chapter. Various other studies have performed the same descriptions. Later, Rubinobich *et al.* [18] evaluated these various radiographic parameters and found that volar tilt was the only parameter that had a direct effect on functional outcome. In 1993, Tsukazaki [19] showed a weak correlation between function and the radiographic parameters already given. These findings demonstrated that as dorsal angulation increased, the resultant flexion of the patient decreased. They showed that grip strength, extension, pronation, and supination did not correlate with the parameters, including dorsal angulation radial shortening or inclination. In a classic 1986 article by Knirk and Jupiter [8], the effect of the articular surface disruption on posttraumatic arthritis was analyzed in 40 young patients. The authors showed that failure to achieve or maintain congruity of the articular surface was the most important factor in reducing the incidence of posttraumatic arthritis and dysfunction. They demonstrated that the die punch classification was an important component of more comprehensive schemes. Regarding radiographic parameters, much controversy has gone on and the answers are probably not known, but dorsal tilt, shortening, and articular congruity have shown some importance in resultant function (or lack of it).

The importance of the articular congruity was also demonstrated by Bradway *et al.* [6] in 1989. Sixteen patients with displaced comminuted intra-articular fractures, classified by the AO group [20] as Type C2 and C3 fractures, were evaluated. The degree of articular incongruity at final healing had a major bearing on outcome. Three quarters of those with incongruity of greater than 2 mm had only fair results. All such patients (four of four) had major arthritis compared with only one of 12 with less than 2 mm of intra-articular incongruity. Overall, the authors noted that functional results dropped dramatically when step-off was greater than 1 mm.

Historically, some orthopedic surgeons have used various eponyms to describe distal radius fractures. Over the past 30 to 40 years, a number of classification schemes have been added to describe these fractures more accurately and some have been more useful than others. In 1950, Cassebaum [21] defined a Colles' fracture as one that occurred within 2 cm of the articular surface. Gartland and Werley [5] were the first to call attention to the finding that many of these fractures were incompletely treated and had poor results. They developed a classification scheme divided into three groups: groups 1 and 2 showed no displacement, group 1 had no articular involvement, and group 2 had articular involvement. Group 3 fractures included those with comminuted displaced articular fragments. Their study showed that many of the distal radius fractures did not do as well as had been proposed earlier. About 88% of the fractures they studied had articular surface involvement and 22% led to posttraumatic arthritis. They averred that closed reduction was inadequate for many of the fractures.

Older *et al.* [22] were the first to combine treatment recommendations with classification. Older's classification divided the fractures into four groups. The first included nondisplaced fractures, and the other three groups involved progressively more displacement and more comminution with attendant shortening. The researchers developed a useful system based on displacement, comminution, shortening, and dorsal angulation. They correlated their study with functional outcome and developed a treatment protocol based on findings within these classification groups. The functional outcome worsened as the injury progressed from group 1 through group 4. Unfortunately, their results, although correlating with functional outcome, were broken down by fracture type and in terms of the treatment used. Therefore, it was not possible to draw conclusions about the type of treatments based on different fracture types.

In 1967, Frykman [23] developed a classification scheme based on a biomechanical study that brought attention to the importance of the distal ulna and the radioulnar joint. However, neither the extent nor the direction of displacement, including comminution and shortening, were included in Frykman's scheme. Through subsequent studies, this classification has not proven to provide prognostication regarding the fractures. More recent classification schemes include those of the AO/ASIF group [20], Melone [24], Rayhack (or Universal) [25], and Mayo [26]. The AO/ASIF classification scheme is the most detailed to date. It was proposed in 1986 and provided an organized fashion to evaluate fractures based on established AO schemes used in other joints, including extra-articular, partially articular, and completely articular fractures. Many studies have addressed different classifications and all have certain drawbacks, including difficulty in observer reproducibility and lack of data regarding the various outcomes.

In 1984, Melone [24] introduced a classification based on the four major components of the radius and recognized that many intra-articular fragments not only had instability but also had specific patterns of displacement. Medial fragments were the most important; displacement altered joint mechanics. Melone classified fractures into four types: Type I included stable minimally comminuted fractures; Type II included comminuted unstable fractures (including the lunate die punch fracture); Type III included fractures with a radial shaft component; and Type IV included fractures with wide separation. Melone also provided an excellent theoretical description of fracture patterns that points toward studying the articular portion of the fracture and categorizing specific patterns of displacement.

Trumble *et al.* [27] performed a retrospective study of 49 patients with comminuted displaced intra-articular fractures treated by open reduction and internal fixation. The authors developed an injury score classification and compared it with the Melone [24], AO/ASIF [20], and Frykman [23] classification schemes. They showed a strong correlation between their proposed injury score and the Melone and AO/ASIF schemes with regard to functional outcome. The Frykman classification scheme did not predict outcome. Trumble *et al.* [27] demonstrated that their injury score was best at predicting outcome based on intra-articular incongruity. Points were assigned for each millimeter of fracture displacement, and additional points were assigned for carpal injury. A significant drop-off in function occurred for patients with an injury score greater than 4. The authors also evaluated several different radiographic parameters and showed that radial tilt was not an important factor in determining outcome but that preoperative articular incongruity, or step-off, and radial shortening did correlate with functional outcome. They concluded that functional outcome correlated with articular congruity and the amount of initial displacement. They also stated that the clinician would need to treat intra-articular distal radius fractures aggressively and recommended treating displaced intra-articular fractures separately from the more usual Colles' [2] fractures.

In 1990, Rayhack [25] developed a simple yet inclusive scheme composed of four groups. Group 1 included nonarticular, nondisplaced fractures. Group 2 included nonarticular, displaced fractures that were either reducible and stable, reducible and unstable, or irreducible. Group 3 included fractures with articular involvement that were not displaced, and group 4 included articular fractures that were displaced with three similar subclassifications. This scheme addressed the entire spectrum of injuries but did not assess the specific regions of fracture as defined by Melone [24]. The Mayo system was described in 1993 by Cooney and Berger [26]. They had previously recognized that the Frykman classification [23] showed relevance to intra-articular patterns and they had changed their treatment based on these findings. They later noticed, however, that it became necessary to recognize the amount of displacement, instability, excessive dorsal angulation, and shortening and that earlier schemes did not address many of these issues. The Rayhack classification [25] was subsequently retermed the Universal classification. It was broad based, simple, and modeled after the Gartland and Werley [5] classification or the subsequent modifications suggested by Solgaard *et al.* [28]. However, Missakain *et al.* [29] showed that several fracture variants did not fit well into the previous schemes, including the Universal classification, and they therefore modified the Universal classification slightly to develop the Mayo classification. This new classification is simple and also divided into four types. Type I are fractures that are extra-articular and either nondisplaced or displaced; the displaced variety are either stable or unstable. Types II, III, and IV are intra-articular fractures that are either nondisplaced, displaced and reducible, displaced and not reducible, or complex. These intra-articular fractures are defined by location; Type II are at the radioscaphoid joint, Type III are at the radiolunate joint, and Type IV include both joints. Jupiter [10] recently wrote a highly informative article that described a useful way of formulating a treatment plan based Müller *et al.*'s [20] AO/ASIF classification system.

Regarding classification schemes, it appears that there are diverse factors involved in defining distal radius fractures. Radiographic parameters such as dorsal tilt and radial length have shown a weak correlation in the literature. Articular incongruity has been shown to be extremely important [6,25,27], as have initial displacement [22,24,27] (which was further quantified by Trumble *et al.* [27]), quality of initial reduction, and shortening and comminution [22,27]. The importance of shortening remains controversial, however. Angular deformities have not proven accurate in providing functional information reproducibly.

These classification schemes and descriptions can benefit the orthopedic surgeon when selecting appropriate treatment for a specific distal radius fracture. Each case should be individualized, however, and emphasis should be on restoring anatomy as closely as possible with any means available.

TREATMENT OPTIONS

In addition to fracture pattern, many other factors influence the choice of treatment. Factors associated with the individual patient, such as lifestyle, psychologic outlook, associated medical conditions, and compliance must be considered [1]. The anticipated functional loading should influence the choice of treatment and stabilization far more than the chronologic age of the patient [30]. Although many papers and book chapters advocate specific surgical techniques, such as external fixation, dynamic external fixation, intrafocal pinning, buttress plating, closed reduction, open reduction, and arthroscopic reduction, we do not think that any one technique is universally appropriate for these fractures. Orthopedic surgeons must have the complete armamentarium of operative techniques and instrumentation available to them as well as nonoperative methods so that they may select the most appropriate treatment for a particular fracture. The goal is not to perform a specific treatment as perfectly as possible but to restore articular integrity as perfectly as possible [31].

Closed Reduction

Closed reduction and immobilization in a rigid cast or splint has remained the accepted method of treatment for 75% to 80% of the fractures of the distal end of the radius and for extra-articular fractures that are minimally displaced or impacted and thus inherently stable [5,32]. One inherent problem with closed treatment and cast immobilization is that, after successful reduction, some orthopedic surgeons will accept the loss of reduction that occurs in the cast or after its removal [33]. Gartland and Werley [5] demonstrated that by the time the patient's fracture had healed, alignment of the fracture had often "returned to [that of the] initial injury." Loss occurred in the normal radial tilt, the normal volar tilt, and, most importantly, in radial shortening with ulnar impaction. Gartland and Werley's treatment program consisted of closed reduction and application of short arm splints with the patient's wrist flexed and ulnarly deviated. They reported a 22% incidence of arthritis and an 18% incidence of wrist stiffness, with attendant loss of radial tilt and shortening, increased radial deviation, and decreased ulnar deviation. Solgaard *et al.* [28] reported their results of 154 patients observed during a follow-up of 3.5 years. They noted a decreased range of motion in patients with malunion. With a dorsal angulation of the distal radius equal to or greater than 10°, good to excellent results decreased. They noted no good or excellent results in patients who had significant radial shortening.

Authors disagree on what adequate reduction means, but a review of the literature suggests that a radial tilt of greater than 10° is important [33]. A volar tilt of at least 0° degrees, or more precisely, no dorsal tilt, and shortening of no more than 2 mm is evidence of a satisfactory reduction. Adequate reduction for intra-articular fractures also allows more than a 2-mm gap at the articular surface, with no step-off [8].

Despite widespread acceptance of immobilization in a rigid cast, questions remain regarding the optimum position, the duration of immobilization, and the need to extend the cast proximal to the elbow. Several prospective studies [12,28,32] have addressed these issues with comparisons of different positions of the hand and wrist, functional bracing with the forearm in supination and short splint, and use of casts above and below the elbow. Neither the position of the forearm in immobilization nor extension of the cast proximal to the elbow appear to influence anatomic outcome to any noteworthy degree [30]. However, immobilization of the fracture with the forearm in supination, as advocated by Sarmiento *et al.* [9], offers the advantage of holding the distal radioulnar joint in a reduced position [30] and minimizing the tendency of the brachioradialis to displace the distal fragment in a radial direction [12].

Redisplacement of the fractures, as already discussed, is common in practice, yet little has been written about the ultimate state of a fracture that has been remanipulated. Two retrospective studies found lasting improvement in 33% and 54% of fractures after remanipulation [34]. In unstable fractures with displacement or extensive dorsal comminution, especially in elderly patients, reduction was lost even after the remanipulation.

Percutaneous Pins

Because of the loss of alignment reported by Gartland and Werley [5], DePalma [35] proposed using a percutaneous pin technique to supplement a closed reduction in which pins were placed through the ulna into the reduced distal radius to maintain alignment. This approach was chosen to avoid injury to the dorsal sensory branch of the radial nerve, as well as to provide stability for the pin by passing it through both cortices of the ulna. DePalma reported good-to-excellent results in 82%, with shortening of less than 2 mm and with minimal loss of alignment [35].

Extra-articular fractures with extensive comminution or fractures with no more than two articular fragments in which anatomic reduction is obtainable are amenable to percutaneous pinning of the fracture fragments and application of a plaster cast [30]. Complications, including loss of reduction, were minimal with each technique. Pin migration or pin tract infection occurred in approximately 10% of cases. Percutaneous pins are still in use today, but to maintain alignment and prevent shortening and deformity, they should, in some cases, be augmented by external fixation (Figure 26-1) [33].

Pins and Plaster

The technique of external fixation using pins incorporated into plaster cast were first introduced by Boehler in 1929 [36]. Indications for this technique included Colles' fractures with dorsal comminution, comminuted Smith's fractures, and comminuted intra-articular fractures. This technique is still in use today although pin tract problems, as well as loss of reduction, have rendered it less popular [33]. Green [37] documented good or excellent results using this technique in 86% of his patients. Green noted a high incidence of both major and minor complications. One third of his patients had some problem associated with the use of pins. Other studies have corroborated the findings of a substantial incidence of complications with this technique [32]. Although pins and plaster offer a method of maintaining reduction in many stable fractures at limited expense, the complications of incorporating pins into circumferential plaster have led to reevaluation of this technique [32].

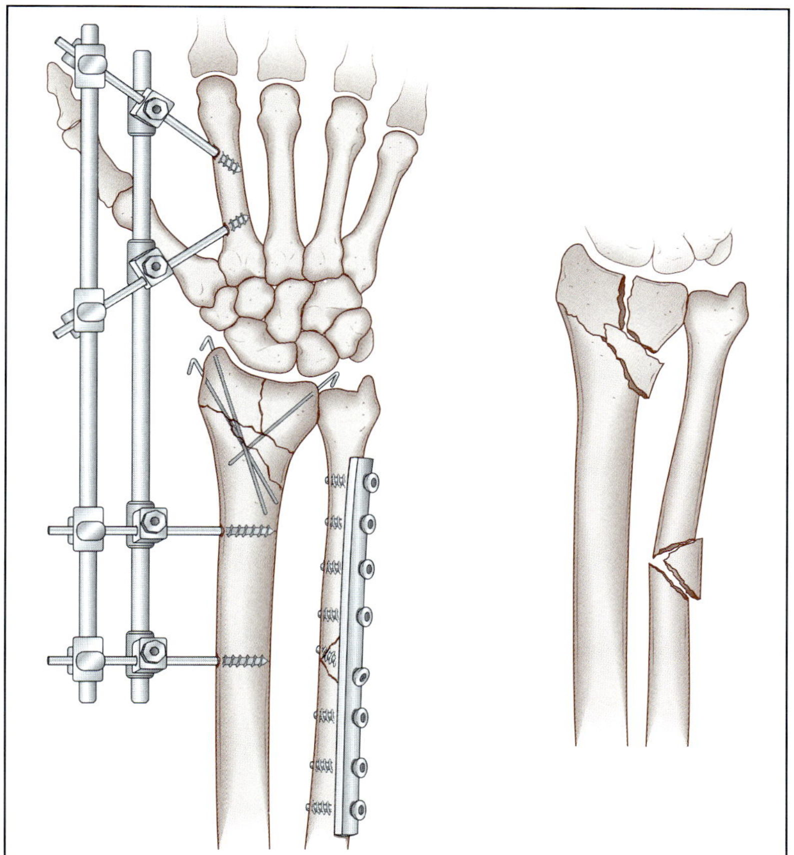

Figure 26-1. Percutaneous pins and external fixation of the distal radius with open reduction and internal fixation of associated ulnar fractures. (*Adapted from* Müller *et al.* [20].)

External Skeletal Fixation

Indirect reduction of distal radius fractures by ligamentotaxis using external fixation was initially designed to be a salvage procedure for extremely comminuted articular fractures that were not amenable to osteosynthesis (Figure 26-1). Application of the technique rapidly expanded to many types of articular and nonarticular distal radius fractures, and favorable initial outcomes were reported [38]. This popularity can be attributed, in part, to recognized problems inherent in previously mentioned techniques and to improvement in design of the frame and in methods of insertion of the pins. Reports of severe wrist stiffness and complications, including reflex sympathetic dystrophy, subsequently tempered initial enthusiasm for the technique.

Deleterious effects of prolonged immobilization of intra-articular cartilage and the surrounding soft tissue structures have been well documented both clinically and experimentally. For these reasons, more and more surgeons are moving toward alternative methods of fixation including open reduction and internal fixation and combined external fixation and distraction with open reduction and internal fixation. Putnam and Fischer [39] studied 26 closed unstable distal radius fractures that were treated using a combination of internal fixation, external distraction (intraoperative), and, in some cases, up to 4 weeks of external fixation (neutralization). This combined technique allowed them to use what they called a comprehensive approach to even the most unstable fractures by merging the advantages of internal and external fixation.

Although radial length and inclination are usually reestablished and maintained with traction (*ie*, ligamentotaxis), the palmar tilt of the radius is rarely restored to normal and reduction of central articular fragments is difficult because such fragments lack ligament attachment. An anatomic study by Bartosh and Saldana [40] suggested that this may occur because stout palmar radiocarpal ligaments reach maximum length before the dorsal ligaments, thus preventing the latter from pulling the dorsal aspect of the distal end of the radius into its normal palmar inclination. Recently, Dienst *et al.* [41] published a paper describing dynamic external fixation for distal radius fractures. They evaluated 30 patients with closed, comminuted, and mostly intra-articular fractures of the distal radius that were treated by closed reduction and immobilization with a dynamic external wrist fixator during a 2-year period. In 13 patients with severely comminuted and unstable fractures, an additional Kirschner wire (K-wire) was used. After 10 to 14 days of rigid fixation in a neutral position, the motion element was unlocked to allow up to 30° of flexion. After 6 weeks, the fixator was removed. The patients were observed for an average of 24 weeks and excellent functional outcome was seen in six patients (20%), a good outcome in 20 patients (67%), and a fair outcome in four patients (13%). Anatomically, 15 patients (50%) had an excellent result, 14 (47%) had good outcome, and one a fair outcome. Only minimal loss of reduction averaging 1° of palmar tilt was seen during mobilization. Two major complications occurred: a deep wire tract infection and an index metacarpal fracture. Minor complications, such as sensory disturbances and pin tenderness, were present but recovered completely after removal of the fixator. This study provided promising data and offered an alternative method in the treatment of distal radius fractures with severe comminution. They recommended that in cases with postreduction unstable fragments, additional K-wires should be used to allow early mobilization of the wrist. The fixator they used was the Hoffman Dynamic Wrist Fixator (Howmedica, Rutherford, NJ), which they found to be more beneficial than static fixation devices; they are currently working on prospective randomized trials to make a comparison. Clyburn [42] also demonstrated the advantages of dynamic external fixation.

Open Reduction and Internal Fixation

For intra-articular fractures with more than a 2-mm displacement after adequate attempts at closed reduction, operative intervention is indicated for all patients irrespective of their age (Figure 26-2).

Combinations of internal and external fixation to reduce the more severely fractured distal radius accurately have been described [39,43]. Axelrod *et al.* [44] reported on their technique of combining external skeletal fixation with open reduction of the displaced lunate facet through a small longitudinal dorsal incision and elevation of the impacted fragment without direct visualization of the surface of the joint. Leung *et al.* [45] reported on 100 complex fractures of the distal end of the radius in which the reduction was augmented with autogenous iliac-crest graft, thus permitting removal of the external fixation frame at 3 weeks and the use of a functional brace for an additional 3 weeks. Bass *et al.* [43] reported combined internal and external fixation techniques for distal radius fractures and a study population of 12 patients. Their results indicated that the surgical strategy, although demanding could be successfully used in the subset of patients that had AO-C3 fractures of the end of the radius.

Because of the need to obtain an anatomic reduction, especially of the articular surface, several authors advocate operative open reduction and internal fixation when necessary. Jupiter [10] asserted that two groups of fractures existed for which open reduction and internal fixation would be advisable. The first group included the two-part shear fracture, which he categorized as a radiocarpal fracture dislocation. The second group included complex articular fractures in which the articular fragments were displaced, rotated, or impacted and thus not amenable to reduction through limited operative exposure.

Operative management of these fractures is difficult and associated with a high rate of early and late morbidity [46]. We recommend that before an incision is made, distraction alone or with the temporary application of an external fixator makes it easier to manipulate the small articular fragments and minimize soft tissue dissection. The anterior approach is believed to be useful for fractures with anterior displacement or rotation of the articular fragments. When the fracture involves multiple small articular fragments, definitive fixation is difficult to accomplish by using open reduction techniques; K-wires with or without external fixation are usually necessary. Although enthusiasm for operative reduction of complex articular fractures of the distal end of the radius is growing, complications include loss of fixation, neuritis of the median nerve, reflex sympathetic dystrophy, infection of the wound, and late posttraumatic arthritis, which can occur even in the practice of an experienced surgeon [31,46].

Carter *et al.* [47] recently published a paper describing fixation of unstable distal radius fractures with the Zimmer Forte low-profile plate (Zimmer, Warsaw, IN). They studied acute dorsally displaced, unstable (high-energy) fractures of the distal radius to determine the safety and efficacy of this new low-profile dorsal plate. No external fixators were used either during or after the operation. Bone grafting was used in 64 of their 71 patients. The system had a special fracture reduction clamp and template preshaped to the normal contour of the dorsal radial metaphysis which assisted in molding the reduction. Using this dorsal plate for comminuted high-energy dorsally angulated fracture, they obtained satisfactory open reduction in 93% of the fractures, which was maintained in 88%. In all, 95% of the fractures demonstrated good or excellent outcomes using a standardized evaluation. Their report provided additional information that acute, unstable, dorsally displaced fractures of the distal radius can be effectively treated with open reduction and internal fixation with a low-profile plate in addition to the techniques mentioned; however, extensive surgical exposure is necessary and this necessity may add to postinjury stiffness or swelling.

Arthroscopically Assisted Reduction of Intra-articular Distal Radius Fractures

The importance of anatomic reduction of the articular surface and the extra-articular alignment of the distal radius has been outlined at some length in this chapter (Figure 26-3). Visualization of the joint through an arthrotomy is troublesome because of the biconcave configuration of the distal radius, which makes restoration

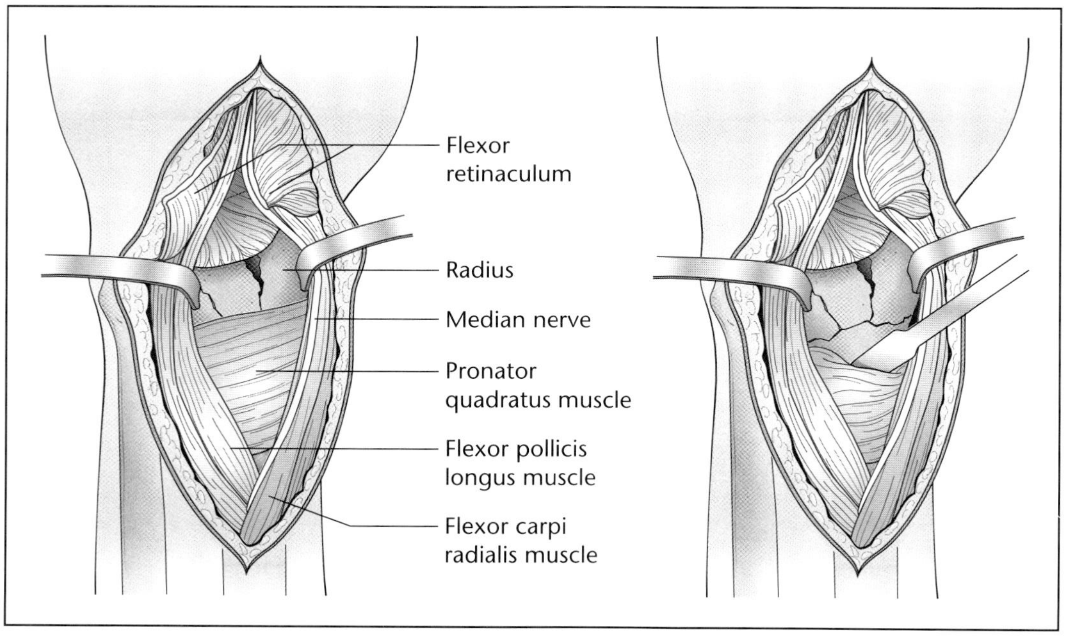

Figure 26-2. Volar approach to the distal radius. (*Adapted from* Müller *et al.* [20].)

difficult [6,8,48,49]. Radial shortening and metaphyseal angulation may be largely corrected by external fixation if ligamentotaxis has been shown not to restore articular congruity in fractures with impacted fragments [8]. Percutaneous and limited open reduction with intraoperative fluoroscopic monitoring allows for reconstruction of the distal radius with a minimum of soft tissue disruption although, with this modality, important associated carpal ligamentous injuries may go undetected [48–50]. Wrist arthroscopy provides an excellent view of the articular surface with minimal soft tissue disruption and it is increasingly recognized as an important adjunct to the management of distal radial fractures (Figure 26-4) [48,49].

Although the importance of restoring bony alignment has been investigated thoroughly, intra-articular ligament injuries associated with these fractures have received surprisingly little attention in the literature [49,51,52]. Hixon *et al.* [53] used wrist arthrograms in a prospective study to investigate the incidence of acute ligamentous injuries in distal radius fractures. These arthrograms were positive in 18 of 22 patients and included various isolated and combined ligament tears. Culp and Osterman [7] discussed their indications for arthroscopic guidance and assistance with distal radius fracture fixation. They stated that arthroscopic guidance is indicated for intra-articular distal radius fractures with an articular displacement of 2 mm or more of the radial carpal and radial ulnar joints after a thorough attempt at closed reduction. Arthroscopic evaluation was considered to be helpful also after open reduction and internal fixation to assess joint congruity in, for example, a volar Barton's fracture. If associated carpal ligament or triangular fibrocartilage injury is suspected, even in a nondisplaced distal radius fracture, wrist arthroscopy may be indicated. Several articles have outlined techniques for using combined arthroscopic assisted techniques for the treatment of distal radius fractures [7,48,49,54].

Our Preferred Method of Treatment

As already discussed, restoration of articular congruency is the most important long-term consideration in the treatment of distal radius fractures. The clinician should also be aware of the high incidence of intra-articular soft tissue injuries to intrinsic ligaments, articular cartilage, and triangular fibrocartilage's complex that are associated with intra-articular distal radius fractures. These soft tissue injuries can heal concurrently with the fracture if they are appreciated early and treated appropriately; they should not be deferred until symptoms arise after the radius fracture has healed. Because many such lesions warrant surgical repair, early diagnosis is justified, and the minimally invasive advantages of arthroscopic examination of the wrist may be indicated earlier.

Arthroscopy therefore enables the treating physician to establish a complete diagnosis of the injury as well as access fracture fragments on the distal radius for accurate reduction and stabilization while paying close attention to restoration of the articular surface (Figure 26-5). Fortunately, the entire distal articular surface of the radius can be visualized well through standard arthroscopic portals, as can most of the articular surface of the sigmoid notch in the distal radioulnar joint. Angular object lenses on smaller arthroscopes enable visualization around the corners through an access portal only 2 mm in diameter, causing minimal surgical disruption of the ligamentous attachments to bone or bone fragments and to the courses of tendons and retinacula. Because the earliest experience with intra-articular fracture reduction of the distal radius assisted by arthroscopic control occurred in 1986, the following techniques have been developed, refined, and used by Whipple in over 300 cases.

Initially, diligent efforts should be used to accomplish closed reduction of the fracture fragments of the distal radius. Arthroscopic intervention is indicated if, after such efforts, joint

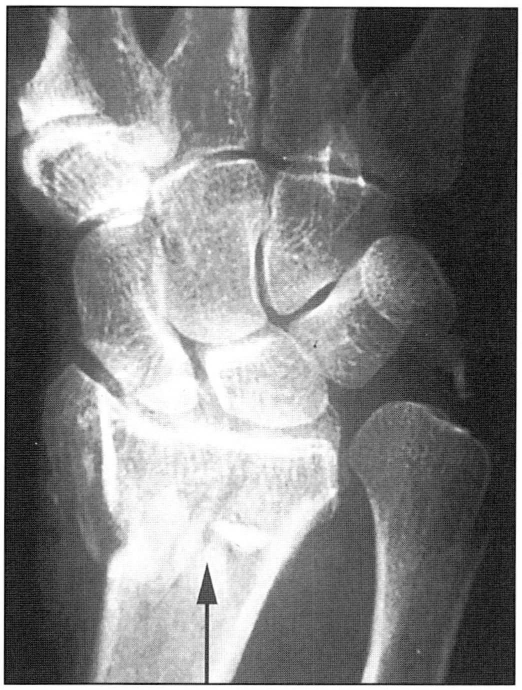

Figure 26-3. Articular fracture of the right distal radius. *Arrow* indicates impacted articular fragments driven into the metaphysis of the bone, leaving unacceptable articular defects. (*Copyright* TL Whipple.)

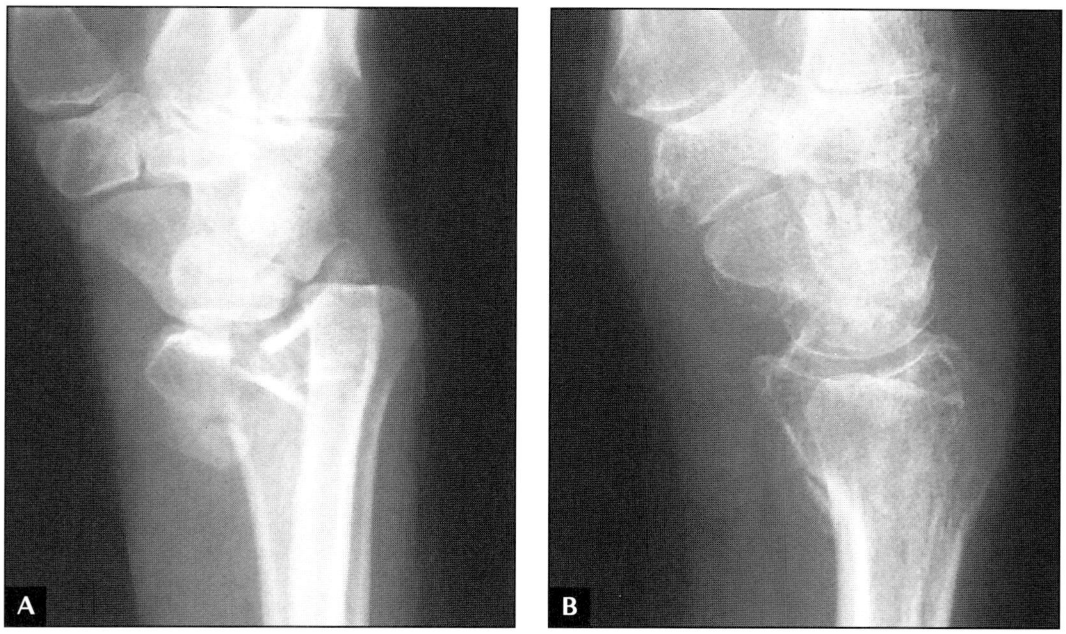

Figure 26-4. A, Lateral radiograph of comminuted distal radius fracture with volar displacement and impaction of subcortical bone fragments. B, Healed fracture after arthroscopic reduction of impacted fragments to restore articular surface. (*Copyright* TL Whipple.)

congruency is compromised by fracture separation, step-off of the articular surface, or significant tilt compared with that seen in the contralateral wrist. Other absolute indications for arthroscopic intervention include extensive articular comminution, small fracture, or cartilage fragments that may be expected to interfere with the smoothness of the radius articular surface, or if radiographs suggest the presence of intercarpal disruption or carpal impaction fractures.

Arthroscopically assisted reduction and stabilization of distal radius fractures should maximize the advantages of minimally invasive surgery techniques. Therefore, interfragmentary fixation with smooth K-wires is effective and placement of the wires can be accomplished in ways that avoid the complications of piercing cutaneous nerves or extensor tendons. Cutaneous nerves traverse basically similar courses to predictable distributions in the skin, but they are difficult to map clinically to avoid tethering or piercing these 1-mm structures.

Readily available 16-gauge hypodermic needles can be used as cannulas through which to drill 0.035-in or 0.046-in K-wires without twisting the subcutaneous tissue and placing inadvertent traction on cutaneous nerve branches. The hypodermic needle is sharp enough to pierce the joint capsule to target carpal bones accurately and also adds stiffness to the thin fixation wires as they are drilled through cortical or subchondral bone.

This technique requires at least four hands to aim the arthroscope, apply external pressure for fracture reduction, steady the hypodermic needle cannula, and drill the fixation wire into place.

Extensor tendons can be readily mapped by palpation or identification of known topographic bony prominences. After pins are inserted, the excursion of tendons can be confirmed by passive manipulation of digits to confirm no accidental incarceration of tendons has occurred with the fixation wires.

During arthroscopic examination of the wrist, fracture debris from excessive comminution or fracture crumbling can be cleared to improve the smoothness of articular surfaces. Similarly, any hemarthrosis present can be evacuated to prevent the formation of postfracture intra-articular adhesions.

Reference is made intraoperatively to preoperative computed tomography (CT) scans to map the fracture lines and to guide the optimal direction of fixation pins. Arthroscopically assisted fracture reduction and stabilization techniques involve several subtle considerations, each of which has been devised for a specific purpose important for optimal fracture treatment. Although these techniques are not mandatory, a surgeon should be adept at their use to maximize the advantages of minimally invasive fracture treatment for patients.

A common need exists for specific surgical equipment on frequent occasions. A small fluoroscopic unit may aid in assessing the depth of pin penetration to avoid irritation of overlying soft tissue structures, and the adequacy of fracture fragment fixation. A Traction Tower (Linvatec, Largo, FL) provides adequate ligamentotaxis with a directional bias toward flexion, extension, radial, or ulnar deviation to facilitate reduction of displaced or impacted fracture fragments (Figure 26-6). A power wire driver that can be operated with one hand and allow adjustment of the fixation pin length is extremely convenient, and of course, smooth K-wires or X-wires up to a diameter of 0.045 in provide optimal fixation.

Arthroscopic portals are selected based on gaining an optimal view of the articular fracture lines visible on transverse CT scans. For example, dorsal rim fractures are better seen from radial or ulnar portals than from middorsal portals where entrance of the arthroscope into the joint capsule will also overlie the fractured portion of the dorsal articular rim. The forearm should be wrapped firmly preoperatively to minimize extravasation of irri-

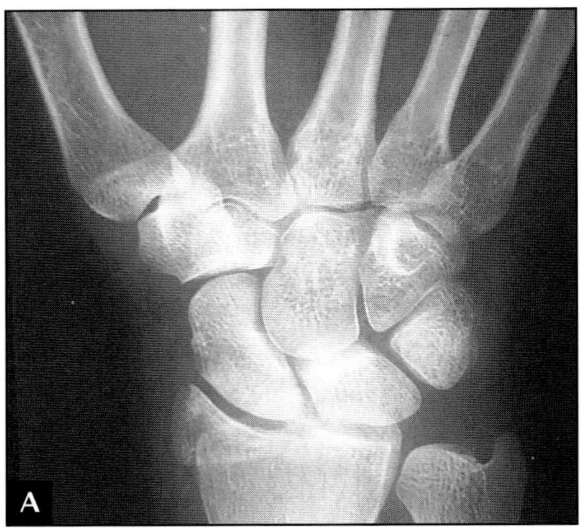

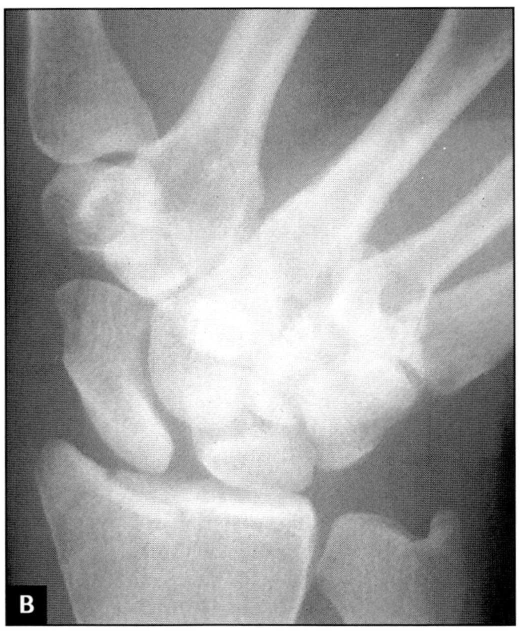

FIGURE 26-5. A, Displaced radial styloid fracture. B, Fracture after arthroscopic reduction of radial styloid displacement. A small step-off remains. (*Copyright* TL Whipple.)

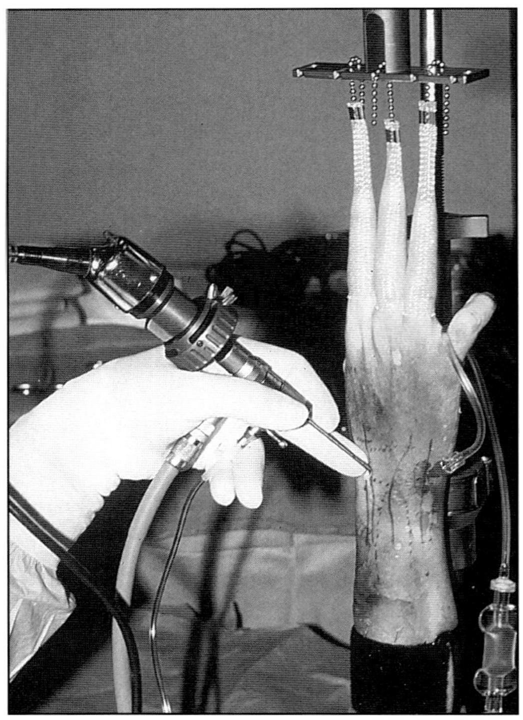

FIGURE 26-6. Fractured right wrist suspended in traction tower with an ulnar inflow portal and the arthroscope introduced between the second and third extensor compartments. (*Copyright* TL Whipple.)

gation fluid through fracture planes into flexor muscles. Development of postoperative compartment syndrome has never been a problem when using physiologic irrigation solutions because they are so readily absorbed by clisis. Compartment syndrome results from the sustained elevation of intracompartmental pressure sufficient to impair arterial or capillary circulation for more than 2 hours, usually a result of blood extravasation into muscle tissues that cannot be readily decompressed.

The optimal time for arthroscopic intervention for fracture fixation is within 2 to 4 days of the injury, before fibrin begins to precipitate from the hemarthrosis, which obscures arthroscopic visualization and may take unnecessarily long to clear and to maintain the visual field.

During diagnostic examination, the physician should attempt to see the fracture lines apparent on radiography or CT scan and assess the mobility of all fracture fragments with intra-articular or external pressure (Figures 26-7 through 26-12). The joint should be thoroughly lavaged to clear fracture debris and blood products. Before fracture reduction, then, attempts should be made to definitively treat nonfracture lesions of the wrist such as carpal instability, torn triangular fibrocartilage complex, or removal of smaller fracture fragments that are likely to displace from articular surfaces.

Next, attention should be turned to the fracture of the distal radius. Through the hypodermic needle cannulas, smooth fixation wires can be drilled between extensor tendon compartments into the cortices of the larger fracture fragments. Fragments are reduced in order of decreasing size so at the conclusion of the procedure, any unreducible fragments will leave minor defects in the articular surface. Fracture fragments are manipulated with the assistance of K-wires introduced and external pressure applied to the fracture cortex. When the fracture line is seen to close anatomically, the fixation wire can be advanced through that fragment into adjacent fragments far enough to engage the opposite cortex. More than one fixation wire may be necessary for larger fragments or those that tend to displace as a result of crumbling of the cancellous bone. Ideally, secondary fixation wires should be introduced at an optimal angle to the first to lock the fragments in place.

Fluoroscopic examination in two or more planes helps guide adjustment of the pins to proper depth. The pins can then be cut superficially to the skin, bent 90° or capped with plastic caps to avoid migration.

Finally, the mobility of digits and their tendons is checked to ensure optimal pin placement. The hand and wrist are then wrapped in a bulky dressing and immobilized with a plaster splint in an intrinsic positive position.

After 3 days, the splint and dressings are removed, using soaking as necessary, and the surgeon or a knowledgeable therapist assists with slight movement of all digits without placing undue pressure on the fracture surface. The pins may be removed after 3 to 6 weeks without anesthesia, and intermittent splinting is prescribed to facilitate resumption of motion without stiffness and without placing excessive pressure on the fracture surfaces. Resumption of strength is a secondary concern and should be postponed until passive mobility has been achieved. Formation of slight granulation tissue around the pin tracks can be easily treated with silver nitrate cauterization.

DISCUSSION AND CONCLUSIONS

Several factors are prognostically related to the function outcome after fractures of the distal radius. These include articular step-off,

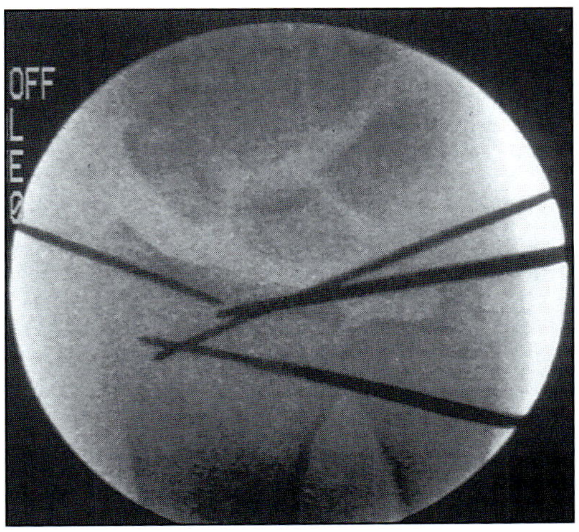

FIGURE 26-7. Intraoperative fluoroscopic view of articular fracture of the distal radius with five Kirschner wires used to transfix articular and metaphyseal fragments. (*Copyright* TL Whipple.)

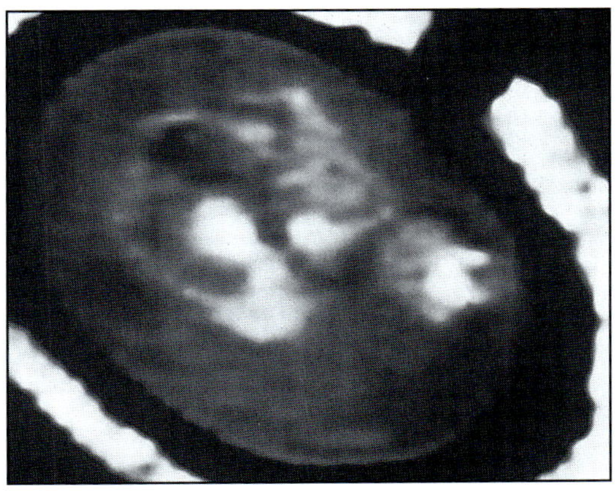

FIGURE 26-8. Transverse computed tomography (CT) scan of distal radius fracture showing three primary articular fragments and smaller densities in the metaphysis representing impacted subchondral bone fragments. (*Copyright* TL Whipple.)

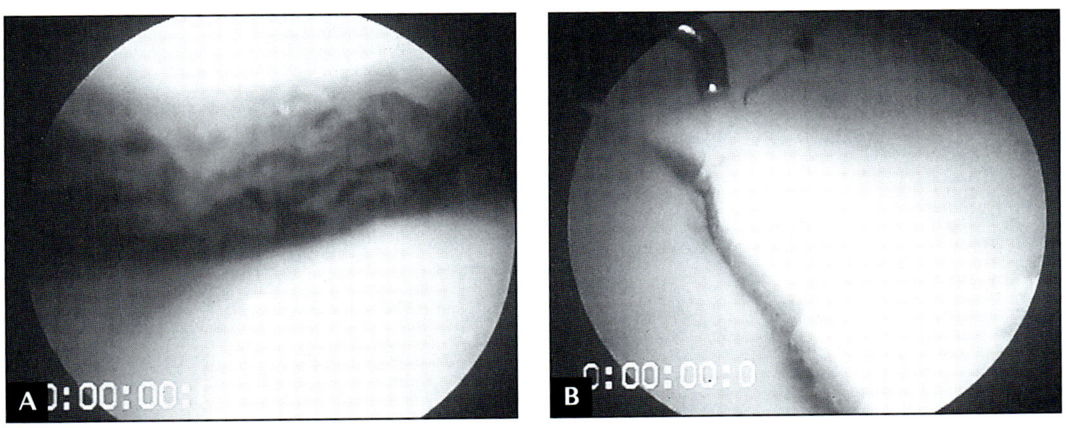

FIGURE 26-9. A, Arthroscopic view of coronal plane fracture displaced and stepped off. B, Arthroscopic view of same fracture from a radial portal to assist with fracture reduction and to visualize the dorsal fragment better. (*Copyright* TL Whipple.)

shortening, angulation, and associated soft-tissue injuries [5,7,8]. Restoration of the articular surface is probably the most important factor in all patients [6,8]. Knirk and Jupiter [8] found that articular depression greater than 1 mm resulted in symptomatic posttraumatic arthritis in 90% of patients. Displaced intra-articular comminuted fractures of the distal radius are often seen in younger patients who have sustained high energy trauma, although they are also seen in elderly patients with less trauma. In the younger patient who has high-energy trauma to create the same fracture, the incidence of associated injuries, both osseous and soft tissue, is greater.

It is important to individualize the method of treatment to the patient's needs as well as the configuration of the fracture. A summary of surgical treatment modalities are shown in Figure 26-13. Arthroscopy offers a technique of evaluating and treating some of the accompanying injuries that are often found with distal radius fractures especially with high-energy trauma in younger patients.

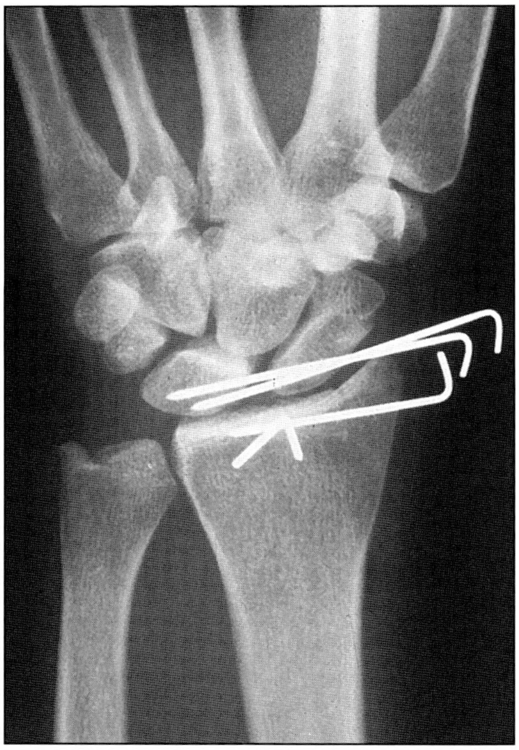

FIGURE 26-10. Postoperative radiograph of reduced articular fracture of the distal radius with concomitant reduction and fixation of displaced scapholunate dissociation under arthroscopic control. (*Copyright* TL Whipple.)

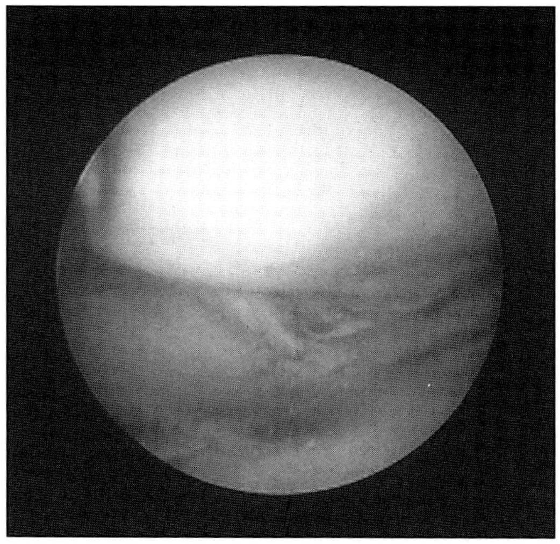

FIGURE 26-11. Arthroscopic view of subchondral contusion of left scaphoid with small articular cartilage fragments from the articular fracture of the radius. (*Copyright* TL Whipple.)

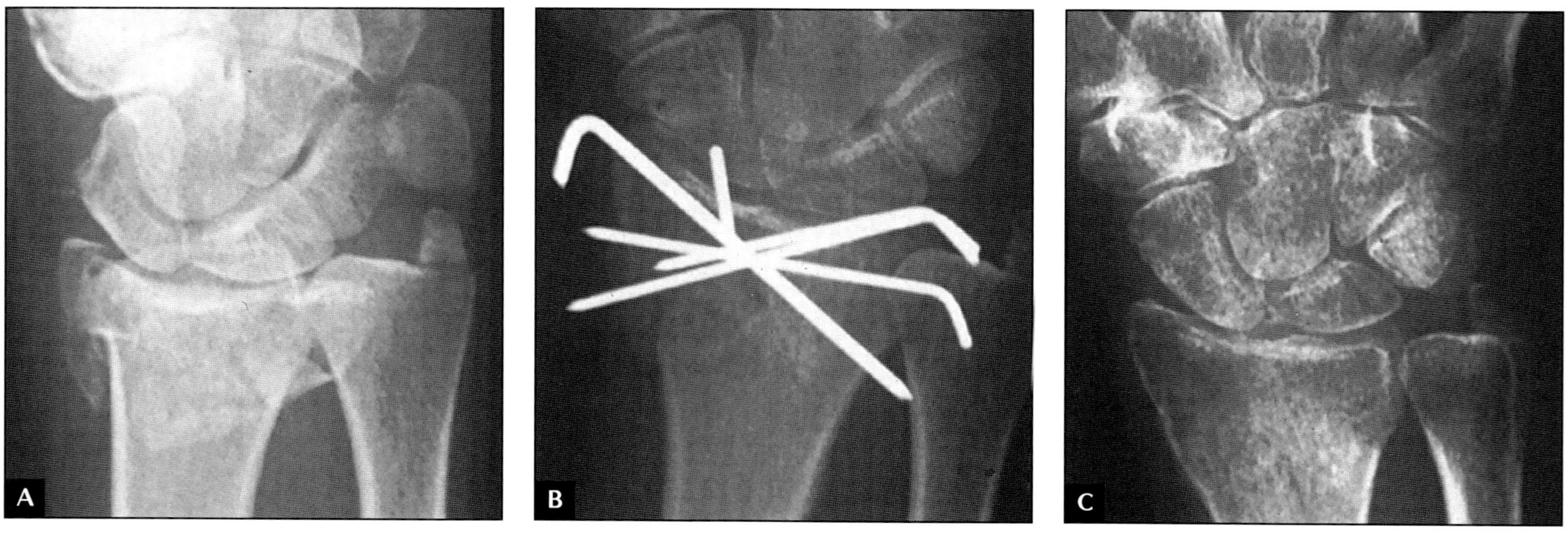

FIGURE 26-12. Comminuted intra-articular fracture of the distal radius seen soon after trauma (A), postoperatively after arthroscopically assisted reduction and fixation (B), and after healing (C). The articular surface has been restored with solid bone union and preserved joint spaces. (*Copyright* TL Whipple.)

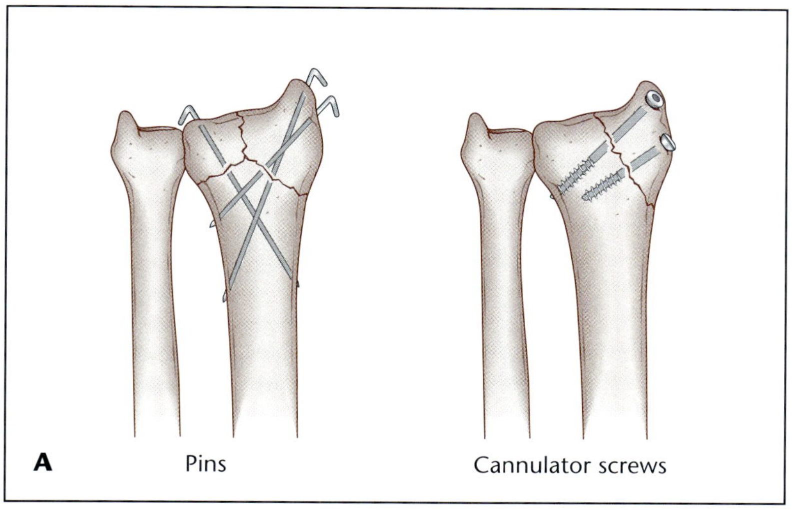

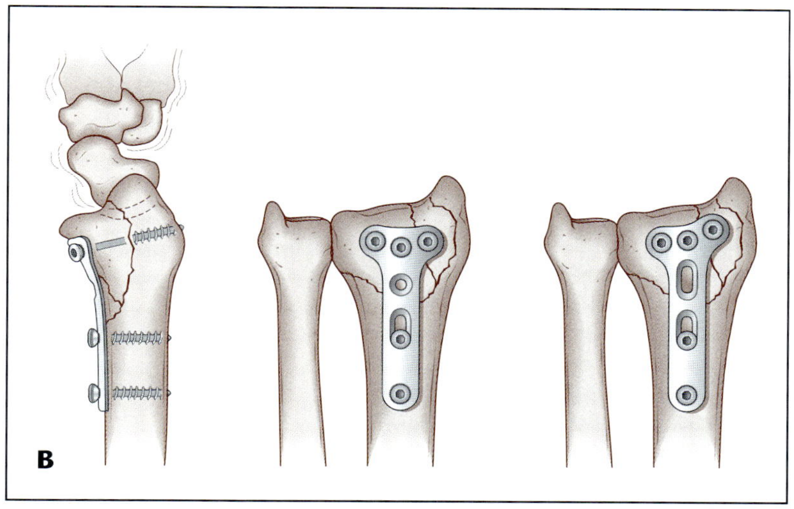

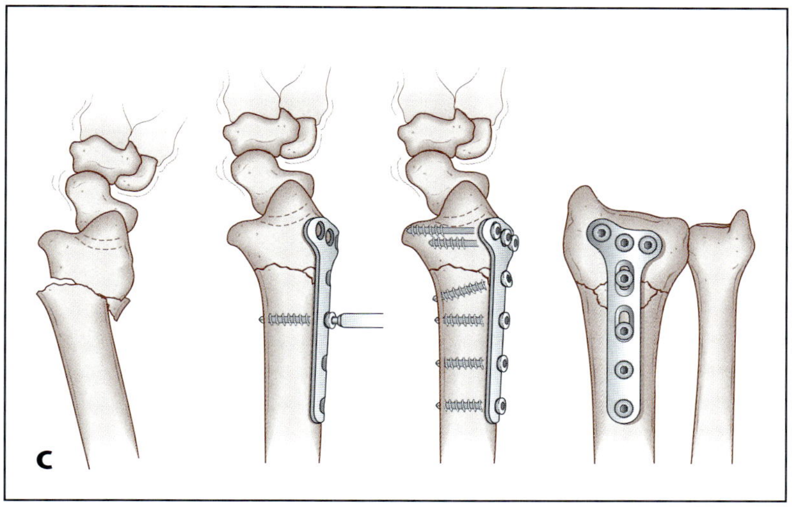

FIGURE 26-13. A, Percutaneous fixation of distal radius fracture. Pins are used in the example on the *right*, and screws in the example on the *left*. B, Open reduction of volar Barton's fractured radius. C, Open reduction and internal fixation with application of dorsal buttress plate. (*Adapted from* Müller *et al.* [20]).

REFERENCES AND RECOMMENDED READING

Recently published papers of particular interest have been highlighted as:
- • Of interest
- •• Of outstanding interest

1. Jupiter JB: Fractures of the distal end of the radius. *J Bone Joint Surg Am* 1991, 73:461–469.
2. The classic: on the fracture of the carpal extremity of the radius. Abraham Colles, Edinburgh Med Surg J. *Clin Orthop* 1972, 83:3–5.
3. Sanders WE: Distal radius fracture. In *Hand Surgery Update*. Edited by Rayhack JM. Base Inglewood, CO: American Society for Surgery of the Hand; 1994:36–42.
4. Cooney WP, Dobyns JH, Linscheid RL: Complications of Colles' fractures. *J Bone Joint Surg Am* 1980, 62:613–619.
5. Gartland JJ, Werley CW: Evaluation of healed Colles' fractures. *J Bone Joint Surg Am* 1951, 33:895–907.
6. Bradway JK, Amadio PC, Cooney WP: Open reduction and internal fixation of displaced, comminuted intra-articular fracture of the distal end of the radius. *J Bone Joint Surg Am* 1989, 71:839–847.
7. Culp RW, Osterman AL: Arthroscopic reduction and internal fixation of distal radius fractures. *Orthop Clin North Am* 1995, 26:739–748.
8. Knirk JL, Jupiter JB: Intra-articular fractures of the distal end of the radius in young adults. *J Bone Joint Surg Am* 1986, 68:647–659.
9. Sarmiento A, Pratt CW, Berry NC, Sinclair WF: Colles' fractures: functional bracing in supination. *J Bone Joint Surg Am* 1975, 57:311–317.
10. Jupiter JB: Complex articular fractures of the distal radius: classification and management. *J Am Acad Orthop Surg* 1997, 5:119–129.
11. Palmer AK: Fractures of the distal radius. In *Operative Hand Surgery* edn 3. Edited by Green DP. New York: Churchill Livingstone; 1993:929–971.
12. Van der Linden W, Ericson R: Colles' fracture: how should its displacement be measured and how should it be immobilized? *J Bone Joint Surg Am* 1981, 63:1285–1288.
13. King RE, Lovell W: Barton's enigma. *J Bone Joint Surg Am* 1959, 41:762–775.
14. Scheck M: Long term follow up of treatment of comminuted fractures of the distal end of the radius by transfixation with Kirschner wires and cast. *J Bone Joint Surg Am* 1962, 44:337–351.
15. Melone CP Jr: Distal radius fractures: patterns of articular fragmentation. *Orthop Clin North Am* 1993, 24:239–253.
16. Hastings H: Symposium: management of intra-articular fractures of the distal radius. *Contemp Orthop* 1990, 21:71–79.
17. Friberg S, Lundstrom B: Radiographic measurements of the radiocarpal joint in normal adults. *Acta Radiol Diagn (Stockh)* 1976, 17:249–256.
18. Rubinovich RN, Rennie WR: Colles' fracture: end results in relation to radiographic parameters. *Can J Surg* 1983, 26:361–363.
19. Tsukazaki T, Takagi K, Iwasaki K: Poor correlation between functional results and radiographic findings in Colles' fractures. *J Hand Surg Br* 1993, 18:588–591.
20. Müller ME, Nazarain S, Koch P, *et al.*: *The Comprehensive Classification of Fractures of Long Bones*. Berlin: Springer-Verlag; 1990.
21. Cassebaum WH: Colles' fracture: a study of end results. *JAMA* 1950, 143:963–965.

22. Older TM, Stabler EV, Cassebaum WH: Colles' fracture: evaluation and selection of therapy. *J Trauma* 1965, 5:469–476.
23. Frykman G: Fracture of the distal radius including sequelae-shoulder-hand-finger syndrome, disturbance in the distal radioulnar joint, and impairment of nerve function. *Acta Orthop Scand Suppl* 1967, 108:1–153.
24. Melone CP Jr: Articular fractures of the distal radius. *Orthop Clin North Am* 1984, 15:217–236.
25. Rayhack JM: Symposium: management of intra-articular fractures of the distal radius. *Contemp Orthop* 1990, 21:71–104.
26. Cooney WP, Berger RA: Treatment of complex fractures of the distal radius: combined use of internal and external fixation and arthroscopic reduction. *Hand Clin* 1993, 9:603–612.
27. Trumble TE, Schmitt SR, Vedder NB: Factors affecting functional outcome of displaced intra-articular distal radius fractures. *J Hand Surg Am* 1994, 19:325–340.
28. Solgaard S, Bunger C, Solund K: Displaced distal radius fractures: a comparative study of early results following external fixation, function bracing in supination, or dorsal plaster immobilization. *Arch Orthop Trauma Surg* 1989, 109:34–38.
29. Missakain ML, Cooney WP, Amadio PC, Glidewell HL: Open reduction and internal fixation of distal radius fractures. *J Hand Surg Am* 1992, 17:745–755.
30. McMurtry RY, Jupiter JB: Fractures of the distal radius. In *Skeletal Trauma*. Edited by Browner B, Jupiter JB, Levine AM, *et al.* Philadelphia: WB Saunders; 1996:1063–1095.
31. Lipton HS, Wollstein R: Operative treatment of intra-articular distal radius fractures. *Clin Orthop* 1996, 327:110–124.
32. Jupiter JB: Fractures of the distal end of the radius. *J Bone Joint Surg Am* 1991, 73:461–469.
33. Herndon JH: Distal radius fractures: nonsurgical treatment options. *Instr Course Lect* 1993, 42:67–72.
34. McQueen MM, MacLaren A, Chalmers J: The value of remanipulating Colles' fractures. *J Bone Joint Surg Br* 1986, 68:232–233.
35. DePalma AF: Comminuted fractures of the distal end of the radius treated by unlar pinning. *J Bone Joint Surg Am* 1952, 34:651–662.
36. Boehler L: *The Treatment of Fractures*. New York: Grune & Stratton;1929.
37. Green DP: Pins and plaster treatment of comminuted fractures of the distal end of the radius. *J Bone Joint Surg Am* 1975, 57:304–310.
38. Seitz WH: External fixation of distal radius fractures: indications and technical principles. *Orthop Clin North Am* 1993, 24:255–264.
39. Putnam M, Fischer MD: Treatment of unstable distal radius fractures: methods and comparison of external distraction and ORIF versus external distraction–ORIF neutralization. *J Hand Surg Am* 1997, 22:238–251.
40. Bartosh RA, Saldana MJ: Intra-articular fractures of the distal radius: a cadaveric study to determine if ligament otaxis restores radiopalmer tilt. *J Hand Surg* 1990, 15A:18–21.
41. Dienst M, Wozasek GE, Seligson D: Dynamic external fixation for distal radius fractures. *Clin Orthop* 1997, 338:160–171.
42. Clyburn TA: Dynamic external fixation for comminuted intra-articular fractures of the distal end of the radius. *J Bone Joint Surg Am* 1987, 69:248–254.
43. Bass RL, Blair WF, Hubbard PP.: Results of combined internal and external fixation for the treatment of severe AO-C3 fractures of the distal radius. *J Hand Surg Am* 1995, 20:373–381.
44. Axelrod T, Paley D, Green J, McMurtry RY: Limited open reduction of the lunate facet in comminuted intra-articular fractures of the distal radius. *J Hand Surg Am* 1988, 13:372–377.
45. Leung KS, Shen WY, Tsang HK, *et al.*: An effective treatment of comminuted fractures of the distal radius. *J Hand Surg Am* 1990, 15:11–17.
46. Axelrod TS, McMurtry RY: Open reduction and internal fixation of comminuted, intra-articular fractures of the distal radius. *J Hand Surg Am* 1990, 15:1–11.
47. Carter PR, Frederick HA, Laseter GF: Open reduction and internal fixation of unstable distal radius fractures with a low-profile plate: a multicenter study of 73 fractures. *J Hand Surg Am* 1998, 23:300–307.
48. Geissler WB: Arthroscopically assisted reduction of intra-articular fractures of the distal radius. *Hand Clin North Am* 1995, 11:19–29.
49. Geissler WB, Freeland AE: Arthroscopically assisted reduction of intra-articular distal radius fractures. *Clin Orthop* 1996, 327:125–134.
50. Fernandez DL, Geissler WB: Treatment of displaced articular fractures of the radius. *J Hand Surg Am* 1991, 16:375–384.
51. Whipple TL: The role of arthroscopy in the treatment of intra-articular wrist fractures. *Hand Clin* 1995, 11:13–18.
52. Mudgal CS, Jones WA: Scapholunate diastasis: a component of fractures of the distal radius. *J Hand Surg Br* 1990, 15:503–505.
53. Hixon ML, Walker CW, Fitzrandolph RL, *et al.*: Acute ligament tears of the wrist associated with Colles' fractures. *Orthop Trans* 1990, 14:164–169.
54. Wolfe SW, Easterling KJ, Yoo HH: Arthroscopic-assisted reduction of distal radius fractures. *Arthroscopy* 1995, 11:706–714.

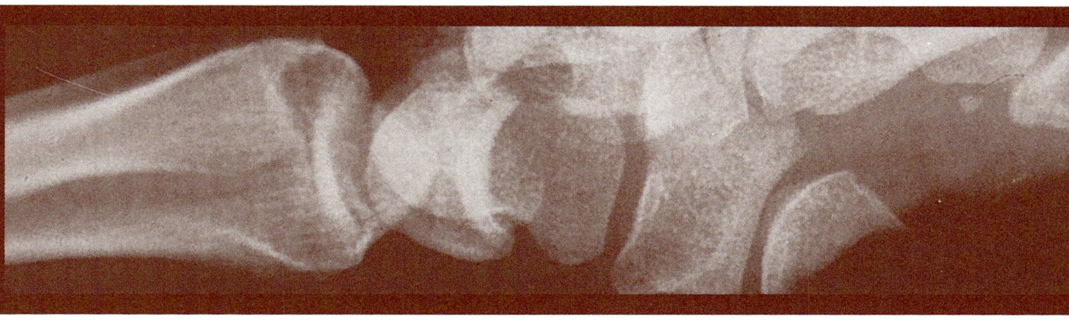

27

Fracture-Dislocations of the Wrist

Robert R. Slater, Jr.

Wrist fractures and fracture-dislocations are common injuries. In major trauma centers, 28.6% of all injuries involve the hand or wrist [1]. Fractures involving the wrist occur most often in the distal radius, but the incidence of scaphoid fractures is a close second [2]. Lunate and perilunate dislocations and fracture-dislocations constitute about 10% of all carpal injuries [3]. Other forms of carpal dislocations are less common but no less important. Missed diagnoses and delays in treatment can have devastating consequences. In this chapter, the anatomic features and the pathomechanics of carpal fractures and fracture-dislocations are reviewed along with specific injury patterns and recommendations for their treatment.

ANATOMY AND BIOMECHANICS: INJURY PATTERNS EXPLAINED

The wrist is a complex arrangement of carpal bones and soft tissue structures. Over the years, many authors have offered conflicting theories that attempt to categorize the carpal bones into functional units [4–7]. Universal among all concepts of carpal mechanics, however, is the importance of a delicate balance inherent throughout the wrist and how easily injuries can disrupt that balance.

Knowledge of the ligamentous anatomy is especially critical in understanding and treating carpal dislocations. The wrist ligaments are intracapsular, which makes them difficult to visualize at surgery because they are covered by a joint capsule. They are best seen arthroscopically. Using current nomenclature [8], there are five important palmar ligaments (Figure 27-1) and two dorsal ligaments (Figure 27-2) [9••]. Palmarly, three principal structures secure the carpus to the radius: the radioscaphocapitate (RSC), long radiolunate (LRL), and short radiolunate (SRL) ligaments. The RSC originates from the radial styloid and inserts on the palmar capitate through a groove in the palmar scaphoid waist. It has two subunits, classified more by their fiber insertion than any discrete anatomic divisions. The radioscaphoid subunit, which runs between the proximal pole of the scaphoid and the distal radius, serves as a prime stabilizer of the proximal pole of the scaphoid. Rotary subluxation and dislocation of the scaphoid cannot occur unless this ligament and the scapholunate interosseous ligament are disrupted [10,11•]. The other subunit is the scaphocapitate ligament, which contributes to the link between proximal and distal carpal rows. The LRL courses from the palmar rim of the distal radius to the radial margin of the palmar horn of the lunate. The SRL originates from the palmar rim of the radius at the level of the lunate facet and inserts on the palmar surface of the lunate, where it blends in with fibers from the triangular fibrocartilage complex (TFCC).

The two remaining important palmar ligaments originate from the ulna as part of the TFCC and insert onto the lunate and triquetrum: the ulnolunate and ulnotriquetral ligaments (Figure 27-1). Just distal to the insertion of the ligaments on the lunate and between the LRL and RSC ligaments is an area of relatively thin areolar tissue palmar to the capitolunate articulation first described by Poirier and Charpy in 1926 [12]. It is through this potential weak spot, the "space of Poirier" that the lunate usually dislocates.

The dorsal wrist ligaments (Figure 27-2) have been described [13,14] as two thickenings of the dorsal wrist capsule. The dorsal radiocarpal ligament originates from the radius, runs obliquely over the lunate, and inserts primarily on the triquetrum. The dorsal intercarpal ligament runs more transversely across the wrist. It has some fibers that insert on the dorsal scaphoid waist, but the bulk of the ligament inserts on the triquetrum and the trapezium.

The intrinsic ligaments in the proximal carpal row, that is, the scapholunate and lunotriquetral interosseous ligaments, allow some rotation and translation between bones. The lunotriquetral interosseous ligament is a thin fibrocartilaginous structure with poor intrinsic vascularity [15]. The scapholunate interosseous ligament (SLIL) has three distinct regions [16•]. The dorsal portion is thickest, with short, transversely oriented collagen fibers; the proximal region is primarily fibrocartilaginous; and the palmar area is thin and composed of obliquely oriented collagen fibers. These morphologic features have implications for tissue repair and healing potential after injury. For example, a dorsal approach to a perilunate dislocation may allow suture repair of the stoutest portion of the SLIL.

The carpal bones of the distal row are aligned in a relatively rigid arch with the convexity positioned dorsally. Only slight rotational motions occur between carpal bones as the wrist moves [17]. The interosseous ligaments in the distal row keep it functioning and moving almost as a single unit [11•,18,19].

The end result of any traumatic force applied to the extended wrist depends on the direction and point of impact of that force, hand position at the time of impact, and the relative strength of the carpal bones and ligaments. Analysis of cadaver loading experiments led Mayfield *et al.* [20–22] to propose a theory of "progressive perilunar instability" (Figure 27-3). Subsequent authors have further clarified the forces likely acting on the hand and wrist and their progression to explain the common injuries seen clinically [23], but the basic concepts originally outlined by Mayfield's team continue to offer a useful framework for conceptualization of injury patterns on the radial side of the wrist. The sequence of ligamentous disruptions begins on the radial aspect of the wrist, progresses distally, and then continues circumferentially around the lunate. There are four stages of instability (Figure 27-3). Stage I includes scapholunate dissociation, caused by disruption of the SLIL and RSC ligaments. Stage II is capitate dislocation, with disruption of the capitolunate joint through Poirier's space (Figure 27-1). Stage III is triquetral dislocation, with disruption of the lunotriquetral ligament. Stage IV is lunate dislocation, with tear-

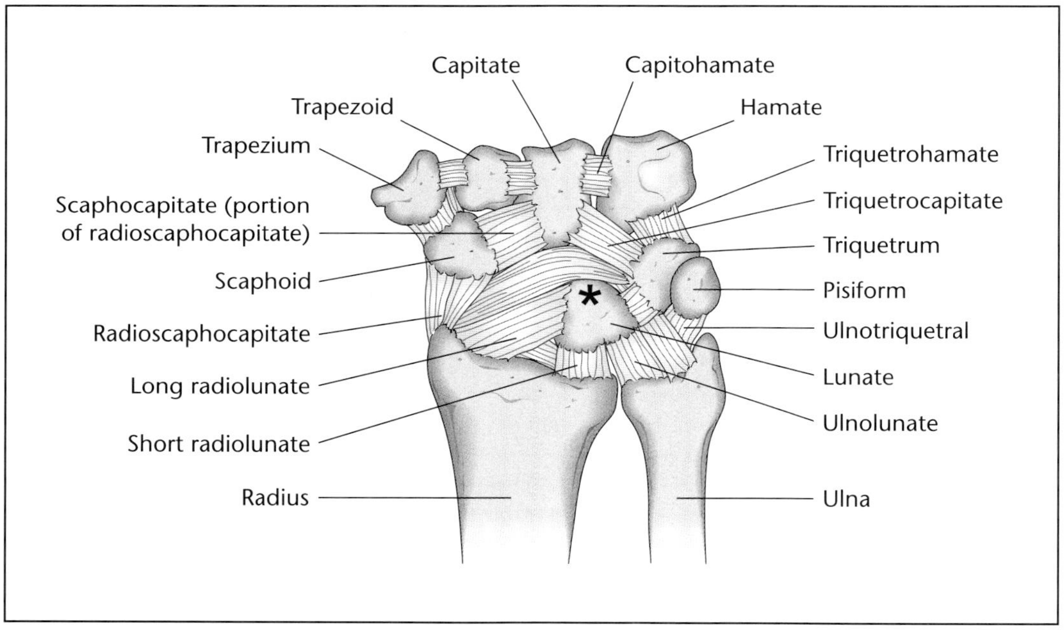

FIGURE 27-1. Extrinsic carpal ligaments from a palmar perspective. The space of Poirier (indicated by *asterisk*) is the area relatively void of ligamentous support on the palmar surface of the lunate between the sweeping arcs of proximal and distal capsular ligaments. (*Adapted from* Berger [9••].)

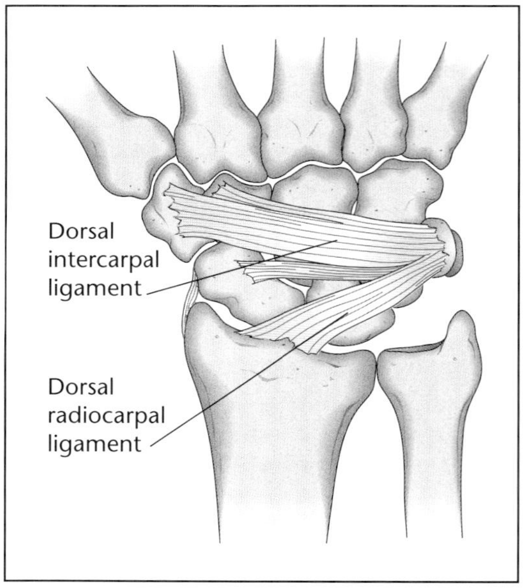

FIGURE 27-2. Extrinsic ligaments on the dorsal side of the wrist. The dorsal radiocarpal ligament originates from the radius and inserts on the triquetrum. The dorsal intercarpal ligament originates from the triquetrum and courses obliquely and distally to insert on the trapezium and trapezoid with a few fibers inserting on the dorsal ridge of the scaphoid as well.

ing of the dorsal capsule and radiocarpal ligament; the lunate may be flipped into the carpal tunnel [24] or, more rarely, displaced into the distal forearm [25].

This concept of progressive perilunar instability is consistent with the most common injury patterns in which the primary dislocation occurs at the midcarpal joint and the capitate is initially displaced dorsal to the lunate. Instability can be limited to the ulnar side of the wrist; however, this finding is not explained by Mayfield's original theory. Therefore, Viegas *et al.* [15] described a staging system for ulnar-sided perilunate instability (Figure 27-4). Stage I of this system involves partial or complete disruption of the lunotriquetral ligament; radiographic evidence of dynamic or static instability may or may not present. Stage II includes complete lunotriquetral ligament tear with clinical and radiographic evidence of *dynamic* volar intercalated segment instability (VISI). Stage III includes *static* VISI deformity.

DIAGNOSIS

Clinical diagnosis of a carpal fracture or dislocation begins with taking the history of the injury mechanism. The key element of the history is a significant force applied to the outstretched hand, usually resulting from a fall or motor vehicle accident. Physical examination after carpal dislocations and fracture-dislocations often reveals diffuse wrist swelling and tenderness. It may be difficult to localize areas of maximal tenderness but specific areas should be palpated, including the radial styloid, scaphoid, lunate, scapholunate joint, triquetrum, and carpal tunnel. Initial clinical evaluation must include a careful assessment of the neurovascular status of the hand, because median nerve injury is present in approximately 40% of these injuries [23,26–28] and other neurovascular structures may also be injured.

DIAGNOSTIC IMAGING

Diagnosis of carpal dislocations and fracture-dislocations is confirmed primarily on the basis of radiographs (Figures 27-5 through 27-9) [29]. Routine posteroanterior (PA), lateral, and oblique views usually suffice. Gilula [30] has stressed the importance of examining the PA views for three smooth arches along the proximal and distal edges of the proximal carpal row and the proximal edge of the distal carpal row. Any break in continuity of any arch suggests an abnormality at the site of the broken arch. Either flexion or extension of the lunate can make it appear more triangular on the PA view and cause a break in Gilula's lines, which suggests an abnormality [30–32]. These lines must be interpreted with cau-

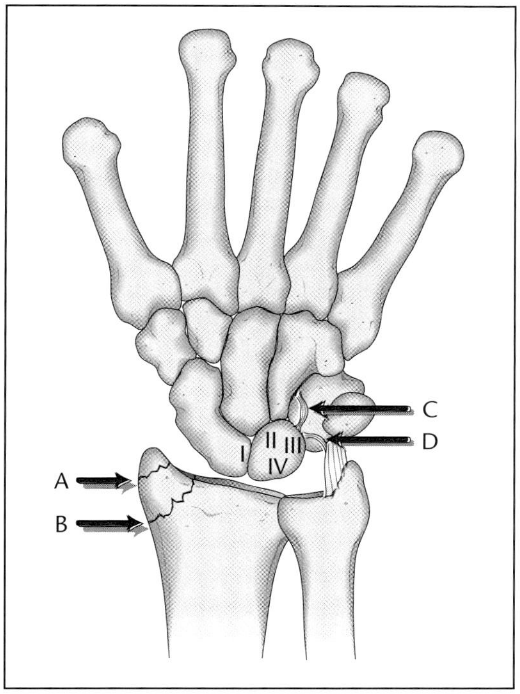

FIGURE 27-3. Progressive lunate instability occurs in four stages. Stage I begins with injury to the scapholunate interosseous ligament. Stage II includes failure of the midcarpal portion of the radioscaphocapitate ligament (or alternatively fracture of the scaphoid). Stage III includes injury of the lunotriquetral and ulnotriquetral ligaments. Stage IV includes rupture of the dorsal radiocarpal ligament allowing palmar dislocation of the lunate. Associated fractures may include: *A*, radial styloid tip; *B*, radial styloid body; *C*, lunotriquetral ligament avulsion; and *D*, ulnotriquetral ligament avulsion. (*Adapted from* Mayfield *et al.* [21].)

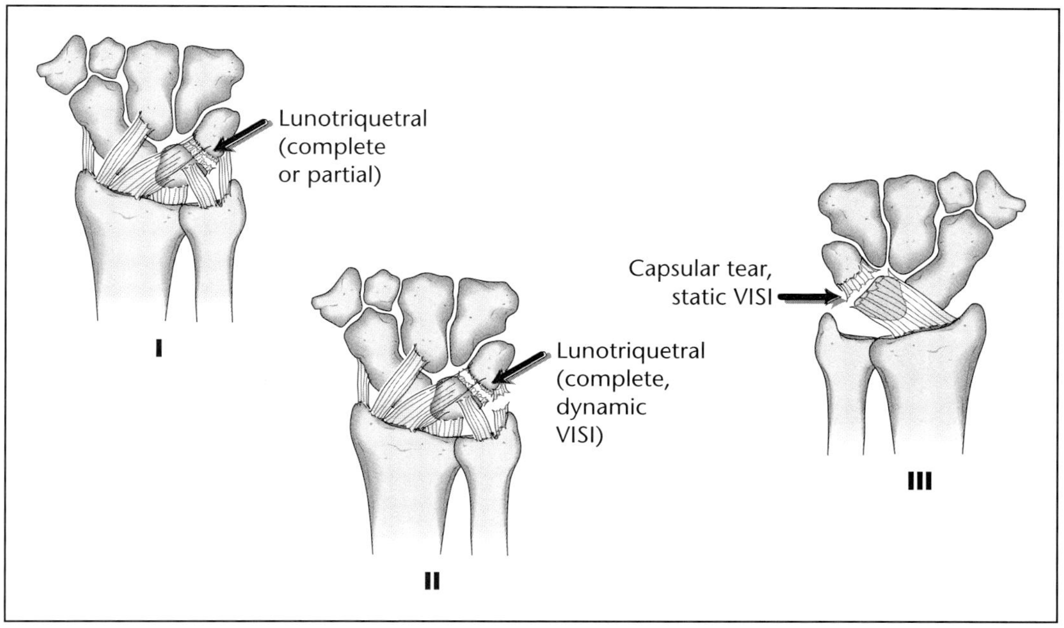

FIGURE 27-4. Classification of ulnar-sided perilunate instability. Stage I—disruption of the lunotriquetral interosseous ligament; Stage II—disruption of the palmar ulnotriquetral in addition to the lunotriquetral ligament; Stage III—disruption of the dorsal radiocarpal ligament. Stages I and II shown from palmar perspective; stage III shown from dorsal perspective. VISI—volar intercalated segment instability. (*Adapted from* Viegas *et al.* [15].)

tion, however, because a more recent study by Peh and Gilula [33•] showed that these arcs are commonly disrupted, even in normal wrists, if the wrist is not in a strictly neutral position.

Carpal bone alignment is best measured on the lateral radiograph. Guidelines for measuring and interpreting the scapholunate, capitolunate, and radiolunate angles have been defined and are considered a routine part of establishing carpal malalignment [32,34,35]. The following guidelines have been established: normal capitolunate angle is 0° and anything greater than 15° is abnormal; normal scapholunate angle is less than 60° and anything greater than 80° is abnormal; normal radiolunate angle is 0° and an angle greater than 15° is abnormal. The values between abnormal and the upper limits of normal are considered "gray zones."

OTHER DIAGNOSTIC TECHNIQUES

Other diagnostic techniques are helpful in some cases. Distraction radiographs can be obtained with the fingers in finger traps and with a 10- to 15-lb counterweight applied to the patient's arm. Usually these views are obtained as a regular part of treatment (*eg*, when preparing to reduce an acute injury) rather than simply for

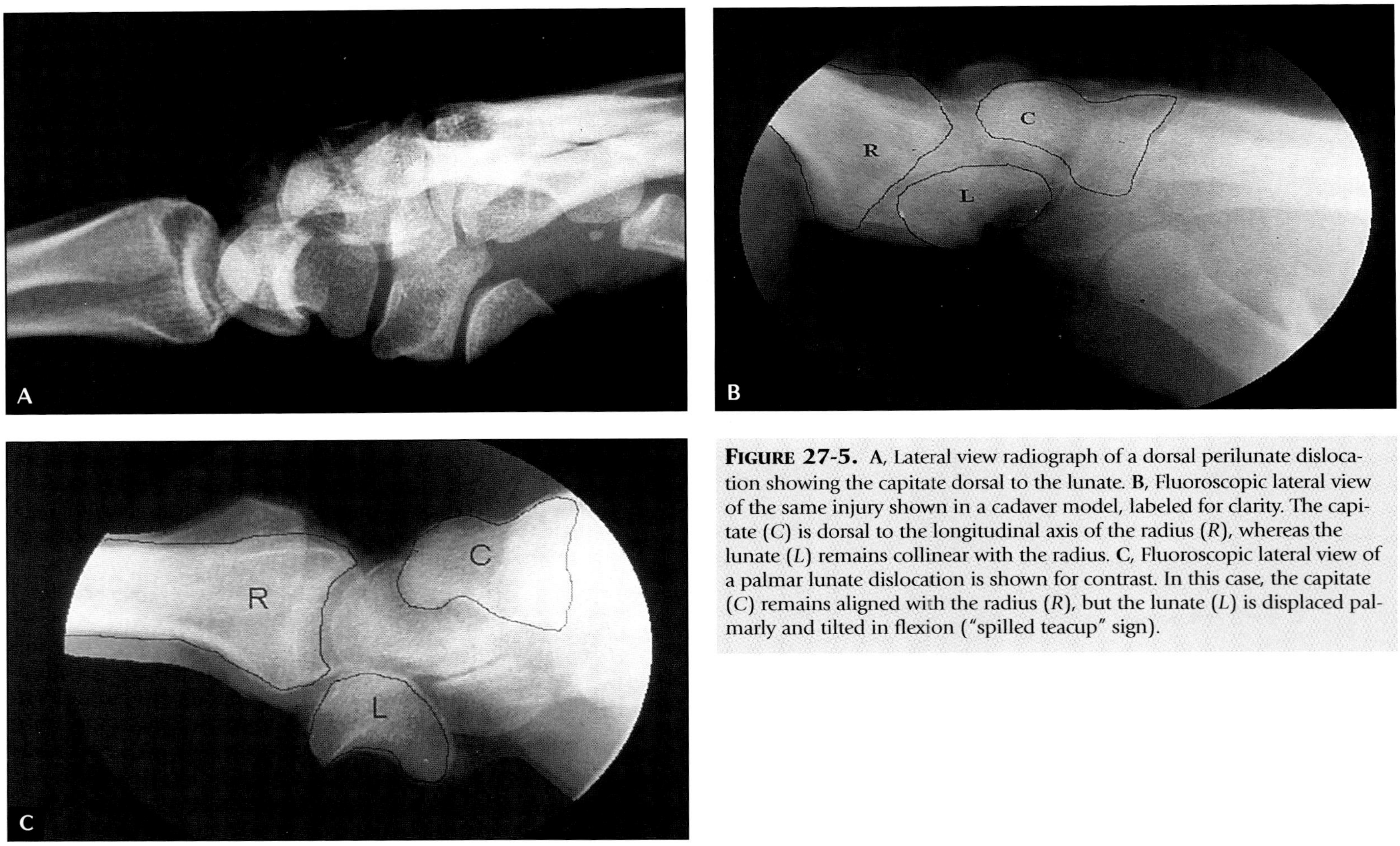

FIGURE 27-5. **A**, Lateral view radiograph of a dorsal perilunate dislocation showing the capitate dorsal to the lunate. **B**, Fluoroscopic lateral view of the same injury shown in a cadaver model, labeled for clarity. The capitate (*C*) is dorsal to the longitudinal axis of the radius (*R*), whereas the lunate (*L*) remains collinear with the radius. **C**, Fluoroscopic lateral view of a palmar lunate dislocation is shown for contrast. In this case, the capitate (*C*) remains aligned with the radius (*R*), but the lunate (*L*) is displaced palmarly and tilted in flexion ("spilled teacup" sign).

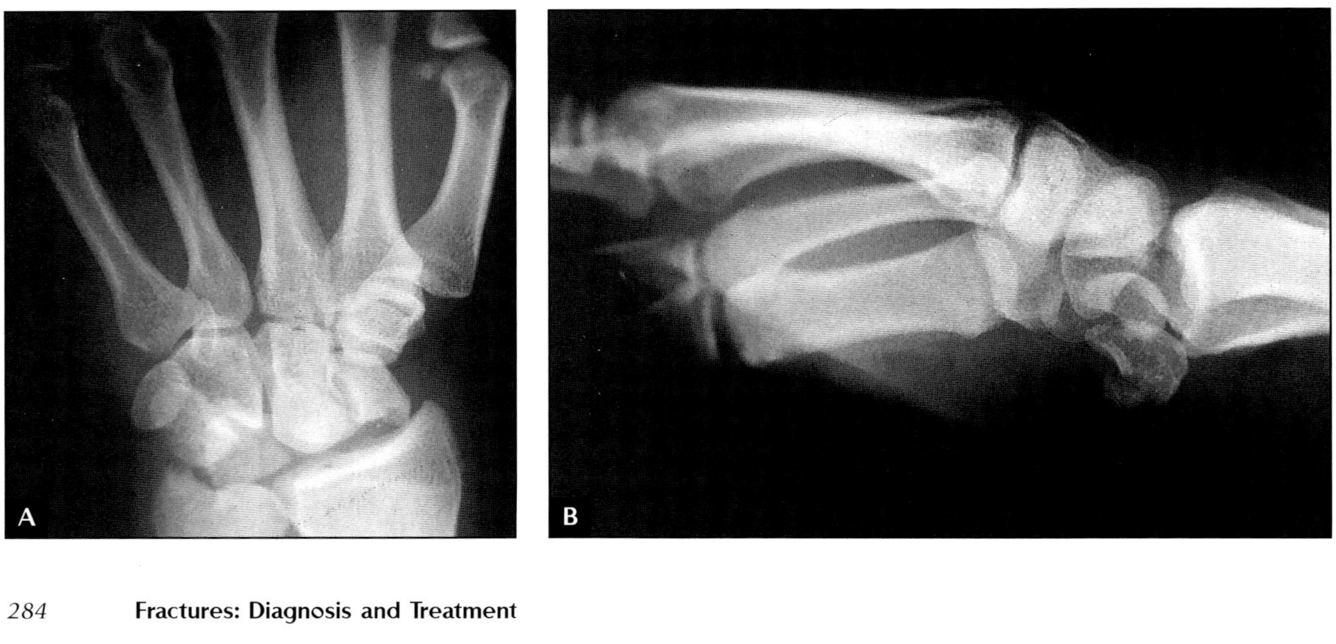

FIGURE 27-6. **A**, Posteroanterior radiograph of a transradial styloid dorsal perilunate dislocation. Carpal overlap, disruption of Gilula's lines, a triangular lunate, and proximal migration of the capitate are shown. **B**, Lateral radiograph of the same injury showing the lunate and proximal pole of the scaphoid together and palmar to the capitate.

diagnosis. Other studies with special indications include examination of the wrist under fluoroscopic control with or without arthrography, bone scans, computed tomography (CT) scans, magnetic resonance imaging (MRI), and arthroscopy.

CLASSIFICATION

To help plan treatment, it is useful to classify carpal fractures and fracture-dislocations according to injury pattern.

Scaphoid Fractures and Dislocations

Isolated scaphoid fractures are common and account for approximately 70% of all carpal bone injuries. Essential to treatment decision making is whether the fracture is displaced (*ie,* greater than 1 mm).

In contrast, true dislocations of the scaphoid (without fracture) occur but are rare. It has been postulated [36] that scaphoid dislocations result from a sequence of ligamentous failures that begins with disruption of the RSC and SLIL ligaments and then progresses to include the LRL and scaphotrapezial ligaments, which results in complete instability of the scaphoid. Displacement of the proximal pole out of the scaphoid fossa is diagnostic for scaphoid dislocation rather than perilunate dislocation.

Dorsal Perilunate Dislocation or Palmar Lunate Dislocation

These entities, once believed separate, are better considered as progressive stages of the same injury [26]. The lateral radiograph is the most revealing (Figure 27-5). In a dorsal perilunate dislocation, the capitate is shown dorsal to the longitudinal axis and the radius. Dorsal rotation of the proximal pole of the scaphoid is also shown. In a lunate dislocation, the forces causing the injury may have resulted in spontaneous reduction of the capitate and the distal carpal row and complete palmar displacement of the lunate. In this case, the lateral radiograph shows the capitate nearly colinear with the longitudinal axis of the radius, and the lunate's distal articular surface faces palmarly to produce the so-called "spilled-teacup" sign [26]. The lateral view also shows dorsal displacement of the triquetrum secondary to the tear in the lunotriquetral ligament.

The PA radiograph continues to show carpal overlap and disruption of Gilula's lines. Because of the disruption between the scaphoid and lunate and the forces acting on the carpal bones, the scaphoid will drop into flexion and the lunate will rotate into extension. This is demonstrated by the presence of the "signet-ring" sign on the PA radiograph, which is the radiographic shadow of the distal pole of the scaphoid seen in cross-section, indicating its flexed posture and a triangular lunate. Typically, a wide gap is also apparent between the scaphoid and lunate. This was once called the "Terry Thomas sign" [37] after the British comedian with a wide front tooth diastasis, but this eponym is perhaps better updated as the "David Letterman sign."

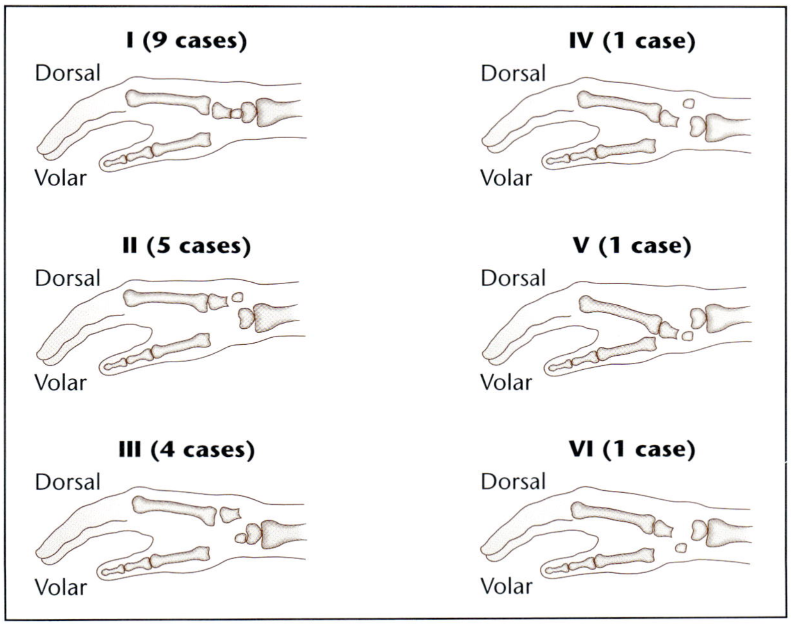

Figure 27-7. Diagram of six patterns of scaphocapitate fracture-dislocations. (*Adapted from* Vance *et al.* [29].)

Dorsal Transcaphoid Perilunate Dislocation

The hallmark of this injury is the displaced scaphoid fracture (Figure 27-6). In this injury, the distal pole of the scaphoid displaces dorsally with the capitate and the lunate remains attached to the proximal pole of the scaphoid. The lunotriquetral ligament may be torn in some cases (*eg,* Mayfield's stage IV equivalent).

Palmar Perilunate Dislocation or Dorsal Lunate Dislocation

This injury pattern is rare. The mechanism of injury remains uncertain and has been much debated; some authors postulate forceful wrist hyperflexion sustained by falling on the back of the hand [38–40]. Others suggest that severe wrist hyperextension can produce this injury as well as the more common dorsal perilunate dislocation [13,38–41]. In one study, Niazi [41] was able to reproduce palmar perilunate dislocations reliably in a series of cadavers by sectioning the scaphotrapezial and palmar radiocarpal ligaments and applying a dorsal shearing force.

Combination Injuries

The most common combination injury is the transradial styloid perilunate fracture-dislocation (Figure 27-9). In this injury, force is dissipated by fracturing through the radial styloid and scapholunate interosseous ligament rather than the scaphoid. Isolated radial styloid fractures are sometimes referred to as "chauffeur's fractures," but if the history suggests a high-velocity fall or axial load, then associated carpal bone fracture and ligamentous instability, specifically of the scapholunate interosseous ligament, must be ruled out. The clinician should have a high index of suspicion for these associated injuries.

Scaphocapitate syndrome (Figure 27-7) is a rare pattern of wrist injury first described by Nicholson in 1940 [42]. Several variants have been described, all of which usually result from severe trauma. Its hallmark is the presence of transverse fractures of both the scaphoid and the capitate with rotation of the proximal pole of the capitate so that its articular surface faces distally [29]. It has been postulated [43] that this syndrome occurs most often in extreme wrist extension when the dorsal rim of the radius impinges on the capitate, thus fracturing it, whereas the scaphoid fractures occur as the result of stress between the proximal and distal carpal rows that is generated by the extreme extension. Midcarpal dislocation then occurs and the proximal pole of the capitate rotates 90° to 180°.

Spontaneous relocation may occur, which leaves only the fractured scaphoid and inverted capitate fragment as evidence of this injury.

Despite displacement of the capitate fragment, this fracture can be missed on routine radiographs and thus mismanaged as a simple scaphoid fracture. The relationship of the radius to the lunate and fractured capitate should be assessed critically on the lateral radiograph. Distraction-view films, sometimes helpful in this situation, will show the squared-off end of the proximal capitate.

Transtriquetral fracture-dislocations occur when the applied force exits through the triquetrum. In such cases, the proximal-radial fragment remains with the lunate through its attachment with the lunotriquetral ligament, whereas the distal-ulnar fragment displaces with the capitate. This can occur in association with perilunate dislocations [26,44] or in association with scaphocapitate syndrome [45].

Longitudinal Disruptions

A constellation of uncommon carpal dislocations and instabilities between the radial and ulnar sides of the carpus can be considered together as longitudinal disruptions. *Axial dislocations of the carpus* fall into this category (Figure 27-8). Rarely seen, they result from blast or crush injuries in which the carpus is separated longitudinally and usually displaced with the respective metacarpals. The hand is flattened with destruction of the normal convex relationship between the metacarpal heads [19]. Because of the mechanism of injury, significant associated soft-tissue injuries and thenar lacerations are frequently noted. Garcia-Elias *et al.* [19,46] have classified these injuries into 3 variants: axial-radial (most common), axial-ulnar, and combined axial-radial-ulnar (least common). In the *axial-radial* type, the radial column is displaced radially and proximally, whereas the ulnar column remains stable with respect to the radius. In *axial-ulnar* disruption, the ulnar column is shifted proximally and ulnarly, whereas the radial column remains relatively stable. In *combined axial-radial-ulnar* injuries, both columns displace proximally.

TREATMENT

Treatment strategy can be determined largely on injury pattern. Although specific treatment must be individualized for each patient, some general guidelines may be useful. A detailed physical examination must be completed first, with attention to identifying and documenting associated injuries and possible neurovascular deficits. If any dislocations are present, particularly if the lunate is displaced in the carpal tunnel such as may occur after perilunate dislocations, they should be reduced immediately to obtain gross carpal alignment and relieve pressure on the median nerve. Beyond these initial steps, the particular treatment must depend on the specific injury and its classification.

Scaphoid Fractures

Nondisplaced fractures of the scaphoid are usually treated nonoperatively. A thumb spica splint or bivalved cast should be applied initially to allow for swelling and converted to a standard thumb spica cast after 5 to 7 days. If a scaphoid fracture is suspected based on history and physical examination but is not evident radiographically, the wrist initially should be immobilized in a thumb spica splint. The patient should then be reexamined after 10 to 14 days to confirm or rule out a fracture. If at that time the physical examination still suggests a fracture but the original radiographs indicate no fracture, a bone scan or MRI should be obtained to evaluate for an occult fracture. Radiographs repeated at that time do not increase diagnostic accuracy, assuming the original films were of adequate quality. I prefer a bone scan because it is less expensive, easily obtained, provides information sufficient to make decisions about treatment, and has reported specificity and sensitivity of 98% and 100%, respectively. If a fracture is confirmed, the wrist should again be immobilized in a thumb spica cast.

It is controversial whether the initial cast should extend above the elbow. Some evidence [47] suggests that duration of time to union may be slightly shorter if the cast extends above the elbow to inhibit forearm rotation, but other studies show no difference. It has also been shown that the institution of early immobilization is more important than the extent of the cast [48,49]. My preference is to treat these injuries in a below-elbow thumb spica cast, because activities of daily living are much easier and elbow stiffness avoided if the elbow has not been not immobilized. Healing can take up to 4 months [47,48]. Because plain radiographs are unreliable for judging union, it should be confirmed with plain tomography or CT scans before the patient is allowed to return to unrestricted activity, particularly if he or she performs physical labor or is an athlete in a contact sport [50].

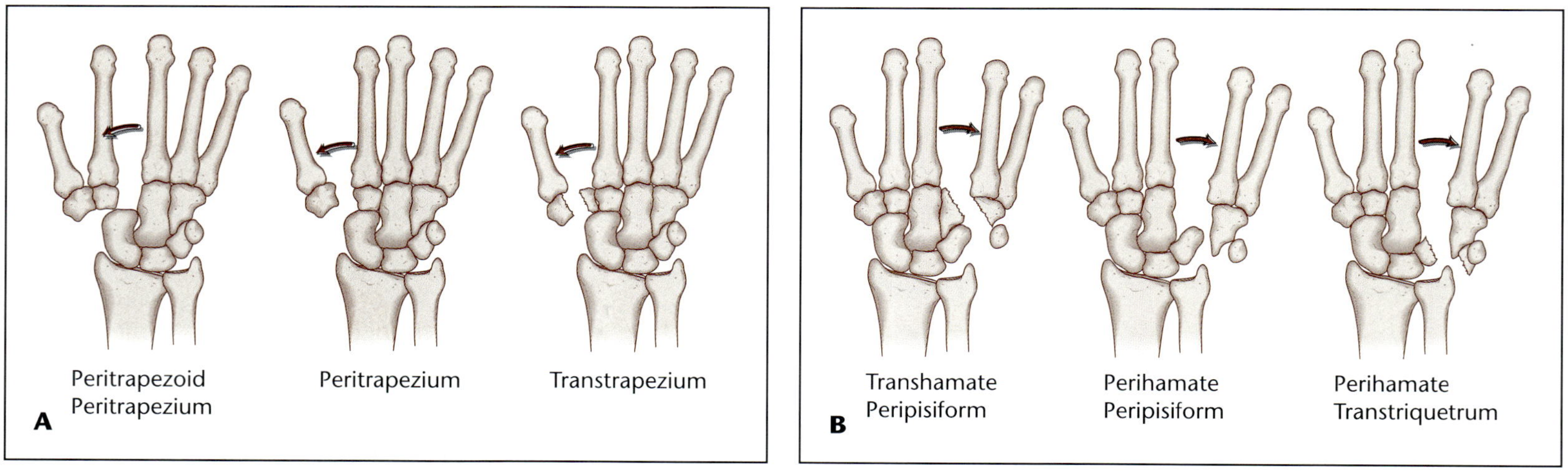

FIGURE 27-8. Longitudinal disruptions of the carpus. The most common types are shown. **A**, Three axial-radial disruptions. **B**, Three axial-ulnar disruptions. Combined injuries also may occur but are rare. (*Adapted from* Garcia-Elias [19].)

Displaced or unstable scaphoid fractures should be treated surgically. Acceptable therapeutic methods include open reduction and internal fixation with Kirschner (K)-wires or screw fixation. Primary bone grafting is indicated in those cases in which extensive comminution has occurred. Delayed unions (*ie,* more than 4 months) and nonunions also indicate operative treatment of scaphoid fractures. Distal pole and waist fractures are often best approached palmarly (as detailed later in this chapter), but proximal pole fractures may be treated from a dorsal approach. Vascularized bone grafts are gaining popularity as a method for treating scaphoid fractures, particularly nonunions, and usually are performed using a dorsal approach [51,52].

Scaphoid dislocations are rare, but the goals of treatment are routine and focus on restoration of the scapholunate relationship. The damaged SLIL should be repaired whenever possible. The role of arthroscopy in managing these injuries is evolving. In a series of three scaphoid dislocations [36], arthroscopy provided useful information about the status of the SLIL and radiocarpal ligaments and allowed thorough joint débridement and removal of loose chondral fragments as part of definitive management.

Perilunate Dislocations

The first step in treating perilunate dislocations is to obtain preliminary reduction. To do so, it is useful to apply traction with finger traps using 10- to 15-lb counterforce at the arm for 10 minutes after appropriately anesthetizing the wrist and sedating the patient. During that time, distraction radiographs may be obtained to delineate the pathology further if any questions about associated injuries remain. The fingertraps should then be removed while longitudinal manual traction is maintained. The clinician should extend the patient's wrist with one hand while using his or her opposite thumb to stabilize the patient's lunate palmarly. The injured wrist should then be flexed gradually, which delivers the head of the capitate back into the lunate concavity, usually with a palpable and audible "clunk." The wrist must be splinted in neutral position and then PA and lateral postreduction radiographs should be obtained.

The scapholunate angle shown on postreduction radiographs should be less than 60° on the lateral view and the scapholunate gap should be less than 2 mm on the PA view. If anatomic reduction is obtained, some researchers have advocated percutaneous pinning using fluoroscopy [13]. In fact, it is highly unlikely that a truly anatomic reduction can be achieved, let alone maintained, by closed means [24,27,53,54]. Therefore, open reduction and fixation are preferred.

One area of controversy in the literature is the preferred surgical approach: dorsal, palmar, or both. Many authors have recommended a dorsal approach because it offers good exposure of the proximal carpal row and midcarpal joint [20,23,55]. Others recommend a palmar approach [24,56], and some recommend using a combined dorsal and palmar approach routinely

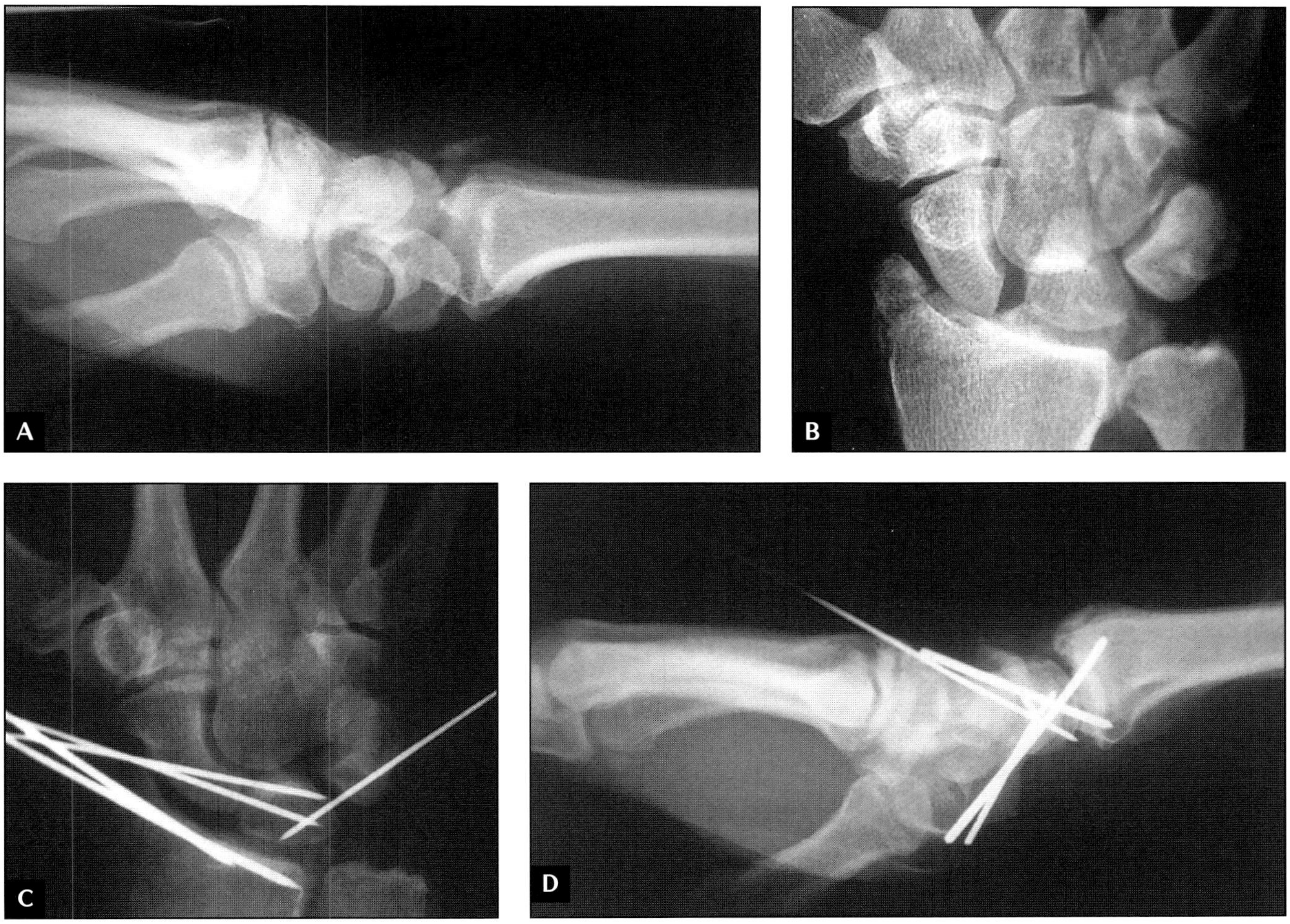

FIGURE 27-9. A, Lateral radiograph of a transradial styloid dorsal perilunate fracture-dislocation. Note the capitate is dorsal to the lunate, which is collinear with the radius. **B**, Posteroanterior (PA) radiograph of the same injury. Note the styloid fracture, pie-shaped lunate, and increased scapholunate gap. **C**, PA radiograph following open reduction and pinning through a dorsal approach. **D**, Postoperative lateral radiograph; note the restoration of collinearity between the radius, lunate and capitate.

[13,44,57,58•,59,60], arguing that the palmar approach provides an opportunity to visualize and repair the palmar ligaments.

A palmar approach is unnecessary for treating most perilunate dislocations. Although the palmar radiocarpal structures are distinct structures when viewed from within the joint, they cannot be distinguished when seen from the palmar side because of the overlying capsule. Traumatic disruption of the normal tissues compounds the problem, making it unlikely that they can be repaired in their correct orientation and under proper tension. It is more likely that attempts to repair the ligaments directly shorten them and thus produce further scarring of the surrounding soft tissues and, ultimately, loss of wrist motion. Recurrent palmar dislocation after a lunate or perilunate dislocation is unlikely; stiffness is far more common. Therefore, a dorsal approach to the wrist is recommended for treating perilunate dislocations with a few exceptions (discussed later in the chapter).

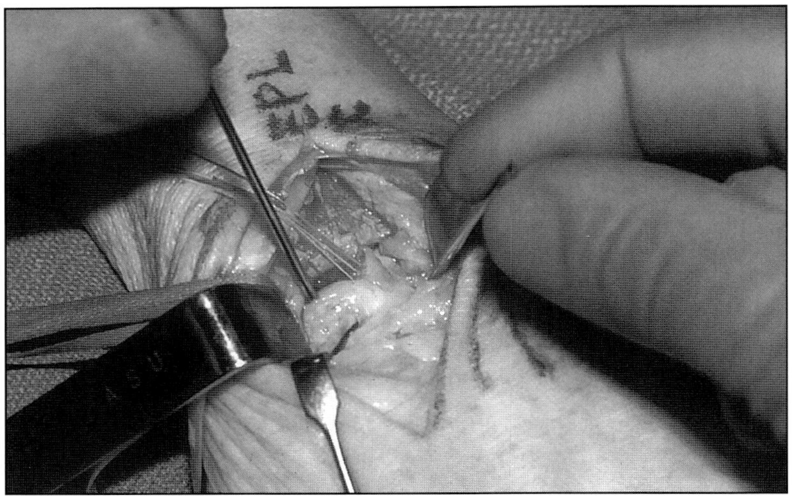

FIGURE 27-10. Dorsal approach to repair a dorsal perilunate dislocation. The interval between the third and fourth extensor compartments is used. Joysticks (0.062-in Kirschner wires) are drilled into the lunate and scaphoid and manipulated to achieve anatomic reduction.

TECHNIQUE

Dorsal Approach

A dorsal longitudinal skin incision should be made, aligned with Lister's tubercle (Figures 27-10 and 27-11). The interval between the third and fourth compartments is developed by dividing the distal portion of the extensor retinaculum and the septum between the compartments. The tendons of the fourth compartment are retracted ulnarly and the extensor pollicus longus radially. The dorsal capsule is incised longitudinally in line with Lister's tubercle; any traumatic rent in the capsule already present should be extended longitudinally. Capsular flaps are elevated by subperiosteal dissection to expose the scaphoid, lunate, triquetrum, and capitate, but the blood supply to the scaphoid entering the dorsal ridge must be carefully avoided.

The scaphoid and lunate can be manipulated with "joysticks" made by drilling 0.062-in K-wires in a dorsopalmar direction, one wire in the lunate and another in the scaphoid (Figure 27-10). These must be drilled deep enough to reach the palmar cortex to provide adequate leverage and control. The scaphoid is manipulated to reduce palmar flexion and the lunate is manipulated to reduce its extension. The joysticks should be used to reduce the interosseous gap. While an assistant maintains the reduction, the clinician should drill two 0.045-in K-wires from the radial side of the carpus percutaneously through the proximal pole of the scaphoid into the lunate and a third wire of the same size percutaneously through the proximal pole of the scaphoid into the capitate. Before placing the third pin (Figure 27-11), the capitolunate joint should be examined to ensure that no chondral fragments or other fracture fragments are present.

The dorsal portion of the scapholunate ligament should be repaired if possible, using 4-0 nonabsorbable suture. If the tear is off bone, the ligament can be tacked down with horizontal mattress sutures passed through drill holes in bone as described by Lavernia *et al.* [61] or through a miniature suture anchor.

Examination must include the lunotriquetral joint to confirm that it is reduced; the bones should be manipulated as necessary to obtain reduction. This reduction is maintained while another 0.045-in K-wire is driven from the ulnar side of the triquetrum into the lunate. Additional pins are usually not necessary.

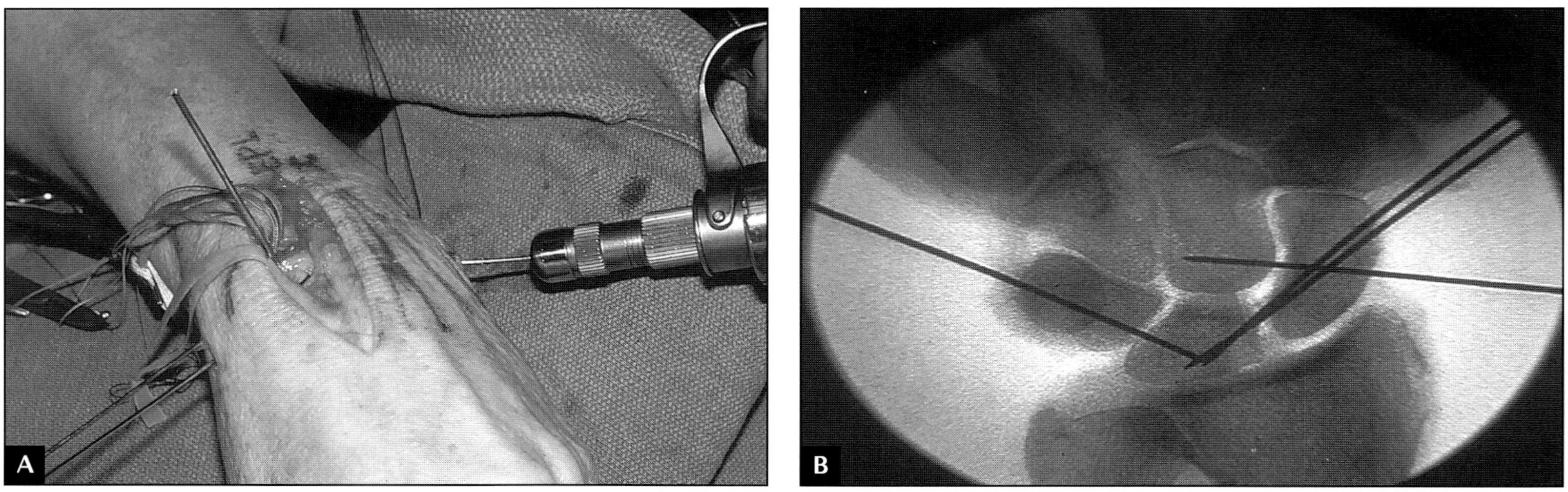

FIGURE 27-11. A, Intraoperative photograph showing technique for treating perilunate dislocations. The scaphoid and lunate have been reduced (the joystick used to manipulate the scaphoid is still in place) and two pins have been placed percutaneously to maintain that alignment while a third pin is being drilled across the triquetrum into the lunate. The superficial branch of the radial nerve has been dissected out and is protected with a rubber dam. B, Fluoroscopic view of the final pin placement including one pin across the scaphocapitate joint.

Placement of pins across the radiocarpal joint should be avoided (Figure 27-11).

A few tips on placing the K-wires should be mentioned. It is possible to injure sensory branches of the superficial radial nerve, the dorsal ulnar nerve, and branches of the radial artery when placing percutaneous pins near the wrist. To minimize this risk, a 3-mm skin incision is made and spread bluntly down to the capsule with a hemostat. Using a blunted 14-gauge angiocather held in a hemostat as a guide, the K-wires are passed through the guide when drilling them into position. The wires beneath the skin are cut to minimize any chance of infection. Intraoperative fluoroscopy is helpful in placing the K-wires to ensure their proper placement with a minimum number of passes through bone and cartilage.

Standard radiographs in the PA and lateral projections should be obtained after final reduction and pin placement have been achieved. The capsulotomy incision as well as any other tears in the dorsal capsule are closed with 4-0 nonabsorbable suture in a routine fashion. A drain is usually unnecessary.

Postoperatively, the extremity is immobilized in a bulky plaster-reinforced thumb spica dressing that extends above the elbow, thus maintaining the forearm in neutral position with the wrist in 15° flexion and 10° radial deviation. This arrangement should be converted to an above elbow (or Muenster's) thumb spica cast after 10 days when the sutures are removed. At 4 weeks, a below-elbow thumb spica cast is applied. The pins may be removed after 8 weeks, at which point a removable splint can be used for patient comfort; range-of-motion exercises should begin.

Palmar Approach

A palmar approach may be added to the dorsal approach for two situations: first, for those cases in which the lunate is dislocated (Mayfield stage IV) and cannot be reduced closed or with the dorsal exposure; and second, for acute carpal tunnel syndrome. To treat the latter, a standard carpal tunnel release extends the incision obliquely and ulnarly across the wrist crease for 1 cm. After complete decompression of the median nerve, the lunate is provisionally reduced through the floor of the radiocarpal joint. Reduction and fixation are then completed in the manner previously outlined.

Transcaphoid Perilunate Fracture-Dislocations

This injury always includes a displaced fracture of the scaphoid for which early open reduction and internal fixation is preferred [27,62,63]. In contrast to a perilunate or lunate dislocation with which a palmar approach is not used routinely, in cases in which the scaphoid is fractured, a palmar approach *is* used routinely to reduce and fix the scaphoid. Bone graft from the distal radius or iliac crest may be added those cases in which extensive comminution is present. Addition of a dorsal approach is usually not necessary.

Technique

Palmar Approach

A standard palmar approach to the scaphoid is used as described by Russe [64] if the carpal tunnel does not need release. If the carpal tunnel does need release, a modified open carpal tunnel release incision is used to carry the proximal portion of the incision more radially than usual. The palmar cutaneous branch of the median nerve must be identified, tagged, and protected when the incision extends across the wrist crease. The radial artery and the flexor carpi radialis (FCR) tendon are identified and retracted radially. The floor of the FCR sheath and the radiocarpal joint capsule should be opened longitudinally to expose the scaphoid and 0.045-in K-wires inserted perpendicular to each fracture fragment to act as joysticks. The fracture is manipulated to achieve reduction and a Freer elevator is placed in the radioscaphoid joint to maintain reduction and apply counterforce. Two smooth 0.045-in K-wires should be drilled percutaneously across the fracture and their position should be confirmed radiographically.

After the scaphoid has been anatomically reduced and fixed, the wrist is examined fluoroscopically. In Mayfield stage IV injuries, the lunotriquetral joint can be reduced and pinned percutaneously by applying palmarly directed pressure to the triquetrum, which is usually displaced dorsally.

The benefits of compression screws, such as the Herbert screw, versus K-wires for fracture fixation remain controversial [65,66]. I prefer K-wires, because they are easier to insert and do not require stripping away the important scaphotrapezial and scaphocapitate ligaments to afford exposure for screw placement. Two K-wires also provide better rotational control of the fracture than a single screw, which can be a problem in the face of comminution, which is frequently encountered. If K-wires are used, they should be cut off under the skin and not removed until the fracture is radiographically united as demonstrated by tomography [11•]. In the small number of cases (5%) [67] in which the scaphoid is fractured through the proximal pole, it may be possible to reduce and fix the fracture using an isolated dorsal approach; in this situation; screw fixation probably provides more stability. A small, cannulated screw is recommended.

Other Combination Injuries

For the transradial styloid perilunate dislocations, fixation of the radial styloid is often possible (Figure 27-9). Because the important radiocarpal ligaments attach here, as much bony stability must be preserved at this corner of the wrist as possible. Single large styloid fragments can be fixed with K-wires, 3.5-mm lag screws, or both in combination.

The scaphocapitate syndrome should be addressed surgically because closed reduction and treatment have been largely unsuccessful [29,43,68]. A dorsal approach is used. Capitate fractures should be fixed anatomically if possible and bone graft added where necessary. Similarly, the transtriquetral fracture-dislocations are best treated surgically using a dorsal approach. Triquetral fractures should be stabilized with additional K-wires as necessary. Postoperative management for these injuries is the same as those for the transcaphoid perilunate fracture-dislocation.

Fractures of the hook of the hamate may occur alone or in combination with other wrist injuries. The hook is prone to injury because of its projection into the palm and its soft tissue attachments. The transverse carpal ligament, pisohamate ligaments, flexor digiti minimi brevis, and opponens digiti minimi all attach to it; it is surrounded by the extrinsic finger flexor tendons on the radial side and the ulnar nerve on the ulnar side. Soft-tissue attachments may also be one reason fractures of the hook present with a variety of symptoms and are prone to nonunion. Acute, nondisplaced fractures may be treated nonoperatively in a cast, but displaced fractures and nonunions are best treated by surgical excision of the hook through its base. Open reduction and internal fixation are more difficult, fraught with complications, and require more time to heal than excision. Furthermore, because of the time required for fractures in this region to heal, surgical excision of the hook may be used even in an acute setting to decrease overall recovery time for patients for whom that is a major consideration.

Longitudinal Dissociations

In longitudinal injuries, the focus of treatment is directed to associated soft-tissue and neurovascular damage, which makes it more difficult to establish generalized treatment guidelines. Certain principles apply to all cases, however. Treatment consists of débridement of nonviable tissues, open reduction and fixation of fractures (usually with K-wires), repair of damaged tendons and neurovascular structures where possible, and application of immediate or delayed skin coverage. Cast immobilization for 6 to 8 weeks is commonly used, after which active hand therapy is begun. Secondary procedures, such as tenolysis and neurolysis, are commonly necessary [11•,19].

Late Recognition and Treatment

Unfortunately, many wrist injuries are misdiagnosed acutely, especially perilunate dislocations and scaphoid subluxations [13,24,44,57,60,69]. In the large series reported by Herzberg *et al.* [67], the diagnosis was missed initially in 25% of cases. Delayed treatment of neglected perilunate or lunate dislocation is difficult and controversial [28,60,70,71]. There is general agreement that results after long delays in treatment or no treatment for perilunate dislocations on fracture-dislocations are poor [27,60,67,72].

A common situation involves a delay in treating scapholunate ligament disruptions in which the scaphoid rotation is not fixed but can be corrected surgically. Various ligament reconstruction and augmentation procedures can be useful in this situation. I prefer the technique described by Lavernia *et al.* [61] that has been modified to include a different capsulodesis technique.

Technique for Scapholunate Ligament Repair and Capsulodesis

A longitudinal skin incision is made, centered over Lister's tubercle. The extensor retinaculum is exposed and incised between the third and fourth compartments. The extensor pollicis longus is unroofed and retracted radially and the fourth compartment dissected subperiosteally to reflect it ulnarly; this should expose the scaphoid and lunate. The remnant of the SLIL is usually avulsed from the scaphoid and remains attached to the lunate. Horizontal mattress sutures are placed in this tissue with 4-0 nonabsorbable sutures. A trough is created in the proximal pole of the scaphoid along its lunate facet to accept the ligament. Holes are drilled in the proximal scaphoid from this trough to the scaphoid waist just distal to the radial styloid; a 0.045-in K-wire works well for this. Two parallel 0.045-in K-wires should be placed percutaneously into the scaphoid in preparation for pinning the reduction. The scaphoid and lunate are reduced, requiring careful attention to raising the scaphoid up out of its flexed posture, and then the K-wires are drilled across into the lunate. Sutures are passed in the SLIL through the drill holes in the scaphoid and tied securely. To correct any residual dorsal intercalated segment instability (DISI) deformity, a third 0.045-in K-wire may be drilled percutaneously across the scaphoid and into the capitate while palmarly directed force is applied manually to the capitate.

The capsulodesis is added next. Different techniques have been described for this step. Lavernia *et al.* [61] use local capsular tissue in a "vest-over-pants" fashion. Another option is the capsulodesis recommended by Blatt [73], in which a 1-cm–wide strip of dorsal capsule is pivoted on its attachment to the radius proximally and sutured to a trough in the scaphoid distal to its axis of rotation. Blatt has recently presented evidence that this transferred capsular tissue may hypertrophy over time [74]. The procedure tethers the distal pole of the scaphoid to the distal radius, in effect reducing wrist flexion, particularly if the tissue becomes hypertrophied rather than attenuated. In Blatt's experience [73,75], patients lose up to 20° of wrist flexion. In a series of patients treated for dynamic scapholunate instability using the capsulodesis, the mean loss of wrist flexion was 12° [76]. In addition, the capsulodesis does not treat the scapholunate gap as occurs in flexion-extension.

Newer soft-tissue procedures may prove to be superior alternatives. One new capsulodesis currently still under investigation is based on the dorsal intercarpal ligament. This ligament, a thickening of the dorsal wrist capsule, normally originates on the dorsum of the triquetrum and inserts on the trapezium and trapezoid (Figure 27-2). To perform the new technique, the dorsal intercarpal ligament is elevated from its insertion onto the trapezium and trapezoid and reflected ulnarly. A bony trough is prepared in the distal pole of the scaphoid, distal to the axis of rotation, and a suture anchor is placed in the base of the trough. The reduced scaphoid is held in a relatively extended posture by applying manual pressure on the palmar side of the wrist or using a K-wire as a joystick and then the prepared ligament is secured to the suture anchor.

Theoretically, the dorsal intercarpal ligament capsulodesis has advantages over others because it may prevent gapping (*ie,* lateral displacement) of the scapholunate articulation by tethering the triquetrum to the scaphoid, keeping the proximal row functioning as a unit. It may also allow more wrist flexion because no tether to the distal radius has been created. The transferred ligament lies over the proximal pole of the capitate like a pulley, which may prevent the scaphoid from dropping into excessive flexion (DISI pattern). Initial biomechanical results in the laboratory look promising [77•].

Regardless of the exact technique used, postoperative management is similar. The extremity is immobilized in a plaster-reinforced above-elbow thumb spica dressing for 10 days, followed by 3 weeks in an above-elbow thumb spica cast and then a below-elbow thumb spica cast for an additional 4 weeks. K-wires are removed after 8 weeks and gentle range-of-motion exercises under supervision are begun; a removable protective splint is worn between exercise sessions. Immobilization is discontinued 3 months after surgery. Forceful axial loading of the wrist, particularly in extension such as with bench pressing, should be avoided for 6 months.

Conclusions

Success in managing carpal dislocations and fracture-dislocations comes from accurate diagnosis based on careful examination of the patients' wrists and radiographs and from early treatment. The goal should always be to restore the anatomy of the injured wrist. For the more common perilunate and lunate dislocations and fracture-dislocations, that means restoring the relationships among three key elements: the scaphoid, the lunate, and the capitate. Some loss of motion and grip strength as well as some degree of pain should be expected after these injuries even with optimal treatment; patients should be counseled about this at an early stage. For example, in a large multicenter study reported by

Herzberg *et al.* [67], outcomes after perilunate dislocations and perilunate fracture-dislocations varied with extent of injury and time to treatment, but in the best situations, patients who had closed injuries treated within 1 week of injury achieved scores averaging 80 out of 100 possible points on a scale evaluating pain, range-of-motion, strength, and function. Similarly, another study by Sotereanos *et al.* [58•] demonstrated that patients lost nearly 30% of wrist range-of-motion and 23% lost grip strength after perilunate dislocations and fracture-dislocations.

It is not possible to render a patient's wrist completely normal again after a fracture or fracture-dislocation. However, if evaluation and diagnosis are diligent and prompt and the principles outlined here are kept in mind, it should be possible to recognize and treat all wrist injuries so that morbidity is minimized and function is maximized.

REFERENCES AND RECOMMENDED READING

Recently published papers of particular interest have been highlighted as:
- • Of interest
- •• Of outstanding interest

1. Angermann P, Lohman M: Hand and wrist injuries: a study of 50,272 injuries. *Ugeskrift for Laeger* 1995, 157:734–737.
2. Amadio PC, Taleisnik J: Fractures of the carpal bones. In *Operative Hand Surgery*. Edited by Green D. New York: Churchill Livingstone; 1993:799–860.
3. Dobyns HH, Linscheid RL: Carpal injuries. In *Fractures in Adults*. Edited by Rockwood CA, Green DP. Philadelphia: JB Lippincott; 1984:451–509.
4. Ruby LK, Cooney WP, An KH, *et al.*: Relative motion of selected carpal bones: a kinematic analysis of the normal wrist. *J Hand Surg* 1988, 13A:1–10.
5. Gilford WW, Bolton RH, Lambrinudi C: The mechanism of the wrist joint with special reference to fractures of the scaphoid. *Guy's Hosp Rep* 1943, 92:52–59.
6. Taleisnik J: Wrist: anatomy, function, and injury. In *American Association of Orthopedic Surgeons Instructional Course Lectures*. Edited by Wissinger HA. St. Louis: CV Mosby; 1978:61–87.
7. Lichtman D, Swafford AR, Mack GR: Ulnar midcarpal instability: clinical and laboratory analysis. *J Hand Surg* 1981, 6:515–523.
8. Berger RA, Landsmeer JMF: The palmar radiocarpal ligaments: a study of adult and fetal human wrist joints. *J Hand Surg* 1990, 15A:847–854.

9.•• Berger RA: The ligaments of the wrist. In *Hand Clinics*. Edited by Nelson DL. Philadelphia: WB Saunders; 1997:63–82.

This is an essential paper for anyone treating wrist injuries. It reviews in detail the important features of the ligamentous anatomy with updated nomenclature.

10. Berger RA, Blair WF, Crowninshield RD, Flatt AE: The scapholunate ligament. *J Hand Surg* 1982, 7:87–91.

11.• Szabo RM, Sutherland TB. Acute carpal fractures and dislocations. In *Surgery of the Hand and Upper Extremity*. Edited by Peimer CA. New York: McGraw-Hill; 1996:711–726.

This is an excellent review of more advanced procedures for wrist fractures and dislocations.

12. Poirier P, Charpy A: *Traite D'Anatomie Humaine*. Paris: Masson; 1926.
13. Green DP: Carpal dislocations and instabilities. In *Operative Hand Surgery*. Edited by Green DP. New York: Churchill Livingstone, 1993:861–928.
14. Mayfield JK, Johnson RP, Kikoyne RF: The ligaments of the human wrist and their functional significance. *Anat Rec* 1976, 186:417–428.
15. Viegas SF, Patterson RM, Peterson PD, *et al.*: Ulnar sided perilunate instability: an anatomic and biomechanic study. *J Hand Surg* 1990, 15A:268–277.

16.• Berger RA: The gross and histologic anatomy of the scapholunate interosseous ligament. *J Hand Surg* 1996, 21A:170–178.

This paper describes anatomic details about ligaments critical for understanding scapholunate instabilities.

17. Ritt MJPF, Berger RA, Kauer JMG: The gross and histologic anatomy of the ligaments of the capitohamate joint. *J Hand Surg* 1996, 21A:1022–1028.
18. Garcia-Elias M: Carpal kinetics. In *Wrist Instability*. Edited by Buchler U. St. Louis: Mosby; 1996:9–13.
19. Garcia-Elias M, Dobyns JH, Cooney WP, Linscheid RL: Traumatic axial dislocations of the carpus. *J Hand Surg* 1989, 14A:446–457.
20. Mayfield JK: Mechanism of carpal injuries. *Clin Orthop* 1980, 149:45–54.
21. Mayfield JK, Johnson RP, Kilcoyne RK: Carpal dislocations: pathomechanics and progressive perilunar instability. *J Hand Surg* 1980, 5A:226–241.
22. Mayfield J: Patterns of injury to carpal ligaments. *J Hand Surg* 1984, 187:36–42.
23. Moneim MS: Management of greater arc carpal fractures. *Hand Clin* 1988, 4:457–467.
24. Hill NA: Fractures and dislocations of the carpus. *Orthop Clin N Am* 1970, 1:275–84.
25. Ekerot L: Palmar dislocation of the trans-scaphoid-lunate unit. *J Hand Surg* 1995, 20B:557–560.
26. Green DP, O'Brien ET: Classification and management of carpal dislocations. *Clin Orthop* 1980, 149:55–72.
27. Campbell RD, Lance EM, Yeoh CB: Lunate and perilunar dislocations. *J Bone Joint Surg* 1964, 46B:55–72.
28. Moneim MS, Hofammann KEI, Omer GE: Transscaphoid perilunate fracture-dislocation: result of open reduction and pin fixation. *Clin Orthop* 1984, 190:227–235.
29. Vance RM, Gelberman RH, Evans EF: Scaphocapitate fractures: patterns of dislocation, mechanism of injury, and preliminary results of treatment. *J Bone Joint Surg* 1980, 62A:271–276.
30. Gilula LA: Carpal injuries: analytic approach and case exercises. *Am J Roentgenol* 1979, 133:503–517.
31. Gilula LA, Destouet JM, Weeks PM: Roentgenographic diagnosis of the painful wrist. *Clin Orthop* 1984, 187:52.
32. Gilula LA, Weeks PM: Posttraumatic ligamentous instability of the wrist. *Radiology* 1978, 129:641–651.

33.• Peh WCG, Gilula LA: Normal disruption of carpal arcs. *J Hand Surg* 1996, 21A:561–566.

This paper indicates the pitfalls of using Gilula's lines if done incorrectly.

34. Garcia-Elias M, An K, Amadio PC, *et al.*: Reliability of carpal angle determinations. *J Hand Surg* 1989, 14A:1017–1021.
35. Linscheid RL, Dobyns JH, Beabout JW, Bryan RS: Traumatic instability of the wrist: diagnosis classification and pathomechanics. *J Bone Joint Surg* 1972, 54A:1612–1632.
36. Szabo RM, Newland CC, Johnson PG, *et al.*: Spectrum of injury and treatment options for isolated dislocation of the scaphoid. *J Bone Joint Surg* 1995, 17A:608–615.
37. Frankel VH: The Terry-Thomas sign [letter]. *Clin Orthop* 1977, 129:321–322.
38. Pournaras J, Kappas A: Volar perilunar dislocation: a case report. *J Bone Joint Surg* 1979, 61A:625–626.
39. Saunier J, Chamay A: Volar perilunar dislocation of the wrist. *Clin Orthop* 1981, 157:139–142.
40. Aitken AP, Nalebuff EA: Volar transnavicular perilunar dislocation of the carpus. *J Bone Joint Surg* 1960, 42A:1051–1057.
41. Niazi TBM: Volar perilunate dislocation of the carpus: a case report and elucidation of its mechanism of occurrence. *Injury* 1996, 27:209–211.
42. Nicholson CB: Fracture-dislocation of the os magnum. *J R Nav Med Serv* 1940, 26:289–291.
43. Stein F, Seigel MW: Noviculocapitate fracture syndrome: a case report. *J Bone Joint Surg* 1969, 51A:391–395.
44. Gellman H, Schwartz SD, Botte MJ, Feiwell L: Late treatment of a dorsal transscaphoid, transtriquetral perilunate wrist dislocation with avascular changes of the lunate. *Clin Orthop* 1988, 237:196–203.

45. Weseley MS, Barenfeld PA: Trans-scaphoid transcapitate, transtriquetral, perilunate fracture-dislocation of the wrist: a case report. *J Bone Joint Surg* 1972, 54A:1073–1078.
46. Garcia-Elias M, Abanco J, Salvador E, Sanchez R: Crush injury of the carpus. *J Bone Joint Surg* 1985, 67B:286–289.
47. Gellman H, Caputo RJ, Carter V, *et al.*: Comparison of short and long thumb-spica casts for non-displaced fractures of the carpal scaphoid. *J Bone Joint Surg* 1989, 71A:354–357.
48. Cooney WP, Dobyns JH, Linscheid RL: Fractures of the scaphoid: a rational approach to management. *Clin Orthop* 1980, 149:90–97.
49. Eddeland A, Eiken O, Hellgren E, Ohlsson NM: Fractures of the scaphoid. *Scand J Plast Recon Surg* 1975, 9:234–239.
50. Dias JJ, Taylor M, Thompson J, *et al.*: Radiographic signs of union of scaphoid fractures: an analysis of interobserver agreement and reproducibility. *J Bone Joint Surg* 1988, 70B:299–301.
51. Zaidemberg C, Siebert JW, Angrigiani C: A new vascularized bone graft for scaphoid nonunion. *J Hand Surg* 1991, 16A:474–478.
52. Sheetz KK, Bishop AT, Berger RA: The arterial blood supply of the distal radius and ulna and its potential use in vascularized pedicled bone grafts. *J Hand Surg* 1995, 20A:902–914.
53. Adkinson JW, Chapman MW: Treatment of acute lunate and perilunate dislocations. *Clin Orthop* 1982, 164:199–207.
54. Campbell RD, Thompson TC, Lance EM, Adler JB: Indications for open reduction of lunate and perilunate dislocations of the carpal bones. *J Bone Joint Surg* 1965, 47A:915–937.
55. Jasmine MS, Packer JW, Edwards GS: Irreducible trans-scaphoid perilunate dislocation. *J Hand Surg* 1988, 13A:212–215.
56. Miller ST, Smith PA: Volar dislocation of the lunate in a weight lifter. *Orthop* 1996, 19:61–63.
57. Minami A, Kaneda K: Repair and/or reconstruction of scapholunate interosseous ligament in lunate and perilunate dislocations. *J Hand Surg* 1993, 18A:1099–1106.
58.• Sotereanos DG, Mitsionis GJ, Giannakopoulos PN, *et al.*: Perilunate dislocation and fracture dislocation: a critical analysis of the volar-dorsal approach. *J Hand Surg* 1997, 22A:49–56.
This is a good review of one treatment philosophy for these injuries and outcome data.
59. Cooney WP, Bussey R, Dobyns JH, Linschied RL: Difficult wrist fractures. *Clin Orthop* 1987, 214:136–147.
60. Howard FM, Dell PC: The unreduced carpal dislocation: a method of treatment. *Clin Orthop* 1986, 202:112–116.
61. Lavernia CJ, Cohen MS, Taleisnik J: Treatment of scapholunate dissociation by ligamentous repair and capsulodesis. *J Hand Surg* 1992, 17A:354–359.
62. White SJ, Louis DS, Braunstein EN: Capitate-lunate instability: recognition by manipulation under fluoroscopy. *Am J Roentgenol* 1984, 143:361–364.
63. Green DP, O'Brien ET: Open reduction of carpal dislocations: indications and operative techniques. *J Hand Surg* 1978, 3:250–265.
64. Russe O: Fracture of the carpal navicular: diagnosis, nonoperative treatment. *J Bone Joint Surg* 1960, 42A:759–768.
65. Herbert TJ, Fisher WE: Management of the fractured scaphoid using a new bone screw. *J Bone Joint Surg* 1984, 66B:114–123.
66. Viegas SF, Bean JW, Schram RA: Transscaphoid fracture: dislocation treated with open reduction and Herbert screw fixation. *J Hand Surg* 1987, 12A:992–999.
67. Herzberg G, Comtet JJ, Linscheid RL, *et al.*: Perilunate dislocations and fracture-dislocations: a multicenter study. *J Hand Surg* 1993, 18A:768–779.
68. Bryan RS, Dobyns JH: Fractures of the carpal bone other than the lunate or navicular. *Clin Orthop* 1980, 149:107–111.
69. Weir IGC: The late reduction of carpal dislocations. *J Hand Surg* 1992, 17B:137–139.
70. Glickel SZ, Millender LH: Ligamentous reconstruction for chronic intercapal instability. *J Hand Surg* 1984, 94A:514–527.
71. Crabbe WA: Excision of the proximal row of the carpus. *J Bone Joint Surg* 1964, 46B:708–711.
72. Stern PJ: Multiple flexor tendon ruptures following an old anterior dislocation of the lunate: a case report. *J Bone Joint Surg* 1981, 63A:489–490.
73. Blatt G: Capsulodesis in reconstructive hand surgery: dorsal capsulodesis for the unstable scaphoid and volar capsulodesis following excision of the distal ulna. *Hand Clin* 1987, 3: 81–102.
74. Blatt G: The case for my capsulodesis method. In *Specialty Day*. San Francisco: American Society for Surgery of the Hand; 1997.
75. Blatt G: Scapholunate instability. In *The Wrist and Its Disorders*. Edited by Lichtman DM. Philadelphia: WB Saunders; 1988:251–273.
76. Wintman BI, Gelberman RH, Katz JN: Dynamic scapholunate instability: results of operative treatment with dorsal capsulodesis. *J Hand Surg* 1995, 20A:971–979.
77.• Slater RR, Szabo RM, Bay BK, Laubach JE: Dorsal intercarpal ligament capsulodesis for scapholunate dissociation: Biomechanical analysis in a cadaver model. *J Hand Surg* 1999, 24A:232–239.
This is a basic-science procedure explaining a new capsulodesis procedure and laboratory test results in a cadaver model.

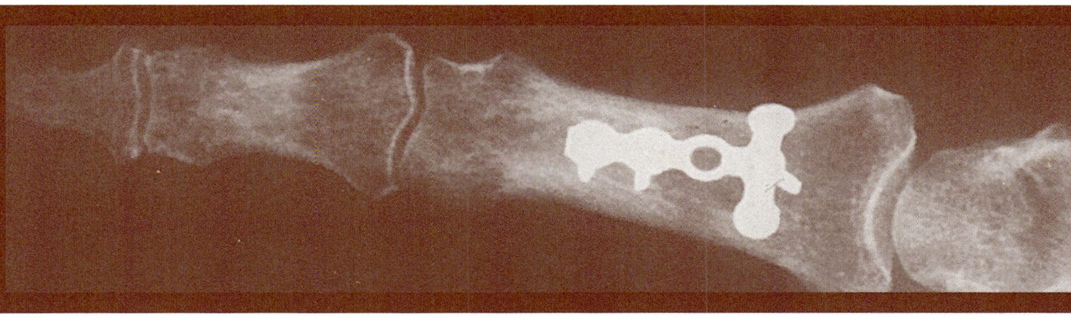

28

Current Management of Selected Problem Fractures of the Phalanges and Metacarpals

Dean S. Louis
Peter J. L. Jebson

The hand is ever susceptible to trauma. Nearly one third of all acute injuries involve the upper extremities. About one fourth of all athletic injuries involve the hand or wrist. Acute upper extremity injuries are responsible for approximately 32 million days of restricted work activity and 10 million days of lost work every year [1]. The total cost of upper extremity disorders in the United States was estimated in 1995 to be $19 billion per year. The exact incidence and cost of fractures of the phalanges and metacarpals are not known because such injuries are typically treated on an ambulatory basis and thus escape the scrutiny and record keeping that accompanies hospitalization.

Although techniques and instrumentation for open reduction and internal fixation have proliferated over the past 25 years, most fractures of the phalanges and metacarpals can be successfully treated by closed means with reduction and splint immobilization. However, some well-established criteria for performing surgical stabilization exist to secure and maintain fracture reduction (Table 28-1).

Prognosis for a good functional result depends on multiple factors. Associated soft tissue injuries, fracture comminution, and open fractures are associated with a poor outcome [2]. In a recent retrospective study, Page and Stern [3••] reported unsatisfactory results in 36% of 105 metacarpal and phalangeal fractures treated with plate and screw fixation. The outcome was most dire in patients with open fractures and phalangeal fractures. Fractures of the metacarpals had a better overall outcome.

It seems clear from the literature that although many new devices are available for fracture reduction and fixation, an inherent risk is present in their use [3••]. It is therefore extremely important that fixation be used for well-defined indications. Of course, many other factors affect the decision-making process, including the patient's age, occupation, avocational interests, general health status, medications, habits (*eg*, use of drugs or alcohol), and the potential for compliance with a mobilization program. An unreliable or poorly motivated patient will only further complicate a demanding postinjury rehabilitation program.

SPECIFIC FRACTURE TYPES

Distal Phalangeal Fractures

Most nonarticular fractures of the distal phalanx are the result of direct trauma, such as a hammer blow or injury caused by a closing door. Frequently, the fingernail and nail bed are also injured and are the major focus of concern to prevent later nail deformity. Following evacuation of the subungual hematoma and repair of the nail bed, these fractures seldom require anything other than splinting.

Intra-articular Fractures of the Distal Phalanx

Most intra-articular fractures of the distal phalanx result from sporting activities. Most mallet finger injuries are amenable to continuous splinting in extension for 6 weeks [4]. After this, full active range of motion should be expected over the ensuing weeks and no long-term sequelae should be expected. Occasionally, the articular component attached to the extensor tendon is so large that the remaining distal phalanx subluxes volarly. This indicates reduction of the distal phalanx so that the articular surface is congruent with the middle phalanx, which thus restores the extensor mechanism (Figure 28-1). Manual reduction and percutaneous pinning are usually sufficient to allow healing of this fracture. Open reduction is rarely indicated [4]. Volar intra-articular fractures involve avulsion of the flexor digitorum profundus and must be reduced to maintain joint congruity and profundus function.

TABLE 28-1. GENERAL INDICATIONS FOR SURGICAL STABILIZATION OF ACUTE FRACTURES OF THE METACARPALS AND PHALANGES
Open fractures
Multiple fractures
Polytrauma
Recurrent deformity secondary to spasticity
Intra-articular fractures
Irreducible fractures
Unstable oblique fractures
Associated soft tissue injury
Bone loss

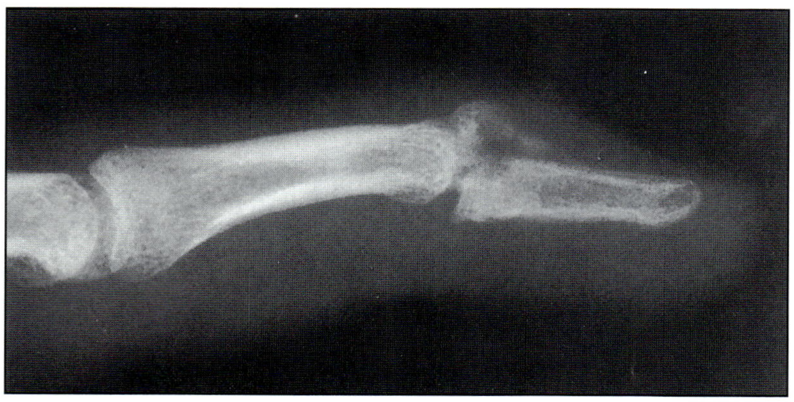

Figure 28-1. Although most distal phalangeal fractures do not require any form of supplemental fixation, this intra-articular fracture dislocation does require reduction and stabilization. In this case, that was accomplished with the use of an axial Kirschner wire after the distal segment was reduced. The pin was removed after 6 weeks and active range-of-motion exercises were begun. (*Copyright* DS Louis and PJL Jebson.)

Condylar Fractures

Fractures of the condyles involve the distal articular surfaces of the metacarpals and the proximal or middle phalanges. Any displacement, angulation, rotation, or shortening is unacceptable (Figure 28-2). Closed reduction and percutaneous pinning are preferred if an acceptable reduction can be achieved. Open reduction may be necessary for bicondylar fractures but can be particularly challenging because of the small size of the fracture fragments and the need to begin mobilization to prevent postoperative joint contractures and the possibility of subsequent tenolysis, capsulotomy, and other soft tissue releases (Figure 28-3). Occasionally, the intra-articular fragment may be so small (Figure 28-4) that judicious splinting with three-point bending is preferable to attempts at open reduction, in which the potential for further fracture fragmentation is a distinct possibility.

Isolated Fractures of the Shafts of the Metacarpals and Phalanges

Many configurations may occur with isolated fractures of the shafts of the tubular bones of the hand. Most transverse fractures may be successfully managed by closed reduction and careful splinting techniques. When satisfactory reduction cannot be obtained and maintained, closed reduction and percutaneous pinning (Figure 28-5) comprise a reliable technique that provides stable fixation and early active motion [5]. Additional alternatives include open reduction with screw or with plate and screw fixation (Figure 28-6). The goal of such fixation is to obtain immedi-

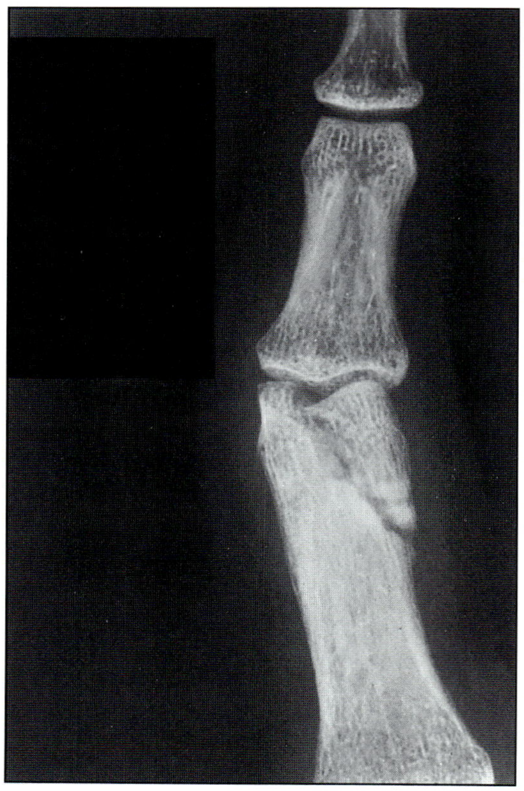

Figure 28-2. The displaced oblique condylar fracture is best treated by reduction and supplemental fixation. (*Copyright* DS Louis and PJL Jebson.)

ate rigid fixation to facilitate early return of range of motion. Such techniques are inherently more invasive and carry with them the potential for extensor tendon adhesions and stiffness. Extreme technical skill is required to carefully reduce these small fractures and to fix them with miniscrews that may be as small as 1.0 mm in diameter (Figure 28-7).

MULTIPLE FRACTURES: POLYTRAUMA

Multiple fractures in the same hand, and cases in which trauma involves not only the hand skeleton, but also the soft tissues, are well-accepted indications for operative reduction and fixation (Figure 28-8). Various techniques are available to accomplish the goals of stable skeletal fixation and early hand motion. The circumstances of the injury dictate which fixation technique is appropriate for initial management. In cases involving severe contamination, definitive fixation may carry a greater risk of infection unless complete decontamination has been achieved. Likewise, in cases in which soft tissue coverage is deficient, definitive stabilization may need to be deferred. The particular technique selected for fixation also depends on the fracture pattern. Temporary fixation usually involves the insertion of Kirschner (K)-wires. Dorsal plating is the preferred technique for achieving rigid fixation, thus facilitating immediate aggressive rehabilitation of the injured hand. Several commercially available plate and screw systems are available. Those that are versatile and feature self-tapping screws are more "user friendly." Clearly, the multiplicity of decisions that apply to each individ-

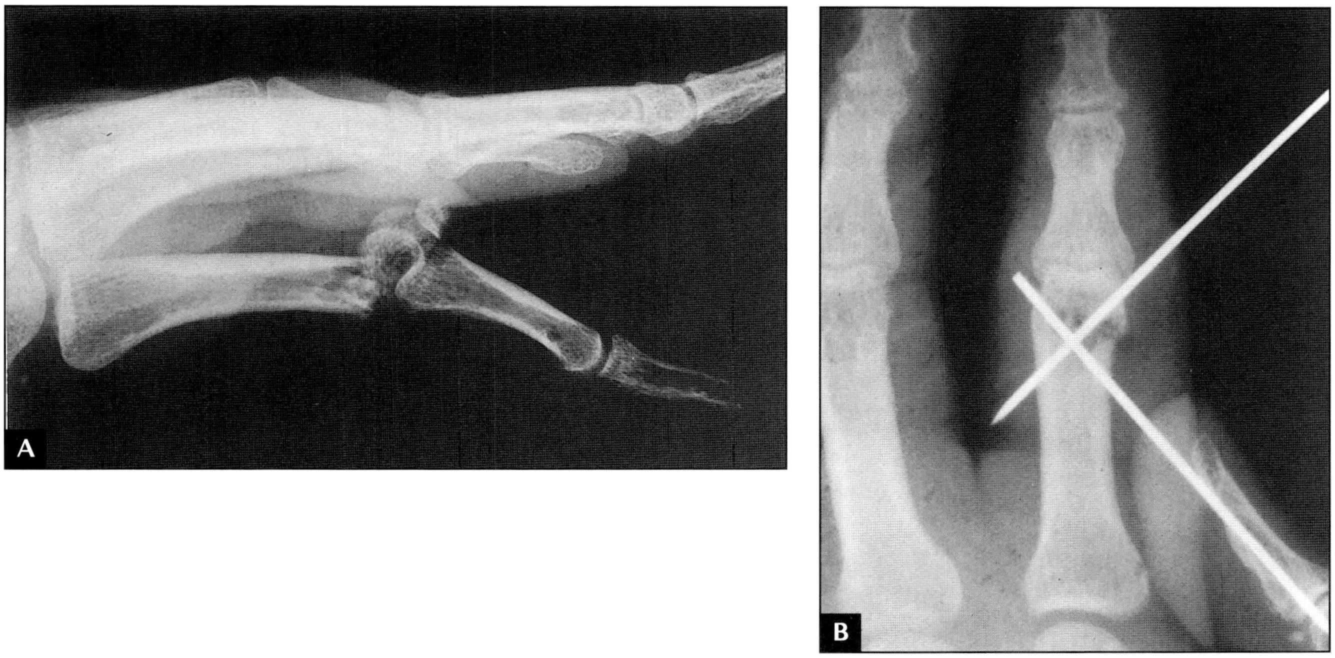

FIGURE 28-3. A and B, This malrotated comminuted condylar fracture requires reduction and stabilization by whatever means seems most appropriate. In this particular case, the intraoperative radiograph (*panel B*) shows a satisfactory position before cutting off the pins. (*Copyright* DS Louis and PJL Jebson.)

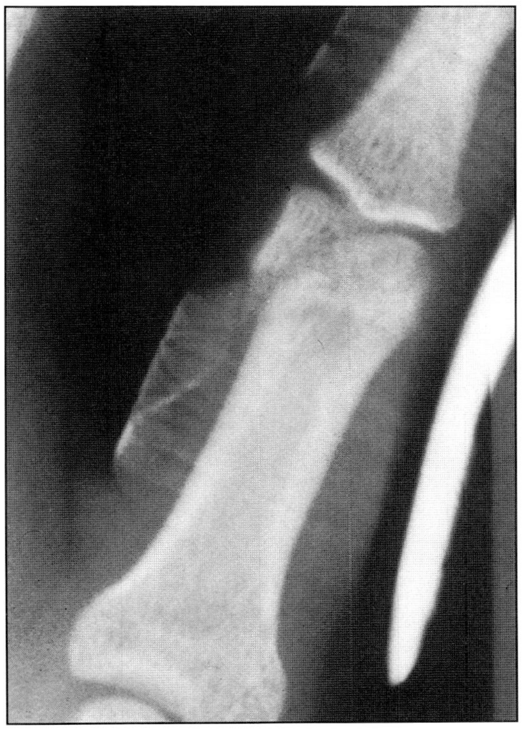

FIGURE 28-4. A minimally displaced intra-articular fracture may be best treated by a three-point bending splint until healing occurs. The results of open reduction of such a fracture include fragmentation, avascular necrosis, and inadequate fixation because of the small size of the fragment. (*Copyright* DS Louis and PJL Jebson.)

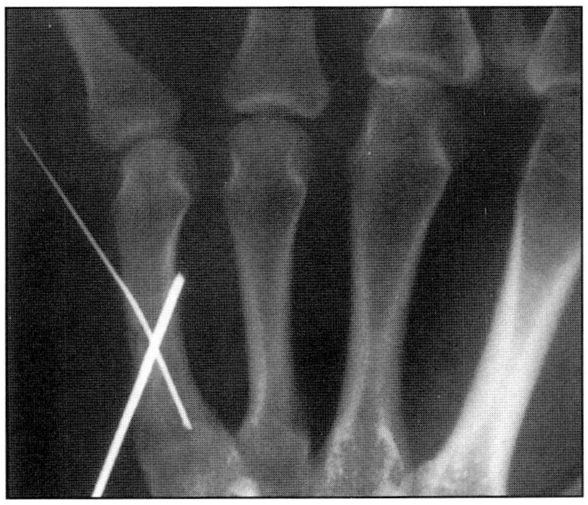

FIGURE 28-5. This transverse fracture of the small finger metacarpal kept deforming after closed reduction and plaster immobilization. Closed reduction and percutaneous pinning was successful as seen in the intraoperative radiograph. (*Copyright* DS Louis and PJL Jebson.)

ual patient requires experienced judgment that cannot be gained by using a cookbook approach.

Bennett's Fracture

Fractures that involve the base of the thumb metacarpal are common (Figure 28-9). Most are extra-articular and amenable to closed treatment. Treatment of Bennett's fracture is usually surgical, because of persistent shaft displacement and articular incongruity with casting alone. Fractures involving less than 25% of the articular surface may be successfully managed using closed reduction and percutaneous pinning of the major fragment to the trapezium or adjacent carpus, and maintaining the fixation for 1 month. For larger fracture fragments, open reduction through a volar approach and interfragmentary screw fixation, if feasible, permits anatomic restoration of the articular surface, rigid fixation, and early motion.

Reverse Bennett's Fracture

An intra-articular fracture at the base of the fifth metacarpal with medial and proximal subluxation of the major fragment is analogous to the Bennett's fracture of the thumb. The insertions of the flexor and extensor carpi ulnaris are responsible for persistent shaft displacement and instability. Closed reduction of the fracture by longitudinal traction and percutaneous pinning to the hamate and adjacent metacarpal are the accepted techniques for management of this condition. Care must be taken to avoid inadvertent iatrogenic malrotation of the small finger.

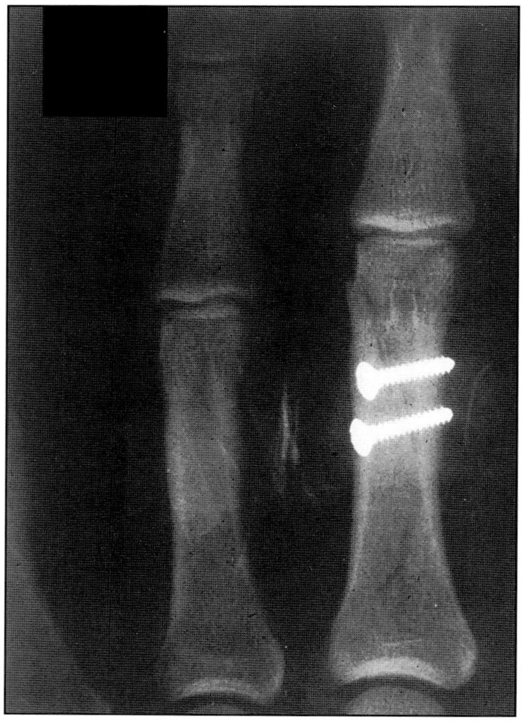

Figure 28-6. This long oblique fracture of the index finger middle phalanx was inherently unstable and continued to shorten and rotate. Open reduction and screw fixation allowed early active motion. (*Copyright* DS Louis and PJL Jebson.)

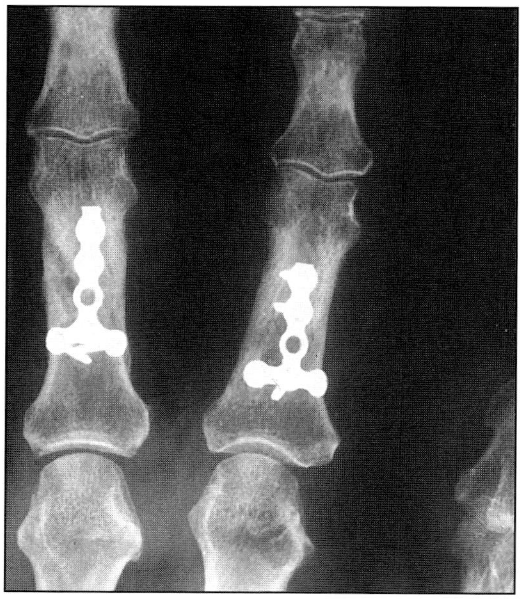

Figure 28-7. Miniplates and screws between 1.0 and 2.0 mm make for low-profile constructs to secure complex shaft fractures. (*Copyright* DS Louis and PJL Jebson.)

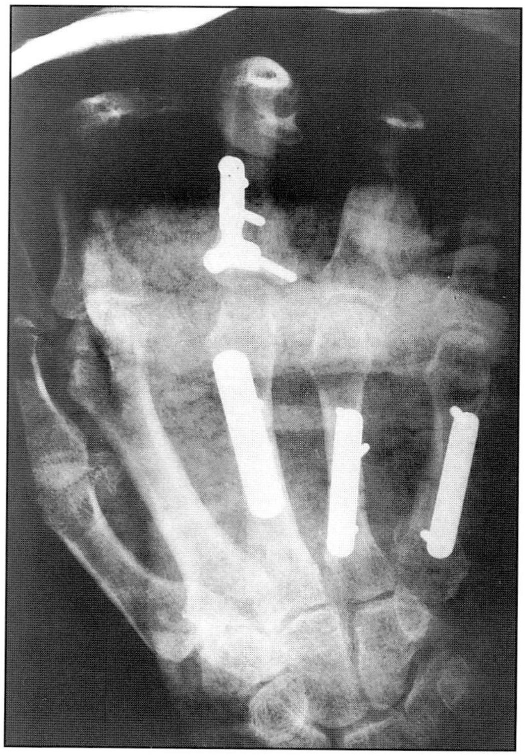

Figure 28-8. Extensive soft tissue injury combined with multiple fractures is a clear indication for operative reduction of the fractures to allow early motion. (*Copyright* DS Louis and PJL Jebson.)

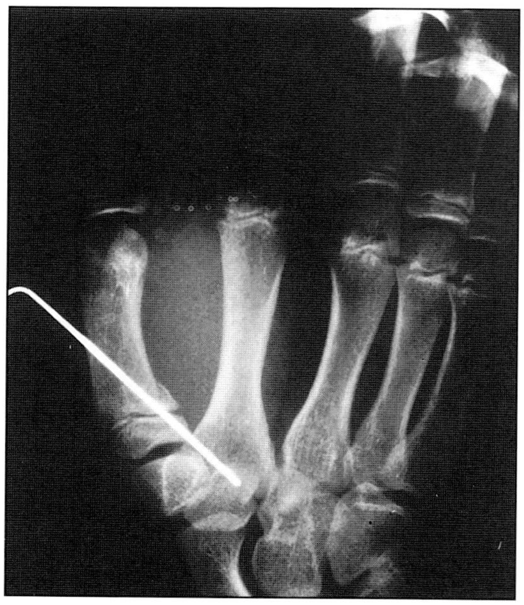

Figure 28-9. This classic Bennett's fracture was reduced and pinned percutaneously. In this case, the fixation was secure with the pin through the base of the second metacarpal. (*Copyright* DS Louis and PJL Jebson.)

Rolando's Fracture

In 1910, Rolando described this fracture, which has perpetuated his name (Figure 28-10) and has come to describe any fracture at the base of the first metacarpal that is intra-articular and comminuted. This fracture is not common, which is fortunate because its treatment is more involved than the relatively simple Bennett's fracture. The alternatives for treatment involve percutaneous K-wire pinning or open reduction and fixation with wires, screws, plates, or a combination of these. For severely comminuted fractures, some authors [6] have advocated the use of a neutralizing miniexternal fixator combined with limited open reduction of the articular surfaces and autogenous bone grafting. The quality of the result is probably dictated more by the severity of the initial injury than by the particular treatment used.

Fractures and Fracture-Dislocations of the Proximal Interphalangeal Joint

Books, chapters, and monographs have been written about these injuries [7]. It would be impossible to adequately cover this topic in this chapter in other than outline form. We have elected, therefore, to cover the basic principles that guide the management of acute injuries.

Failure of appropriate management of a fracture of the distal interphalangeal joint may lead to a stiff or arthrodeses joint. The functional loss from such a situation is minimal. By contrast, a stiff proximal interphalangeal joint can have a devastating impact on the function of the entire hand. Because no totally satisfactory joint replacement has been developed for this joint, it is imperative that every reasonable attempt be made to restore articular congruity, maintain reduction of the joint, and provide early mobilization for the various combinations of fractures and dislocations that affect the proximal interphalangeal joint.

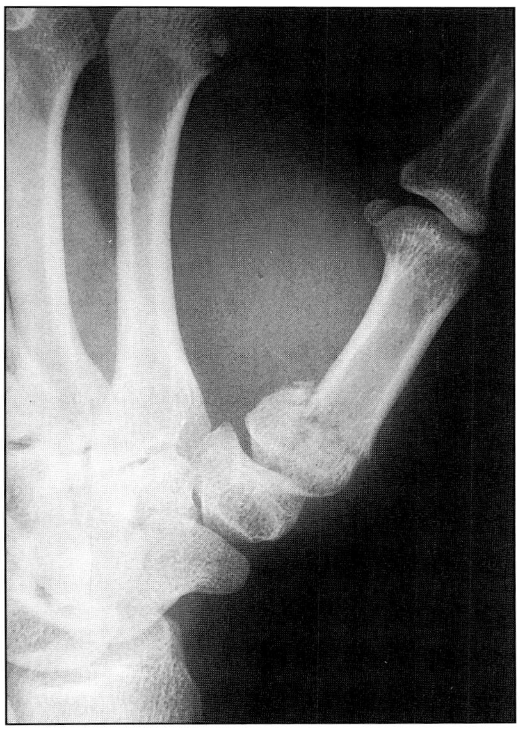

Figure 28-10. This is a classic example of Rolando's fracture. In this case, the intra-articular component is minimally displaced and the longitudinal alignment is satisfactory. This was treated successfully by cast immobilization alone. In most circumstances, the displacement is such that open reduction is indicated. (*Copyright* DS Louis and PJL Jebson.)

Initial evaluation of the injured proximal interphalangeal joint involves obtaining a history of the injury, followed by evaluation of the patient's active range of motion and extent of existing deformity. Further physical evaluation is contraindicated at this time because of pain. Radiographs of the involved finger should be obtained. Depending on the severity of the injury, a more extensive evaluation of range of motion may be indicated. This is best performed under digital block anesthesia to eliminate pain, preserve intrinsic muscle function, and allow the physician the opportunity to assess both active and passive motion and joint stability. This is particularly important because the findings dictate subsequent management. Fractures that are small (generally less than 30% of the articular surface) are usually stable (Figure 28-11) and may be treated by early active motion after acute swelling and pain have diminished. It should be remembered that even a joint that has only been jammed, without fracture, may be stiff and painful for many weeks or months after the acute episode. Patients with these injuries should be observed carefully during follow-up to be sure that motion is restored and that a flexion contracture does not develop.

Those noncomminuted fracture dislocations that are unstable may be treated by various techniques, including extension block splinting, as described by Dobyns and McElfresh [8]. This technique is the least invasive way of managing these difficult situations. Dynamic force couple techniques [9] also have a role in the management of some of these injuries, but the technique is demanding and requires persistence on the part of both patient and surgeon.

Beyond these two types of fracture dislocations is a vast spectrum of injuries that challenge even the experienced surgeon. Those representing such challenges are the severely comminuted fracture at the base of the middle phalanx or those fractures with central depression of the articular surface (Figure 28-12). These have been termed "pilon fractures." Options for management of these severe injuries are multiple. They include open reduction and pin fixation, open reduction with plates and screws, or various combinations thereof, with the option of using supplemental bone grafting. Postoperative management of these complex injuries should involve early active motion when feasible. Traction with early motion has also been extensively used by Schenck [10] as a means of maintaining reduction while instituting early active range of motion. Other extensive protocols have been developed that attest to the need for aggressive management of these complex injuries [11].

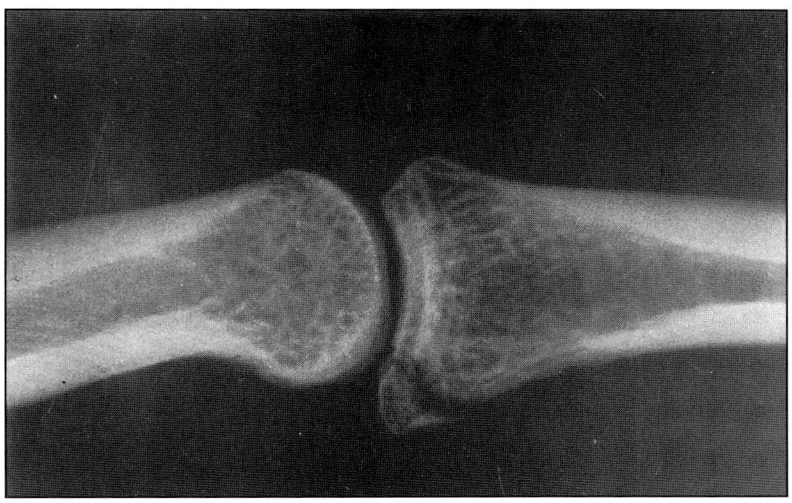

Figure 28-11. Nondisplaced fractures such as this at the base of the middle phalanx are usually stable, but the proximal interphalangeal joint should be evaluated for stability. (*Copyright* DS Louis and PJL Jebson.)

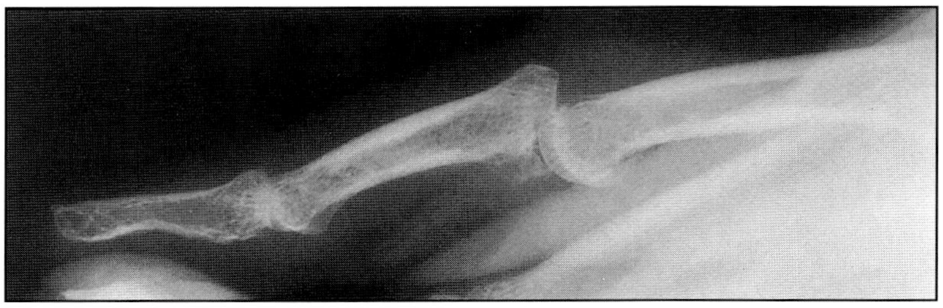

FIGURE 28-12. This comminuted fracture-dislocation of the proximal interphalangeal joint with fragmentation and depression of the articular surface is one of the most challenging yet most common problems in hand surgery. Some form of joint reduction, fixation, and articular reconstruction is mandatory. (*Copyright* DS Louis and PJL Jebson.)

CONCLUSIONS

Although most fractures of the phalanges and metacarpals can be managed by closed means, there are specific situations in which this is not sufficient. Evolving techniques using various internal fixation techniques have helped to improve management of many complex fractures of the hand. The cost for this improvement in fracture reduction has been a series of complications relating to the techniques themselves. Postoperative hand therapy has become an absolutely necessary part of the management of patients with these severe problems.

REFERENCES AND RECOMMENDED READING

Recently published papers of particular interest have been highlighted as:
- • Of interest
- •• Of outstanding interest

1. Kelsey J, Proemer A, Nelson L, *et al.*: *Upper Extremity Disorders: Frequency, Impact, and Cost.* New York: Churchill Livingstone; 1997.
2. Pun WK, Chow SP, So YC, *et al.*: A prospective study on 284 digital fractures of the hand. *J Hand Surg* 1989, 14A:474–481.
3. •• Page SM, Stern PJ: Complications and range of motion following plate fixation of metacarpal and phalangeal fractures. *J Hand Surg* 1998, 23A:827–832.

The authors of this article point out the pitfalls of plate fixation in healing fractures of the hand skeleton.

4. Schneider LH: Fractures of the distal interphalangeal joint. *Hand Clin North Am* 1994, 10:277–285.
5. Stern PJ: Fractures of the metacarpals and phalanges. In *Operative Hand Surgery* edn 4. Edited by Green DP. Philadelphia: WB Saunders; 1999:741–746.
6. Buchler U, McCollam SM, Oppikofer C: Comminuted fractures of the basilar joint of the thumb: combined treatment by external fixation, limited internal fixation and bone grafting. *J Hand Surg* 1991, 16A:556–560.
7. Molerich MM, Eaton RG: The volar plate reconstruction for fracture-dislocation of the proximal interphalangeal joint. *Hand Clin North Am* 1994, 10:251–260.
8. Dobyns JH, McElfresh EC: Extension block splinting. *Hand Clin North Am* 1994, 10:229–237.
9. Buchanan RT: Mechanical requirements for application and modification of the dynamic force couple method. *Hand Clin North Am* 1994, 10:221–228.
10. Schenck RR: The dynamic traction method. *Hand Clin North Am* 1994, 10:187–198.
11. Oyama M, Kimo Y, Mochida M, *et al.*: Postoperative management of the dorsal fracture-dislocation of the proximal interphalangeal joint. *Tech Hand Upper Extrem Surg* 1999, 3:66–73.

INDEX

Italics indicate figures; *t* indicates tables.

Acetabulum, anatomy of, 24–25, *25*
fractures of, 79–87
classification of, 24–26, *26t*, 80, *80*
complications of, 87
computed tomography of, 8, *8*, 26, *27*
diagnosis of, 79–80
postoperative care of, 87
prognosis of, 87
radiography of, *25*, 25–26
treatment of, 80–82, *81*, *82t*, *83–86*, 87
Acromioclavicular joint, fracture of, imaging of, 39
Adult respiratory distress syndrome, in thoracic trauma, 127
Advanced Trauma Life Support Program protocol, in pelvic ring fractures, 73, *74*
Age, in femoral neck fractures, 94–*95*
in humeral head and neck fractures, 218–219, 222, *222*
Amputation, in pilon fractures, 178
in tibial shaft fractures, 171, *171*
Ankle, anatomy of, 186, *186*, 189–190, *190*
dislocations of, *194*, 194–195
fractures of, 185–194
classification of, 29
computed tomography of, 8, 29
evaluation of, 186
lateral malleolar, 186, *186–187*, 188
magnetic resonance imaging of, *10*
medial malleolar and bimalleolar, 189–191, *191–192*
open, 192–194, *194*
radiography of, 29
trimalleolar, 191–192, *193*
syndesmosis injuries of, 188–189, *188–189*
Anterior capsule, anatomy of, 250, *250*, *263*
Anterior capsulotomy, in femoral neck fractures, 92–94
Anterior cruciate ligament graft harvest, patellar fracture after, 150, *151*
Anterior decompression, in thoracolumbar burst fractures, 63–64, *65*
Antibiotics, in femoral shaft fractures, 125
in tibial shaft fractures, 170
AO classification, of acetabular fractures, 80, *80*
of ankle fractures, 29, 185
of distal radius fractures, 271
of pilon fractures, 176
of supracondylar femoral fractures, 131, *132*
of supracondylar humeral fractures, *244*
AO tension-band wires, of patellar fractures, 144, *145–146*, 147
Arbeitsgemeinschaft für Osteosynthesefragen classification *See* AO classification
Arm, fractures of, 217–279 *See also* specific structures and fracture types
radiography of, 36–37, *37*
Arterial avulsion, in acetabular fractures, *84*
Arthodesis, in pilon fractures, 178
Arthroplasty, total hip, in acetabular fractures, *86*
total knee, patellar fractures in, 151
Arthroscopy, in distal radius fractures, 274–278, *275–278*
in patellar fractures, *146*, 147, 151
in tibial plateau fractures, 157–158
Arthrosis, after elbow fractures, 252
after pilon fracture, 182
Association for the Study of Internal Fixation classification *See* AO classification
Atlantoaxial instability, in cervical spinal subluxation, 51, *51*
Atlantoaxial spondylolisthesis, 55, *56*
Atlantodens interval, cervical instability and, 50, *50*
Atlas injury, imaging of, 15, *15*
Avascular necrosis, in femoral neck fractures, 94
in humeral head and neck fractures, 221, *222*
Avulsion, in tear-drop fracture, 54
Avulsion fractures, patellar, 147–149, *148*
supracondylar humeral, 245

Bar fixation, of pelvic ring fractures, 77, *77*
Bennett's fracture, 296, *296*
Bicondylar tibial plateau fractures, *156*, 157, 161, *161*
Bilateral facet dislocation, cervical spinal, 52, *53*
Bimalleolar fractures, 189–191, *192*
Biodegradable fixation, of patellar fractures, 147
Blade plate fixation, of supracondylar femoral fractures, 136–137, *137*
Bleeding, in acetabular fractures, 87
in femoral shaft fractures, 121
in pelvic ring fractures, 74
Blood supply, femoral neck, 91–92, *92*
humeral head and neck, 217–218
Blumensaat's line, in supracondylar femoral fractures, 136, *136*
Böhler's angle, in calcaneal fractures, 30, *30*
Bone bridging, imaging of, *44*, 44–45
Bone bruises, magnetic resonance imaging of, 43
Bone grafting, in burst fractures, 54, *54*
in forearm fractures, 264
in humeral fractures, 234
in humeral head and neck replacement, 223
in subtrochanteric femoral fractures, 115
in supracondylar femoral fractures, 137
in supracondylar humeral fractures, *247*
in tibial plateau fractures, 158
Bone–tendon–bone autograft, patellar, 150, *151*
Bracing, of humeral fractures, 225–230, *226–229*
of tibial shaft fractures, 168
Broden's radiographic view, in foot fractures, 198, *199*
Brooks fusion, in odontoid fracture, *53*
Bruises, bone *See* Bone bruises
Burst fractures, cervical spinal, 51, 54–55, *54–55*
thoracolumbar spinal, 60, *60*, *60t–62t*, *62*, 63–64, *64–65*, 67
imaging of, *16*, *16–19*, *19*
Buttress plating, of supracondylar femoral fractures, 135, *135*, *138*, 139
of tibial plateau fractures, 158–159

Cable fixation, of patellar fractures, 147
Calcaneus, fractures of, 198, *199*
computed tomographic evaluation of, 8
imaging of, 29–30, *30*
Calcar femorale, 100, *100*
Cancer, metastases to bone of, *37*
Capitellum, in elbow anatomy, 250, *250*
Capsulodesis, in scapholunate ligament repair, 290
Capsulotomy, in femoral neck fractures, 92–94
Carpal dislocations, 281–291 *See also* Wrist
Carpal fractures *See* Wrist, fractures of
Cast immobilization, in foot fractures, 198, 200–201
in tibial shaft fractures, 168
Cathode ray tubes, in computed radiography, 35
Cement augmentation, in femoral neck fractures, 95
Central depression tibial plateau fractures, 156, *156*, 159
Cervical spine, anatomy of, 50
dislocation of, 50, 52, *52–53*
imaging of, 16, *16*
fracture-dislocation of, 54–55
fractures of, 49–55
anterior, 50–51
burst, 51, 54–55, *54–55*
classification of, 50–51, *51*
compression, 50, 53–54
evaluation of, 49
instability in, 50–51, *50–51*, 51*t*
lateral, 56
odontoid, 52–53, *53 See also* Odontoid fractures
posterior, 51, 55–56, *56*
tear-drop, 54
treatment of, 49
fracture-subluxation of, imaging techniques in, 13, *14*
imaging of, computed tomographic, 7–8, *8*, 14–15, *14–15*
radiographic, 4, *4*, 14–15, *15*
spinal cord injury in, 56–57
subluxation of, 5–51
Chance fracture, imaging of, 17
radiographic, 4, *5*, 17, *18*
tomographic, 14

Childress' pin, in ankle fractures, *187*, 194, *194*
Chopart's joint, in midfoot fractures, 200
Clavicle, fractures of, imaging of, *38*, 39, *40*
Clay-shoveler's fracture, radiographic evaluation of, 4, *5*
Closed reduction, of distal radius fractures, 272
Colles' fractures, 271
Comminuted fractures, acetabular, *86*
forearm, 264
hand and finger, *295*, *298*
humeral, *228*, *237–238*, 240, *240*
intertrochanteric hip, 100
pilon, 178
subtrochanteric femoral, *108*
supracondylar femoral, 139–140, *140*
supracondylar humeral, 244–246, *247*
thoracolumbar spinal, *62*, 63
imaging of, *16*, 16–17
Compartment syndromes, in distal radius fractures, 277
in femoral shaft fractures, 121
in forearm fractures, 258
in tibial plateau fractures, 157
in tibial shaft fractures, 172
Compression fractures, cervical spinal, 50, 53–54
distal radius, 270
thoracolumbar spinal, 60, 60*t*–62*t*, 62–63
in osteoporosis, 62–63
Compression screws, in glenoid process fractures, 210, *210*
in intertrochanteric hip fractures, 104
in patellar fractures, 144–145, *145*, 147, 149
in subtrochanteric femoral fractures, 111, *113*
in wrist fracture-dislocations, 289
Computed radiography, principles of, 34–35
upper extremity, 34, *34*
Computed tomography, in fractures, 7–8, *7–8*
healing and, *44*, 44–45
helical *See* Spiral computed tomography
limited cone-beam, 22
pelvic and lower extremity, 21–30, *22–23*, *27*, *30*, 74, *75–76*, 176
shoulder and upper extremity, 33–36, *36*, 39–41, *39–41*, 44–45, 276–277
spinal, 7–8, *7–8*, 13–19, *14–16*
thoracolumbar, 59–60, 66
spiral, 13, 22, *22* *See also* Spiral computed tomography
Condylar fractures, metacarpophalangeal, 294, *294–295*
Continuous passive motion, in supracondylar femoral fractures, 141
Coronoid process, in elbow anatomy, 249–250, *250*
fractures of, 251–252, *251–252*, 254–255
radiographic evaluation of, *5*
Critical injury, femoral shaft fractures in, 127
Crosby and Fitzgibbons classification, of calcaneal fractures, 30
Crucial angle of Gissane, in calcaneal fractures, 29–30, *30*
Cuneiform bone, fractures of, 200
magnetic resonance evaluation of, *10*

Danis-Weber classification, of ankle fractures, 29, 185
Débridement, in femoral shaft fractures, 125
in patellar fractures, 150
in tibial shaft fractures, 170
Decompression, in spinal cord injury, 56
in thoracolumbar burst fractures, 63–64, *65*
Deep venous thrombosis, in acetabular fractures, 87
in supracondylar femoral fractures, 141
in tibial plateau fractures, 162
Deforming muscular forces, in femoral shaft fractures, 123, *124*
in supracondylar femoral fractures, 133, *134*
Diagnosis of fractures, imaging in, 3–10, *4–10*
Diaphyseal humeral fractures, 225–230, *226–229*
Digital radiography, upper extremity, 34, *34*
Disk herniation, in cervical spinal facet dislocation, imaging of, 16, *16*
in thoracolumbar flexion-distraction injuries, 66
Dislocations, ankle, *194*, 194–195
cervical spinal, *42*, 50, 52
fractures and, elbow, *251*, 251–252
imaging of, 16, *16*, *52*
wrist, 281–291
Displaced fractures, patellar, 144
Distal phalangeal fractures, 294, *294*
Distal radius *See also* Wrist
anatomy of, 270
fractures of, 269–270
classification of, 270–272
mechanism of injury in, 270
treatment of, 272–277, *273–279*
Distraction injury, thoracolumbar spinal, imaging of, 17, *18*
Dynamization, of tibial shaft fractures, 169

Elbow, anatomy of, 243–244, *244*, 249–251, *250*
in diaphyseal humeral fracture bracing, 227
fracture-dislocations of, *251*, 251–252
fractures of, 249–255
computed tomography of, 40, *40*
coronoid, 251–252, *251–252*, 254–255
olecranon, *251*, *251–252*, *255*, *255*
radial head, 251–253, *251–253*
radiography of, *5*, *5*, 36–37, *37*
ulnohumeral, *251*, 251–252
Elderly patients, femoral neck fractures in, *94–95*
humeral fractures in, 230
humeral head and neck fractures in, 222, *222*
intertrochanteric hip fractures in, 99
pelvic ring fractures in, 71, 78
subtrochanteric femoral fractures in, 108
Electromyography, in diaphyseal humeral fractures, 229
Ender nails, in humeral fractures, 235–236
in subtrochanteric femoral fractures, 111–112
Essex-Lopresti classification, of foot fractures, 29
Essex-Lopresti fracture-dislocations, 265, *265*
Evans' staple fixation, of humeral head and neck fractures, 220
Exercise, after diaphyseal humeral fractures, 227
Extended iliofemoral approach, in acetabular fractures, 81, *81*, 82*t*
Extension injury, supracondylar humeral, 245
External fixation, of distal radius fractures, *273*, 273–374
of humeral fractures, 239–240, *240*
of pilon fractures, 177, *177*, *179*
of tibial shaft fractures, 169, 171–172
Eye sign, in hamate fractures, 6

Facet dislocation, cervical spinal, 52, *52–53*
imaging of, 16, *16*, *52*
Facet fractures, cervical spinal, 55–56
Falls, foot fractures from, 198, *199*, 200
Fast spin echo magnetic resonance imaging, defined, 22
Fat–blood interface, in knee fractures, 6, *7*
Fat-pad sign, in elbow and forearm fractures, 37
Femoral condyle, fractures of, *10*
Femoral head, anatomy of, 91, *92*
in femoral neck fractures, 95
fracture of, acetabular fracture and, *84*, *86*
Femoral neck, anatomy of, 91, *92*
fractures of, 91–96
classification of, 26
imaging of, 26
pathophysiology of, 92
treatment of, 92–96, *93–94*, *96*
Femoral shaft, fractures of, 121–127
in critical injury, 127
evaluation of, 121–122
femoral neck fractures and, 94, *94*
open, 125
segmental, 124–125
surgical treatment of, *122–126*, 122–127
Femur *See also* Femoral head; Femoral neck; Femoral shaft

anatomy of, intertrochanteric, 99–100, *100*
supracondylar, 132–133, *133*
fractures of, imaging of, 26, *28*
intertrochanteric, 99–105 *See also* Intertrochanteric hip fractures
shaft, 121–127 *See also* Femoral shaft, fractures of
subtrochanteric, 107–119 *See also* Subtrochanteric femoral fractures
supracondylar, 131–141 *See also* Supracondylar femoral fractures
replacement of, in comminuted fractures, 140
Fibula, fractures of, computed tomographic evaluation of, *8*
in pilon fractures, 178
Fingers, fractures of, 294–298, *294–298*
Fixation *See also* specific fixation types
in acetabular fractures, 81–82, *83–86*, 87
in femoral neck fractures, 92–94, *93–94*
in femoral shaft fractures, 121–127, *125–126*
Flexion injury, supracondylar humeral, 245
Flexion-distraction injury, thoracolumbar spinal, 60, 60t–61*t*, *66*, 66–67
imaging of, 17, *18*
types of, 66
Flexion-rotation injury, thoracolumbar spinal, imaging of, 17, *17*
Flip trochanteric osteotomy, in acetabular fractures, 81, *85*
Fluoroscopy, in distal radius fractures, 276–277, *277*
in femoral neck fractures, *93*
in femoral shaft fractures, 122–124, *125*
Foot, fractures of, 197–203 *See also* specific structures
calcaneal, 198, *199*
imaging of, 29–30, *30*, 198
Lisfranc's, 200–201, *202*
metatarsal, 201
midfoot, 200
phalangeal, 201, 203
talar, 198–200
Forearm, anatomy of, 258, *259*, 270
fractures of, 257–279 *See also* specific structures and fracture types
radiography of, 36–37, *37*
Fracture blisters, in pilon fractures, 177
Fracture fragments, imaging of, *40*, 42, *42*
tibial shaft, 170
Fracture table, in acetabular fractures, 81, *83*
in femoral neck fractures, 92
in femoral shaft fractures, 122
Fracture-dislocations, Monteggia, 260–261, 261*t*, *262–264*
olecranon, *251*, 251–252
talar, *199*
thoracic spinal, imaging of, 17, *17–18*
thoracolumbar spinal, 60, 60*t*–61*t*, 67, *67*
ulnohumeral, *251*, 251–252
wrist, 281–291
Fractures *See also* specific fractures and fracture sites
classification of, acetabular, 24–26, 26*t*, 80, *80*
ankle, 29, 185
calcaneal, 29–30
distal radius, 270–272
intertrochanteric hip, 101, *103*
Monteggia, 261*t*, *262*
patellar, 143
pelvic, 23, *24*, 24*t*
pelvic ring, 73–75, *73–77*, 77–78
pilon, 176
shoulder, 41
subtrochanteric femoral fractures, *108–109*, 109, 109*t*
supracondylar femoral, 131, *132*
supracondylar humeral, *244*, 244–245, 245*t*
thoracolumbar spinal, 60, 60*t*–62*t*, *60–61*, 62
tibial plateau, 28, 156, *156*
tibial shaft, 166–167, *166–167*, 168*t*
wrist, 285–286, *285–286*
comminuted *See* Comminuted fractures
healing of, imaging in, 43–45, *44*
imaging of, 3–10, *4–10*
pelvic and lower extremity, 21–31, *22–30*, 24*t*
shoulder and upper extremity, 33–45, *34–44*
spinal, 13–19, *14–19*
occult *See* Occult fractures
stress *See* Stress fractures
Functional bracing, of diaphyseal humeral fractures, 225–230, *226–229*
Fusion, Brooks, in odontoid fracture, *53*

Galeazzi fracture-dislocations, 264–266, *265*
Gamma nails, in subtrochanteric femoral fractures, 114–115, *115–119*, 117
Garden classification, of femoral neck fractures, 26
Ghost sign, in spinal fractures, 4, *5*
Gilula's lines, in wrist fracture-dislocations, 283, *284*, 285
Gissane, crucial angle of, in calcaneal fractures, 29–30, *30*
Glenoid process, fractures of, 209–213, *210–213*
Grashey view, in shoulder radiography, *39*
Gunshot injury, humeral fracture as, *233*, *240*
subtrochanteric femoral fracture as, *116*
Gustilo and Anderson classification, of tibial shaft fractures, 167, 168*t*

Hackethal nails, in humeral fractures, 236, *237–238*
Halo brace, for burst fracture, 54
for cervical fracture-dislocation, 55
Hamate hook, fractures of, computed tomography of, 36, *36*
radiography of, 6, *6*, 36, *36*
in wrist injuries, 289–290
Hand, digital radiography of, *34*
fractures of, 293–298, *294–298*
indications for surgery of, 294*t*
magnetic resonance imaging of, *42*, 42–43
multiple, 295–296, *296*
radiography of, 35–36, *36*
Hanging cast, in humeral fractures, 226
Hangman's fracture, 55, *56*
Hawkins' classification, of talar fractures, 198
Healing of fractures, imaging in, 43–45, *44*
Helical computed tomography *See* Spiral computed tomography
Hematoma, in femoral neck fractures, 92
in pelvic ring fractures, 71
in pilon fractures, 177
Hemiarthroplasty, in femoral neck fractures, 93–95
Hemodynamic stability, in pelvic ring fracture management, 73–75, *74–77*, 76–77
Hemorrhage, in acetabular fractures, 87
in pelvic ring fractures, 74
Henry approach, in elbow fractures, 258, *260*
in forearm fractures, 265–266
Hip *See also* specific structures
biomechanics of, 100–101, *101–102*
fractures of, 89–120
anatomy of, 99–100, *100*
classification of, 101, *103*
computed tomographic evaluation of, 8, *8*
incidence of, 99
intertrochanteric, 99–105, *101–104*
Hip arthroplasty, in acetabular fractures, *86*
Humeral head and neck, fractures of, 217–223
anatomic considerations in, 218, *219*
surgical indications in, 217–218, *218*
treatment of, 219–223, *220–223*
in glenoid process fractures, 210–211
replacement of, 222–223, *222–223*
Humerus, anatomy of, *231*, 231–232, 243–244, *244*
fractures of, 225–240
humeral head and neck, 217–223 *See also* Humeral head and neck, fractures of
nonoperative treatment of, 225–230, *226–229*
open, 230
operative treatment of, 230–239, *232–240*
shaft, 230–239, *232–240*
supracondylar, 243–248 *See also* Supracondylar humeral fractures

Hybrid external fixation, of pilon fractures, 181
Hyperextension injury, tear-drop fracture as, 54

Iliac crest, imaging of, 23, 26
Ilioinguinal approach, in acetabular fractures, 81, *81*, 82*t*
Imaging, 1–45 *See also* specific imaging techniques and anatomic structures
  in fracture evaluation, choice of methods in, 13
    computed tomographic, 7–8, *7–8*
    magnetic resonance, 9–10, *9–10*
    radiographic and tomographic, 3–6, *4–7*
    scintigraphic, 8–9, *9*
  in fracture healing, 43–45, *44*
Immobilization, cast *See* Cast immobilization
Infections, in femoral shaft fractures, 125
  in humeral head and neck fractures, 219
  in pilon fracture, 181–182
  in tibial shaft fractures, 172
Instability, elbow, 252
  spinal *See* Spinal instability
  wrist, 282–283, *283*
Interlocking nail fixation, of humeral fractures, 237, *238–239*, 239
  of tibial shaft fractures, 169, *170*, 171
Internal fixation, of distal radius fractures, 274, *278–279*
  of femoral neck fractures, 92–95, *93–94*
  of humeral head and neck fractures, 219–221, *219–222*
  of intertrochanteric hip fractures, 101–102, *102*, *104*, 104–105
  of metatarsal fractures, 201
  of patellar fractures, 144–145, *145–146*, 147, 150, *151*
  of pelvic ring fractures, 74
  of pilon fractures, 177–178, *179–180*, 180–181
  of subtrochanteric femoral fractures, 110–115, *111–115*
  of supracondylar humeral fractures, 245, *246*
  of tibial shaft fractures, 169–172, *170*, *172*
Intertrochanteric hip fractures, 99–105
  anatomy of, 99–100, *100*
  classification of, 101, *103*
  clinical signs of, 101–102
  complications of, 105
  epidemiology of, 99
  postoperative care of, 104
  prosthetic replacement in, 104–105
  radiography of, 102
  treatment of, 102, 104, *104*
Intramedullary nail fixation, of femoral shaft fractures, 121–127, *125–126*
  of forearm fractures, 264
  of humeral fractures, 231, *231–232*, 234–237, *237*
  of subtrochanteric femoral fractures, 111–115, *114–115*
  of supracondylar femoral fractures, 139*t*, 139–140, *140*
  of tibial shaft fractures, 169–172, *170*, *172*
Ischial tuberosity, imaging of, 23, 26

Jefferson's fracture, radiographic evaluation of, 4, *4*, *15*
Johner and Wruhs classification, of tibial shaft fractures, *166*, 166–167
Judet views, in acetabular fracture evaluation, 25, *25*

Kaneda device, in thoracolumbar burst fractures, 64
Kelikan technique, of patellar fracture treatment, *148*
Kirschner wires, in foot fractures, 198, 201, *202*
  in glenoid process fractures, *210*, 213
  in patellar fractures, 144
  in supracondylar femoral fractures, 137, *137*
  in wrist fracture-dislocations, 287–290
Knee, arthroplasty of, patellar fractures in, 151
  fractures of, 129–163
    computed tomography of, *8*, *28*, 28–29
    magnetic resonance imaging of, *9–10*, 29, *29*
    patellar, 143–153 *See also* Patella, fractures of
  radiography of, 6, *7*, 28, *28–29*
  supracondylar femoral, 131–141 *See also* Supracondylar femoral fractures
  tibial plateau, 155–163 *See also* Tibial plateau, fractures of
Kocher-Langenbeck approach, in acetabular fractures, 81, *81*, 82*t*, *85*, 87

Lag screw fixation, of supracondylar humeral fractures, 246–247, *246–247*
Lamina fracture, cervical spinal, 55
Laparotomy, in pelvic ring fractures, 74
Lateral collateral ligament, in elbow anatomy, 250, *250*
Lateral epiphyseal artery, in femoral neck anatomy, 91, *92*
Lateral malleolar fractures, 186, *186–187*, 188
Lateral mass fractures, cervical spinal, 56
Lauge-Hansen classification, of ankle fractures, 29, 185
Lavage, in tibial shaft fractures, 170
Leg, amputation of, 171, *171*, 178
  fractures of, 99–203 *See also* specific structures and fracture types
Letournel and Judet's classification, of acetabular fractures, 24–26, 26*t*, 80
Ligamentotaxis, in tibial plateau fractures, 158, *158*
Ligaments, ankle, 186, *186*, 189–190, *190*
  anterior cruciate, patellar fracture after harvest of, 150, *151*
  pelvic, *72*
  in tibial plateau fractures, 156
  wrist, 270, 281–283, *282–283*
Limb salvage, in tibial shaft fractures, 171
Limited cone-beam computed tomography, defined, 22
Lipohemarthrosis, in knee fractures, 6
Lisfranc's fracture-dislocation, 200–201, *202*
  radiographic evaluation of, 6
Longitudinal fractures, patellar, 149
Lower extremity *See also* specific structures
  imaging of fractures of, *28–30*, 28–31
Lumbar spine *See also* Thoracolumbar spine
  imaging of, 4, *5*, 16–19, *16–19*
Lunate dislocations, *284*, 285

Magnetic resonance imaging, fast-spin-echo, 22
  in fracture evaluation, 9–10, *9–10*
  pelvic and lower extremity, 22, 26, 28–29, *28–29*, 102
  principles of, 22
  shoulder and upper extremity, 33–35, *38*, 41–43, *42–43*, 45
  spinal, 9, 13–17, *17*, 19, *19*
  thoracolumbar, 59–60, 66
Malunion, of tibial shaft fractures, 171
Mayo classification, of distal radius fractures, 272
Medial collateral ligament, in elbow anatomy, 249–250, *250*
Medial condyle epicondyle, in elbow anatomy, 249–250, *250*
Medial malleolar fractures, 189–191, *191*
Medial tibial plateau fractures, *156*, 157, 159, *160*
Mehne and Matta's classification, of supracondylar humeral fractures, 244–245, 245*t*
Metacarpal head, fracture of, nonunion of, *44*
Metastatic cancer, osseous, *37*
Metatarsal fractures, 201
Methylprednisone, in spinal cord injury, 57
Midfoot fractures, 200
Minimally invasive plate osteosynthesis, in supracondylar femoral fractures, 132, 140
Miyakawa patellectomy technique, 15, *152*
Monteggia fracture, *251–252*, 252, 260–261, 261*t*, *262*
  radiography of, *37*
Moore radiographic view, in tibial plateau fractures, 157
Motor vehicle accidents, foot fractures in, 197–198, 200–201, *202*
  pelvic ring fractures in, 71, *75–76*

Müller's classification, of supracondylar humeral fractures, 244, *244*
Muscular deforming forces, in femoral shaft fractures, 123, *124*
in supracondylar femoral fractures, 133, *134*

Nail fixation, of femoral shaft fractures, 121–127, *125–126*
of forearm fractures, 264
of humeral fractures, 235–237, *238–239*, 239
of subtrochanteric femoral fractures, 111–115, *114–119*, 117
of tibial shaft fractures, 169–172, *170*, *172*
National Acute Spinal Cord Injury Study, steroids and, 57
Navicular fractures, 200
Necrosis, avascular *See* Avascular necrosis
Neer classification, of humeral head and neck fractures, 217–218
of shoulder fractures, 41
Neurologic deficit, in thoracolumbar burst fractures, 63, *65*
in thoracolumbar flexion-distraction injuries, 66
Neurologic examination, in forearm fractures, 258
in pelvic ring fractures, 72
in thoracolumbar injury, *59*
Neuropathy, after supracondylar humeral fractures, 244
Night-stick fractures, ulnar, 260, *261*
Nonabsorbable suture, of patellar fractures, 147
Nondisplaced fractures, pilon, 177–178
Nonunion of fractures, diaphyseal humeral, 230
forearm, 266
imaging of, *44*
intertrochanteric hip, 105
patellar, 153
tibial plateau, 162
tibial shaft, 169–172, *172*

Occipital condyle, fractures of, computed tomographic evaluation of, 7, *7*
Occipitocervical injury, imaging of, 15, *15*
Occult fractures, defined, 33
magnetic resonance imaging in detection of, 42, *42*
Odontoid fractures, imaging of, computed tomographic, 7, *7*, 15, *15*
magnetic resonance, 15
radiographic, 4, *4*
trispiral tomographic, 14, *15*
treatment of, *52–53*, *53*
Olecranon, in elbow anatomy, *250*, 251
fracture-dislocations of, *251*, 251–252
fractures of, *251*, *251–252*, *255*
Olecranon osteotomy, in supracondylar humeral fractures, 246, *246*
Open fractures, ankle, 192–194, *193*, *194*
femoral shaft, 125
humeral, 230
patellar, 150
pilon, 177
Open reduction, of ankle fractures, 190–192
of distal radius fractures, 274, *274*, *278–279*
of femoral neck fractures, 92–93, *93*, 95–96, *96*
of patellar fractures, 144, 150, *151*
of pelvic ring fractures, 74
of pilon fractures, 177, 180–181
of subtrochanteric femoral fractures, *116*
of supracondylar humeral fractures, 245
in tibial shaft fractures, 169
Open-book pelvic fracture, management of, 74, *75*
Orthopedic Trauma Association classification, of tibial shaft fractures, 167, *167*
Osteochondral fractures, patellar, 150
Osteology, humeral, *231*, 231–232
Osteomyelitis, after forearm fractures, 266
after pilon fractures, 181
Osteonecrosis, in femoral neck fractures, 92
humeral head, *43*
Osteoporosis, hip fractures in, 26, 100, 102, 104
prevention of, 96
thoracolumbar fractures in, 62–62
tibial plateau fractures in, 159
Osteosynthesis, minimally invasive plate, in supracondylar femoral fractures, 132
Osteotomy, olecranon, in supracondylar humeral fractures, 246, *246*
tibial tubercle, in patellar fractures, 149, *150*

Pain, in tibial plateau fractures, 162
Palsy, in humeral fractures, 228, *228*, 230, 232, 234
Patella, fractures of, 143–153
after anterior cruciate ligament graft harvest, 150, *151*
classification of, 143
displaced, 144
evaluation of, 143–144
longitudinal, 149
minimally displaced, 144
nonoperative treatment of, 144
nonunion of, 153
open, 150
operative treatment of, 144–153
osteochondral, 150
patellectomy in, 150–153, *152*
periprosthetic, 151
polar, 147–149, *148*
stellate, 149–150, *149–150*
transverse, 144–145, *145–146*, 147
in supracondylar femoral fractures, 133, *134*
Patellectomy, 150–153, *152*
Patellofemoral contact, after patellar fracture treatment, 149, *149*
Pathologic fractures, subtrochanteric femoral, 108
Pelvic ring *See also* Pelvis
fractures of, 71–78
classification of, 72, *72–73*
diagnosis of, 71–73
management of, 73–75, *74–77*, *77–78*
stabilization of, 73–74
Pelvis *See also* Pelvic ring
anatomy of, 22
fractures of, acetabular fractures and, *84*
classification of, 23, *24*, 24*t*
imaging of, 21–27, *22–28*
ligaments of, *72*
Percutaneous fixation, of acetabular fractures, 82, *85*
of distal radius fractures, 272–273, *273*, *279*
of humeral head and neck fractures, 219–220, *220*
Perilunate dislocations, *284*, 285, *287–288*, 287–289
Periprosthetic fractures, patellar, 151
Pfannansteil incision, in pelvic ring fractures, 74
Phalangeal fractures, 294–298, *294–298*
lower extremity, 201, 203
Physical therapy, after scapular fractures, 215
in supracondylar femoral fractures, 141
Picture archiving and communication system, computed radiography in, *34–35*
Pilon fractures, 175–182
characterization of, 177
classification of, 29, 176
defined, 175
imaging of, 29, 176, *176*
injuries associated with, 176, *176*
nondisplaced, 177–178
open, 177
soft tissues and, 177, *177*
treatment of, operative, 178, *179–182*, 180–182
principles of, 175
unreconstructable, 178
Pin fixation, of distal radius fractures, 272–273, *273*, *279*
in intertrochanteric hip fractures, 102, 104, *104*
Plate fixation, of ankle fractures, *187*, 188, 190, *191–192*, *194*
of burst fracture, 54, *54–55*
of elbow fractures, 254–255, *255*
in forearm fractures, 261–266, *263–266*, *279*
of glenoid process fractures, *210*, 213, *213*
of humeral fractures, 232, *232–233*, 234, *235–236*
of humeral head and neck fractures, *219*, 221, *222*

Plate fixation, *continued*
of pelvic ring fractures, 75, *76–77*
of pilon fractures, 178, *180*, 180–181
of subtrochanteric femoral fractures, 110–111, *110–113*
of supracondylar femoral fractures, *135*, *135–137*, *137–138*, 139
of supracondylar humeral fractures, 246–247, *247*
of tibial plateau fractures, 158–159, *160–162*, 161
of tibial shaft fractures, 169
Polar fractures, patellar, 147–149, *148*
Posterior capsule, anatomy of, *250*, 251, *263*
Posterior decompression, in thoracolumbar burst fractures, 63–64
Pronation, in forearm fractures, 263, *263*
Prosthesis, hip, 104–105
humeral head and neck, 222–223, *222–223*
radial head, *253*, 254
Proximal interphalangeal joint, fractures of, 297, *298*
Pseudosubluxation, cervical spinal, 14
Pulmonary complications, of acetabular fractures, 87
of femoral shaft fractures, 127

Radial head, anatomy of, 250, *250*, 259
dislocation of, radiography of, *37*
fractures of, 251–253, *251–253*
radiography of, 5, 37
prosthetic replacement of, *253*, 254
Radial nerve palsy, in humeral fractures, 228, *228*, 230, 232, 234
Radiography, in cervical spinal instability, *51t*
computed, principles of, 34–35
upper extremity, 34, *34*
digital, 34, *34*
in fractures, 3–6, *4–7*
femoral shaft, 122
pelvic and lower extremity, 6, *7*, 21–31, *23*, *25*, *27–30*, 72–73, 176
shoulder and upper extremity, 5–6, *5–6*, 33–40, *34–43*
spinal, 3–5, *4–5*, 13–18, *15–19*, 59–60
Radionuclide bone scanning, in stress fracture evaluation, 8, *9*
Radioulnar synostosis, 266
Radius, anatomy of, 243, *244*, 258, *259*, 270
fractures of, 257–258, *260–261*, 262–267
distal, 269–279 *See also* Distal radius, fractures of
in Monteggia fracture-dislocations, 260–262, 261*t*, *262–264*
Range of motion, after diaphyseal humeral fractures, 227, 230
after patellar fractures, 147, 149
after patellectomy, 152–153
after scapular fractures, 215
Reduction, of acetabular fractures, 81, *83–86*
of femoral neck fractures, 92–93, *93*, 95–96, *96*
Rehabilitation, after scapular fracture, 215
after scapular fractures, 215
Retrograde intramedullary nailing, in femoral shaft fractures, *126*, 126–127
of supracondylar femoral fractures, 139*t*, 139–140
Rheumatoid arthritis, tibial plateau fractures in, *160*
Rolando's fracture, 297, *297*
Rotary subluxation, cervical spinal, imaging of, 15
Rotation, in forearm fractures, 263–264, *263–264*
Rüedi and Allgöwer classification, of ankle fractures, 29
of pilon fractures, 176
Rush pins, in humeral fractures, 235–236

Sacrum, fractures of, management of, 73
Scaphocapitate syndrome, *285*, 285–286, 289
Scaphoid bone, fractures of, 285–287
computed tomography of, 45
magnetic resonance imaging of, 45
nonunion of, 44, *44*
radiography of, 6, *6*, *35*
Scapholunate ligament repair, 290
Scapula *See also* Shoulder
fractures of, 207–215
diagnosis of, 208, *208*
imaging of, *38*, 39–40
incidence of, 207, *208*
nonoperative treatment of, 208–209
operative treatment of, 209–214, *210–215*
rehabilitation after, 215
Schatzker classification, of tibial plateau fractures, 156, *156*
Scintigraphy, in fracture evaluation, 8–9, *9*
Screw fixation, of acetabular fractures, 82, *83–86*
of ankle fractures, *187*, 188, 190, *191–192*, 192, *194*
of elbow fractures, 254–255, *255*
of femoral neck fractures, 92–93, *93*
of humeral head and neck fractures, *219*
of intertrochanteric hip fractures, 100–102, 104
of odontoid fractures, 53, *53*
of patellar fractures, 150
of pelvic ring fractures, 75, *76–77*
of subtrochanteric femoral fractures, 110–111, *110–114*
of supracondylar femoral fractures, 136–137, *138*
of supracondylar humeral fractures, 246–247, *246–247*
of syndesmosis injuries, 188–189, *189*
of tibial plateau fractures, 158–159, *158–159*
of tibial shaft fractures, 169
Seat belt injury, diagnosis and treatment of, 60, 60*t*–61*t*, *66*, 66–67
radiographic evaluation of, 4, *5*, 17, *18*
Segmental fractures, femoral shaft, 124–125
Seinsheimer's classification, of subtrochanteric femoral fractures, *108–109*, 109, 109*t*
Shear injury, in distal radius fractures, 270
thoracolumbar spinal, 17, *18*
Shoulder *See also* Scapula
in diaphyseal humeral fractures, 227, *227*, 230
fractures of, classification of, 41
computed tomography of, 39–41, *39–41*
digital radiography of, *34*
healing of, 44–45
magnetic resonance imaging of, *38*, 41–43, *43*
radiography of, 37, *38–40*, 39–40
skeletal scintigraphy of, 40
ultrasonography of, 43
Side plate fixation, of supracondylar femoral fractures, 136–137, *138*
Single photon emission computed tomography, in fracture evaluation, 8–9
Skeletal scintigraphy, in fracture evaluation, 8–9, *9*, 40
Skin necrosis, after pilon fracture, 181, *181*
Sliding devices, in hip fractures, 100–101, *101–102*
Slings, in diaphyseal humeral fractures, 226, *226*, 228
Soft tissue, in ankle fractures, 192–194
in foot fractures, 198
in forearm fractures, 263
in pilon fractures, 177, *177*, 181, *181*
in tibial shaft fractures, 167–168, 170, *171*
Space of Poirier, in wrist anatomy, 282, *282*
Spica cast, in wrist fracture-dislocations, 286, 289–290
Spinal cord compression, magnetic resonance imaging of, 13, *14*
Spinal cord injury, evaluation of, 56
treatment of, 56–57
Spinal fractures, 49–67 *See also* Cervical spine; Thoracolumbar spine
cervical, 49–55
imaging of, 13–19
computed tomographic, 7–8, *7–8*, 13–14, *14*
conventional tomographic, 13, *15*
general principles of, 13–14, *14–15*
magnetic resonance, 9, 13–14
radiographic, 3–5, *4–5*, 13
thoracolumbar, 59–67
Spinal instability, cervical, 50–51, *50–51*, *51t*
imaging of, cervical, 15
thoracolumbar, 16–17
thoracolumbar, 60
Spinous process fractures, cervical, 55

Spiral computed tomography, advantages of, 13, 22
pelvic, 23
principles of, 22, *22*
Splinting, of diaphyseal humeral fractures, 226, 229
of forearm fractures, 264
in supracondylar femoral fractures, 132
Split tibial plateau fractures, 156, *156*, 158, *159*
Split-central depression tibial plateau fractures, 156, *156*, 158–159, *160*
Spondylolisthesis, atlantoaxial, *55*, *56*
stress fractures in, radiographic evaluation of, 4–5
thoracolumbar burst fractures in, *64*
Spur sign, in acetabular fracture, *27*
Stabilization, of pelvic ring fractures, 73–74
of supracondylar humeral fractures, 246–247, *247*
Staple fixation, of humeral head and neck fractures, 220, *220*
Stellate fractures, patellar, 149–150, *149–150*
Sternoclavicular joint, fracture of, imaging of, 39, *39*
Steroids, in spinal cord injury, 56–57
Straight lateral approach, in acetabular fractures, 81, *81*, 82*t*
Stress fractures, magnetic resonance evaluation of, 9–10, *10*
patellar, 151
skeletal scintigraphy in evaluation of, 8, *9*
in spondylolisthesis, radiographic evaluation of, 4–5
Subaxial subluxation, cervical spinal, 50–51
Subluxation, cervical spinal, 50–51
rotary cervical spinal, imaging of, 15
Subtrochanteric femoral fractures, 107–119
biomechanics of, *108*, 108–109
classification of, *108–109*, 109, 109*t*
diagnosis of, 109
epidemiology of, 108
imaging of, 109–110
open, 115, *116*
treatment of, 110–118, *110–119*
Superior shoulder suspensory complex, double disruptions of, 214, *214*
Supination, in forearm fractures, *263*, 263–264
Supracondylar femoral fractures, 131–141
classification of, 131, *132*
complications of, 141
treatment of, *134–138*, 134–141, 139*t*, *140*
history of, 132
surgical anatomy in, 132–133, *133*
Supracondylar humeral fractures, 243–248
classification of, *244*, 244–245, 245*t*
injuries associated with, 244
treatment of, *246–247*, 246–248
Surgical treatment *See also* specific fracture types
Suturing, of patellar fractures, 147
Symphysis pubis, imaging of, 22, 26
open reduction and internal fixation of, 74
Syndesmosis injury, ankle, 188–189, *188–189*
Synostosis, radioulnar, 266

Talus, fracture-dislocations of, *199*
fractures of, 198–200
computed tomography of, 8
Tarsometatarsal joint, fractures of, 200–201, *202*
Tear-drop fracture, cervical spinal, 54
Tendon rupture, in pilon fractures, *176*
Tension-band wires, of patellar fractures, 144–145, *145–146*, 147–149, *148*, 151
Tension-band wiring, of humeral head and neck fractures, *221*
Terrible triad, in elbow fracture-dislocations, 250, 252, *253*
Thompson approach, in elbow fractures, 258, *261*
in forearm fractures, 266
Thoracolumbar spine, flexion-distraction injury of, 60, 60*t*–61*t*, *66*, 66–67
fracture-dislocations of, 60, 60*t*–61*t*, 67, *67*
fractures of, 59–67
burst, 60, *60*, 60*t*–62*t*, *62*, 63–64, *64–65*, 67
classification of, 60, 60*t*–62*t*, *60–61*, 62
compression, 60, 60*t*–62*t*, 62–63
diagnosis and treatment of, 62–67, *64–67*
evaluation of, 59–60
imaging of, 4, 16–19, *17–19*
distraction injury of, 17, *18*
of fracture-dislocations, 17, *17–18*
Thrombosis, deep venous *See* Deep venous thrombosis
Thumb, fractures of, 296–297, *296–297*
Tibia *See also* Tibial plateau
anatomy of, 165–166
fractures of, fragmented, *42*
incidence of, 165
magnetic resonance imaging of, *9–10*, 29, *29*
pilon, 175–182 *See also* Pilon fractures
shaft, 165–174 *See also* Tibial shaft fractures
Tibial plateau, anatomy of, 155–156, *156*
fractures of, 155–163
arthroscopy in, 157–158
classification of, 28, *156*, 156–157
clinical evaluation of, 157
complications of, 162
computed tomography of, *8*, *28*, 28–29, 157
magnetic resonance imaging of, *10*, 29, *29*
radiography of, 6, *7*, 28, *28–29*, 157
treatment of, 157–162, *158–162*
type I (split), 156, *156*, 158, *159*
type II (central depression), 156, *156*, 159
type II (split-central depression), 156, *156*, 158–159, *160*
type IV (medial plateau), *156*, 157, 159, *160*
type V (bicondylar), *156*, 157, 161, *161*
type VI, *156*, 157, 161, *162*
Tibial shaft fractures, 165–174
classification of, 166–167, *166–167*, 168*t*
closed, 168–170
complications of, 171–172, *172*
initial assessment of, 167–168
open, 170–171, *170–171*
Tibial tubercle osteotomy, in patellar fractures, 149, *150*
Tile classification, of pelvic ring fractures, 72, *73*
Toes, fractures of, 201, 203
Tomography *See also* Computed tomography
in fracture evaluation, 3–6, *4–7*
in hamate fractures, 6, *6*
in odontoid fractures, 14, *15*
in tibial plateau fractures, 6, *7*
trispiral *See* Trispiral tomography
Total hip arthroplasty, in acetabular fractures, *86*
Traction, in femoral shaft fractures, 122–123, *124*
in intertrochanteric hip fractures, 102
in subtrochanteric femoral fractures, 110
in supracondylar femoral fractures, 132, 134, *134*, 134*t*
temporary fixation in, 140
Transradial styloid perilunate fracture-dislocations, *284*, 285, *287*, 289
Transtriquetral fracture-dislocations, 286
Transverse fractures, patellar, 144–145, *145–146*, 147
Triangular fibrocartilage complex, 258, 266, 282
Trimalleolar fractures 191–192
Trispiral tomography, in hamate fractures, 6, *6*
in odontoid fractures, 14, *15*
in tibial plateau fractures, 6, *7*
Trochanteric osteotomy, in acetabular fractures, 81, *85*
Trochlea, in elbow anatomy, 243–244, 251

Ulna, in elbow anatomy, 251, 258, *259–260*
fractures of, 257–264, *260–264*, 266
radiography of, *37*
neuropathy of, after supracondylar humeral fractures, 244
Ulnohumeral dislocation-fractures, *251*, 251–252
Ulnohumeral fractures, *251*, 251–252
Ultrasonography, tibial, *42*
upper extremity, 43

Unilateral facet dislocation, cervical spinal, 52, *52*
Universal classification, of distal radius fractures, 272
Unreconstructable fractures, pilon, 178
Upper extremity *See also* specific structures
Upper extremity fractures *See also* specific structures
imaging of, 33–37, *34–37*, *40–44*, 40–45

Varus deformity, after diaphyseal humeral fractures, 227, *227*, 230
Vascular examination, in forearm fractures, 258

Watson-Jones incision, in femoral neck fractures, 92
Weight bearing, after patellar fractures, 147, 149
after patellectomy, 152
after pilon fracture, 181
in supracondylar femoral fractures, 141
Wiring, in cervical spinal dislocation, 52, *52–53*
in cervical spinal subluxation, 51, *51*
of patellar fractures, 144–145, *145–146*, 147–149, *148*, 151
Wrist *See also* Distal radius
anatomy and biomechanics of, 270, 281–283, *282–283*
digital radiography of, *34*
fractures of, 281–291
classification of, 285–286, *285–286*
computed tomography of, 40–41, *41*
diagnosis of, 283–285, *284*
injury patterns in, 281–283, *283*
magnetic resonance imaging of, *42*, 42–43
radiography of, 6, *6*, 35–36, *35–36*, *42*
treatment of, 286–291, *287–288*

Zickel nails, in subtrochanteric femoral fractures, 113–114